# Lesbian, Gay, Bisexual, and Transgender Healthcare

Kristen L. Eckstrand  •  Jesse M. Ehrenfeld
Editors

# Lesbian, Gay, Bisexual, and Transgender Healthcare

A Clinical Guide to Preventive, Primary, and Specialist Care

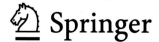 Springer

*Editors*
Kristen L. Eckstrand, MD, PhD
Program for LGBTI Health
Vanderbilt University Medical Center
Nashville, TN, USA

Department of Psychiatry
University of Pittsburgh
Pittsburgh, PA, USA

Jesse M. Ehrenfeld, MD, MPH
Program for LGBTI Health
Vanderbilt University Medical Center
Nashville, TN, USA

ISBN 978-3-319-79287-3        ISBN 978-3-319-19752-4    (eBook)
DOI 10.1007/978-3-319-19752-4

Springer Cham Heidelberg New York Dordrecht London
© Springer International Publishing Switzerland 2016
Softcover reprint of the hardcover 1st edition 2016

Printed on acid-free paper

Springer International Publishing AG Switzerland is part of Springer Science+Business Media (www.springer.com)

# Foreword

## LGBT Health in a Changing World

A decade ago, there were few options for serious study of the health needs of LGBT people. There were no texts in the United States, there was no official recognition by the federal government, and providers with interest in caring for the needs of LGBT people were most notably found practicing in a handful of health centers mainly located in large cities around the country as well as in private practice. GLMA: Health Professionals Advancing LGBT Equality, formerly the Association of Physicians for Human Rights, held an annual conference that provided some anchoring and sustenance for clinicians interested in caring for the community who there were able to feel as if they had some collegial connections from across the nation.

How things have changed! This is now the second text on LGBT health care in the United States, following the publication of the Fenway Guide to LGBT Health by the American College of Physicians in 2008. Healthy People 2020 contained a section on the health disparities experienced by LGBT people in the United States and put them on an agenda for eradication in this second decade of the twenty-first century. The National Institutes of Health commissioned the Institute of Medicine of the National Academy of Sciences to write a report on the state of LGBT health and to delineate a research agenda aimed at learning more about the etiology of and barriers to overcoming disparities in care. This publication "Lesbian, Gay, Bisexual and Transgender Healthcare: A Clinical Guide to Preventative, Primary, and Specialist Care" has become an invaluable resource for anyone wanting to read what is and is not known about the LGBT population and gather ideas for study and education. Changes in federal policies have been legion and coming in rapid sequence with the legalization of same-sex marriage. The Affordable Care Act protects LGBT against discrimination for policies purchased through the marketplace. There are new regulations prohibiting discrimination in nursing home admissions.

Perhaps the most important reason to use this readily available text is that care of LGBT people is now seen as a critical offering of many mainstream healthcare providers across the nation. It is not just happening in pockets or large cities, but across the nation and increasingly the world. Despite personal politics, most healthcare providers believe in providing equitable care for all, including LGBT people. This places great importance on the easy availability of standards of care on just the topics covered in the chapters of this book. It is important to understand unique clinical needs, but just as important to be able to ask questions to understand one's identity, behavior, and desires and how to systemize what should be routine screenings and immunizations based on that information. It is important not only to recognize the need to learn about one's gender identity but also how to appropriately and sensitively approach those who have and may not have had any significant surgery in order to assure that necessary cancer screening is carried out correctly. These are but a few examples of why we need more resources on the healthcare needs of LGBT people. In addition, we have to create programs for care that do outreach to the very diverse people who are L, G, B, and/or T as well as others who may not readily identify as such but who engage behaviors and have desires that warrant exploration by caring and sensitive clinicians who work in inclusive and affirming care environments holistically providing medical and behavioral health needs optimally in an integrated setting.

The challenges ahead are great. Many states which chose not to extend Medicaid are in the South where there is a high incidence of HIV among young MSM, a group which may be a proxy for a larger circle of LGBT people who may still be uninsured. We need to find those who are uninsured, or simply not accessing care, engage them in discussion to help them overcome possible negative experiences with the health care system, work with them on understanding the importance of seeking care, and help them find places where they can receive appropriate care. I end this introduction with the hope that it will not only an introduction to a new resource but an introduction to a new generation of providers who will enlarge the circle of clinicians caring and teaching about caring for LGBT people in the years ahead.

Boston, MA                                                                    Harvey J. Makadon

# Preface

Individuals identifying as lesbian, gay, bisexual, and transgender (LGBT) experience disparities in access and receiving health care, as exemplified in foundational reports including the Institute of Medicine's *The Health of Lesbian, Gay, Bisexual, and Transgender People: Building a Foundation for Better Understanding* and the National Center for Transgender Equality's *Injustice at Every Turn: A Report of the National Transgender Discrimination Survey.*

As a result, striking advances have been made over recent years to address disparities in the quality of care and health outcomes of individuals who identify LGBT. These improvements address all aspects of personhood and across the healthcare system from the clinic environment, patient-provider interactions, and quality medical care. The result is improving access to and receipt of quality care by LGBT individuals. The breadth of information available for health care practitioners is exciting; however, synthesizing emerging research and new guidelines into the patient care encounter can be overwhelming to healthcare providers unfamiliar with the health needs of LGBT patients. Furthermore, challenges arise when defining what is core clinical knowledge for all practitioners and what is specific to different clinical specialties. For example, what information do all healthcare providers need to know to provide quality care for LGBT individuals versus what information do Pediatricians needs to know? Surgeons? Dermatologists?

The purpose of this book is to serve as a guide for LGBT preventive and specialty medicine that can be utilized within health professions education from students, residents, and healthcare practitioners. The book begins with core information on providing care to LGBT individuals relevant to all healthcare practitioners. Subsequent chapters address best practices in specialty and subspecialty care, providing depth beyond core clinical concepts. Across chapters are threads of information related to healthcare systems, patient advocacy, and sociopolitical climate as they relate to clinical care. Specific attention is paid throughout the text to how we can ensure our healthcare systems are better designed to accommodate the needs of LGBT patients. Each chapter is accompanied by learning objectives linked to the Association of American Medical Colleges' *Professional Competencies to Improve Health Care for People Who Are or May Be LGBT, Gender Nonconforming, and/or Born With DSD.* This text is thus aligned with emerging best practices in education and training to facilitate the understanding and acquisition of key concepts.

It is our hope that this text will inform quality health care for LGBT patients, ultimately reducing the inequities in health care faced by LGBT individuals and improving the health of LGBT communities.

Nashville, TN, USA                                                      Kristen L. Eckstrand
                                                                        Jesse M. Ehrenfeld

# Acknowledgements

This book would not have been possible without the support of our families, our colleagues, and most importantly our LGBT patients from whom we have learned so much. Special thanks to Irene Eckstrand, Steve Eckstrand, Nathan Eckstrand, and Laurel Eckstrand, Judd Taback, David Ehrenfeld, and Katharine Nicodemus. Additionally, we would like to thank our Vanderbilt Team—Drs. Andre Churchwell, Kim Lomis, Amy Fleming, and Bonnie Miller—for their encouragement in the development of this book and the Vanderbilt Program for LGBTI Health.

# Contents

# Contributors

**Kellan Baker, M.P.H., M.A.** Senior Fellow, LGBT Research and Communications Project, Center for American Progress, Washington, DC, USA

**Ignatius Bau, J.D.** Independent Consultant, San Francisco, CA, USA

**Keisa Fallin-Bennett, M.D., M.P.H.** Department of Family and Community Medicine, University of Kentucky, Lexington, KY, USA

**Gregory S. Blaschke, M.D., M.P.H.** Department of Pediatrics, Oregon Health and Science University, Doembecher Children's Hospital, Portland, OR, USA

**Derek R. Blechinger, M.D.** Department of Internal Medicine and Preventive Medicine, Kaiser Permanente San Francisco and University of California San Francisco, San Francisco, CA, USA

**Edwin Bomba, B.A., M.B.A.** LGBT Elder Initiative, Philadelphia, PA, USA

**Benjamin N. Breyer, M.D., M.S.** Department of Urology, University of California San Francisco, San Francisco, CA, USA

**Daniel Calder, M.P.H.** Perelman School of Medicine, University of Pennsylvania, Philadelphia, PA, USA

**Edward J. Callahan, Ph.D.** University of California, Davis School of Medicine, Sacramento, CA, USA

**Scott R. Chaiet, M.D., M.B.A.** Division of Otolaryngology—Head and Neck Surgery, Department of Surgery, University of Wisconsin School of Medicine and Public Health, Madison, WI, USA

**Michael Clark, Dr.N.P., A.P.N.-B.C., D.C.C.** Rutgers School of Nursing-Camden, Camden, NJ, USA

**John A. Davis, M.D., Ph.D.** Department of Infectious Diseases, Ohio State University College of Medicine, Columbus, OH, USA

**Kristen L. Eckstrand, M.D., Ph.D.** Vanderbilt Program for LGBTI Health, Vanderbilt University Medical Center, Nashville, TN, USA

Department of Psychiatry, University of Pittsburgh, Pittsburgh, PA, USA

**E. Kale Edmiston, Ph.D.** Vanderbilt Program for LGBTI Health, Vanderbilt University Medical Center, Nashville, TN, USA

**Randi Ettner, Ph.D.** New Health Foundation Worldwide, Evanston, IL, USA

**Sarah C. Fogel, Ph.D., R.N., F.A.A.N.** School of Nursing, Vanderbilt University, Nashville, TN, USA

**Stephen E. Gee, M.D.** Department of Obstetrics and Gynecology, Ohio State University College of Medicine, Columbus, OH, USA

**Brian Ginsberg, M.D.** The Ronald O. Perelman Department of Dermatology, NYU Langone Medical Center, New York, NY, USA

**Samantha J. Gridley, A.B.** Vanderbilt University School of Medicine, Nashville, TN, USA

**Scott N. Grossman, M.D.** Department of Neurology, NYU Langone Medical Center, New York, NY, USA

**Christopher E. Harris, M.D.** Department of Pediatrics, Cedars Sinai Medical Center, Los Angeles, CA, USA

**Catherine A. Henderson, B.A.** University of California, Davis, Davis, CA, USA

**Shelly L. Henderson, Ph.D.** Department of Family and Community Medicine, University of California Davis, Sacramento, CA, USA

**Abbas Hyderi, M.D., M.P.H.** Department of Family Medicine, University of Illinois at Chicago, Chicago, IL, USA

**Vishesh Kothary, B.S.** Vanderbilt University School of Medicine, Nashville, TN, USA

**Michael B. Leslie, M.D.** Department of Psychiatry, McLean Hospital/ Harvard Medical School, Belmont, MA, USA

**Keith Loukes, M.D., M.H.Sc., F.C.F.P.** Department of Family Medicine, University of Toronto, Toronto, ON, Canada

**Scott MacDonald, M.D.** Department of Primary Care Network and Information Technology, University of California, Davis Health System, Sacramento, CA, USA

**Harvey J. Makadon, M.D.** The National LGBT Health Education Center, The Fenway Institute, Boston, MA, USA

**Matthew A. Malouf, Ph.D.** Connecticut Children's Medical Center, Hartford Hospital, University of Connecticut Health, Hartford/Farmington, CT, USA

**Christopher A. McIntosh, M.Sc., M.D., F.R.C.P.C.** Centre for Addiction and Mental Health, University of Toronto, Toronto, ON, Canada

**Henry H. Ng, M.D., M.P.H.** Center for Internal Medicine-Pediatrics, The MetroHealth System/Case Western Reserve University School of Medicine, Cleveland, OH, USA

**Giang T. Nguyen, M.D., M.P.H., M.C.S.E.** Department of Family Medicine and Community Health and Student Health Service, University of Pennsylvania, Philadelphia, PA, USA

**Carolina Ornelas, B.A.** Department of Human Biology, Stanford University, Stanford, CA, USA

**Christopher M. Palmer, M.D.** Department of Psychiatry, McLean Hospital/ Harvard Medical School, Belmont, MA, USA

**Andrew J. Para, M.D.** Department of Medicine, Northwestern University Feinberg School of Medicine, Chicago, IL, USA

**Jennifer Potter, M.D.** Harvard Medical School, Boston, MA, USA

Beth Israel Deaconess Medical Center, Boston, MA, USA

The Fenway Institute, Boston, MA, USA

**Laura Potter, B.A.** Lesbian, Gay, Bisexual and Transgender Medical Education Research Group (LGBT MERG), Stanford University, Stanford, CA, USA

**Asa E. Radix, M.D., M.P.H.** Callen-Lorde Community Health Center, New York, NY, USA

**Tulsi Roy, M.Sc., M.D.** University of Chicago Medical Center, Chicago, IL, USA

**Craig A. Sheedy, M.D.** Department of Emergency Medicine, Vanderbilt University Medical Center, Nashville, TN, USA

**Alan W. Shindel, M.D., M.A.S.** Department of Urology, University of California, Davis, Sacramento, CA, USA

**Carl G. Streed Jr., M.D.** School of Medicine, Johns Hopkins Bayview Medical Center, Baltimore, MD, USA

**Hendry Ton, M.D.** Department of Psychiatry and Behavioral Sciences, University of California, Davis School of Medicine, Davis, Sacramento, CA, USA

**Matthew D. Truesdale, M.D.** Department of Urology, University of California, San Francisco, San Francisco, CA, USA

**Amy B. Wisniewski, Ph.D.** University of Oklahoma Health Sciences Center, Oklahoma City, OK, USA

**Baligh R. Yehia, M.D., M.P.P., M.Sc.** Perelman School of Medicine, University of Pennsylvania, Philadelphia, PA, USA

**Heshie Zinman, B.A., M.B.A.** LGBT Elder Initiative, Philadelphia, PA, USA

# Part I

# The LGBT Population and Health

# Understanding the LGBT Communities

Derek R. Blechinger

## Purpose

The purpose of this chapter is to provide an overview of the lesbian, gay, bisexual, and transgender (LGBT) communities, persons affected by differences in sex development (DSD-affected), and the unique health needs of these populations.

## Learning Objectives

- Define key sexuality and gender terminology used by and for LGBT patients (*KP1*)
- Discuss key differences between gender vs. sexuality, gender vs. anatomic sex, gender identity vs. gender expression, transgender vs. gender non-conforming, and the various sexual orientations (*KP1*)
- Identify frameworks for approaching the unique health needs and disparities experienced by LGBT & DSD-affected patients (*KP3, KP4*)
- Discuss the impact of minority stress on sexual and gender minorities' health outcomes (*KP3, ICS3, SBP4*)

D.R. Blechinger, M.D. (✉)
Department of Internal Medicine and Preventive Medicine, Kaiser Permanente San Francisco and University of California San Francisco,
2425 Geary Blvd, San Francisco, CA 94115, USA
e-mail: drblech@uw.edu

## Do You Have Sex with Men, Women or Both?

Medical practitioners are often ready and willing to ask about sex to round out a solid social history. This dialogue often begins with the question, "Do you have sex with men, women, or both?" The rote expectation is that patients will report opposite sex partners. But what do you do when the patient says something less expected, such as "both"?

While medical schools across the nation are increasingly teaching future physicians to ask this important question, a 2011 study published in JAMA showed that 132 schools spent a median of 5 h of teaching lesbian, gay, bisexual and transgender (LGBT)-related content [1]. This content was broken down into 16 clinically relevant topics and, when asking what was actually taught, only 8 % of schools reported teaching all 16 topics. For most schools, topics like HIV and STDs topped the list as "LGBT-specific" while important issues such as LGBT adolescent health, transgender hormone management, suicide and coming out were left in the proverbial academic dust.

It is noteworthy that providers are being better equipped to ask the question "Do you have sex with men, women, or both?" but the art of medicine goes well beyond data gathering. It is not enough to simply elicit with whom a patient has sex; providers must use this question and others to build therapeutic alliance, reduce risk, and improve clinical outcomes. Nearly every LGBT

© Springer International Publishing Switzerland 2016
K.L. Eckstrand, J.M. Ehrenfeld (eds.), *Lesbian, Gay, Bisexual, and Transgender Healthcare*,
DOI 10.1007/978-3-319-19752-4_1

patient (97 %) in the U.S. accesses health care at non-LGBT affiliated medical facilities [2], making this an important question even in spaces not specific to LGBT healthcare. The Kaiser Family Foundation recently released a report showing nearly half of all gay and bisexual men have never discussed their sexual orientation with a physician [3]. This has important consequences. All providers, regardless of specialty, must know how to identify LGBT patients, understand their unique health needs, and know how to be not just culturally competent, but culturally excellent. It is our hope that, regardless of specialty, this book will help you achieve just that—excellence.

## An Introduction for the Busy Practitioner

The turn of the twenty-first century has been an auspicious time for advancing lesbian, gay, bisexual, transgender (LGBT) health. This historically stigmatized, highly hidden, diverse, underserved population has a variety of unique health needs and health disparities, many secondary to discrimination and minority stress [4–10]. In contrast, individuals affected by differences in sex development (DSD) still have not received the publicity and consideration that recent decades have afforded the LGBT community (the history of DSD-affected persons and health is discussed in detail in Chap. 23). Regardless of specialty or geographic location, we all work with LGBT and DSD-affected patients (whether they go recognized as such or not). Sexual and gender minority patients are youth, adults, elderly, rich, middle class, poor, employed, unemployed, disabled, able-bodied, citizens, immigrants and of every religious, ethnic and racial background that exists in every corner of the world. The health needs of sexual and gender minorities span the entire spectrum of medicine. Efforts are underway to better serve LGBT patients and address a variety of health disparities as highlighted by Healthy People 2020:

- LGBT individuals have the highest rates of tobacco, alcohol and other drug use [11–15].

- LGBT youth are more likely to be homeless and are two to three times more likely to attempt suicide [16–19].
- LGBT elders face barriers to health because of isolation and a lack of social services and culturally competent providers, often having to "go back into the closet" [20].
- Lesbian women are less likely to get preventive services for cancer [21, 22].
- Lesbian and bisexual women are more likely to be obese [23].
- Gay and bisexual men, while making up only 4 % of men in the U.S., account for 61 % of new HIV infections annually, 44 times that of other men [24].
- Transgender people experience high rates of victimization, HIV/STDs, mental health issues, suicide and lower rates of health insurance [25–29].

These and many other disparities have also been outlined by the 2011 Institute of Medicine's Report "The Health of LGBT People" funded by the NIH. Numerous professional associations including the American Medical Association, American Nurses Association, American Academy of Family Physicians, American Academy of Pediatrics, American Psychiatric Association, American Cancer Society, GLMA: Health Professionals Advancing LGBT Equality, and others have written position statements in support of a variety of LGBT issues (see Appendix C). Our nation and leading medical associations have heard the call to better serve LGBT people, and providers across all medical fields are being called to respond.

## Terminology for the Busy Practitioner

Sexuality and gender are at the core of our experience as human beings. They are complex and multidimensional, and do not conform to traditional binaries (ex. masculine versus feminine, straight versus gay). It is the aim of this chapter to make the material approachable for all practitioners. Like many things in medicine, broadening your differential for "gender" and "sexuality" will help you better understand your patients and

**Table 1.1** LGBT and DSD-affected medical terminology in the clinical encounter

| Acronym | Possible associated identities[a] | Examples of usage |
|---|---|---|
| MSM | • Gay man<br>• Queer<br>• Homosexual<br>• Can include bisexual men | • Pt is a 41 year old MSM presenting w/…<br>• Pt is a gay man w/hx of…<br>• Pt identifies as a queer man w/… |
| MSMW | • Bisexual man<br>• Queer<br>• Can include straight-identified men | • Pt is a 32 year old MSMW in a primary relationship w/…<br>• Pt identifies as a queer man, reports sex with men and women |
| WSW | • Lesbian<br>• Gay woman<br>• Queer<br>• Can include bisexual women | • Pt is a 89 year old WSW presenting w/…<br>• Pt identifies as lesbian<br>• Pt self-identifies as a queer woman who only has sex with women |
| WSWM | • Bisexual woman<br>• Queer<br>• Can include straight-identified women | • Pt is a 20 year old WSWM in a primary relationship w/…<br>• Pt identifies as a queer woman, reports sex with women and transmen |
| MTF | • Transgender woman<br>• Transwoman<br>• Genderqueer<br>• May be pre- or post-op | • Pt is a 52 year old MTF transgender woman presenting w/history of…<br>• Pt identifies as an MTF woman w/intermittent hx of estrogen use.<br>• Pt identifies as genderqueer, assigned male at birth, preferred pronouns "they/them" |
| FTM | • Transgender man<br>• Transman<br>• Transsexual man<br>• May be pre- or post-op | • Pt is a 24 year old FTM transman<br>• Pt identifies as man now s/p top surgery, continuing gender-affirming hormones now presenting w/…<br>• Pt identifies as trans (FTM, pre-op), interested in pursuing GRS in July |
| GRS | • SRS (sex reassignment surgery)<br>• Gender reassignment surgery (less accurate description)<br>• Post-op | • Pt is a 29 year old transman s/p GRS 4 years ago continuing on gender-affirming hormone therapy<br>• Pt identifies as an MTF woman, now s/p SRS × 1 year continuing on estrogen therapy |
| DSD-affected | • Intersex | • Pt is a 35 year old woman assigned female at birth s/p genital surgery 2/2 congenital adrenal hyperplasia<br>• Pt identifies as DSD-affected s/p corrective surgery at birth w/hx of…<br>• Pt is a 19 year old woman w/hx of infertility 2/2 androgen insensitivity syndrome presenting with… |

[a]These identities may be associated with a preferred sexual or gender identity, but these are not universal associations. Rather than make assumptions, always let patients self-identify their preferred terminology

improve your clinical acumen (see Table 1.1 for examples of how to incorporate terminology into clinical practice).

**Helpful Hint**

Gender identity, gender expression, and sexuality are not binary concepts—thinking of them as having two ends on a linear spectrum artificially limits understanding of their complexities.

## Beginner Level

Many practitioners without much experience with sexual and gender minorities have likely already heard the terms "lesbian", "gay", "bisexual", and "transgender". These four terms are often combined into the acronym "LGBT". While this acronym contains both identifiers of sexuality *and* gender, they are not the same. In order to understand the complexities of LGBT healthcare, an understanding of basic terminology is required:

*"Gender"*—a highly complex biopsychosocial concept often reduced to a binary set of identities and behaviors that are either masculine or feminine, male or female. Gender is multifacited and can be quite fluid throughout the lifetime, including concepts such as identity and expression. Gender is often confused for biologic sex, however gender is independent of anatomy.

*"Gender identity"*—an internalized concept of self as a particular gender, regardless of external appearance. Because gender identity is internally defined, it is separate from a person's physical anatomy—male genitalia does not mean one's gender identity is that of a man, nor does female genitalia or breasts identify someone as a woman.

*"Gender expression"*—describes a set of behaviors that have been socially assigned as masculine or feminine. Remember that the simple binary of "male" vs. "female" behavior belies the myriad, complex, often overlapping nature of these behaviors independent of actual gender identity. A person may express a particular gender at any given time without changing their gender identity.

*"Sex"*—a descriptor of a person's anatomical state, most often reduced to two phenotypes of male (e.g., penis, scrotum, testicles) vs. female (e.g., breasts, vagina, uterus, ovaries). Medically, we know that there are a multitude of natural variations on anatomical sex not just limited to different shapes and sizes but also presence, absence and extent of differentiation of various structures. Regardless of function, phenotypes incongruent with the male vs. female binary are often identified by medical practitioners as differences of sex development (DSD).

*"Sexual orientation"*—a set of sexual attractions, behaviors and/or romantic feelings for men, women or both. Sexual orientation is often reduced to specific terms like homosexual vs. bisexual vs. heterosexual, however there is a broad spectrum of sexual orientations that can vary depending on the gender identity of the person and that person's various attractions, which may include attractions to certain sexes, gender identities, gender expressions and combinations thereof. The first attempts to quantify sexual orientation were made in the Kinsey scale, ranking people as 0 (exclusively heterosexual) to 6 (exclusively homosexual), or "X" for asexual. More sophisticated, contemporary models of sexuality have since been developed, recognizing it's breadth of natural variation and fluidity throughout a lifetime.

**Helpful Hint**

At the risk of over-simplification: Gender is between the ears. Sex is between the legs. Sexual orientation refers to attraction to either of these things (see Fig. 1.1).

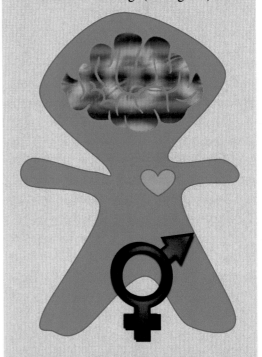

**Fig. 1.1** The modified gender gingerbread person model, which can be used as an aid to explain gender (image courtesy, J. Ehrenfeld)

*"Lesbian"*—used to describe women who are primarily attracted to women. This identifier of sexual orientation notably describes attraction vs. behavior. Identifying as lesbian implies sexual activity with women but does not exclude them from having attractions or sexual experiences with men, and it is important to clarify with your

patient not only who they are primarily attracted to, but also whether or not they have sex with men. "Homosexual woman" is antiquated and can be depersonalizing for your patient.

*"Gay"*—used to describe both men and women who have same-sex attractions. Historically, this has been used to refer to men who are primarily attracted to and sexual with men but can also refer to women who are primarily attracted to and sexual with women. If you are unsure of whether a woman identifies as "gay" or "lesbian", ask how they self-identify. "Homosexual" is antiquated and can be depersonalizing for your patient.

*"Bisexual"*—used to describe a person who is attracted to both men and women. This can encompass a wide spectrum of individuals who may have leanings toward a particular gender, or equal attraction to all genders, or attraction to specific aspects of various genders. Being in a relationship with a same-sex partner does not make a bisexual person gay. Being in relationship with an opposite-sex partner does not make a bisexual person straight. Bisexual people sometimes experience a unique type of disownment from both the straight and gay communities, rejected for not being "straight enough" or "gay enough." Others can experience a sense of invisibility (e.g. "bi-invisibility"), feeling lost or ignored within the LG(B)T communities.

*"Differences of sex development"*—refers to a group of phenotypes where there is a variation of sex, either chromosomal, hormonal, or anatomical, such that one's sex is not congruent with society's male versus female anatomical binary. This term does not define a person's identity, rather someone is affected by differences in sex development (DSD-affected). Prior terms for this group have, and still, include "differences of sex development" or "intersex", and their usage depends on the patient or medical society using them. The latter term is considered antiquated by some, but still in use by many, including the addition of the "I" to LGBT to form LGBTI. For further detail, see Chap. 23.

*"LGBTI"*—aforementioned acronym "LGBT" with the addition of "intersex". While the intention of this acronym is to be inclusive of all sexual and gender minorities and the often overlooked "I", not all DSD-affected individuals identify as intersex, and not all intersex individuals identify themselves as part of the "LGBTI" community. The experiences and needs of DSD-affected individuals are unique and may not fit under the wide umbrella cast by "LGBTI".

## Intermediate Level

*"MSM"*—men who have sex with men, an epidemiologic term describing a man who has sex with men regardless of how he self-identifies. MSM includes not only men who identify as gay or bisexual, but also men who self-identify as straight but are sexual with men. This term is helpful when trying to categorize health risks and behaviors at a population level, though MSM would be unlikely to refer to themselves as MSM, but more likely as gay, straight or bisexual.

*"MSMW"*—men who have sex with men and women, an epidemiologic term exclusively describing a man who has sex with both men and women. A person does not need to identify as bisexual to be categorized as MSMW.

*"WSW"*—women who have sex with women, an epidemiologic term described a woman who has sex with women, regardless of how she self-identities. WSW includes not only women who identify as lesbian, gay or bisexual, but also those who self-identify as straight but are sexual with women. This is a useful epidemiologic term, especially when trying to categorize health risks and behaviors at a population level, though WSW would be unlikely to refer to themselves as WSW, but more likely as lesbian, gay, straight or bisexual.

*"WSWM"*—women who have sex with women and men, an epidemiologic term exclusively describing a woman who has sex with both men and women. A person does not need to identify as bisexual to be categorized as WSWM.

*"Cis-gender"*—a person whose anatomical birth sex is congruent with their gender identity. The majority of humans would be considered cis-gendered, though many may not have given much thought to this identification given society's designation of cis-gender as default, or "normal".

"*Transgender*"—a person whose anatomical birth sex is incongruent with their gender identity. Transgender people often exhibit cross-gender behavior at an early age. If their designated sex is female, their gender identity is male (often shorted to "trans man" or "female to male" or "FTM"). Conversely, if their birth sex is designated male, their gender identity is female (often shorted to "trans woman" or "male to female" or "MTF"). Note that using the word "trans-" prior to a patient's identifier as a man or a woman can be perceived as belittling and should only be used if the patient identifies that way. For more detail, see Part V.

> **Helpful Hint**
> When considering cis- vs. trans-gender, think back to organic chemistry and recall cis- vs. trans-isomerism (on the same side vs. on the other side!).

"*Genital reassignment surgery*"—often shortened GRS, an intervention that surgically changes the genital anatomy of an individual to better fit their gender identity with society's corresponding anatomic expectations. "Sex reassignment surgery" (SRS) refers to surgeries affecting genitals as well as secondary sex characteristics. For more detail, see Chap. 20.

"*Transsexual*"—in the past, this term referred to a transgender person after sexual reassignment surgery. Notably, this is an adjective and not a noun. For example, a MTF transwoman who is now post-op would be medically described as a transsexual woman, as opposed to a transsexual. When used as a noun, the word "transsexual" is often perceived as a highly medical term and is considered pejorative by patients who would otherwise identify as their gender.

## Advanced Level

"*Queer*"—an umbrella term that encompasses a wide range of sexualities and genders that are outside the societal "norm". This may include lesbian, gay, bisexual, transgender individuals and allies who don't ascribe to being "normal". Historically a term used to denigrate LGBT individuals, this term has been reclaimed in the twenty-first century as a term of empowerment. Some LGBT individuals, especially those of older generations, find this word to be hate speech and too painful or disturbing to use. Self-identifying as queer has become more common in younger generations of sexual and gender minorities.

"*Pansexual*"—an individual who has a diverse set of attractions to a variety of anatomies, gender expressions and gender identities. While at first glance similar to bisexuality, the self-designation as pansexual is an intentional rejection of the gender binary and encompasses the whole spectrum of sexuality and genders.

> **Helpful Hint**
> During the clinical encounter, reflect the terminology used by your patient. If you are uncertain about terms or preferred pronouns, ask.

"*Drag*"—a type of cross-gender expression, often done as performance art. The art of drag has received national attention via the television show "RuPaul's Drag Race". Men who perform as women are called drag queens and women who perform as men are called drag kings. A transman is not a drag king and similarly a transwoman is not a drag queen. Drag is a performative act of gender expression, not a gender identity.

"*Genderqueer*"—an umbrella term that encompasses a wide range of genders. This term can include those who feel like they fit outside of a gender binary of male vs. female, as well as individuals who consider themselves to have multiple genders or no gender at all. Genderqueer subverts the simple distinction between cisgender vs. transgender people, as well as blurring the distinctions between gender identity and gender expression. A person who identifies as genderqueer may use gender neutral pronouns such as "they", "them", "their" or fluidly change between "she/her" or "he/him".

*"Trans\*"*—the addition of the asterisk (\*) to trans (ex. trans\*) is meant to be inclusive of gender queer and gender non-conforming individuals that don't think of themselves as on a cis- or transgender binary (ex. FTM transman versus MTF transwoman). Trans\* can be used to describe any person not identifying as a cis-man or cis-woman, encompassing the entirety of non-cis gender identities and expressions.

*"Gender dysphoria"*—the most recent Diagnostic and Statistical Manual of Mental Disorders (DSM-5) [30] designation for individuals who experience clinically significant distress associated with their gender associated with their gender identity for 6 months or greater. Gender dysphoria replaces "gender identity disorder" as an attempt to better characterize the experiences of gender non-conforming individuals. Notably, the DSM-5 has an additional diagnostic code for individuals who have already transitioned and are continuing medical treatment (e.g. ongoing hormone therapy, supportive counseling, surgeries) to ensure treatment access (and insurance coverage) without terming their gender or anatomic sex status as "disordered". Gender dysphoria has been intentionally separated from chapters including paraphilic and sexual dysfunction disorders to help address the stigma produced by our previous attempts at medically coding transgender, intersex and genderqueer individuals. For more detail, see Chap. 13.

*"Heteronormativity"*—a subjective world view that heterosexuality is normal and measuring any variations in human sexuality from the heterosexual "norm". Heteronormativity is similar in concept to "ethnocentric", as pertaining to sexuality. It is a term that addresses the concept of heterosexual privilege, or the advantages in social, political, and economic arenas granted to heterosexuals that are acquired by default given their status as a valued, preferred sexual orientation in society. Exclusive recognition of heterosexuality and constant depictions of heterosexual acts in public, media and graduate medical education are mainstays of heteronormativity, contributing to LGBT discrimination and stigma. See Fig. 1.2.

**Helpful Hint**
Try to avoid gendered or heteronormative language during the clinical encounter. For example, try using "partner" instead of boyfriend, girlfriend, husband, wife, or spouse. Remember that your clinic forms can make this mistake before the patient even meets you.

*"Coming out"*—an act by which a sexual or gender minority discloses their identity to another person. Coming out to family and other loved ones are often particularly formative experiences for LGBT people ranging from profoundly affirming to violent rejection. When asking a LGBT patient when they came out, you are asking them the first time they disclosed their identity as a sexual or gender minority. However, all LGBT people are constantly having to come out in large and small ways throughout their life time—every time they meet a new person, start a new job, join a new church, and even when deciding to hold hands with their loved one while walking in a park. As a result of heteronormativity, LGBT people are often in a constant state of vigilance around the words they use, their body language and the gender pronouns they use about themselves or their loved ones lest they come out unintentionally. This hypervigilance can be a significant source of stress and likely contributes to a number of LGBT health disparities. For more detail, see Chap. 4.

## Exercise: Reflections on LGBT Terminology

Now that you understand some of the basic differences between sexuality and gender, let's dive deeper. Take the term "lesbian", for example. Notice that this word describes not only sexual orientation but also gender identity. For someone

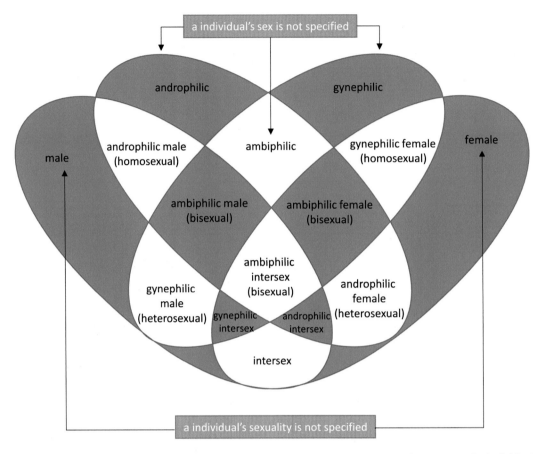

**Fig. 1.2** A diagram showing the relationships between sexual orientation and assigned sex. Some prefer to use the terms androphilia and gynephilia, because homo- sexual and heterosexual assign a sex to the individual (image courtesy J. Ehrenfeld)

to identify as a lesbian, they most likely have a gender identity that is female and a sexual attraction to women. This distinction is subtle but important. For example, a transgender woman whose gender identity is female and their attraction is to other women makes them perceived as "straight" by some if only their birth sex is being considered. This, however, would not be honoring the person's autonomy in self-determining their gender and their sexuality. Remember that anatomy does not equal gender identity, making anatomic sex irrelevant. A transwoman attracted to other women would most likely self-identify as a lesbian. A transman attracted to other men would most likely self-identify as gay. Ultimately, every patient has the right to self-identify and it is up to us as medical professionals to learn to ask questions that help us understand the unique health needs and stratify risks for each and every patient we serve.

Deconstructing LGBT terminology can be difficult even for experienced LGBT health care providers. Continuing to struggle with the content and asking questions is a sign of a healthy, curious, well-intentioned practitioner. When approaching this material at an advanced level, it is also helpful to recognize your own place of privilege, whatever it may be, regarding sexuality and gender. Privilege, as mentioned above in the definition of "heteronormativity", is a set of unearned social, political and economic advantages obtained by virtue of a person's identity being valued by society. While the focus of this chapter is on sexuality and gender, certainly race, age, religious affiliations, economic status, mental health, class, profession and other factors come with their own set of privileges and interact with sexual and gender identity in a variety of ways. Below are some starting places accompanied by a hypothetical reflection to help consider sexuality and gender privilege:

- Perhaps you are straight, and you've never had to decide whether or not to tell your family, friends, employer, or government officials your sexual orientation for fear of rejection, discrimination or violence.
- Perhaps you are a gay man who has never had to grapple with the idea of being attracted to both sexes and not fully belonging to either the gay community or the straight community.
- Perhaps you are a cis-gendered lesbian who has never considered what it would be like to have a penis instead of a vagina.
- Perhaps you are a transwoman who, while feeling you have body parts incongruent with your gender, have never had your genitals surgically altered without your consent as a child.
- Perhaps you are bisexual, and have not considered your increased potential to marry in every state in America and improved possibility of having children without reproductive assistance if paired with an opposite sex partner.

These reflections are by no means meant to shame or discourage practitioners of various walks of life, but rather begin the exploration of how one fits (or does not fit) in various communities and gain greater insight into the experiences of those different from you. Being a gay man does not automatically provide insight into the experiences of a transwoman. Nor does being a transgender person provide someone with special knowledge of the bisexual community. Regardless of our sexuality, gender or sex, we all should objectively assess our own privileges and limitations without guilt and continue to be curious about ourselves and others.

## LGBT Demographics (Table 1.2)

Sexual and gender minorities are a unique demographic as they cut across all other demographics. LGBT & DSD-affected people can be very

**Table 1.2** LGBT demographics

| | U.S. population estimate (%) |
|---|---|
| LGBT | 3.8 |
| LGB | 3.5 |
| LG | 1.7 |
| B | 1.8 |
| T | 0.3 |
| Lesbian women | 1.1 (of women) |
| Gay men | 2.2 (of men) |
| Bisexual women | 2.2 (of women) |
| Bisexual men | 1.4 (of men) |
| Have engaged in same-sex sexual behavior | 8.2 |
| Acknowledge some same-sex sexual attraction | 11 |

rich or very poor. Lesbian women can be African American. Bisexual men can be Muslim. Transwomen can be found in rural communities. Gay men can be elderly. DSD-affected people can be Southeast Asian immigrants. Bisexual women can be disabled. Notably, the vast majority of LGBT children are born and raised by cis-gendered, heterosexual parents. This limits the vertical transmission of culture and histories from older to newer generations enjoyed by other cultures. The shared experiences of stigma, discrimination and having to come out as a sexual or gender minority is what ties this complex, sometimes highly hidden demographic together. Same-sex couples are found in 99 % of counties across America [31]. Regardless of specialty or practice location, all providers care for sexual and gender minority patients. See Fig. 1.3.

**Helpful Hint**
Same-sex couples are found in 99 % of U.S. counties. You have sexual and gender minority patients.

There have been many attempts over the decades to estimate the number of LGBT people in the U.S. Alfred Kinsey, famed for his work in sexuality and the development of the "Kinsey Scale", noted in his research that 10 % of men

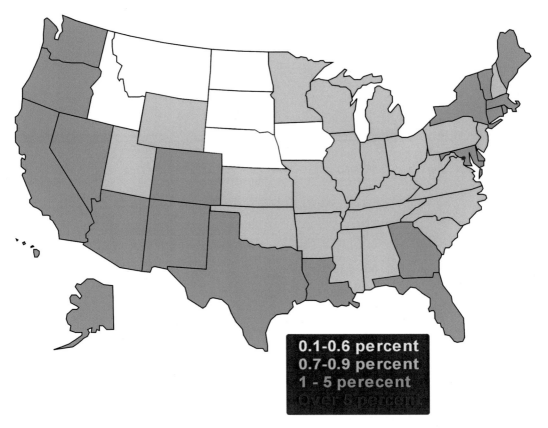

**Fig. 1.3** Percentage of households with same-sex couples 2010 (adapted from the U.S. Census Bureau)

between 16 and 55 engaged in same-sex behavior exclusively for 3+ years. This led to the popularization of the "10 %" estimate for LGB prevalence. Since then, lower estimates have been made by the National Epidemiological Survey on Alcohol and Related Conditions (2004–2005), the National Survey of Family Growth (2006–2008), the General Social Survey (2008), the California Health Interview Survey (2009), and the National Survey of Sexual Health and Behavior (2009). Challenges in successfully integrating the data can be found in differing survey methodology, consistent ways of asking about sexual orientation vs. attraction vs. behavior, and changes in who is included as a sexual or gender minority. More contemporary data analysis utilizing population-based data by the Williams Institute at the UCLA School of Law has become the current standard, estimating 3.5 % of adults in the U.S. identify as LGB (over 8 million people) and 0.3 % Americans identify as transgender (700,000 peo-

ple) [32]. Gates' review of state and national surveys also delineated identity from behavior and attraction, finding 8.2 % of Americans have same-sex sexual behavior and 11 % of Americans have same-sex sexual attraction.

## Demographics by Sexual Orientation

In 2014, the CDC released its first National Health Interview Survey on sexual orientation and health. The study which interviewed more than 33,500 people ages 18–64 found that approximately 96 % of Americans described themselves as straight, 1.6 % gay, or lesbian, 0.7 % said they were bisexual, and just over 1 % identified as "something else." This equates to approximately 1.4 million lesbian women and 2.5 million gay men. Interestingly, gay men make up a greater percent of MSM than bisexual men (2.2 % vs. 1.4 %), in contrast to the trend noted in WSW. Notably, bisexual people make up the majority subgroup within the LGBT community but are often subject to "bi-invisibility" given their perception as either gay when with a same-sex partner or straight when with an opposite-sex partner.

## Demographics by Gender Identity

Population estimates for transgender individuals remains elusive, largely because population surveys such as the Decennial Census or American Community Survey do not directly ask about gender identity. Attempts at estimating the prevalence of transgender have instead focused on transsexualism, given at least the raw prevalence data from sex reassignment surgery (SRS) clinics throughout Europe from decades ago. A reanalysis by Olyslager and Conway [33] using mathematical modeling from those earlier reports found a most likely prevalence to be between 1:1000 and 1:2000. Using more recent incidence data and alternative estimation methods, they found that the rate is at least 1:500 (0.2 %), and possibly even higher. Their results were presented at the WPATH 20th International Symposium in Chicago, but not adopted by the APA. Incidentally, more contemporary researchers working with population data have found similar rates. By averaging the data from the Massachusetts and California surveys, Gates [34] estimates the number of Americans who identify as transgender to be 0.3 %—nearly 700,000 transgender U.S. citizens.

Transgender people can be found throughout America, from places both urban and rural and participating in society in every way imaginable. Increased trans visibility in the media include remarkable individuals such as Isis King (*America's Next Top Model*), Thomas Beatie (transman who publically came out as pregnant in 2008), Laverne Cox (*Orange is the New Black*), Chaz Bono (*Becoming Chaz*), Dr. Marci Bowers (pioneer and first transwoman GRS surgeon) and the brilliant and inspiring Janet Mock (author and staff editor at *People Magazine*). Kristin Beck, the first openly transgender Navy SEAL, told her story in her autobiography *Warrior Princess* in 2013. Notably, she retired from the military prior to coming out as

transgender, as the repeal of "Don't Ask, Don't Tell" in 2011 only applied to the LGB portion of the LGBT communities, leaving the "T" unaddressed. The military still officially forbids openly transgender people from serving, but the results of the National Transgender Discrimination Survey showed us that 20 % of trans people had served in the military—two times that of the general population [35]. This discriminatory policy continues to be under pressure for change by civil rights advocates, and may hopefully see change even by the time of publishing this text.

## Differences of Sex Development/Intersex

There is a remarkable lack of epidemiologic data when it comes to DSD-affected people. While sometimes lumped with transgender people, DSD-affected experiences and health care needs as detailed by the clinical guidelines published by the Intersex Society of North America that are different from those of transgender people [36]. Most often, DSD-affected individuals have intersected with the medical field at birth, perhaps experiencing unnecessary procedures, diagnostic testing or unwanted surgeries. The Intersex Society of North America has endorsed the review of medical literature ranging from 1955 to 1998 by Anne Fausto-Sterling et al. [37] that found the total number of people with bodies different from standard male or female anatomy was 1:100 births and people receiving corrective genital surgery was 1–2 per 1000 births. Complete gonadal dysgenesis is estimated to happen in 1:150,000 and hypospadias in 1:770. Klinefelter (XXY) was found to be 1:1000, androgen insensitivity syndrome 1:130,000, and congenital adrenal hyperplasia in 1:13,000 births. For more detail, see Chap. 23.

## Youth

While it is probably true that rates of sexual and gender minorities are very similar in youth as in adult LGBT populations, efforts are underway to better describe this highly vulnerable population. Estimates from the CDC's Youth Risk Behavior

Survey conducted from 2001 to 2009 in nine states that assessed sexual identity found 1.0–2.6 % identified as gay or lesbian and 2.9–5.2 % identified as bisexual. Students unsure of their sexual identity ranged from 1.3 to 4.7 % [38].

## LGBT Parents

Using U.S. Census 2010 data and Gallup Daily Tracking Survey data, Gates [34] estimates that of the 650,000 same-sex couples in the U.S., 19 % of same-sex households have children under age 18 and 37 % of LGBT adults have had a child. Gates also estimates that nearly half of LGBT women and a fifth of LGBT men are raising children. Notably, the U.S. regions with the highest rates of same-sex childrearing are in the Midwest, the Mountain West and the South. In support of transgender estimates in this analysis, National Transgender Discrimination Survey data shows 38 % of transgender respondents self-identified as parents [35].

## Immigrants

Confidently estimating the number of documented and undocumented LGBT immigrants in the U.S is a daunting but not impossible task. In a report by the UCLA Law School's Williams Institute, Gates [34] does so by using same-sex couple data gathered by Gates and Konnoth [39], Pew Research Hispanic Center data, Gallup Daily Tracking Survey and the U.S. Census Bureau's 2011 American Community Survey:

- 267,000 LGBT undocumented adult immigrants (2.7 % of undocumented adults)
  - 71 % are Hispanic, 15 % are Asian or Pacific Islander
- 637,000 LGBT documented adult immigrants (2.4 % of documented adults)
  - 30 % are Hispanic, 35 % are Asian or Pacific Islander.

Certainly, it is even more difficult to estimate the number of transgender individuals who are immigrants. The National Transgender Discrimination Survey [29] found that, of 6450 transgender and gender non-conforming study participants, 4 % identified as undocumented non-citizens.

## History Highlights of LGBT Communities (Table 1.3)

Over the decades, the "LGBT" community alphabet has seen changes, additions, subtractions and positioning of the various letters in attempts to continue to describe this diverse set of sexual and gender minorities. Indeed, it is entirely impossible to capture everyone that exists outside of the cis-gendered, 100 % heterosexual experience. Together, sexual and gender minorities are brought together by a shared experience of discrimination and "otherness". And while LGBT people are together a community, they have separate needs. Each of the LGBT letters comes with its own unique set of histories—together a community, but with separate needs. The following are highlights of historical information you may find useful in better understanding each letter of the LGBT alphabet and establishing rapport.

## Gay and Lesbian

The medicalization and cultural definitions of "homosexuality", "sexual inverts" and "gays" did not come until the nineteenth and twentieth centuries, from the work of historical figures such as Sigmund Freud to Alfred Kinsey. However, evidence of same-sex behavior dates back throughout ancient history across cultures. A key component to understanding sexual minorities in the twenty-first century is the not-so-distant past medicalization and criminalization of consensual same-sex behaviors and relationships. Homosexuality as a mental illness wasn't removed from the American Psychiatric Association's Diagnostic and Statistical Manual (DSM) until 1973. Prior to that, aversion therapy using chemicals, mechanical violence and electricity

**Table 1.3**  Highlights of LGBT history

| |
|---|
| 630 BC: Greek lyric poet Sappho born on the island of Lesbos, famous for her lesbian-themed poetry |
| 326 BC: Alexander the Great is first bisexual to conquer most of the known Western world |
| 1786: Pennsylvania repeals death penalty for sodomy |
| 1895: Irish author and playwright Oscar Wilde convicted and imprisoned for gross indecency for same-sex behavior |
| 1937: Pink triangle is used in Nazi concentration camps to identify gay men |
| 1948: Alfred Kinsey publishes the Kinsey Scale |
| 1948: Alfred Kinsey brings a transgender girl to Dr. Harry Benjamin, who uses estrogen for the first time as treatment for MTF transgender patients |
| 1952: Dr. Harry Benjamin's first SRS patient Christine Jorgensen makes front page of New York Daily News as first American to undergo SRS |
| 1962: Notable author and bisexual African American publishes his novel "Another Country" |
| 1966: Dr. Harry Benjamin first uses the term transsexual |
| 1968: University of Minnesota begins "Bi Alliance" group |
| 1969: Stonewall Riots, an uprising against police harassment of LGBT people at Stonewall Inn, NYC; basis of annual Pride Festival celebrations across the country (June 27th) |
| 1973: American Psychiatric Association removes homosexuality from the DSM-II |
| 1978: San Francisco city supervisor Harvey Milk assassinated |
| 1978: Rainbow flag is crafted as a symbol for LGBT pride |
| 1980: First set of Harry Benjamin Standards produced for transgender patient providers |
| 1981: First documented case of AIDS by the CDC |
| 1990: U.S. census includes same-sex household data. |
| 1993: Intersex Society of North America founded |
| 1993: "Don't Ask, Don't Tell" signed into law banning LGBT people from serving openly in the military |
| 1993: Transman Brandon Teena was raped and murdered, became subject of film "Boys Don't Cry" |
| 1994: Olympic gold swimmer Greg Louganis comes out |
| 1996: "Defense of Marriage Act" (DOMA) enacted into law non-recognition of same-sex marriages for federal purposes |
| 1998: Matthew Shepard, a gay student at University of Wyoming, was tortured and murdered |
| 2001: Netherlands first country to legalize same-sex marriage |
| 2002: U.S. Dept of Health and Human Services publishes Healthy People 2010, identifying sexual minorities as having disparate health concerns |
| 2003: Remaining state sodomy laws in U.S. struck down by Supreme Court |
| 2004: Massachusetts first state to issue marriage licenses to same-sex couples |
| 2004: American Academy of Pediatrics reports on the state of LGBT youth health disparities |
| 2007: Janice Langbehn denied access to her dying partner Lisa Pond by Jackson Memorial Hospital despite power of attorney paperwork, Pond passed away without her partner or three young children |
| 2010: Healthy People 2020 includes addressing LGB and T health disparities as a special topic for national public health goals |
| 2010: Hospital visitation rights for same-sex couples established by presidential order to DHHS |
| 2011: Directed by the National Institutes of Health, the Institute of Medicine releases consensus report on LGBT health, demographics, data collection and research recommendations |
| 2011: Repeal of "Don't Ask, Don't Tell", allowing LGB service members to serve openly |
| 2011: "Bisexual Invisibility: Impacts and Regulations" released by San Francisco's Human Rights Commission |
| 2012: California law bans reparative therapy, the discounted pseudoscientific practice of converting sexual minorities to heterosexual lifestyles |
| 2013: DSM-5 eliminates the stigmatizing designation "gender identity disorder" in favor of "gender dysphoria", highlighting only those distressed by their gender identity |
| 2013: DOMA (Section 3 barring same-sex marriage recognition) repealed, ruled unconstitutional by the Supreme Court |
| 2014: by July, 19 U.S. states have marriage equality laws |
| 2015: Supreme Court rules in favor of marriage equality, making same-sex marriage legal across the U.S. |

were used on sexual minorities in unsuccessful efforts to change their orientation [40]. Despite widespread renouncement of this pseudoscientific, barbaric practice, it continues in many parts of the U.S. The end of the twentieth century saw increased political efforts to decriminalize same-sex behavior, but it wasn't until 2003 when the remaining state sodomy laws in the U.S. were struck down by the Supreme Court. It is in this context—a society that considers the way a whole community of people find sex, love and relationships to be diseased and criminal—that gay and bi men and women were forced to build community.

Urban centers were optimal places for both the sheer numbers and anonymity required for sexual and gender minorities to congregate and cultivate culture. Many LGBT communities across the nation today center around bar culture, as these were the first places where sexual and gender minorities could find each other. Gay bars were only marginally safe, however, as they often were raided by police and others. An historic moment for LGBT rights occurred on June 27th, 1969 at the Stonewall Inn, a gay bar in New York City. During a police raid, Stonewall patrons as well as their neighbors stood up to the police and rioted. The 1970s became a prolific time for LGBT civil rights and organizations, with Stonewall now a rallying cry for LGBT civil rights and the basis for annual Pride Festival celebrations across the country.

Bar culture provided a space for the development of the LGBT communities. Unfortunately, relying on institutions that promote alcohol, tobacco and sometimes other drug use has likely played a strong role in the health disparities seen in LGBT patients. Perhaps the most defining event for the LGBT community was the HIV epidemic. It is beyond the scope of this chapter to review in detail the deep and multilayered impact HIV has had on the LGBT communities. But to better understand LGBT patients it is important to have a basic understanding of how it has ravaged the LGBT community, further stigmatized sexual and gender minorities and left many with complicated relationships to medical care.

In 1981, the first cases of AIDS were diagnosed in gay men, mistakenly called gay-related immune deficiency (GRID) until HIV was further understood. During this time, thousands of gay and bi men died, entire swaths of men cut from the fabric of the LGBT communities. Important work by Levine [41, 42] and other scholars pointed out the sense of individual and communal trauma experienced by the LGBT communities through this ongoing epidemic. Government inaction under the Reagan administration led to incredible losses and the subsequent community-based responses to the HIV epidemic. Lesbian women came to the aid of their dying friends abandoned in hospitals, sometimes filling the role of family and even nurses [43]. AIDS service organizations (ASOs) across the country sprang up and into action. Led by LGBT activists, ASOs pressed the government and biomedical industries to respond to the AIDS crisis. Many of these ASOs continue to advocate for HIV prevention and care services throughout the nation and created an infrastructure from which LGBT health efforts could emerge. Advances in HIV antiretroviral therapies, post-exposure prophylaxis (PEP), and pre-exposure prophylaxis (PrEP) have changed the landscape of HIV treatment and prevention, but in 2010, the CDC reports MSM accounting for two-thirds of new HIV infections in the U.S., an increase of 12 % from 2008. Kaiser Family Foundation research shows that gay and bisexual men see HIV as the top health issue facing their community, but most are not personally worried about getting infected and are not testing regularly [3]. The HIV epidemic persists. Notably, the LGBT communities have shown a remarkable amount of resilience in the face of a modern-day plague, as well as enduring centuries of criminalization and medicalization of their identities.

LGBT communities are unique in that members of the community are most often not born to LGBT parents. In most groups (ex. race, ethnicities, religious groups, etc.) history and culture are passed from grandparents to parents to children both explicitly and implicitly. When considering the histories being brought to the table by your patients, it is important to realize that LGBT people that lived through the beginning of the HIV epidemic have often profound, intimate understanding of HIV and its impact on their lives.

It is not hard to imagine how devastating an epidemic like HIV has been to a community of people that relies on prior generations outside of their biological family to pass on history and culture to new generations. Those born in 1982 and onward have never known a world without HIV and may not have the same personal or historical relationship with HIV as important or even relevant to their lives—an example of the importance and power of vertical transmission of histories to subsequent generations.

## Bisexual

While present in nearly every important LGBT moment in history, bisexual people have often been either overlooked or excluded as participants in the LGBT histories. Interestingly, bisexual people actually are the majority population within the LGBT community [44] but have a markedly decreased visibility. Despite their majority, a challenge often faced by bisexual people is the sense that they belong to both the straight and gay communities but often feel excluded based on their otherness from both straight and gay communities. When participating in straight culture, their same-sex attractions place them in the same stigmatized category as gay people, and may be perceived as simply gay. When participating in gay culture, bisexual people may be perceived as "not gay enough" or "going through a phase" (a particularly hurtful but all-too common opinion of lesbian and gay people). Throughout the history of the LGBT communities, they have experienced a phenomenon called "bi-invisibility".

---

**Helpful Hint**

To avoid bi-invisibility, don't forget the "B" in LGBT as a healthy, normal aspect of human sexuality. Indeed, bisexuals make up the majority subgroup of the LGBT communities!

---

Bi-invisibility can be noted when a bisexual person marries an opposite-sex partner and is subsequently seen as straight. The same is true of bisexual people who marry a same-sex partner—they are often perceived as gay because of the gender of their primary partner. An example of bi-invisibility can be seen in our own field. If researchers do studies on sexual minorities, it's often on gay men and women. . If bisexual people get included, they tend to get lumped into "MSM" or "WSW", and sometimes their own unique health needs as bisexual people get lost in the milieu. Both epidemiologically and socially, we are taught to think in binaries, and having a range between and outside of exclusively heterosexual and exclusively homosexual requires additional thoughtfulness that sometimes is lacking, often due to limitations of survey data.

Since the turn of the century, there has been increased attention to bisexual people as having unique health disparities and needs from gay men and women. The sense of otherness from both straight and gay communities seems to contribute to many of the health disparities seen in both bisexual men and women, often at greater rates than those experienced by their gay and lesbian peers [45–49]. Bisexual people have developed their own Bi Pride flag, their own organizations, and continue to fight bi-invisibility both in the straight and LGBT communities.

## Transgender

While included in "LGBT", transgender and gender non-conforming individuals have histories and experiences unique from sexual minorities. Transgender people may identify as lesbian, gay, bisexual or otherwise and thus share in the experiences of LGB people. However, trans individuals can also be straight. Gender identity is not sexual orientation and comes with its own unique set of histories that transect other histories.

Ultimately, transgender history is marked by experiences in the context of their gendered "otherness", and often saw both legal and medical advances well after those achieved by sexual minorities. In regards to the HIV epidemic, it wasn't until well into the 1990s that transgender individuals were even included as risk populations at the federal level [25]. This trend of lagging behind LGB rights and medical inclusion has continued and is often a source of contention within LGBT advocacy organizations and between LGBT civil rights activists.

While transgender people have been involved in all of the LGB history such as the Stonewall riots, there are other individuals and events specific to the transgender experience. Dr. Harry Benjamin is a widely known figure in transgender history as the first to use cross-gender hormone therapy in the U.S. in the late 1940s. Christine Jorgensen was his first patient to undergo GRS and received national attention. Dr. Benjamin went on to write "The Transsexual Phenomenon" in 1966. His namesake was attached to the first international association of transgender care professionals (Harry Benjamin International Gender Dysphoria Association) and their set of clinical standards for transgender health were dubbed the Harry Benjamin Standards of Care. This organization is now the World Professional Association for Transgender Health (WPATH) and continues to set standards for transgender care.

In addition to Sylvia Rivera and other trans activists' participation in the Stonewall Riots of 1969, trans women also took a stand against police harassment and discrimination in the less-well-known Compton Cafeteria Riots in 1966 [49]. It wasn't until 1978 that the first state law was passed allowing transsexual individuals to change their birth certificate to their new name and designated sex. The turn of the twenty-first century saw the formation of important trans agencies such as the Sylvia Rivera Law project (2002) and the National Center for Transgender Equality (2003). And while Minneapolis was the first city to pass transgender civil rights protections, it wasn't until 2012 that the Equal Employment Opportunity Commission (EEOC) stated that it was a violation of the Civil Rights Act to discriminate against transgender Americans. Growing pains even in the LGBT communities over trans inclusion and language can be seen in RuPaul's Drag Race, a popular TV show about drag queens competing for the crown of "America's Next Drag Superstar". Despite the show's revolutionary exposure of Americans via mass media to gay men, drag performance art, and gender identities and expression outside of the mainstream "norm", heated controversy over

the use of the word "tranny" and "You've Got She-mail" has shown how difficult it has been for the LGBT communities to come together and move forward on such divisive issues. Like the term "queer", both of these terms have been used as derrogatory hate language and as terms of affection between different people, and their ongoing use has been challenged. Overall, transgender patients continue to have complicated relationships with social and medical institutions of all types. Whether seeking out gender affirming hormone therapy, GRS or just basic primary care services, transgender patients continue to experience discrimination and violence even in their doctor's office [50].

## LGBT in the Twenty-First Century

Federally, there have been great strides toward recognizing the rights of LGBT citizens since the turn of the century. Through the Affordable Care Act in 2010, new legal protections against discrimination based on sexual orientation and gender identity were unrolled. Studies have shown LGBT individuals have lower rates of health coverage, an important contributor to health disparities that will in part be addressed by expanded coverage through the ACA. In 2010, the Presidential Memorandum on Hospital Visitation made it illegal to prevent same-sex partners from visiting their loved ones in the hospital. This came after the heart-wrenching story from Miami, Florida that drew national attention when Janice Langbehn was denied access to her dying partner Marie Pond even after providing power of attorney documentation. Marie died while Janice was barred from the hospital. With the repeal of "Don't Ask, Don't Tell" in 2011, our LGB military members and veterans are not only being recognized but provided the protections and benefits they've earned during their service. The Department of Health and Human Services under the leadership of Secretary Kathleen Sebelius has been actively working since 2010 to improve the health of LGBT Americans as shown in their 2013 annual report highlighting various efforts encompassing LGBT youth, adults and elderly in arenas like anti-bullying, violence, homelessness, suicide and health workforce cultural competency.

In the summer of 2013, the Defense of Marriage Act (DOMA) was struck down by the Supreme Court, validating relationships across the country in a both profoundly personal, social, and legal way. In 2015, the Supreme Court ruled same-sex marriage a constitutional right, making marriage equality the law of the land.

## Understanding LGBT Health

The Institute of Medicine's 2011 report "The Health of Lesbian, Gay, Bisexual and Transgender People: Building a Foundation for Better Understanding" [51] is a superb road-map for more deeply understanding the health needs of LGBT patients. They propose a life-course framework for healthcare researchers and providers. Issues of mental health, physical health, risk/protective factors, health services and contextual influences are considered in three life stages: childhood/adolescence, adulthood and later adulthood.

The life-course framework proposed by the 2011 IOM report is included below (Table 1.4) for your reference as you prepare to continue on to other chapters and more deeply explore the unique health needs of the LGBT communities.

**Table 1.4**  Life-course framework

| | |
|---|---|
| Childhood and adolescence | • The burden of HIV falls disproportionately on young men, particularly young black men, who have sex with men<br>• LGB youth are at increased risk for suicidal ideation and attempts as well as depression. Small studies suggest the same may be true for transgender youth<br>• Rates of smoking, alcohol consumption, and substance use may be higher among LGB than heterosexual youth. Almost no research has examined substance use among transgender youth<br>• The homeless youth population comprises a disproportionate number of LGB youth. Some research suggests that young transgender women are also at significant risk for homelessness<br>• LGBT youth report experiencing elevated levels of violence, victimization, and harassment compared with heterosexual and non-gender-variant youth<br>• Families and schools appear to be two possible focal points for intervention research |
| Early and middle adulthood | • As a group, LGB adults appear to experience more mood and anxiety disorders, more depression, and an elevated risk for suicidal ideation and attempts compared with heterosexual adults. Research based on smaller convenience samples suggests that elevated rates of suicidal ideation and attempts as well as depression exist among transgender adults; however, little research has examined the prevalence of mood and anxiety disorders in this population<br>• Lesbian women and bisexual women may use preventive health services less frequently than heterosexual women<br>• Lesbian women and bisexual women may be at greater risk of obesity and have higher rates of breast cancer than heterosexual women<br>• HIV/AIDS continues to exact a severe toll on men who have sex with men, with black and Latino men being disproportionately affected<br>• LGBT people are frequently the targets of stigma, discrimination, and violence because of their sexual- and gender-minority status<br>• LGB adults may have higher rates of smoking, alcohol use, and substance use than heterosexual adults. Most research in this area has been conducted among women, with much less being known about gay and bisexual men. Limited research among transgender adults indicates that substance use is a concern for this population<br>• Gay men and lesbian women are less likely to be parents than their heterosexual peers, although children of gay and lesbian parents are well adjusted and developmentally similar to children of heterosexual parents |
| Later adulthood | • Limited research suggests that transgender elders may experience negative health outcomes as a result of long-term hormone use<br>• HIV/AIDS impacts not only younger but also older LGBT individuals. However, few HIV prevention programs target older adults, a cohort that also has been deeply affected by the losses inflicted by AIDS<br>• There is some evidence that LGBT elders exhibit crisis competence (a concept reflecting resilience and perceived hardiness within older LGBT populations)<br>• LGBT elders experience stigma, discrimination, and violence across the life course<br>• LGBT elders are less likely to have children than heterosexual elders and are less likely to receive care from adult children |

The previous sections highlight the history of the LGBT communities, including the legal, social, cultural, and economic barriers they face. A common language to discuss LGBT and DSD-affected patients and their experiences has been outlined. The concept of minority stress has been introduced and how these factors contribute to LGBT health disparities. In the following chapters, we will further explore these disparities and how to improve the health and well-being of your sexual and gender minority patients. It is our hope that this text will not only help you achieve clinical excellence, but will excite you to seek out opportunities to serve these unique, diverse, resilient communities.

## References

1. Obedin-Maliver J, et al. Lesbian, gay, bisexual, and transgender-related content in undergraduate medical education. JAMA. 2011;306(9):971–7.
2. Ng H, Sudano J. Health centers in the United States. Presented at American Public Health Association meeting, 2012.
3. Kaiser Family Foundation. HIV/AIDS in the lives of gay and bisexual men in the United States. 2014. http://kff.org/hivaids/report/hivaids-in-the-lives-of-gay-and-bisexual-men-in-the-united-states/. Accessed Sept 2014.
4. Cochran S, Keenan C, Schober C, Mays V. Estimates of alcohol use and clinical treatment needs among homosexually active men and women in the U.S. population. J Consult Clin Psychol. 2000;68:1062–71.
5. Gilman S, Cochran S, Mayx V, Hughes M, Ostrow D, Kessler R. Risk of psychiatric disorders among individuals reporting same-sex sexual partners in the National Comorbidity Survey. Am J Public Health. 2001;91:933–9.
6. Mays V, Yancey A, Cochran S, Weber M, Fielding J. Heterogeneity of health disparities among African American, Hispanic and Asian American women: unrecognized influences of sexual orientation. Am J Public Health. 2002;92:632–9.
7. Drabble L, Trocki K. Alcohol consumption, alcohol-related problems, and other substance use among lesbian and bisexual women. J Lesbian Stud. 2005;9:19–30.
8. Hughes T, Wilsnack S, Szalacha L, Johnson T, Bostwick W, Seymour R, et al. Age and racial/ethnic differences in drinking and drinking-related problems in a community sample of lesbian women. J Stud Alcohol. 2006;67:579–90.
9. Kripke M, Weiss G, Ramirez M, Dorey F, Ritt-Olson A, Iverson E, Ford W. Club drug use in Los Angeles among young men who have sex with men. 2007. Club drug use in Los Angeles among young men who have sex with men. Subst Use Misuse. 2007;42: 1723–43.
10. Cochran S, Mays V. Physical health complaints among lesbian women, gay men, and bisexual and homosexually experienced heterosexual individuals: results from the California Quality of Life Survey. Am J Public Health. 2007;97:2048–55.
11. Lee GL, Griffin GK, Melvin CL. Tobacco use among sexual minorities in the USA: 1987 to May 2007: a systematic review. Tob Control. 2009;18:275–82.
12. Xavier J, Honnold J, Bradford J. The health, health-related needs, and lifecourse experiences of transgender Virginians. Virginia HIV Community Planning Committee and Virginia Department of Health. Richmond, VA: Virginia Department of Health; 2007. Available from: http://www.vdh.virginia.gov/epidemiology/DiseasePrevention/documents/pdf/THISFINALREPORTVol1.pdf.
13. Hughes TL. Chapter 9: Alcohol use and alcohol-related problems among lesbian women and gay men. Annu Rev Nurs Res. 2005;23:283–325.
14. Lyons T, Chandra G, Goldstein J. Stimulant use and HIV risk behavior: the influence of peer support. AIDS Educ Prev. 2006;18(5):461–73.
15. Mansergh G, Colfax GN, Marks G, et al. The circuit party men's health survey: findings and implications for gay and bisexual men. Am J Public Health. 2001;91(6):953–8.
16. Garofalo R, Wolf RC, Wissow LS, et al. Sexual orientation and risk of suicide attempts among a representative sample of youth. Arch Pediatr Adolesc Med. 1999;153(5):487–93.
17. Conron KJ, Mimiaga MJ, Landers SJ. A population-based study of sexual orientation identity and gender differences in adult health. Am J Public Health. 2010;100(10):1953–60.
18. Kruks G. Gay and lesbian homeless/street youth: special issues and concerns. J Adolesc Health. 2010; 12(7):515–8.
19. Van Leeuwen JM, Boyle S, Salomonsen-Sautel S, et al. Lesbian, gay, and bisexual homeless youth: an eight-city public health perspective. Child Welfare. 2006;85(2):151–70.
20. Cahill S, South K, Spade J. Outing age: public policy issues affecting gay, lesbian, bisexual and transgender elders. Washington, DC: National Gay and Lesbian Task Force; 2009.
21. Buchmueller T, Carpenter CS. Disparities in health insurance coverage, access, and outcomes for individuals in same-sex versus different-sex relationships, 2000–2007. Am J Public Health. 2010;100(3): 489–95.
22. Dilley JA, Simmons KW, Boysun MJ, et al. Demonstrating the importance and feasibility of including sexual orientation in public health surveys: health disparities in the Pacific Northwest. Am J Public Health. 2010;100(3):460–7.

23. Struble CB, Lindley LL, Montgomery K, et al. Overweight and obesity in lesbian and bisexual college women. J Am Coll Health. 2010;59(1):51–6.
24. Centers for Disease Control and Prevention (CDC). HIV and AIDS among gay and bisexual men. Atlanta: CDC; Sept 2010. Available from:http://www.cdc.gov/nchhstp/newsroom/docs/2012/CDC-MSM-0612-508.pdf.
25. Herbst JH, Jacobs ED, Finlayson TJ, et al. Estimating HIV prevalence and risk behaviors of transgender persons in the United States: a systematic review. AIDS Behav. 2008;12:1–17.
26. Whitbeck LB, Chen X, Hoyt DR, et al. Mental disorder, subsistence strategies, and victimization among gay, lesbian, and bisexual homeless and runaway adolescents. J Sex Res. 2004;41(4):329–42.
27. Diaz RM, Ayala G, Bein E, et al. The impact of homophobia, poverty, and racism on the mental health of gay and bisexual Latino men: findings from three US cities. Am J Public Health. 2001;91(6):141–6.
28. Kenagy GP. Transgender health: findings from two needs assessment studies in Philadelphia. Health Soc Work. 2005;30(1):19–26.
29. National Gay and Lesbian Taskforce. National transgender discrimination survey: preliminary findings. Washington, DC: National Gay and Lesbian Taskforce; Nov 2009. Available from: http://www.thetaskforce.org/downloads/reports/fact_sheets/transsurvey_prelim_findings.pdf.
30. American Psychiatric Association. Diagnostic and statistical manual of mental disorders. 5th ed. Washington, DC: American Psychiatric Publishing; 2013.
31. Gates G, Ost J. Estimating the size of the gay and lesbian population. The gay and lesbian atlas. Washington, DC: Urban Institute Press; 2004. p. 17–21.
32. Gates G. How many people are lesbian, gay, bisexual, and transgender? A Report of the Williams Institute. Los Angeles, CA: Williams Institute, UCLA School of Law; 2011.
33. Olyslager F, Conway L. On the calculation of the prevalence of transsexualism. Paper presented at WPATH 20th international symposium, Chicago, USA, 2007.
34. Gates G. LGBT adult immigrants in the United States. Los Angeles, CA: Williams Institute at UCLA Law School; 2013.
35. Grant J, et al. Injustice at every turn: a report of the national transgender discrimination survey. Washington, DC: National Gay and Lesbian Task Force and National Center for Transgender Equality; 2011.
36. Consortium on the Management of Disorders of Sex Development. Clinical guidelines for the management of DSD in childhood. Intersex Society of North America. 2006.
37. Fausto-Sterling A, et al. How sexually dimorphic are we? Review and synthesis. Am J Hum Biol. 2000;12:151–66.
38. Centers for Disease Control and Prevention. Sexual identity, sex of sexual contacts, and health risk behaviors among students in grades 9–12 in selected sites—youth risk behavior surveillance, United States, 2001–2009. MMWR Surveill Summ. 2011;60(7):1–133. Early Release.
39. Gates G, Konnoth C. Same-sex couples and immigration in the United States. Los Angeles, CA: Williams Institute, UCLA School of Law; 2012.
40. Feldman M. Aversion therapy for sexual deviations: a critical review. Psychol Bull. 1966;65:65–79.
41. Levine M. The impact of AIDS on the homosexual clone community in New York City. Paper presented at 5th international conference on AIDS, Montreal, 1989.
42. Levine MP, et al. In changing times: gay men and lesbian women encounter HIV/AIDS. Chicago, IL: University of Chicago Press; 1997.
43. Hereck G. AIDS and stigma. Am Behav Sci. 1999;42:1106–16.
44. Herbenick D, Reece M, Schick V, Sanders SA, Dodge B, Fortenberry JD. Sexual behavior in the United States: results from a national probability sample of men and women aged 14–94. J Sex Med. 2010;7 Suppl 5:255–65.
45. Koh AS. Use of preventive health behaviors by lesbian, bisexual and heterosexual women: questionnaire survey. West J Med. 2000;172(6):379–84.
46. Koh AS, Ross LK. Mental health issues: a comparison of lesbian, bisexual and heterosexual women. J Homosex. 2006;51(1):33–57.
47. Wilsnack SC, et al. Drinking and drinking-related problems among heterosexual and sexual minority women. J Stud Alcohol Drugs. 2008;69(1):129–39.
48. American Lung Association. Smoking out a deadly threat: tobacco use in the LGBT community. 2010.
49. Diamant AL, et al. Health behaviors, health status and access to and use of health care: a population-based study of lesbian, bisexual and heterosexual women. Arch Fam Med. 2000;9(10):1043–51.
50. Grant J, Mottet L, Tanis J, Herman J, Harrison J, Keisling M. National Transgender Discrimination Survey: findings of a study by the National Center for Transgender Equality and the National Gay and Lesbian Task Force. National Center for Transgender Equality; 2010.
51. Institute of Medicine. The health of lesbian, gay, bisexual, and transgender people: building a foundation for better understanding. Washington, DC: National Academies Press; 2011.

# Access to Care

2

Keisa Fallin-Bennett, Shelly L. Henderson,
Giang T. Nguyen, and Abbas Hyderi

## Purpose

The purpose of this chapter is to review access to health care for LGBT persons, specifically the barriers to care faced by LGBT patients, as well as how providers can establish a medical home with LGBT patients and assess their identity as part of patient-centered care.

K. Fallin-Bennett, M.D., M.P.H. (✉)
Department of Family and Community Medicine, University of Kentucky, 2195 Harrodsburg Road, Ste. 125, Lexington, KY 40504, USA
e-mail: keisa.bennett@uky.edu

S.L. Henderson, Ph.D.
Department of Family and Community Medicine, University of California Davis, 4860 Y Street, Suite 2300, Sacramento, CA 95817, USA
e-mail: shelly.henderson@ucdmc.ucdavis.edu

G.T. Nguyen, M.D., M.P.H., M.S.C.E.
Department of Family Medicine & Community Health and Student Health Service, University of Pennsylvania, 3535 Market Street, Suite 100, Philadelphia, PA 19104, USA
e-mail: GNguyen@upenn.edu

A. Hyderi, M.D., M.P.H.
Department of Family Medicine, University of Illinois at Chicago, M/C 785, 1819 Polk Street, Chicago, IL 60657, USA
e-mail: ahyder2@uic.edu

## Learning Objectives

- List the barriers that could cause difficulties in communication between LGBT patients and providers and identify facilitators to overcome these barriers (*ICS2, ICS3, PPD1*).
- Describe how social and medical institutions contribute to health care access disparities for LGBT patients (*KP4, ICS3*).
- Discuss the role of training of health care providers in health care access issues for LGBT patients (*Pr3, Pr4*).
- Identify at least three opportunities to support a patient-centered medical home or patient-centered practice to facilitate access for LGBT patients (*Pr3, PPD1*).

## Barriers to Care

Many LGBT patients may avoid or delay accessing healthcare. Though historically few studies on health care access have included questions on sexual identity, sexual behavior, or gender identity, studies mainly on cervical cancer screening offer some evidence. In one large, national survey conducted in the mid 1990s, lesbian women were less likely to report routine Pap tests despite having higher risk sexual practices [1]. In a similar sample of adolescents and young adults, women who identified in a sexual orientation category other than completely heterosexual were significantly less likely to have had a Pap test in their lifetimes and in the last year [2]. A smaller study examined reasons for lack of screening and found that fear of discrimination, low knowledge about screening, and lower likelihood to have disclosed sexual orientation were significantly related to not receiving routine Pap tests [3].

The reasons behind delay in or avoidance of care are not completely understood but are likely multifactorial. Studies consistently demonstrate lower proportions of health insurance coverage among sexual minority women (SMW), likely related to the fact that women in general earn less than men and have a higher tendency to be covered under a male partner's insurance [4] As insurance coverage for domestic partners grows in popularity and the Affordable Care Act takes effect (also see Chap. 24), SMW may make gains in insurance coverage; however, current trends in income have not relieved the gender gap [5], leaving households without men at a disadvantage in terms of health care access. It is widely accepted that transgender people have even less access to health insurance. Several studies support this disparity, including one conducted in San Francisco (N=515) in which 52 % of male-to-female (MTF) and 41 % of female-to-male (FTM) persons lacked insurance [6]. The National Transgender Discrimination Survey in Health Care found that 19 % of respondents were uninsured, higher than the national rate of 15 % at the time. Rates were even higher in ethnic minorities and MTFs [7]. Although the ACA eliminates the barrier of coverage denial for transgender patents based on a "pre-existing condition," the degree to which medical care for transgender-related diagnoses are covered by insurance is variable, leaving trans patients personally responsible for a significant proportion of their medical bills.

**Helpful Hint**
Sexual minority women and transgender patients are at higher risk of not having health insurance. Transgender-related care such as hormone therapy and surgery is not covered under many plans.

Stigma and discrimination also play a role. There is substantial evidence that LGBT patients perceive discrimination in the health care environment [8, 9]. In the National Transgender Discrimination survey, 28 % of transgender and gender nonconforming respondents reported postponing or avoiding acute care and 33 % did the same for preventive care, with discrimination and disrespect most commonly cited as causes [7]. Kitts et al. [10] surveyed 464 resident and attending physicians and found that the majority of physicians did not routinely discuss sexual orientation, attractions, or gender identity with sexually active adolescents, even in the setting of depression or suicidal ideation. Nearly half did not know the association between LGBT identity, those questioning their identity, and suicide [10].

Lack of health care provider training correlates with patient experiences. Providers may knowingly create an unwelcoming environment on the basis of upholding religious or cultural beliefs. Perhaps more commonly, they can unknowingly express stigma or discriminate even with the best of intentions. They may lack awareness of sexual minority health issues or lack training in terminology and patient communication. Even recent studies have found that providers feel unprepared to give quality care for LGBT patients. In the Kitts [10] study, only 44 % of physicians agreed that they had the skills needed to address sexual orientation with patients and 75 % agreed that sexual orientation should be covered more often during training. The results of a 2010 GLMA–American Medical Association Collaborative Survey on Physician Experiences Caring for LGBT Patients (Survey on Physician Experiences) reveal the lack of current physician training on LGBT issues and LGBT discrimination in health care settings. Almost 40 % of physicians participating in the survey reported they had no formal training in medical school, residency or from continuing medical education on LGBT health issues, while 50 % reported receiving fewer than 5 hours of training on LGBT health. Of those who received some training in LGBT health, most found that the training was "not very" or "not at all" useful in preparing them to care for LGBT patients. Fifteen percent had witnessed discriminatory care for LGBT patients and nearly 20 % had witnessed disrespect toward the partner of an LGBT patient. 5 % of physicians in this survey said they referred an LGBT patient to another provider because they felt uncomfortable treating them [11].

**Helpful Hint**
Discomfort discussing sexuality and gender exists for both providers and patients. Providers may not receive training and are often not prepared to ask about and respond to these issues. Learning and practicing communication regarding sexuality facilitates these encounters and then builds trust that can help patients be more open in their communication as well.

Research on the extent and quality of LGBT health training for medical trainees has focused primarily on undergraduate medical education [12–15]. In a large recent survey assessing LGBT curriculum in undergraduate medical education, Deans from a majority of existing medical schools reported a median of 5 hours of time devoted to LGBT training overall, and a median of 2 hours during clinical years. When asked about the content, 26 % said the content was "poor" or "very poor" [13]. The only recent study of LGBT health inclusion in residency found similar results among Family Medicine residency directors. 16 % had no content and the majority had 1–5 hours, but only a minority of directors rated the curriculum as "adequate." In addition, 11 % had major concerns or would not rank a transgender applicant, revealing a residency climate that might not promote diversity [16].

Some medical schools have begun to integrate LGBT health in their curriculum with associated increases in knowledge and more positive attitudes. Sanchez et al. [17], for example, found that students having more interactions with LGBT patients were more likely to ask about sexual orientation, hold more positive attitudes toward LGBT issues, and demonstrate objective LGBT health knowledge. In this cross-sectional study, students with more positive attitudes might have been more likely to ask about orientation and

therefore report more experiences with LGBT patients [17]. Nonetheless, additional small studies evaluating specific LGBT health training curricula have demonstrated some positive outcomes [18–20]. Only a few curricular innovations in LGBT health during residency exist in the literature (e.g. [21, 22]) Anecdotally, many more medical schools, residency programs, and other health professional training programs have added LGBT health curricular content in recent years. These programs, however, have rarely been evaluated or published, so little is known about the quantity and quality of training needed to improve knowledge and skills, much less about specific topics or modalities that are effective in achieving learning and practice outcomes.

**Helpful Hint**
Having a reputation for respect and open communication with all patients will help LGBT patients find and trust you as a provider.

## Finding a Medical Home

Despite the importance put on having a personal medical home, in most health systems it is up to the patient to find one. Many patients stay with a primary care provider or practice that they already feel is their medical home, but those who need a new primary care provider (PCP) or want to switch doctors or practices face obstacles. Due to primary care physician/provider shortages in many regions of the country [23], the number of providers not accepting public insurance, and limitations on practice choice as a cost control imposed by insurance companies, many PCP's no longer accept new patients or have very long waits for a new patient appointment [24].

Finding a PCP who is knowledgeable about LGBT issues and welcoming to this diverse clientele can be even more challenging. *GLMA: Healthcare Professionals Advancing LGBT Equality*, a national LGBT advocacy organization for health professionals, suggests a number of strategies employed by practices successful at providing LGBT patients with competent care in a patient-centered environment. These strategies include featuring LGBT persons and families in the materials available in the waiting room or exam rooms and posting non-discrimination policies including sexual orientation and gender identity prominently in public areas. GLMA also recommends actions compatible with the welcoming displays, including having gender-neutral restrooms and registration forms inclusive of diverse genders and relationships [25, 26]. These types of practices are perceived as important to patients in choosing and staying in a practice [9, 27]. The GLMA guidelines are available through a URL in the helpful hints [26]. GLMA also operates a national list of providers who have identified themselves as LGBT-affirming [28]. Providers can designate themselves as allies (non-LGBT persons who are supportive of the community) if desired and are only asked for name, specialty, and some form of office contact information. The GLMA provider directory is free—both for providers to list themselves and for patients to access. Most non-LGBT patients are unaware of this resource, so it provides a particularly helpful and powerful method for providers in more conservative communities to let LGBT patients know of them without overt advertising or symbols. The listing can be accessed by interested patients through the privacy of their own computers and thus avoid any sense of being "outed" by actively asking about welcoming providers, while providers can use this list in cases where more overt signs of LGBT solidarity might not be as well received by the community at large. Nevertheless, most LGBT patients who have a trusted PCP find that person through word-of-mouth and through scanning the safety and competency of the practice environment, as well as implicitly or explicitly assessing the attitudes and competency of the individual provider [29–31]. The best thing that a provider can do to become a medical home for LGBT patients is to be respectful, patient-centered, and competent with regard to the care of all patients.

> **Helpful Hint**
> Health professional schools are beginning to teach LGBT Health. One repository of peer-reviewed LGBT health education resources for students is shared through the Association of American Medical Colleges LGBT/DSD Affected Patient Care Project of MedEdPORTAL: https://www.mededportal.org/

To add yourself to the GLMA Provider Directory or access the GLMA Guidelines for Care of LGBT patients, go to: http://www.glma.org/

## Assessing Identity (Table 2.1)

One of the challenges for the PCP attempting to be welcoming to LGBT patients is that of identifying who they are. Historically, sexual orientation and gender identity were almost universally guarded due to high levels of societal stigma and discrimination. Health care providers often adopted the practice of specifically not documenting patient identification as a confidentiality issue [32]. Unfortunately, that stigma and discrimination also translated into providers not assessing sexual or gender identity at all. As noted in the section on provider training above (under "Barriers to Care"), health professionals generally are not trained to assess identity. Often training consists of learning to ask in a sexual history, "Have you had sex with women, men or both?," a question which is helpful in assessing behavior but incomplete. It also reveals little about a person's identification, can lead to erroneous assumptions when used to ascertain identity, and is not always appropriate for the clinical situation.

A fundamental principle of assessing sexual identity is the recognition that attraction, behavior and identity are not the same. (See Chap. 1 for more details on the definitions and differences. See Chaps. 5 and 7 on intake for details and electronic health records). Behavior can be assessed

**Table 2.1** Model questions for a primary care interview

Note that the following questions are not meant to be exhaustive. Some would be used in different situations than others. They are examples that you could use or adapt for the appropriate time in the clinical interview. You would often consider prefacing many of these questions with a normalizing remark, such as, "In order to better understand all the things that affect my patients health, I ask about ..." (identity, sexual history, exposure to violence, etc.). Reminders about confidentiality are also helpful. Remember that the most important elements of the clinical interview with all patients are to avoid assumptions, ask open ended questions first, and always demonstrate respect for the patient and the truth of the patient's own experience

*Directly assessing identity*
- How do you define your gender?
- What pronouns do you use for yourself, for example she/her, he/him, or something different?
- How do you define your sexual orientation?
- Do you feel attracted to men, women, both, or neither?

*Taking a social history*
- Who have you brought with you to the visit?
- Do you have a significant other?
- Are you in a relationship?
- Can you tell me a little about your partner or significant other?
- What do you call your partner?
- Tell me about who makes up the people you consider your family?
- Who are the people that you turn to for support?
- Are there people in your life who are not supportive?

*Taking a sexual history*
- Do you have any concerns or questions about your sexuality, sexual orientation, or sexual desires?
- Can you describe the sexual aspect of your life with your partner(s)?
- Have you had any sexual contact with others in the last year, (meaning, have you had any contact that involves the mouth, vagina, penis or anus)?
- When was the last time you were sexually active?
- Have you had any sexual contact in your lifetime?
- Can you tell whom you are attracted to?
- How many partners do you have now? (how many partners have you had in your lifetime?)
- Have your sexual partners been men, women, or both?
- What kind of sexual activities are a part of your relationship?
- What kind of sexual activities are a part of your sex life with partners that you are not involved with romantically?
- Do you use sex toys or other items as part of your sex life?
- In what ways do you practice safer sex?

in a fairly straightforward manner as part of a sexual history when such a history is appropriate. Sexual identity, while clearly related to inherent attractions and behavior, is a more complex social construct that can change over time and with a change in environment. In a patient-centered approach, the patient's self-identification as straight, gay, lesbian, bisexual, queer, questioning, asexual, something else, or no identification at all, should be respected regardless of whether that identification seems to the provider to match attractions or behaviors of the patient. Open-ended questions are the most patient-centered way to ascertain patient sexual orientation while deriving accurate information [26, 33]. Because identity can be a sensitive issue for some patients, it is common that patients might need several visits with a provider in order to feel comfortable discussing identity [34, 35]. Nevertheless, we agree with the finding of the Institute of Medicine Board of Select Populations that best practice for holistic, patient-centered care dictates that the provider know enough about the patient to understand how the patient identifies, and that communication to that effect should occur within a few preventive or chronic care visits or as needed during acute visits when it might relate directly to behavioral risks or mental health concerns [32]. A number of sample questions for ascertaining identity in an open-ended manner appear in the box above. It is recommended that health professionals and students practice these questions in simulated patient visits or professional trainings in order to become more comfortable using them. Curriculum guidelines for medical student education and residency education from the Association of American Medical Colleges (AAMC) and the American Academy of Family Physicians (AAFP), respectively, detail these and other recommendations [36, 37].

Assessing gender identity can be just as challenging. As noted in Chap. 1, people may identify as transgender as an umbrella concept of not identifying as a single, clear gender all of the time. Patients may use the term transgender to mean that their sense of gender does not exactly match the sex of their birth, or that they have already taken steps to live in a gender different than the sex assigned at birth. Others identify as bigender, transsexual, genderqueer, or even reject the notion of gender entirely [38, 39]. The word used academically for the majority of people whose gender identity matches their sex assigned at birth, "cisgender," is not generally used by the people it describes (in contrast to the words "heterosexual" or "straight," which are widely understood and used in casual language). Given the variety of gender identities, the changing landscape of gender identity terms, and a particular lack of provider training in this area, it is especially crucial to approach gender identity in an open-ended manner. Cisgender people might be confused about being asked for a gender identity that they perceive as evident, so asking for gender identification requires practice and finesse. Using multiple options for gender on registration forms (as noted in Chaps. X and Y on intake and EHR), is a particularly good way to have some transgender-spectrum patients identify in a more comfortable way while simultaneously training other patients and staff to be comfortable with such questions. In addition to identity terminology, transgender persons may also have particular preferences in terms of referring to body composition that providers should be aware of. Questions to use during a primary care interview are listed above and body specific terminology is covered in Chap. 18 [26, 32].

It is also important to emphasize again that sexual orientation does not indicate or predict gender identity, and vice-versa. Several studies on the sexual identity of transgender persons find a large diversity of identifications spanning straight, gay, lesbian, bisexual, and other identities [38, 39]. A gender transition for someone already in a relationship may also complicate sexual identity identification terms and how to communicate those to others. Ultimately, it is important for patients to be able to identify both sexual and gender identities for themselves, even when that includes nontraditional labels or no labels at all. It is also to be expected that these identity labels could change over time and does not indicate instability in mental health [39–42].

Similarly, it is important to remember that LGBT persons may have multiple other identities that influence their feelings about gender or orientation, as well as the labels they use for themselves. It is vital that the PCP and the medical home as a whole view patients in the multiple cultural contexts in which they exist, where culture ranges from race/ethnicity to age to occupation to neighborhood.

**Helpful Hint**
A patient-centered approach is key. Not every visit is appropriate for discussions of sexual and gender identity, but practice in ascertaining identity and responding to disclosures is important for trust-building that allow patients to receive tailored care and work in collaboration to improve their own health.

**Helpful Hint**
Terms to avoid

- Sexual preference (use the term *sexual orientation* or *sexual identity* instead)
- Homosexual (use the words *gay* or *lesbian* instead; use the words the patients use to describe themselves)
- Transvestite (use *transgender* or the words the patients use for themselves)

Portions adapted from: 1. Policy Brief: How to Gather Data on Sexual Identity and Gender Identity in Clinical Settings. The Fenway Institute. 2012. Available via: http://thefenwayinstitute.org/documents/Policy_Brief_HowtoGather..._ v3_01.09.12.pdf AND 2. Guidelines for Care of Lesbian, Gay, Bisexual and Transgender Patients. GLMA. 2006. Available via: http://glma.org/_data/n_0001/resources/live/GLMA%20guidelines%202006%20FINAL.pdf

# References

1. Matthews AK, Brandenburg DL, Johnson TP, Hughes TL. Correlates of underutilization of gynecological cancer screening among lesbian and heterosexual women. Prev Med. 2004;38(1):105–13.

2. Charlton BM, Corliss HL, Missmer SA, Frazier AL, Rosario M, Kahn JA, et al. Reproductive health screening disparities and sexual orientation in a cohort study of U.S. adolescent and young adult females. J Adolesc Health. 2011;49(5):505–10.

3. Tracy JK, Lydecker AD, Ireland L. Barriers to cervical cancer screening among lesbians. J Womens Health. 2010;19(2):229–37.

4. Heck JE, Sell RL, Sheinfeld GS. Health care access among individuals involved in same-sex relationships. Am J Public Health. 2006;96:1111–8.

5. Salam R. Which gender gap? Natl Rev. 2014;66(1): 19–20.

6. Clements-Noelle K, Marx R, Guzman R, Katz M. HIV prevalence, risk behaviors, health care use, and mental health status of transgender persons: implications for public health intervention. Am J Public Health. 2001;91(6):915–21.

7. Grant JM, Mottet LA, Tanis J. National Transgender Discrimination Survey Report on Health and Health Care. 2010.

8. Sinding C, Barnoff L, Grassau P. Homophobia and heterosexism in cancer care: the experiences of lesbians. Can J Nurs Res. 2004;36(4):170–88.

9. Saulnier CF. Deciding who to see: lesbians discuss their preferences in health and mental health care providers. Soc Work. 2002;47(4):355–65.

10. Kitts RL. Barriers to optimal care between physicians and lesbian, gay, bisexual, transgender, and questioning adolescent patients. J Homosex. 2010;57(6):730–47.

11. Allison R et al. GLMA-AMA collaborative survey on physician experiences caring for LGBT patients (survey on physician experiences) 2010.

12. Tamas RL, Miller KH, Martin LJ, Greenberg RB. Addressing patient sexual orientation in the undergraduate medical education curriculum. Acad Psychiatry. 2010;34(5):342–5.

13. Obedin-Maliver J, Goldsmith ES, Stewart L, White W, Tran E, Brenman S, et al. Lesbian, gay, bisexual, and transgender-related content in undergraduate medical education. JAMA. 2011;306(9):971–7.

14. Tesar CM, Rovi SL. Survey of curriculum on homosexuality/bisexuality in departments of family medicine. Fam Med. 1998;30(4):283–7.

15. Wallick MM, Cambre KM, Townsend MH. How the topic of homosexuality is taught at U.S. medical schools. Acad Med. 1992;67(9):601–3.

16. Nguyen G, Bennett K, Herbitter C, Hyderi A, Bennett A, Player M. LGBT health in family medicine education: results from a national survey of residency program directors. Unpublished manuscript.

17. Sanchez NF, Rabatin J, Sanchez JP, Hubbard S, Kalet A. Medical students' ability to care for lesbian, gay, bisexual, and transgendered patients. Fam Med. 2006;38(1):21–7.

18. Dixon-Woods M, Regan J, Robertson N, Young B, Cordle C, Tobin M. Teaching and learning about human sexuality in undergraduate medical education. Med Educ. 2002;36(5):432–40.

19. Kelley L, Chou CL, Dibble SL, Robertson PA. A critical intervention in lesbian, gay, bisexual, and transgender health: knowledge and attitude outcomes among second-year medical students. Teach Learn Med. 2008;20(3):248–53.

20. McGarry KA, Clarke JG, Cyr MG, Landau C. Evaluating a lesbian and gay health care curriculum. Teach Learn Med. 2002;14(4):244–8.

21. McGarry K, Clarke J, Cyr MG. Enhancing residents' cultural competence through a lesbian and gay health curriculum. Acad Med. 2000;75(5):515.

22. Townsend MH. Gay and lesbian issues in graduate medical education. N C Med J. 1997;58(2):114–6.

23. Petterson SM, Phillips RL, Bazemore AW, Koinis GT. Unequal distribution of the U.S. primary care workforce. Am Fam Physician. 2013;87(11).

24. Gindi RM, Kirzinger WK, Cohen RA. Health insurance coverage and adverse experiences with physician availability: United States, 2012. NCHS Data Brief. 2013;(138):1–8.

25. Levitt N. Creating a welcoming and safe environment for LGBT people and families. GLMA. 2013.

26. GLMA. Guidelines for care of lesbian, gay, bisexual and transgender patients. 2006.

27. Hoffman ND, Freeman K, Swann S. Healthcare preferences of lesbian, gay, bisexual, transgender and questioning youth. J Adolesc Health. 2009;45(3):222–9.

28. GLMA. Find a provider [25 Apr 2014]. Available from: http://www.glma.org/index.cfm?fuseaction=Page.view Page&pageId=939&grandparentID=534&parentID=93 8&nodeID=1.

29. Boehmer U, Case P. Sexual minority women's interactions with breast cancer providers. Women Health. 2006;44(2):41–58.

30. Ginsburg KR, Winn RJ, Rudy BJ, Crawford J, Zhao H, Schwarz DF. How to reach sexual minority youth in the health care setting: the teens offer guidance. J Adolesc Health. 2002;31(5):407–16.

31. Klitzman RL, Greenberg JD. Patterns of communication between gay and lesbian patients and their health care providers. J Homosex. 2002;42(4):65–75.

32. Institute of Medicine Board on the Health of Select Populations. Collecting sexual orientation and gender identity data in electronic health records: workshop summary. Washington, DC; 2013.

33. Bradford J, Cahill S, Grasso C, Makadon HJ. Policy focus: how to gather data on sexual orientation and gender identity in clinical settings. Boston, MA: Fenway Health; 2012.

34. Levine DA. Office-based care for lesbian, gay, bisexual, transgender, and questioning youth. Pediatrics. 2013;132(1):e297–313.

35. Mravcak SA. Primary care for lesbians and bisexual women. Am Fam Physician. 2006;74(2):279–86.

36. American Academy of Family Physicians. Lesbian, gay, bisexual, transgender health: recommended curriculum guidelines for family medicine residents. In: Physicians AAoF, editor. 2013.

37. Association of American Medical Colleges. LGBT & DSD-affected individuals—competency domains and objectives for medical student education. MedEdPORTAL; 2012.

38. Meier S, Pardo S, Labuski C, Babcock J. Measures of clinical health among female-to-male transgender persons as a function of sexual orientation. Arch Sex Behav. 2013;42(3):463–74.

39. Kuper LE, Nussbaum R, Mustanski B. Exploring the diversity of gender and sexual orientation identities in an online sample of transgender individuals. J Sex Res. 2012;49(2/3):244–54.

40. Policy Brief: How to gather data on sexual identity and gender identity in clinical settings. The Fenway Institute. 2012. Available from http://thefenwayinstitute.org/documents/Policy_Brief_HowtoGather..._v3_01.09.12.pdf.

41. Guidelines for Care of Lesbian, Gay, Bisexual and Transgender Patients. GLMA. 2006. Available from http://glma.org/_data/n_0001/resources/live/GLMA%20guidelines%202006%20FINAL.pdf.

42. Brooks KD, Quina K. Women's sexual identity patterns: differences among lesbians, bisexuals, and unlabeled women. J Homosex. 2009;56(8):1030–45.

# Culture, Climate, and Advocacy

**3**

Baligh R. Yehia, Scott N. Grossman,
and Daniel Calder

## Purpose

The purpose of this chapter is to examine the impact of LGBT health-related institutional climate, culture, and advocacy on patient care and health education. This chapter will also provide practical suggestions for improving institutional climate.

## Learning Objectives

After reading this chapter, learners will be able to:

- Identify at least three national resources for improving culture and climate in academic medicine (*SBP1, SBP3*)
- Discuss the current barriers to an inclusive climate for LGBT students, staff, and faculty (*Pr4*)
- Discuss at least three specific tools for improving culture and climate within an academic institution (*IPC1, Pr4*)

B.R. Yehia, M.D., M.P.P., M.Sc. (✉)
D. Calder, M.P.H.
Perelman School of Medicine, University of
Pennsylvania, Philadelphia, PA, USA
e-mail: byehia@upenn.edu; dcalder@upenn.edu

S.N. Grossman, M.D.
Department of Neurology, NYU Langone Medical
Center, New York, NY, USA
e-mail: sgrossma@alumni.upenn.edu

- Understand the importance of using organization change models to promote LGBT inclusion and climate change (*IPC1, Pr4*)
- Understand the impact of culture and climate on establishing a safe learning environment for students and trainees within health-care institutions (*Pr4*)

## Growing National Recognition of the Unique Health Needs of LGBT Populations

Over the past decade, progress has been made towards understanding the health needs of LGBT populations. Federal bodies, including the Department of Health and Human Services and the Agency for Healthcare Research and Quality, have released guidance and reports addressing health disparities in the LGBT community. In addition, several non-governmental organizations, including the Human Rights Campaign and GLMA: Health Professionals Advancing LGBT Equality, have developed resources for improving the climate for LGBT patients and trainees in healthcare settings. Several of these reports and resources are reviewed below.

*Institute of Medicine (IOM)/National Academy of Medicine (NAM)* The IOM/NAM is one of America's premier professional organizations with

© Springer International Publishing Switzerland 2016
K.L. Eckstrand, J.M. Ehrenfeld (eds.), *Lesbian, Gay, Bisexual, and Transgender Healthcare*,
DOI 10.1007/978-3-319-19752-4_3

the purpose of providing national advice on matters of science, medicine, and public health. In 2011, the National Institutes of Health (NIH) asked the IOM/NAM Committee of Lesbian, Gay, Bisexual and Transgender Health Issues to assess the current state of knowledge about the health of LGBT people and to "identify research gaps and formulate a research agenda that could guide NIH in enhancing and focusing its research in this area."

In response to the NIH request, the IOM/NAM produced the report "The Health of Lesbian, Gay, Bisexual, and Transgender People: Building a Foundation for Better Understanding." This broad document takes several approaches in its study and emphasizes four conceptual frameworks: *the life-course framework, the minority stress model, intersectionality, and social ecology*. It also stresses the importance of historical context for understanding the health status of LGBT individuals in the current period.

The report acknowledges that the LGBT community is diverse and its members have commensurately diverse health needs. It identifies the many challenges to conducting LGBT research including establishment of the definitions of sexual orientation and gender identity, the fear of disclosure on the part of LGBT individuals, and the problems associated with attracting research participation in a relatively small population. Moreover, the report addresses "health status over the life course" of LGBT people as divided into three stages: *childhood/adolescence, early/ middle adulthood, and later adulthood*. Within each stage, the committee evaluated mental health, physical health, risks and protective factors, health services and contextual influences.

The IOM/NAM report concludes with specific recommendations on implementing a research agenda to advance knowledge and understanding of LGBT health. These recommendations include: (1) collection of data on sexual orientation and gender identity in federally-funded surveys and electronic health records; (2) development and standardization of sexual orientation and gender identity measures to facilitate comparison and combination of data across large studies; (3) support for methodological research aimed at developing new methods for conducting research within small populations; and (4) development of a comprehensive research training program to raise awareness of LGBT health among researchers.

*Healthy People 2020* Healthy People is a federally-funded initiative with the goal of providing science-based national objectives for improving the health of all Americans. The program aims to attain high-quality health status for all citizens, create social and physician environments that promote good health, and achieve health equity and eliminate disparities. Healthy People 2020 included an LGBT Health component with the goal of improving "the health, safety, and well-being of lesbian, gay, bisexual and transgender individuals." The program notes that LGBT individuals face many health-related disparities linked to societal stigma, discrimination, and denial of civil and human rights. To begin addressing these issues, Healthy People 2020 established the following objective: increase the number of population-based data systems used to monitor Healthy People 2020 objectives that include in their core a standardized set of questions that identify LGBT populations.

*Agency for Healthcare Research and Quality (AHRQ)* The AHRQ National Healthcare Disparities Report is an annual report that tracks "prevailing disparities in health care delivery as it relates to racial factors and socioeconomic factors in priority populations". In 2011, for the first time, the National Healthcare Disparities Report added a section on LGBT populations, with an emphasis on transgender individuals. The Report highlighted disparities LGBT individuals experience in access to health care, postponement of health care, and discrimination by medical providers.

*The Human Rights Campaign (HRC)* The HRC Health Equity Index (HEI) is a valuable resource for healthcare organizations seeking to provide equitable, inclusive care to LGBT Americans. HRC developed this resource to be used by hospitals and clinics to ensure they provide LGBT patient-centered care in compliance with legal, Centers for Medicare and Medicaid Services (CMS), and Joint Commission requirements;

improve quality and safety; enhance patient satisfaction ratings; and receive benchmark assessment of their performance with regard to the HRC HEI Core Four criteria: *patient non-discrimination policies; equal visitation policies; employment non-discrimination policies; and training in LGBT patient-centered care.* The HEI report is released annually and offers individuals and prospective patients the opportunity to learn about facilities and their performance relative to others within specific geographic areas.

*The Joint Commission (TJC)*  The Joint Commission is an independent not-for-profit organization that accredits and certifies more than 20,000 health care organizations and programs in the United States. In 2011, TJC published a field guide titled "Advancing Effective Communication, Cultural Competence and Patient- and Family-Centered Care for the LGBT Community." This guide explicitly aims to improve the effectiveness of patient-provider communication for LGBT individuals and cites the general neglect of LGBT-related communications tools from official authorities. It is divided into five content-driven chapters and several appendices with resources for health care agencies. The five chapters are: *Leadership, Provision of Care, Workforce, Data Collection and Use* and *Patient, Family and Community Engagement.* Each chapter contains information on both the driving forces underlying the need for change in LGBT health as well as practical tools for improving performance within that content area. The guide also includes 'recommended issues to address' and 'practice examples' for each of the topics. The appendices to the document include checklists to be used by organizations to ensure that they have taken all TJC-supported steps to optimize the environment and provision of care for LGBT patients.

*GLMA: Health Professionals Advancing LGBT Equality*  GLMA is a leading association of LGBT healthcare professionals. In their report *Guidelines for Care of Lesbian, Gay, Bisexual, and Transgender Patients*, GLMA recognizes that many LGBT individuals avoid or delay care and receive inappropriate or inferior care because of perceived or real judgment and discrimination

by health care providers and institutions. The Report provides succinct and informed recommendations on how to foster a welcoming physical environment, add or change intake and health history forms, improve provider–patient communication, and increase staff's knowledge to meet the needs of LGBT patients.

*American Medical Association (AMA) LGBT Advisory Committee*  The AMA is the largest association of physicians in the United States. The AMA's LGBT Advisory Committee works to improve the health of LGBT persons through policy and advocacy. In addition, the committee provides access to a wide variety of LGBT resources relating to the clinical care of LGBT populations, how to create an LGBT-friendly medical practice, enhancing communication with LGBT patients, understanding LGBT health disparities, and increasing awareness of LGBT health issues.

*Association of American Medical Colleges (AAMC)*  The AAMC, which represents accredited U.S. and Canadian medical schools, recently released guidelines for training physicians to care for people who are LGBT, gender nonconforming, or born with differences of sex development. The report identifies 30 competencies that physicians must master. These competencies fall under eight domains of care critical to training physicians, including patient care, knowledge for practice, practice-based learning and improvement, interpersonal and communication skills, professionalism, systems-based practice, interprofessional collaboration, and personal and professional development.

*The Fenway Institute*  The Fenway Institute is an interdisciplinary center for research, training, education and policy development whose mission targets access to quality, culturally competent medical and mental health care for LGBT people and those affected by AIDS. The Fenway Institute is well known for several signature initiatives, including its clinical program, Fenway Health, which first began caring for Boston-area gay men and lesbians in 1971. In 1980, Fenway first began its program in research and community education—this effort has grown to include the Center for Population Research in LGBT Health and active participation in HIV Vaccine Trials. The National Center for LGBT Health Education at Fenway provides education, resources and consultation to health care organizations on issues related to LGBT health. Moreover, The Fenway Guide to Lesbian, Gay, Bisexual, and Transgender Health is the first American medical textbook dedicated to LGBT health and remains an invaluable reference for healthcare professionals. First published in 2008, it has since been updated to reflect evidence-based changes in care guidelines. The Fenway Guide is broadly delineated into six sections: Understanding LGBT Populations, The Life Continuum, Health Promotion and Disease Prevention, Transgender and Intersex Health, Patient Communication and the Office Environment and Legal Issues and the LGBT Community.

## Impact of Culture and Climate on Patient Care and Health Education

Institutional culture and climate are key elements for providing a safe environment for inclusive and equitable patient care. In addition, culture and climate are important for establishing a welcoming learning environment for LGBT trainees.

### Patient Care

LGBT patients face particular challenges in health care settings. They struggle with being open about their sexuality and gender identity due to the fear of judgment and discrimination. In a Lambda Legal Study, 73 % of transgender patients and 29 % of LGB patients believed medical personnel would treat them differently if they disclosed their LGBT status. As a result, LGBT patients either avoid seeing a provider or do not divulge their sexual orientation and/or gender identity, which further contribute to LGBT health disparities. Compared to their heterosexual counterparts, LGBT individuals are more likely to delay or not seek medical care, in part due to the fear of dis-

crimination and hostility. Relatedly, data from the National Center for Transgender Equality indicates that 19 % of the approximately 6000 gender non-conforming individuals sampled reported that they had been refused medical care due to their gender expression and 50 % had to teach their medical providers about transgender care. In addition, 28 % of surveyed individuals reported that they had postponed medical care when they were sick or injured out of fear of discrimination.

If the climate and culture of a health care setting is unwelcoming towards the LGBT community, optimal patient care isn't possible. Therefore, providers and staff should ensure that LGBT patients feel welcomed and understood during their healthcare experience. Creating a welcoming environment can include (1) have "sexual orientation" and "gender identity and expression" in patient's bill of rights and non-discrimination policy; (2) develop or adopt a policy ensuring equal visitation; (3) post rainbow flags, pink triangles, or other LGBT-friendly symbols or stickers in the waiting room and providers office; (4) exhibit posters showing racially and ethnically diverse same-sex couples or transgender people; (5) make available LGBT health resources such a brochures and pamphlets; and (6) train staff and providers on how to communicate with and welcome LGBT patients.

### Health Education

Establishing welcoming environments benefits not only LGBT patients and communities, but also individual trainees.

In a 2008 diversity survey of 261 medical, physician assistant, and physical therapy students at one academic medical school, 90 % of respondents found education value in a diverse faculty and student body. In addition, students endorsed the value of a diverse and inclusive climate and its role in a medical school's educational and clinical care missions. However, despite these beliefs, one quarter of respondents reported witnessing other students or residents make disparaging remarks or exhibit offensive behaviors toward LGBT groups. In 2013, the AAMC sends a questionnaire to all second year medical students in the United States to better understand student satisfaction, empathy, and well-being. In addition, for the first time, the questionnaire included a question on sexual orientation. In total, 3466 students responded (18 % response rate), with 5.9 % identifying as LGB. Compared to their counterparts, LGB students reported higher stress levels, less social support, increased financial concerns, and greater levels of social isolation.

Prior research indicates that LGB medical students and residents experience significant challenges during training, and that the safety of the learning environment impacts both decisions about identity disclosure and future career paths. Residents use the presence of identifiable supports, curricula inclusive of LGBT health issues, and effective non-discrimination policies to assess the professional and personal risks during training.

Institutions with an emphasis on respect and diversity are likely to enhance the experiences of LGBT trainees. Creating a welcoming and inclusive learning environment may include: (1) clinical and simulated patient problems that include LGBT identity as a normal part of the human range; (2) enhanced medical school and residency curricula in sexuality; (3) institution-sponsored support groups that recognize and allow the stresses of being LGBT during medical training;

(4) explicit faculty role models and mentors for LGBT trainees; (5) written, broadly distributed policies condemning discrimination against LGBT persons with effective reporting and enforcement mechanisms; and (6) practical institutional measures to address homophobia and heterosexism.

## Use of Organizational Change Models to Promote LGBT Inclusion and Climate Change

Organizational change models guide the transition of an institution from its present to a desired future state, helping them address why change should occur, how it should happen, and what actions and resources are required to produce the intended outcomes. These models have been used effectively to increased access to care and improve self-efficacy among racial/ethnic minorities. More recently, the use of organizational change models had been applied to the promotion of LGBT inclusion and climate change.

The Eckstrand, Lunn, and Yehia *Organizational Change Model of LGBT Inclusion* (Fig. 3.1) highlights elements necessary for initiating LGBT organization change (LGBT organization priority and resources, organization champions, depth of

**Fig. 3.1** Organizational change model of LGBT inclusion (source: K. Eckstrand)

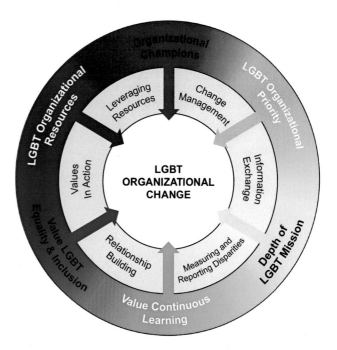

LGBT mission, value continuous learning, value LGBT equality and inclusion) and processes to accelerate the change process (values in action, leveraging resources, change management, information exchange, relationship building, measuring and reporting disparities) (Fig. 3.1).

Through the use of this and similar models, health organizations can initiate and sustain meaningful organizational climate and culture change to improve the health and healthcare of the LGBT communities.

## Practical Tools for Improving Culture and Climate

The first steps towards improving institutional climate and culture are often to create practical tools that can be used by trainees and faculty. Tables 3.1 and 3.2 contain several suggestions and resources that can be used to improve institutional climate. This is not an exhaustive list but merely a series of suggestions to be deployed within individual institutions.

## Conclusions

Institutional climate and culture contribute in essential ways to the experience of LGBT patients and trainees. Although much has been written in recent years regarding the improving environment for LGBT people within the healthcare space, there clearly remains room for further development in this area. Institutions and individuals aiming to maximize their commitment to diversity now have a broad array of practical tools to employ in their efforts. As has been discussed, LGBT patients still face many barriers to equitable care and inclusive healthcare environments. With further efforts on the part of both private and governmental actors, our healthcare system can transform to better serve LGBT patients and their families.

**Table 3.1** Improving climate for students, faculty, and staff

| Action | Description |
| --- | --- |
| Identify advocates | Having advocates both within an institution and in the community is a key element of fostering a safe and welcoming environment for LGBT trainees, faculty, and staff |
| Celebrate LGBT holidays | The LGBT community has several prominent dates on the calendar that could be celebrated. Such dates include National Coming Out Day, National Trans Day of Remembrance, and Pride |
| Create an outlist | One important way to foster positive institutional climate is through the creation and maintenance of an "outlist." Outlists are resources composed of out LGBT-identified individuals within an institution who volunteer to have their name and position posted online and are willing to serve as a resource for students |
| Implement a SafeZone workshop | The SafeZone program was developed to enhance and maintain environments in workplaces, schools and other social settings that are culturally competent and supportive to LGBT individuals, as well as straight identified people who care about diversity, equality and inclusion |
| Create a LGBT group | LGBT student, faculty, and/or staff groups can bring together members of the community and allies. The group can serve as support for LGBT individuals and increase visibility |

(continued)

**Table 3.1** (continued)

| Action | Description |
| --- | --- |
| Recruit LGBT students, faculty, and staff | Developing targeted LGBT outreach materials and recruiting at LGBT events and organizations can attract a greater number of LGBT individuals to the institution and improve climate and visibility |
| Include "sexual orientation" and "gender identity and expression" in nondiscrimination policies | An explicit policy against LGBT discrimination protects LGBT students, faculty, and staff. It also sends a clear message that LGBT individuals should feel welcomed and comfortable at the institution |

**Table 3.2** Improving climate for patients

| Action | Description |
| --- | --- |
| Include "sexual orientation" and "gender identity and expression" in patient's bill of rights and non-discrimination policy | In any written policies prohibiting non-discrimination against patients, include sexual orientation and gender identity and expression as a personal characteristic not to be discriminated again. This will protect LGBT patients and make them feel welcomed and understood at the institution |
| Develop or adopt a policy ensuring equal visitation | The visitation policy should allow the patient to designate visitors, including, but not limited to, a spouse, domestic partner (including a same-sex partner), children (regardless of legal recognition), other family member or friend |
| Create a welcoming atmosphere | Post rainbow flags, pink triangles, or other LGBT-friendly symbols or stickers. Exhibit posters showing racially and ethnically diverse same-sex couples or transgender people |
| Display LGBT health materials | There are many brochures and posters with LGBT health material. Make these available to inform LGBT patients about their particular health needs. These materials will also send a message to LGBT patients that the institution cares for their health |
| Communicate with LGBT patients with understanding and compassion | Listen to patients and how they describe their own sexual orientation, partner(s) and relationship(s), and reflect their choice of language. Ask non-judgmental questions about sexual practices and behaviors, and respect the gender identity of a patient by using the patient's preferred pronouns (e.g., he/him/his, she/her) |
| Stay informed about LGBT health issues | Seek information and stay up to date on LGBT health topics. Be prepared with appropriate information and referrals for LGBT patients |

## Resources

1. Advancing effective communication, cultural competence and patient- and family-centered care for the LGBT community. The Joint Commission; 2011.
2. Dhaliwal JS, Crane LA, Valley MA, Lowenstein SR. Perspectives on the diversity climate at a US medical school: the need for a broader definition of diversity. BMC Res Notes. 2013;6:154.
3. The Fenway Institute: About. http://thefenwayinstitute.org/about/.
4. Healthy People 2020. Lesbian, gay, bisexual, and transgender health. http://www.healthypeople.gov/2020/topicsobjectives2020/overview.aspx?topicid=25.
5. Human Rights Campaign Healthcare Equality Index. www.hrc.org/hei.
6. Gay and Lesbian Medical Association (GLMA). www.glma.org.
7. Grant JM, Mottit LA, Tanis J. Injustice at every turn: a report of the national transgender discrimination survey. 2011.
8. Krehely J. How to close the LGBT health disparities gap. Washington, DC: Center for American Progress; 2009.
9. National Healthcare Disparities Report: 2011. US Department of Health and Human Resources. Agency for Healthcare Research and Quality; 2011.
10. Risdon C, Cook D, Willms D. Gay and lesbian physicians in training: a qualitative study. CMAJ. 2000;162(3):331–4.
11. Robb N. Fear of ostracism still silences some gay MDs, students. CMAJ. 1996;155(7):972–7.
12. Snowdon S. Equal and respectful care for LGBT patients. The importance of providing an inclusive environment cannot be underestimated. Healthc Exec. 2013;28(6):52, 54–5.
13. The health of lesbian, gay, bisexual, and transgender people: building a foundation for better understanding. Institute of Medicine (US) Committee on Lesbian, Gay, Bisexual, and Transgender Health Issues and Research Gaps and Opportunities. Washington, DC: National Academies Press; 2011.
14. When health care isn't caring: Lambda Legal's survey of discrimination against LGBT people and people with HIV. New York: Lambda Legal; 2010.

# Internalized Homophobia, Disclosure, and Health

# 4

## Sarah C. Fogel

## Purpose

The purpose of this chapter is to identify personal and community characteristics that may impact the provision of, or access to, healthcare for LGBT patients.

## Learning Objectives

This chapter will prepare you to:

- Differentiate between homophobia and internalized homophobia (*ICS3*)
- Identify at least three ways that heterosexism may affect your daily practice and the health of LGBT people (*Pr3, SBP4*).
- Identify at least two opportunities and two barriers to disclosure of sexual orientation and gender identity in your practice (*ICS1, ICS4, PLBI1*).
- Develop an environment that will elicit disclosure of sexual orientation and gender identity in a safe and appropriate manner (*PBLI2, Pr4, ICS3, ICS4*).

S.C. Fogel, Ph.D., R.N., F.A.A.N. (✉)
School of Nursing, Vanderbilt University,
307 Godchaux Hall, 221 21st Avenue South,
Nashville, TN 37240, USA
e-mail: sarah.fogel@vanderbilt.edu

## Internalized Homophobia vs. Internalized Heterosexism

Homophobia is a construct that represents negative feelings about LGBT people, ranging from a general lack of understanding, to fear and loathing or hate [1]. Homophobia will be referred to as inclusive of biphobia and transphobia (equivalent constructs applied to bisexual and transgender persons, respectively) when discussed in this chapter. It is important to note that, all too frequently, bisexuals and transgender people are overlooked in the literature and in the minds of many straight, lesbian and gay people, including healthcare providers. This chapter is to be read with the acknowledgment of all of the populations represented in the LGBT acronym (lesbian, gay, bisexual, transgender, queer/questioning and intersex). It is also important to note that many people who identify as part of this population do not label themselves with any of these descriptors. Perhaps the most important thing healthcare providers can do is to invite patients to tell you who they are and to acknowledge what they have told you.

Although homophobia has been, and continues to be, a major issue for the health and well-being of LGBT people, a more current phenomenon that may be replacing outright homophobia is that of heterosexism (see Table 4.1). Heterosexism is an "ideological system that denies, denigrates,

**Table 4.1** Examples of heterosexism and microaggressions

| Heterosexism | Microaggressions |
|---|---|
| • Assuming that all of your patients are heterosexual and that everyone has or is interested in having an opposite-sex partner<br>• Assuming that all children have opposite-sex parents<br>• Assuming all sexually active women need birth control<br>• Using language that presumes heterosexuality in others, such as husband or wife, instead of gender neutral language such as partner<br>• Using forms that allow for acknowledgment of only *marital status* as opposed to *relationship status* | • Asking someone if they are a woman or a man (male or female)<br>• Endorsing heteronormative culture or language<br>• Referring to bisexual people as *confused*<br>• Assuming that all LGBT are the same; telling someone that they are not a typical lesbian<br>• Assuming that all LGBQ people want to engage in sex with anyone if bisexual or with anyone of the same gender if lesbian, gay or queer |

and stigmatizes any nonheterosexual form of behavior, identity, relationship, or community" [2]. One difference between homophobia and heterosexism is demonstrated through the use of legal terms; qualification of actions based on homophobia are *hate crimes* while heterosexism results in *crimes of omission* [3]. Heterosexism, heteronormativity and gender normativity permeate society and most cultures in an insidious manner that is not unlike institutionalized racism [2], and more recently microaggression [4–6]. Shavers et al. [7] describe institutionalized racism as discrimination through long-standing policies, practices, structures, and regulations. Microaggression, too, has its origins in racism, but applies just as easily to matters of sexual orientation and gender identity/expression. Microaggressions are verbal, behavioral or environmental demonstrations of prejudice and discrimination that may appear to be harmless on the surface (see Table 4.1) [5, 8]. There is no seemingly overt intention of harm with institutionalized racism, microaggressions or with the most common forms of heterosexism. However, the results are frequently similar and harm is ultimately perpetrated.

This chapter will discuss the resulting disparities of access and provision of healthcare to LGBT people when homophobia, biphobia, transphobia and/or heterosexism becomes internalized. Internalized homophobia, or self-stigmatization, incorporates society's negative views into the self-concept and results in negative feelings about one's own non-heterosexual identity [9]. Not uncommonly, this internalization contributes to health issues including emotional, mental and

physical self harm. The effects of internalized heterosexism, with its more deceptive presentation, are not as evident to LGBT people or to their healthcare providers. Heterosexism is so thoroughly entrenched in daily life that it effects everyone, LGBT or straight, and without conscious effort. Internalized homophobia may be as insidious as heterosexism.

**Helpful Hint**
Although internalized heterosexism has yet to be considered by many healthcare providers or LGBT people, it has likely impacted the way LGBT people view the world and how others, including healthcare providers, perceive them.

## Relevance to Health

There is a strong association between health access and outcomes for any group of people who experience a perception of stigma and marginalization [10, 11]. There is an extensive literature that supports negative health outcomes in the presence of fear [12]. There are also several policy-impacting documents (i.e. Healthy People [HP] 2010, LGBT Companion Document, HP 2020 and the 2011 IOM report) that substantiate the problems associated with lack of healthcare access and of poor health outcomes in LGBT populations. Fear among LGBT people, and among healthcare providers, results from what is not known, or from past experiences among providers and LGBT people (either their own or that of others) that continue to reinforce negative reactions. This frequently develops a circular pattern of fear for the LGBT patient; lack of access because of avoidance that results in poorer health outcomes that leads back to increased fear and vulnerability. Fear on the part of the provider has consequences that also impact the LGBT patient, as the patient is dependent on care from that provider. The provider may restrict his or her practice from accepting LGBT patients to reduce their own experience of fear or of being uncomfortable, but that perpetuates the cycle of fear and increases lack of access for an entire population of people.

## Fear and Hate

No one likes to think of healthcare providers as harbingers of hate, but unless there is adequate screening of all involved personnel (in the office, hospital, surgical area…), the potential is there. If we examine the word *hate* and include its synonyms (animosity, revulsion, disgust, abhorrence and dislike), it is easier to imagine it entering our practices. The potential for hate to have an impact on practice, just like heterosexism, may be insidious. Impact on practice will be more thoroughly discussed later in this chapter in the section on *Disclosure in the Healthcare Environment.*

Fear, on the other hand, is the primary emotion experienced by most people when they approach an unknown situation. Some people may experience excitement and a feeling of empowerment from the unknown, but many experience fear. It is not uncommon for anyone, regardless of sexual or gender identity, to have a fear of healthcare providers. This fear is from what is not known; are we going to be told that we have an incurable disease, that the family curse of diabetes has finally gotten us or that we are overweight or obese and then be subject to that fear turning into shame? Healthcare providers are in a position of power and authority over patients; it is assumed that we have the talent,

knowledge, information and medicine that can fix myriad problems. Fear may also be a result of the tendency of healthcare providers to universalize human health and to minimize sexual and gender differences, thus creating a feeling of invisibility among LGBT people.

Fear is also a valid emotion for providers. It can be intimidating to be expected to know everything while faced with an unfamiliar clinical problem. Likewise, there can be a fear of misguided diagnoses and treatment if not familiar with particular health risks facing LGBT people, leading to potential accusations of clinical misjudgment.

> **Helpful Hint**
> LGBT people are at a higher risk for several diseases related to not only sexual behaviors, but other health sequellae related to obesity, higher rates of drinking alcohol and smoking, nulliparity as discussed in other chapters.

## Implicit Bias

There is a growing body of evidence examining and measuring implicit bias, also known as unconscious bias, among healthcare providers. This type of bias is, like heterosexism and microaggression, somewhat hidden and insidious. These are the biases that we do not like to acknowledge, but are there affecting our attitudes and behaviors in the clinic and other health healthcare settings (see Fig. 4.1). Again, this phenomenon grows out of studying racism and other culturally-based prejudices [13]. It is also applicable to the care of LGBT people, as any characteristic in someone else that triggers a negative reaction in a healthcare provider (consciously or not) has the potential to negatively impact patient care. Blair, Steiner and Havranek [14] have provided a "roadmap" for future research on implicit bias by identifying three goals. These goals are to

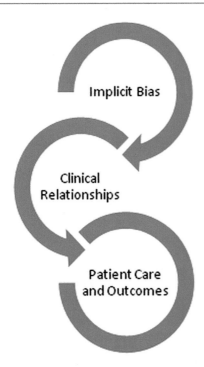

Implicit Bias

Clinical
Relationships

Patient Care
and Outcomes

**Fig. 4.1** Impact of implicit bias on patient care

"determine the degree of implicit bias with regard to the full range of social groups for which disparities exist", to understand "the relations between implicit bias and clinical outcomes" and to test interventions to reduce effects of implicit bias on processes of care and clinical outcomes. Meanwhile, providers must recognize and consider their own triggers and not ignore them so that they are not unconsciously compromising care. Other potential deflectors include considering the patient's perspective, challenging the recognizable cues to bias and reaffirming egalitarian goals as a provider.

## Current Policy

The Presidential Memorandum on Hospital Visitation was developed to help improve the lives of LGBT people by ensuring "the rights of hospital patients to designate visitors regardless

of sexual orientation or gender identity" ([15], ¶ 4). This document summarizes Acts, rules and provisions developed over the past several years to safeguard human rights for all Americans. The policies include:

- The Affordable Care Act
- The Centers for Medicare & Medicaid Services (CMS) rules (requiring all hospitals that participate in Medicare and Medicaid) to respect the rights of all patients to choose who may visit them, and that same-sex couples have the same rights as other couples for naming a representative who can make informed care decisions on a patient's behalf if incapacitated. CMS has also clarified that individual states have the flexibility to extend rights for long-term care under Medicaid to LGBT couples and to protect the couple's home. This is federal law for married couples
- Strengthened internal policies at the USDHHS to help ensure that LGBT individuals have equal access to HHS programs and employment opportunities

The Better Health and Well-being document also provides a listing of increased resources and plans for increasing knowledge related to health disparities in the LGBT population.

The Affordable Care Act (ACA) is considered a triumph by many LGBT people and communities. Although it has been criticized by many, acknowledgment of LGBT people, health disparities and consideration, for the first time on this level, gave many people a feeling of *arrival* or acceptance by the federal government. Some of the easily identified benefits of the ACA include the ability to be insured without having a recognized domestic partner, a job or a pre-existing condition. Research indicates that LGBT people have higher rates of being uninsured because of the inability to have coverage by their partner's plan in many places, higher rates of unemployment and higher rates of chronic disease, including HIV/AIDS, than the general public [16, 17].

## Beyond Sexual Orientation and the into Conflagration of Sex and Gender

We live and practice in a binary world. Kinsey's work in the 1940s was the first time the comfort of the binary was openly challenged. Since then, the concept of the *scaling* of sexual orientation has been pretty much accepted with many scholars, and the general public, recognizing that attraction is more complicated than simply hormones [18]. With the exception of individuals affected by differences in sex development (DSD-affected)/intersex people, gender has also existed in the binary (either/or female or male). This is currently being challenged in the same way that heterosexuality was in the 1940s. Sex and gender were largely considered to be the same, but today we know that sex is biologic and that one of the main theories on gender proposes that gender is socially constructed [19, 20]. This section will dissect gender without compounding it with sexual orientation. Please note that any sexual orientation may be integrated within any gender identification.

**Gender Normativity**   Just as heteronormativity affects LGBT people, gender normativity affects people who do not identify with a specific gender or people who identify as a gender not congruent with their physical body. This effect is evident in language (pronoun use), history and intake forms (relevant to identification other than male or female), health examinations and treatment needed and received (e.g., does your patient who presents as a male need a gynecological exam and hormones because he still has a uterus and ovaries?) and relationships with healthcare providers (providers are used to interacting with the binary on all levels). More recently, how do the differences in the sexes and the reactions to medications play out in prescribing for transgender people? Scientists are just beginning to recognize potential biological differences necessary in medication prescribing for male and female patients [21]. This becomes even more complicated and important when we expand the binary structure of sex *and* gender to include other

options that support transsexual bodies and transgender identities.

**Gender Typical/Atypical**   Many LGBT people present characteristics that do, or do not, align with their biologic sex. Among lesbian women, for example, many lesbian females are completely comfortable in their female bodies. These women will present anywhere from very feminine to androgynous to even quite masculine in their appearance. The term *lesbian female* may seem to contain redundancy, but there are many lesbian women who do not identify with the female or *feminine* parts of their anatomy (or similarly, females may not identify with the term lesbian). The same is true for gay men. People who identify as gender atypical or gender nonconforming do not necessarily consider themselves transgender.

> **Helpful Hint**
> Using visual cues and assessment in the LGBT population may lead to assumptions and not be as trustworthy as asking and listening. Always "listen to your patient", understand their chosen terminology, and replicate this in all settings.

## Disclosure in the Healthcare Environment

Disclosure is a behavior or action that informs a healthcare provider of the sexual and/or gender identity of an LGBT person. This section will provide language and other options that will allow providers to elicit this type of sensitive information. It will also explain how internalized homophobia, heteronormativity and gender normativity may prevent disclosure, thus limiting providers' ability to provide appropriate care and support.

**Why?**   Although disclosure of sexual orientation is possibly crucial for providing population-based healthcare, the development of patient/

provider relationships and meeting the objectives of Healthy People 2020, little is known about the phenomenon. It is, therefore, important to examine both facilitators and barriers to disclosure.

**Facilitators** Facilitators of disclosure consist of: (a) positive healthcare provider behaviors including inclusive language in health histories, being supportive, showing respect, and calm acknowledgment of identity; (b) a welcoming clinical environment including reading material of interest to LGBT people in the waiting area and exam rooms, affirming posters or artwork and culturally aware office staff; and (c) healthcare provider knowledge of LGBT health issues [22, 23]. Similar, but considered to be predictors of disclosure of sexual orientation are healthcare provider familiarity with the LGBT community and certain personal characteristics or demographic characteristics of LGBT people. However, the LGBT community is extremely diverse so what may be a facilitator to one culture or group may be a barrier to another [24]. Providers must be aware and familiar with their communities.

**Barriers** Although there has been little attention focused on facilitators of disclosure, barriers to disclosure have been examined more extensively. Four distinct sets of problems related to disclosure in the healthcare environment have emerged, along with the realization of internalized homophobia [25]. Many barriers to the act of disclosure are subsumed within these problem areas. The four main problem areas encompass negative healthcare provider (HCP) reactions to disclosure, potential and actual consequences to disclosure, cultural and political influences that have hindered healthcare access for LGBT people, and consequences of nondisclosure. The ensuing sections will present each of these barriers related to the major problem areas.

*Negative HCP Reactions to Disclosure* Fear of, and actual negative reactions from healthcare providers continue to be a part of the disclosing experience for lesbian women and gay men [26]. Barriers that emerge from negative healthcare provider reactions stem from homophobia and include: (a) ignoring the disclosure [27]; (b) dismissal, "There is always the chance that doctors will treat us differently, you know, dismiss us, be less concerned…" ([27], p. 223); (c) intrusion or invasion of privacy [28]; (d) curiosity and anxiety [28]; (e) stereotyping; and (f) shock, pity, fear, and embarrassment [29]. Homophobia is one of the primary barriers that lesbian women and gay men cite when hesitating to access healthcare [26, 30]. Although negative HCP reactions, or the fear of negativity, may or may not affect the medical treatment of the patient, both the fear and actual experience of mistreatment may indeed impact the healthcare experience in a negative way and result in the avoidance of care in the future.

*Potential and Actual Consequences to Disclosure* The distinction between potential and actual consequences is the same as the distinction between fear of and actual experiences of negative healthcare provider reactions—that is, what may happen and what has happened. Negative consequences to disclosure have included: (a) inappropriate behavior (e.g., referral to a mental health provider, voyeuristic curiosity) [30]; (b) rejection [31]; (c) rough physical handling [32]; (d) misdiagnosis and inappropriate healthcare teaching [33]; and (e) breached confidence [22, 27]. Negative consequences to disclosure set up barriers to future disclosure and healthcare access. Fear of mistreatment and lack of trust with disclosure are, perhaps, the most damaging barriers as they impede good relationships in the healthcare setting. Impedance of good relationships may decrease healthcare satisfaction and impact outcomes such as increased cost, decreased access and advanced stages of disease upon diagnosis [34].

*Cultural and Political Influences That Have Hindered Healthcare Access* Perhaps the most devastating influence of the twentieth century on LGBT healthcare was acceptance of the practice of diagnosing homosexuality as a treatable mental illness. Even though the American Psychiatric Association removed homosexuality from the diagnostic criteria in 1973, the influence of that earlier era on politics and American culture has persisted into the twenty-first century. Stevens [35] addressed the problem of heterosexist structure in healthcare as a macrolevel, or, a delivery system problem. Heterosexism, heteronormativity and gender normativity represent systems level influences that *maintain* individual prejudice and homophobia/bi/transphobia as the individual level prejudices. Political and societal environments contribute to heterosexist structuring. Heterosexist structuring implies an assumption that all people are heterosexual and that delivery of healthcare centers around typical gender roles. This practice results in LGBT people feeling "invisible, uninformed, and alienated from the health care process" [35]. Heterosexism has been a major issue in healthcare and continues to be a major barrier to disclosure.

*Consequences of Nondisclosure*  Because LGBT people are at risk for several health-related problems based on identity and behavior, it is imperative that healthcare providers be able to identify people in this higher risk group for preventive and primary healthcare. Consequences to nondisclosure include: assumptions of heterosexuality (therefore, potential risks may be overlooked); invisibility of self and sources of support such as a partner or other chosen family; irrelevant healthcare teaching; insensitive questioning; sexism; improper treatment; and misdiagnosis [10, 34]. Each of these consequences impacts practice, resulting in less than optimal and potentially dangerous healthcare.

In summary, few facilitators of, and several barriers to disclosure have been identified. Barriers to disclosure, and therefore barriers to appropriate healthcare, are heterosexism, homophobia and discrimination, misinformation about health risks related to sexual and life-style behaviors, invisibility in the healthcare environment, fear and past experiences of healthcare providers and of LGBT people. These barriers, as well as facilitators, may impact disclosure of LGBT people differently. Constant surveillance of these phenomena impacting practice is warranted.

**Your Motives as a Provider** It is well-documented that culturally competent care for LGBT patients includes an examination of the motives of the practitioner, and in some cases the environment, for eliciting personal information. Curiosity is never a reason to engage in the type of dialogue that would prompt disclosure of gender or sexual identity. Curiosity is frequently translated as voyeurism and further interpreted as fear-provoking and as a threat [36]. However, if you are providing primary care and risk assessments for an LGBT patient and trying to establish a medical home, knowing personal characteristics of your patient is important not only for physical and mental health, but also to identify social support mechanisms and primary relationships in the case of an emergency. This is also appropriate in the tertiary care setting to ensure proper treatment of a patient's family of choice and appropriate informed consent and advance directives.

> **Helpful Hint**
> Always be able to explain to a patient why you are asking for confidential information.

## Healthcare Advantages and Disadvantages

The advantages and disadvantages of healthcare provider's being aware of a person's sexual and gender orientation are numerous. The American Medical Association (AMA), indicated that competent care can be best provided with the knowledge of the patient's sexual orientation [37]. Yet, there still remains pervasive fear and ill effects of that disclosure. The disadvantages include failure to screen, diagnose and treat. There are also disadvantages to the partnership/relationship between the provider and the patient when an important aspect of a person's life is withheld. As discussed earlier (in the section facilitators and barriers), there are negative consequences socially, emotionally and physically when health-impacting information is withheld.

Conversely, when sexual orientation and/or gender identity is known, the relationship and environment deemed *safe* by the LGBT patient and problems or stressors identified, appropriate care can be provided and issues addressed at an earlier stage of disease, thereby, improving health outcomes. These include improved physical, mental and emotional health.

## Physical and Social Responsibility

As healthcare providers, it is our duty to provide a safe environment for all patients. Although there is a right to refuse a patient care based on availability or other reasons outlined in the codes of ethics for respective healthcare disciplines, there is never a right to discriminate or participate in discriminatory practices toward any patient. By virtue of the power relationships within medical or other healthcare practices, the responsibility of a safe and welcoming environment, including other office personnel, becomes that of the office management and care providers. There are innumerable resources available to assist with creating this environment (see Chaps. 3 and 7). A few suggestions include: demonstration of all kinds of diversity (posters of different ethnicities, types of families, groups of friends, etc.); an assortment of reading material that includes more than family journals and bible stories; intake forms that provide an opportunity to identify more than two genders or marital status (relationship status is an alternative) with options for married or partnered, single, etc. (this will also provide insight into support systems and sexual practices of heterosexual people); history forms that ask about sexual practices other than the assumption of heterosexuality; language used by staff and providers that does not make assumptions about gender or relationships. Providing an opportunity to disclose information will yield much better results than having patients walk in and walls go up around their identity or sexual practices (see Helpful Hint box for references and resources). As for social responsibility, being aware of appropriate referrals and resources for LGBT patients is also important.

**Helpful Hint**
Being prepared to make informed and appropriate referrals will contribute to a trusting relationship with LGBT clients.

## Summary

Homophobia and heterosexism continue to impact the health and well-being of LGBT people. Health consequences are sometimes compounded by the internalization of these phenomena by LGBT people making the development of positive healthcare relationships difficult. Several studies and articles have indicated that the impact of the relationship with healthcare providers, the healthcare environment, and other access issues that support disclosure, play a vital role in health-seeking behaviors [24, 29, 31, 37–42]. LGBT people who have positive relationships with healthcare providers seek to actively participate in health promoting behaviors. The establishment of a relationship of trust between healthcare providers and patients promotes favorable healthcare outcomes and is increasingly important for many regulatory, financial and personal reasons.

## References

1. Sears JT, Williams WL, editors. Overcoming heterosexism and homophobia: strategies that work. 1st ed. New York: Columbia University Press; 1997.
2. Herek GM. The context of anti-gay violence: notes on cultural and psychological heterosexism. J Interpers Violence. 1990;5:316–33.
3. Herek GM, Cogan JC, Gillis JR, Glunt EK. Correlates of internalized homophobia in a community sample of lesbians and gay men. J Gay Lesbian Med Assoc. 1998;2(1):17–26.
4. Balsam KF, Molina Y, Beadnell B, Simoni J, Walters K. Measuring multiple minority stress: the LGBT People of Color Microaggressions Scale. Cultur Divers Ethnic Minor Psychol. 2011;17(2):163–74. doi:10.1037/a0023244.
5. Sue DW, Capodilupo CM, Torino GC, Bucceri JM, Holder AM, Nadal KL, Esquilin M. Racial micro-

aggressions in everyday life implications for clinical practice. Am Psychol. 2007;62(4):271–86. doi:10.1037/0003-066X.62.4.271.

6. Platt LF, Lenzen AL. Sexual orientation microaggressions and the experience of sexual minorities. J Homosex. 2013;60(7):1011–34. doi:10.1080/00918369.2013.774878.

7. Shavers VL, Fagan P, Jones D, Klein WMP, Boyington J, Moten C, Rorie E. The state of research on racial/ethnic discrimination in the receipt of health care. Am J Public Health. 2012;102(5):953–66. doi:10.2105/AJPH.2012.300773.

8. Shelton K, Delgado-Romero EA. Sexual orientation microaggressions: the experience of lesbian, gay, bisexual, and queer clients in psychotherapy. J Couns Psychol. 2011;58(2):210–21. doi:10.1037/a0022251.

9. Thoits P. Self-labeling processes in mental illness: the role of emotional deviance. Am J Sociol. 1985;91(2):221–49.

10. Hatzenbuehler ML, Nolen-Hoeksema S, Dovidio J. How does stigma get under the skin? The mediating role of emotion regulation. Psychol Sci. 2009;20(10):1282–9. doi:10.1111/j.1467-9280.2009.02441.x.

11. Hatzenbuehler ML, Phelan JC, Link BG. Stigma as a fundamental cause of population health inequalities. Am J Public Health. 2013;103(5):813–21. doi:10.2105/AJPH.2012.301069.

12. Risher K, Adams D, Sithole B, Ketende S, Kennedy C, Mnisi Z, Baral SD. Sexual stigma and discrimination as barriers to seeking appropriate healthcare among men who have sex with men in Swaziland. J Int AIDS Soc. 2013;16(3 Suppl 2):18715. doi:10.7448/IAS.16.3.18715.

13. Moskowitz GB. On the control over stereotype activation and stereotype inhibition. Soc Pers Psychol Compass. 2010;4(2):140–58.

14. Blair IV, Steiner JF, Havranek EP. Unconscious (implicit) bias and health disparities: where do we go from here? Perm J. 2011;15(2):71–8.

15. USDHHS. Better health and well-being. 2012. http://www.hhs.gov/lgbt/health-update-2011.html. Retrieved 14 Jan 2014.

16. Buchmueller T, Carpenter CS. Disparities in health insurance coverage, access, and outcomes for individuals in same-sex versus different-sex relationships, 2000–2007. Am J Public Health. 2010;100(3):489–95.

17. Ponce NA, Cochran SD, Pizer JC, Mays VM. The effects of unequal access to health insurance for same-sex couples in California. Health Aff. 2010;29(8):1–10.

18. Giles J. Sex hormones and sexual desire. J Theory Soc Behav. 2008;38(1):45–66. doi:10.1111/j.1468-5914.2008.00356.x.

19. Alsop R, Fitzsimons A, Lennon K. Theorizing gender. Malden, MA: Blackwell; 2002.

20. Herek GM. On heterosexual masculinity: some psychical consequences of the social construction of gender and sexuality. Am Behav Sci. 1986;29(5):563–77. doi:10.1177/000276486029005005.

21. Soldin OP, Chung SH, Mattison DR. Sex differences in drug disposition. J Biomed Biotechnol. 2011;20(1):14. doi:10.1155/2011/187103.

22. Fogel SC. Identifying facilitators and barriers to disclosure of sexual identity to healthcare providers. Kans Nurse. 2005;80(9):1–3.

23. St Pierre M. Under what conditions do lesbians disclose their sexual orientation to primary healthcare providers? A review of the literature. J Lesbian Stud. 2012;16(2):199–219. doi:10.1080/10894160.2011.604837.

24. Durso LE, Meyer IH. Patterns and predictors of disclosure of sexual orientation to healthcare providers among lesbians, gay men, and bisexuals. Sex Res Soc Policy. 2013;10(1):35–42. doi:10.1007/s13178-012-0105-2.

25. Austin EL. Sexual orientation disclosure to health care providers among urban and non-urban southern lesbians. Women Health. 2013;53(1):41–55. doi:10.1080/03630242.2012.743497.

26. Ranji U, Beamesderfer A, Kates J, Salganicoff A. Health and access to care and coverage for lesbian, gay, bisexual, and transgender individuals in the U.S. The Henry J. Kaiser Family Foundation. 2014. http://kaiserfamilyfoundation.files.wordpress.com/2014/01/8539-health-and-access-to-careand-coveragefor-lesbian-gay-bisexual-and-transgender-individuals-in-the-u-s.pdf. Accessed 3 Mar 2014.

27. Stevens PE. Protective strategies of lesbian clients in healthcare environments. Res Nurs Health. 1994;17:217–29.

28. Reagan P. The interaction of health professionals and their lesbian clients. Patient Couns Health Educ. 1981;28:21–5.

29. Smith EM, Johnson SR, Guenther SM. Health care attitudes and experiences during gynecologic care among lesbians and bisexuals. Am J Public Health. 1985;75:1085–7.

30. Cochran SD, May VM. Disclosure of sexual preference to physicians by black lesbian and bisexual women. West J Med. 1988;149:616–9.

31. Tiemann K, Kennedy S, Haga M. Rural lesbians' strategies for coming out to health care professionals. J Lesbian Stud. 1998;2(1):61–75.

32. Stevens PE, Hall JM. Stigma, health beliefs and experiences with health care in lesbian women. Image J Nurs Sch. 1988;20(2):69–73.

33. Lehmann JB, Lehmann CU, Kelly PJ. Development and health care needs of lesbians. J Womens Health. 1998;7:379–87.

34. IOM (Institute of Medicine). The health of lesbian, gay, bisexual, and transgender people: building a foundation for better understanding. Washington, DC: National Academies Press; 2011.

35. Stevens PE. Structural and interpersonal impact of heterosexual assumptions on lesbian health care clients. Nurs Res. 1995;44:25–30.

36. Leninger M, McFarland M. Transcultural nursing: concepts, theories, research and practice. 3rd ed. New York: McGraw-Hill; 2002.

37. American Medical Association. AMA policy H-160.991, health care needs of the homosexual population. http://www.ama-assn.org/ama/pub/about-ama/our-people/member-groups-sections/glbt-

advisory-committee/ama-policy-regarding-sexual-orientation.shtml. Accessed 27 Jan 2014.

38. Cole SW, Kemeny ME, Taylor SE, Visscher BR. Elevated health risk among gay men who conceal their homosexual identity. Health Psychol. 1996;15:243–51.

39. Dardick L, Grady KE. Openness between gay persons and health professionals. Ann Intern Med. 1980; 93:115–9.

40. Simkin RJ. Lesbians face unique health care problems. Can Med Assoc J. 1991;145:1620–3.

41. Taylor B. 'Coming out' as a life transition: homosexual identity formation and its implication for health care practice. J Adv Nurs. 1999;30:520–5.

42. Trippet SE, Bain J. Reasons American lesbians fail to seek traditional health care. Health Care Women Int. 1992;13:145.

# Part II

# The LGBT-Inclusive Clinical Encounter

# Clinic and Intake Forms

**5**

Craig A. Sheedy

## Purpose

The purpose of this chapter is to advise on ways to create an inclusive and welcome clinic environment for members of the lesbian, gay, bisexual, and transgender (LGBT) community.

## Learning Objectives

- Discuss the importance of creating a safe and welcoming environment for LGBT patients in the healthcare setting (*KP4, PBLI1, SBP5*).
- Describe at least three strategies for improving components of the structural and interpersonal environments based on the needs of LGBT patients (*PBLI1, SBP5, ICS3, ICS4*).
- Identify at least three strategies for staff training and patient engagement to support a safe and welcoming medical home (*PBLI2, Pr4, ICS3, ICS4*).
- Discuss opportunities to connect and provide outreach to members of the LGBT community (*SBP4*).

The delivery of healthcare is a complex process that involves determining patient needs, planning and providing care, and coordinating therapy and additional services. Within this process, the environment surrounding a clinical encounter is an integral component of any healthcare visit, and can be a significant factor in overall patient satisfaction [1]. Creating an inclusive and welcoming environment for LGBT patients takes thought and effort by healthcare providers and organizations. Furthermore, having a well-planned clinical environment can lay the foundation for developing a successful therapeutic relationship between a provider and the LGBT patient. The clinical environment can be broken down into three broad categories as described by Wilkerson: the physical, systemic, and interpersonal environments [2]. Special attention should be given to each of these areas in order to improve on care provided to members of the LGBT community.

## Physical Environment: Create a Welcome Space

The first impression an LGBT patient has regarding a visit with a healthcare provider is of the clinic space itself. The structural components that affect a patient's experience include welcoming décor, the physical facilities, and patient flow.

C.A. Sheedy, M.D. (✉)
Department of Emergency Medicine, Vanderbilt University Medical Center, 1313 21st Ave. S., 703 Oxford House, Nashville, TN 37232, USA
e-mail: craig.a.sheedy@vanderbilt.edu

© Springer International Publishing Switzerland 2016
K.L. Eckstrand, J.M. Ehrenfeld (eds.), *Lesbian, Gay, Bisexual, and Transgender Healthcare*,
DOI 10.1007/978-3-319-19752-4_5

## Décor and Materials

Given the historic marginalization of the LGBT community, LGBT patients often search an office for signs that the provider is friendly towards LGBT individuals [1–3]. A clinic that primarily serves the LGBT community will include many relevant LGBT materials, but even clinics with a diverse patient population can show that they are LGBT-friendly by including even a few elements. Once a specific sign or material suggesting the establishment is LGBT friendly has been identified, patients are likely to feel more comfortable with the clinic environment. Many different options are available for inclusion in the clinic space, and examples include:

- Post a rainbow flag sticker, the Human Rights Campaign (HRC) logo, or other similarly identifiable symbol of the LGBT community in the waiting area [1, 2].
- Include posters that show diverse same-sex couples or transgender people, or posters from non-profit LGBT or HIV/AIDS organizations [1, 4].
- Include brochures discussing LGBT health concerns such as mental health, hormone therapy, substance use, safe sex, and cancer awareness. These can be posted in the waiting area, but also consider posting in the exam room where they are available in privacy from other patients (Fig. 5.1, see "Resources" section at the end of this chapter for more information) [1, 3].
- Wear a rainbow pin on the healthcare provider's white coat (Fig. 5.2).
- Include LGBT specific media such as national or local magazines or newsletters.
- Acknowledge relevant days of observance [5]:
  - National LGBT Health Awareness Week (Last week of March)
  - LGBT History Month (October)
  - National Coming Out Day (October 11th)
  - National Transgender Day of Remembrance (November 20th)
  - World AIDS day (December 1st).

> **Helpful Hint**
> LGBT-inclusivity can be enhanced by posting materials reflective of LGBT lives, such as a rainbow flag, poster of same-sex couple, or LGBT health brochures in the clinic waiting room.

## Gender-Inclusive Restrooms

Another aspect of the physical space to consider is the available restrooms. Transgender and other people not conforming to gender stereotypes have been harassed for entering the "wrong" bathroom when only dichotomous "Men" and "Women" options are available [6]. Offering at least one labeled unisex, gender-inclusive restroom is a way to help create a safer and more comfortable atmosphere for patients [2, 3] (Fig. 5.3). In addition, such a restroom also better serves parents caring for opposite sex children, and disabled persons with opposite sex caregivers [5]. It should be noted that while offering a unisex restroom can be an important signal of acceptance, patients should still be allowed to use restrooms with respect to their gender identity, and not be required to use the unisex restroom.

## Patient Flow

Patient flow is defined as the systematic process of caring for patients, starting from the time they enter the medical facility to the time when they check out. It includes both medical and administrative functions. Flow can be one of the most difficult components of the physical environment to successfully address for LGBT patients [2]. It is complicated by the number of individual points of contact the patient has with members of the healthcare team, support staff, and other patients, especially in public areas such as the waiting room. Communication about sexual orientation or gender identity can be challenging for LGBT patients because of a fear of discrimination by

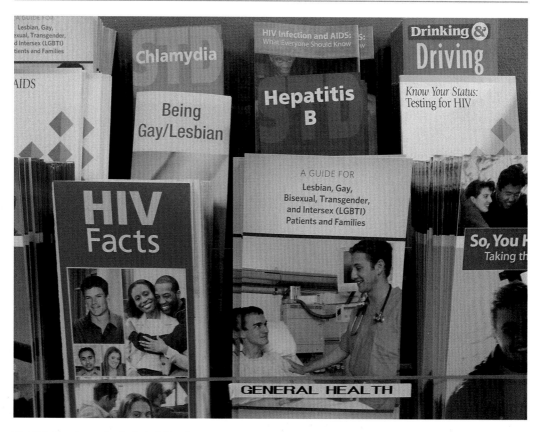

**Fig. 5.1** Brochures that include LGBT health topics placed in the clinic waiting area

**Fig. 5.2** A rainbow
caduceus and rainbow
button which may be
worn on a healthcare
provider's white coat or
ID badge

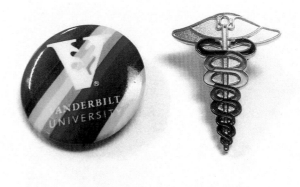

providers, staff or other patients, a misunderstanding of the reason for the clinic visit, or an outright denial of care. For example, transgender patients have described situations where other patients or staff have stared at them uncomfortably or began laughing at their appearance [2].

**Fig. 5.3** Sign for a gender-inclusive restroom

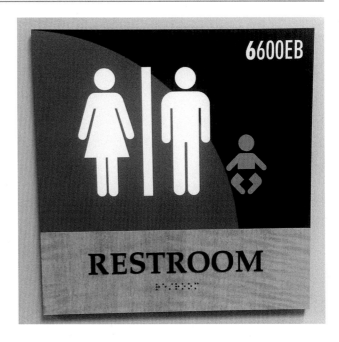

LGBT individuals have described being asked questions that forced them to out themselves as being LGBT in front of other patients or staff who did not need such information. Similarly, HIV-positive patients have been put in situations during which their HIV-status was disclosed to individuals who did not need access to such information [2].

Many of these problematic situations occur in the waiting area. Providers commenting on this topic have recognized that poor patient flow is a problem, but have experienced difficulty addressing many such problems. In an ideal patient setting, patient flow supporting LGBT patients should include a special focus on the following:

- Maintaining privacy at all steps of the patient–provider interaction [1, 3, 7].
- Avoid collecting sensitive information in public areas.
- Provide staff sensitivity training as discussed later in this chapter [1, 4, 7].
- Make adjustments to the physical space and include LGBT décor and materials as described above—this will let LGBT patients know that you are attempting to create a culturally relevant space.

## Systemic Environment

In addition to structural environment, elements of the clinic system and operations as a whole are crucial to the patient experience. Considerations that fall into this realm include the mission statement, operational policies, and patient intake forms. Careful attention to these elements will serve as a foundation, allowing the healthcare organization to address the unique needs of the LGBT population.

## Comprehensive Mission Statement, Non-discrimination and Visitation Policies

### Mission Statement

As a starting point, the healthcare facility should have a mission statement that assures the organization's commitment to respect individual diversity, which is inclusive of LGBT persons [2, 4, 5]. This mission statement will serve as a foundation for specific policies that will ensure the equal and fair treatment of all patients. Most important amongst such policies are patient and employee non-discrimination and visitation policies, which are premier on the list for creating a safe clinical environment according to the Healthcare Equality Index.

## Non-discrimination Policy

A comprehensive non-discrimination policy needs to be carefully drafted and implemented. This policy should explicitly state that equal care will be given to all patients regardless of age, race, sex, ethnicity, physical ability or attributes, religion, socioeconomic status, sexual orientation, and gender identity/expression [1, 3, 4]. The Joint Commission mandates that all hospitals prohibit discrimination on the basis of personal characteristics, which includes sexual orientation and gender identity or expression [3]. Furthermore, many states and some cities similarly have made discrimination on the basis of sexual orientation or gender identity or expression illegal. The non-discrimination policy should be posted in an easily visible location (including print material and on the facility website) for all staff and patients to view, helping to demonstrate a dedicated commitment to serve all patients with high quality and equitable care.

### Sample Non-discrimination Policy

Our hospital does not discriminate against individuals on the basis of their sexual orientation, gender identity, or gender expression in our provision of care to patients, employment, hiring practices, programs, or hospital activities.

## Visitation Policy

The healthcare facility/hospital should develop a written policy to outline visitation rights and procedures. Each patient should be granted the right to receive visitors as designated by the patient, including a spouse, domestic partner, family member, or friend [3, 4]. The importance of this originated following the Langbehn vs. Jackson Memorial Hospital case where, even with proper legal documentation, Lisa Pond's partner and children were denied medical information and kept in the waiting room for eight hours while she lay dying (see Lambda Legal's Report). Despite a presidential mandate, many hospitals still do not have inclusive visitation, healthcare proxy, or next-of-kin policies, the results of which are devastating for patients.

## Assure Confidentiality

Patient information is protected by the Health Insurance Portability and Accountability Act of 1996. When a patient chooses to disclose being LGBT, this information should be treated as sensitive and confidential. Furthermore, it is essential to assure patients of this confidentiality so they are comfortable disclosing personal information that is pertinent to their health, knowing that it is protected [1, 7]. This should include information contained in the medical record, on all documents, and conversations with a provider.

Healthcare facilities should develop and distribute a written confidentiality statement. The key components of such a policy should include the information covered, which office personnel has access to the medical record, how test results are kept confidential, the policy on sharing information with insurance companies, and any specific instances where confidentiality is not possible [1]. The policy should be provided to every patient in writing, and all staff must agree to this statement.

> **Helpful Hint**
> Special consideration should be given to creating policies for non-discrimination, visitation, and patient confidentiality, to help foster trust during the clinical encounter.

## Intake Forms

Similar to the structural environment, filling out an intake form is also one of the earliest impressions that a patient will have concerning a healthcare practice [1, 7]. Intake forms are often described as "unfriendly" by members of the

LGBT community [2, 8]. Therefore, intake forms should be modified to have more inclusive choices so that they are applicable to a diverse patient population [3, 4]. Whenever possible it is best to use open-ended questions, and in many cases it is preferred to offer a blank space for the patient to fill in an answer instead of check boxes that only offer a limited number of responses [1, 3]. In addition, the intake form should explain why the information is being collected, and should be tailored to the needs of each facility's patient population [2]. Certain questions can be interpreted as unnecessary or intrusive when the patient does not understand how the information will be used by the health practitioner.

Intake forms are also a component of patient flow. To better protect patient privacy, consider having an option for online completion of the intake form before coming to a scheduled appointment. This allows the patient to complete such forms in a private setting which can help to minimize any concerns of private information being discovered by other individuals in the waiting area.

**Helpful Hint**
Intake forms should have LGBT inclusive choices. Whenever possible use a blank space for the patient to fill in an answer to allow for self-identification… life is a spectrum and no one should be excluded!

Additional specific recommendations for LGBT sensitive intake forms are included below. Please also see Table 5.1 for sample intake form questions.

### Gender Identity
Understanding a patient's gender identity will help the provider to avoid making assumptions, will allow the provider to use the correct pronoun to address the patient, and will help guide the healthcare visit. Adding transgender options to the male/female selection on the intake from will help to better collect information on such indi-

viduals, and also offers a sign of acceptance to that person [1, 6]. This can include options for Female-to-Male (FTM)/Transgender Male, Male-to-Female (MTF)/Transgender Female, gender queer, or Additional Gender Category.

### Sexual Orientation
Incorrect assumptions about a patient's sexual orientation can interfere with establishing trust and lead to inappropriate care [1, 3, 7]. The intake form should offer a wide range of choices to signal acceptance, including: bisexual, gay, heterosexual/straight, lesbian, queer, and an option for unsure/do not know. It may be preferred to offer a fill in the blank answer as opposed to a check box since many individuals prefer not to conform to a specific label. It is important not to use the term "other", as this term suggests that a patient's identity is not worth listing or not part of the LGBT community.

### Relationship Status
Intake forms should use the term "relationship status" in the place of "marital status," as this is more reflective of the spectrum of possibilities [1, 3, 7]. Also as a general rule, intake forms should employ use of the word "partner" in place of the word "spouse." Ensure that staff is trained to know how to respond to the possible options. Possibilities can include: single, partnered, married, domestic partnership, separated, divorced, involved with multiple partners, and open or polyamorous relationships.

### Living Environment
Asking about the living environment may help provide information about social needs and potential stressors. Particular topics may include if the patient lives alone, with a roommate, with guardian(s) or family, with a significant other, and whether there are children or dependents in the household.

### Parent/Guardian
On intake forms for children, it is preferred to have labels for "parent/guardian" instead of listing "Mother" and "Father." These terms are inclusive of same-sex parents who may or may not be the biological parents [7].

**Table 5.1** Sample intake form questions

| | |
|---|---|
| Legal Name _____<br>Preferred Name _____<br>Preferred Pronoun<br>□ He<br>□ She<br>Gender Identity _____<br>OR<br>Gender Identity<br>□ Male<br>□ Female<br>□ Transgender<br>　　　　□ Male to female<br>　　　　□ Female to male<br>□ Additional gender _____<br>Current Sexual Partner(s) (last 6 months)<br>□ Men<br>□ Women<br>□ Transgender (please specify)<br><br>　_____<br>□ None/abstinent<br>Use of Birth Control<br>□ No<br>□ Yes<br>　What type? _____<br>□ I would like more information about options<br>Relationship Status<br>□ Partner<br>□ Married<br>□ Multiple partners<br>□ Separated/Divorced<br>□ Single<br>□ _____<br>Living Environment<br>□ Live alone<br>□ Live with spouse or partner<br>□ Live with roommate(s)<br>□ Live with parents/guardian(s) or family<br>□ Live with children/dependents<br>Children/Dependents<br>Name　　　　　　　　Relationship<br>_____　　_____<br>_____　　_____<br>_____　　_____<br>_____　　_____<br>Parent(s)/Guardian(s)<br>Name　　　　　　　　Relationship<br>_____　　_____<br>_____　　_____ | Sexual Orientation Identity<br>　□ Bisexual<br>　□ Gay<br>　□ Heterosexual/straight<br>　□ Lesbian<br>　□ Queer<br>　□ _____<br>　□ Not sure<br>Would you like information/recommendations on safer-sex techniques?<br>　□ No<br>　□ Yes<br>　　□ With men<br>　　□ With women<br>　　□ With both men and women<br>Have you used hormones (current or past) such as testosterone or estrogen?<br>　□ No<br>　□ Yes<br>　　Which? _____<br>　□ I would like more information about<br>　　hormone use<br>Have you been tested for HIV?<br>　□ No<br>　□ Yes<br>　　Date _____<br>　　Result _____<br>Have you been diagnosed with/treated for the following infections? (Mark all that apply.)<br>　□ Bacterial vaginosis<br>　□ Chlamydia<br>　□ Gonorrhea<br>　□ Herpes<br>　□ Hepatitis A<br>　□ Hepatitis B<br>　□ Hepatitis C<br>　□ HPV (human papillomavirus<br>　□ Syphilis<br>　□ Trichomonas<br>　□ None<br>Have you been vaccinated against any of the following infections? (Mark all that apply.)<br>　□ Hepatitis A<br>　□ Hepatitis B<br>　□ HPV (Gardasil or Cervarix vaccinations) |

## Hormone Therapy

Knowing whether a transgender patient is currently or has ever been on hormone therapy is an important piece of information when considering the overall health of such a patient [7, 8]. This should be included on the intake form for clinics that serve a high volume of LGBT patients. Asking whether the patient has questions regarding hormone therapy will allow the healthcare provider to consider this topic and be able to discuss it during the provider interview.

## Safer Sex Techniques

The intake form should inquire as to whether the patient would like more information about safer sex techniques, and can include asking whether information is requested for techniques with men, women, or both [1, 7]. This can serve as a starting point for a meaningful patient–provider conversation that may otherwise get overlooked during a busy clinical interaction.

## HIV Testing/Status

Given the increased prevalence of HIV within the LGBT population, it is recommended to ask if the patient has been tested for HIV, and the date of the most recent test if known [1, 7]. This should include asking if the result of the test was positive or negative. For a positive result, ask if the patient is currently being treated or followed for HIV infection.

## History of Transmissible Infections

Inquiring about a history of additional sexually transmitted infections (STIs) or other transmissible infections can potentially help the provider with risk stratification, and can also identify those with specific infections beyond HIV that can cause chronic disease and pose a risk of transmission to partners [1, 3, 7]. Infections to ask about include: bacterial vaginosis, chlamydia, gonorrhea, herpes, human papillomavirus (HPV), syphilis, hepatitis A, B, or C virus.

## Vaccinations

Ask whether the patient has received vaccination for hepatitis A, B and HPV. Members of the LGBT community, especially gay and bisexual men, are at increased risk for contracting these vaccine preventable diseases [1, 8]. Universal vaccination for hepatitis A and B is recommended, as well as vaccination for HPV for individuals younger than 27 years old.

## Interpersonal Environment

The interpersonal environment includes the interactions that occur between people, namely the LGBT patient and those involved in providing care. These interactions are additional factors that affect how healthcare providers and patients interact, build trust, and feel safe as coming out as LGBT.

## Staff Sensitivity Training

Training should be provided to ensure that both nursing and support staff are comfortable communicating with LGBT patients and follow office standards of respect [1, 2, 4, 5]. Ideally, staff would include individuals who are openly lesbian, gay, bisexual or transgender. Such individuals are an incredible asset and will provide first-hand knowledge about serving the LGBT public, and will help LBGT individuals to feel represented in their care. For those less familiar with LGBT topics, guidelines should be created to guide patient interactions. This can help reduce anxiety that staff may possibly have in regards to interacting with LGBT patients when they do not have familiarity with such a population. Training should be periodic to address staff changes and keep staff up-to-date [1]. Particular areas of focus for staff training are presented by GLMA: Health Professionals Advancing LGBT Equality, and include using appropriate language, being aware of relevant LGBT health issues, overcoming personal discriminatory beliefs, and having knowledge of additional LGBT resources [1].

**Helpful Hint**
Staff sensitivity training should be provided, with focus on the following topics:
- Using appropriate language when addressing LGBT patients
- Being aware of relevant LGBT health issues
- Overcoming personal discriminatory beliefs
- Having knowledge of additional LGBT resources

## Language

Staff must learn the appropriate language to use when addressing or referring to patients or significant others. This is particularly relevant to transgender individuals, and includes such topics as using their chosen name and referring to them by their chosen pronoun [6, 7]. When communicating with patients, staff is advised to follow the patients' lead [1] (see Chap. 1). It is therefore important to pay attention to how patients describe themselves, their partners, specific body parts, etc. If there is any doubt, you can also ask the patient what they prefer. It is better to be curious and to try to learn about your patient, than to not ask due to worry about causing offense.

## LGBT Health Issues

Sensitivity training should include a basic understanding of the most commonly encountered concerns in the area of LGBT health [1, 3, 8]. Such topics include the impact of discrimination and violence, the prevalence of depression and mental health issues, substance abuse, and safer sex practices. The topics addressed should be tailored to the needs of each individual healthcare practice to best suit the needs of its population.

## Potential Obstacles

One of the keys to staff training is that individuals must able to identify and overcome any personal discriminatory beliefs about LGBT people. Some employees may have pre-existing prejudices or negative feelings about LGBT patients due to ignorance or lack of exposure to LGBT issues [1, 8]. Some may also have religious beliefs that they feel require them to denounce members of this community. However, all employees must understand that discrimination against LGBT patients and coworkers is unethical and equally unacceptable as any other type of discrimination. Employers will need to make it clear that discrimination will not be tolerated in the workplace. Further training or individual counseling may be necessary to overcome these potential barriers to providing safe and equitable care.

## Knowledge of Healthcare Resources

The final piece of sensitivity training should include knowledge of additional healthcare resources available to LGBT community members, when available. Your practice should have a way to provide referral to LGBT-identified or friendly providers outside of your practice [1, 7]. To facilitate this goal, consider developing a reference list containing LGBT-friendly community resources and organizations as an aid for staff referral.

## The Clinical Interview

When interviewing a member of the LGBT community, as with any patient encounter, the healthcare provider should approach the interview with empathy, open-mindedness, and without passing judgment. LGBT individuals are more likely to have had traumatic past experiences with doctors and healthcare providers causing anxiety or mistrust [1, 6]. The provider's reaction as surprise or discomfort when learning a patient is LGBT will likely alienate these patients and result in lower quality or inappropriate care [2]. Therefore, it is particularly important to develop rapport and trust, which may take longer and require additional sensitivity from the provider [1]. To achieve this goal, advanced thought and preparation is helpful.

During the interview it is best to ask open-ended questions and avoid making assumptions [3, 1]. Whenever possible, explain why the questions you are asking are necessary. In addition to

LGBT status, the provider must also be aware of additional barriers caused by differences in socio-economic status, culture, race/ethnicity, religion, age, physical ability, and geography [1, 7]. Do not make assumptions about literacy, language capacity, and comfort with direct communication. Becoming skilled in the area of taking a medical history takes awareness and constant refinement. Here we offer only a brief overview, but this topic will be addressed in greater detail in Chap. 6.

## Reporting Discrimination

The ultimate goal is to eliminate discrimination from the healthcare system, not just for the LGBT population but for all individuals. However, when discrimination or disrespectful behavior does occur there must be an organized process for both patients and staff to report an event, and it must be accessible and easy to utilize [3, 7]. The organization is then tasked with completing a thorough and timely evaluation of such instances of discrimination or disrespectful behavior. The goal is to address and prevent recurrence of such situations, through additional staff training or changes in policy.

## Request Feedback for Improvement

After implementing new changes to better serve the LGBT population, healthcare providers should then engage patients to discuss whether the changes, available services, and programs are meeting the needs of LGBT patients [3, 7]. Being flexible and making adjustments is critical since the needs and demographics of patients, families, and the LGBT community is continually changing. By actively engaging members of the LGBT community, the healthcare provider will be better situated to understand and respond to experiences and healthcare needs.

## Addressing Patient Concerns

Every healthcare organization should have a method for patients and employees to file and resolve concerns and complaints. Each organiza-

tion or provider should create a reporting system where patients or employees can voice their concerns or suggestions for improvement, either as an online or via paper system [5]. The patient should have the option to submit a report anonymously if desired. However, if the patient provides his or her contact information this will allow an administrator to contact to the patient to provide feedback on how the complaint or concern was addressed and the process improved. It is good practice to have one individual in the workplace serve as a point of contact for evaluating and responding to patient complaints.

## Patient Satisfaction Surveys

Routine requests for feedback can be implemented via survey. A confidential or anonymous patient satisfaction survey is a great method to assess how patients are served by your practice. The survey content should address the patient's overall experience with services, which services were used, if all their needs are being met, and additional suggestions for improvement [3]. Surveys can be conducted by mail, phone, or in person.

> **Helpful Hint**
> Request feedback from LGBT patients about staff responsiveness and whether their needs are being addressed in your practice.

## Additional Considerations: Ways to Promote and Connect

One way to let patients know that your practice is LGBT friendly before they even walk in the door is to conduct patient outreach and marketing in LGBT venues, websites, and media. There are many organizations on both the national and local level that are involved in connecting LGBT members to healthcare services.

## The Referral Network

As a starting point, consider listing your practice in a provider referral program. For example, the non-profit organization GLMA: Health Professionals Advancing LGBT Equality maintains a national provider directory of culturally-competent physicians, therapists, nurses, dentists, and other providers (www.glma.org) [1]. This online directory allows patients to search by location for providers that are self-identified as serving members of the LGBT community. This service is free to join. Within your local organization, advertise your LGBT-focused services and make them publicly available on any electronic/online materials.

## Community Outreach: Organizations and Media

The role of LGBT community as a source of support cannot be understated for most LGBT individuals. A history of social stigma and discrimination has strengthened the sense of cohesiveness within the LGBT community. Similarly, the link between this community and the HIV/AIDS epidemic means that healthcare already holds a prominent role without this group [8]. This has created a culture where individuals may feel more accepted and have more support from their community than from their family of origin or religious affiliation.

Most cities offer local organizations for the LGBT community. Finding a local community center would be a great place to advertise or meet members of the community [3]. To find a local LGBT community center near to your hospital or practice, try searching at the following address: http://www.lgbtcenters.org. Similarly, advertisement in local media such as a newspaper or magazine would also be a great way to start connecting with the LGBT environment [2].

For those providers really wanting to engage the LGBT community, offering educational outreach programs is ideal [3]. An educational series could be arranged at one of the local community centers. The additional benefit of such programs is that they can help improve the health of the community by reaching people outside of traditional healthcare settings [4]. Topics can include any of the healthcare topics discussed in this text, such as:

- Support for the psychosocial and mental health needs of LGBT youth.
- Aging and end of life concerns of LGBT seniors.
- Programs for transgender patients, such as on the process of transition.
- Education and counseling on HIV/AIDS.
- Presentation from well-known LGBT community members offering personal thoughts on healthcare issues.

## Evaluating Success: The Healthcare Equality Index

Consider participating in the Healthcare Equality Index (HEI) [5]. The HEI, organized by the Human Rights Campaign, was established as a resource for healthcare organizations that desire to provide exceptional care to LGBT individuals (www.hrc.org). The HEI is an online survey that allows healthcare organizations to assess their policies and practices with respect to LGBT patient-centered care as outlined by The Joint Commission requirements [3]. In addition, it provides additional support to such healthcare facilities through supplemental training and resources. Finally, it also allows organizations to receive public recognition for their commitment to equality and LGBT health.

## Resources

## Brochures

### American Cancer Society
- Cancer Facts for Gay and Bisexual Men
- Cancer Facts for Lesbians and Bisexual Women
- Tobacco and the LGBT community

Free brochures and be ordered by phone: 800-ACS-2345.

They can also be viewed online:
http://www.cancer.org/healthy/findcancerearly/
menshealth/cancer-facts-for-gay-and-bisexual-
men
http://www.cancer.org/healthy/findcancerearly/
womenshealth/cancer-facts-for-lesbians-and-
bisexual-women

## American College Health Association

- Man to Man: Tips for Healthy Living for Men Who Have Sex with Men
- Women to Women: Tips for Healthy Living for Women Who Have Sex with Women
  These can be located at http://www.acha.org/
  Topics/lgbtq.cfm

## Centers for Disease Control and Prevention

Fact sheets can be found by searching the Centers for Disease Control and Prevention (CDC) website at http://www.cdc.gov

## Safe Schools Coalition

Provides online links and ordering information for brochures from many different LGBT-friendly organizations.
http://www.safeschoolscoalition.org/RG-brochures.
html

## Helpful Internet Resources

Center Link—LGBT community center directory.
http://www.lgbtcenters.org

Centers for Disease Control and Prevention (CDC)—General information is available on many topics specific to the LGBT population including mental health, cancer screening, substance abuse, HIV, STIs, and also recommendations for preventative health.
http://www.cdc.gov

Gay, lesbian, Bisexual, and Transgender Health Access Project—Community based program offering training and materials to help providers learn about the health needs of LGBT populations.
www.glbthealth.org

GLMA: Health Professionals Advancing LGBT Equality—Association of lesbian, gay, bisexual and transgender healthcare professionals working towards LGBT healthcare equality. Maintains a national LGBT provider directory.
www.glma.org

Human Rights Campaign—Healthcare Equality Index (HEI); an online survey for healthcare organizations to assess their policies and practices with respect to LGBT patient-centered care.
www.hrc.org

Lambda Legal—Nonprofit legal organization pursuing full recognition of the civil rights of lesbians, gay men, bisexuals, transgender people and those with HIV.
http://www.lambdalegal.org/

The Joint Commission—Health care accreditation and certification organization, including standards for patient-centered care and specific considerations for the LGBT community.
http://www.jointcommission.org

The Penn Program for LGBT Health
http://www.pennmedicine.org/lgbt/

Vanderbilt Program for LGBTI Health
https://medschool.vanderbilt.edu/LGBTI

## References

1. GLMA: Health professionals advancing LGBT equality. Guidelines for care of lesbian, gay, bisexual, and transgender patients. 2006. http://www.glma.org/_data/n_0001/resources/live/Welcoming%20Environment.pdf.
2. Wilkerson JM, Rybicki S, Barber C. Results of a qualitative assessment of LGBT inclusive healthcare in the twin cities. Minneapolis, MN: Rainbow Health Initiative; 2009.
3. The Joint Commission: advancing effective communication, cultural competence, and patient- and family-centered care for the lesbian, gay, bisexual, and transgender (LGBT) community: a field guide. Oak Brook, IL; October 2011. LGBTFieldGuide.pdf.
4. Gay and Lesbian Medical Association: healthy people 2010: companion document of lesbian, gay, bisexual, and transgender (LGBT) health. April 2011. http://

www.glma.org/_data/n_0001/resources/live/HealthyCompanionDoc3.pdf.

5. Snowdon S. Recommendations for enhancing the climate for LGBT students and employees in health professional schools: a GLMA white paper. Washington, DC: GLMA; 2013.

6. Feldman J, Bockting W. Transgender health. Minn Med. 2003;86(7):25–32.

7. Kaiser Permanente. Provider's handbook on culturally competent care: LGBT population. 2004. http://kphci.org/downloads/KP.PHandbook.LGBT.2nd.2004.pdf.

8. Dean L, Meyer IH, Robinson K, et al. Lesbian, gay, bisexual, and transgender health: findings and concerns. J Gay Lesbian Med Assoc. 2000;4(3):101–51.

# 6

## Carl G. Streed Jr.

## Purpose

The purpose of this chapter is to provide guidance on completing a thorough, competent, and culturally appropriate health history with details specific to the care of LGBT individuals and communities.

## Learning Objectives

- Identify at least three ways that the medical history can create and foster the patient–provider relationship with LGBT patients (*PC1, PBL11, ICS2*)
- Discuss ways that language can be used in the medical history to avoid assumptions about a patient's sexual orientation, gender identity, or relationship to other individuals (*KP1, ICS1, ICS2*).
- Identify at least five strategies to engage in an open dialogue with patients to address sensitive issues in the medical history (*ICS1, Pr1, PC1*)
- Identify at least three opportunities to adapt health messages and counseling efforts to address high-risk behaviors to meet the needs

of patients with diverse sexual orientations, gender identities, and sex and gender histories (*PC3, PC4, PC5, PC6*).

## (Re)Building the Therapeutic Relationship

To provide complete and appropriate care for patients requires an open dialogue built on trust. However, health care providers have an uphill climb to creating such a trusting relationship with their LGBT patients. A 2010 report by Lambda Legal[1] and a 2011 report by the National Center for Transgender Equality[2] outline where the health care professions have failed to maintain the trust and confidence of those it is meant to treat [1, 2]. Appropriately titled "When Health Care Isn't Caring" and "Injustice at Every Turn," respectively, the surveys highlight the discrimination LGBT[3]

---

[1] Lambda Legal (Lambda Legal Defense and Education Fund) is an American civil rights organization that focuses on lesbian, gay, bisexual, and transgender(LGBT) communities as well as people living with HIV/AIDS (PWAs) through impact, societal education, and public policy work.

[2] The National Center for Transgender Equality (NCTE) is a social justice organization dedicated to advancing the equality of transgender people through advocacy, collaboration and empowerment.

[3] Patients affected by differences in sex development were not explicitly included in this survey.

C.G. Streed Jr., M.D. (✉)
School of Medicine, Johns Hopkins Bayview
Medical Center, Baltimore, MD, USA
e-mail: cjstreed@gmail.com

© Springer International Publishing Switzerland 2016
K.L. Eckstrand, J.M. Ehrenfeld (eds.), *Lesbian, Gay, Bisexual, and Transgender Healthcare*,
DOI 10.1007/978-3-319-19752-4_6

patients have experienced from the health care establishment:

- Nearly 8 % of LGB individuals, over 25 % of transgender and gender-nonconforming individuals, and 19 % of people living with HIV reported that they had been denied needed health care outright.
- Approximately 50 % of transgender respondents reported having to *teach* their health care providers about transgender care.
- Over 10 % of LGB individuals and over 20 % of transgender and gender-nonconforming respondents reported being subjected to harsh or abusive language from a health care professional.
- Approximately 11 % of LGBT individuals and almost 36 % of people living with HIV reported that health professionals refused to touch them or used excessive precautions.
- More than 12 % of LGB individuals, over 20 % of transgender and gender-nonconforming individuals, and over 25 % of people living with HIV reported being blamed for their health status.
- Almost 8 % of transgender and gender-nonconforming individuals reported experiencing physically rough or abusive treatment from a health care professional.

Not surprisingly, LGBT individuals report a high degree of anticipation and belief that they will face discrimination when seeking health care, and such concerns are a barrier to seeking care. Overall, 9 % of LGB individuals are concerned about being refused health services when they need them and 20 % of people living with HIV and over half of transgender and gender-nonconforming respondents share this same concern [1, 2]. As LGBT individuals are less likely to seek health care, there are fewer opportunities to offer care, conduct screenings, provide education, and other health promotions [3]. In addition to effectively scaring LGBT patients away from seeking health care, nearly two-thirds of transgender patients who have been refused care on the basis of their transgender identity report a lifetime suicide attempt [4]. There is obviously significant room for improving the relationship between LGBT and gender non-conforming patients and the health professions.

It is beyond the scope of this chapter to provide strategies to connect patients with the health care system. However, successful and positive interactions between LGBT patients and health care providers in which providers have awareness of and demonstrated commitment to the needs of LGBT patients will attract new and loyal patients, reduce their risk of complaints and negative publicity, and achieve higher patient satisfaction scores while improving the health outcomes [5–7]; such LGBT competent care is in alignment with Centers for Medicare & Medicaid Services and The Joint Commission Requirements [8]. Chapter 5 of this text addresses the importance of the pre-encounter experience and provide guidance for how to create welcoming reception areas, train staff to be LGBT friendly and competent, and provide examples of intake forms that are LGBT inclusive [9–11].

## Interviewing Techniques; One Size Does Not Fit All (Table 6.1)

Assuming the clinic staff and intake process are culturally competent and appropriately matched to the patient, it then falls to the health care provider to ensure adequate and complete care for the LGBT patient. For any of their patients, health care providers should be aware of how personal bias can affect the patient–provider relationship. Heterosexist attitudes and homophobic beliefs inculcated by the majority culture influence interactions between patients and providers from either's perspective; heterosexist bias affects how providers communicate and internalized homophobia may prevent patients from disclosing their sexual orientation and/or gender identity in even the most welcoming of clinics.

Though it may seem unnecessary to mention, greeting the patient and whomever may be accompanying them sets the tone for the entire clinical encounter. First, the gender identity or sexual orientation of the patient should never be assumed based on name or outward appearances or even name in the medical chart; transgender

**Table 6.1** Interviewing techniques

| Use preferred name | This should be addressed on intake and noted in all future visits |
| --- | --- |
| Do not assume gender | Do not refer to the patient as "Mr. Smith" or "Ms. Smith" <br> Use the patient's preferred full name or preferred first name |
| Be aware of pronouns | If the patient notes that they are not single, do not assume the gender of their significant other <br> Avoid "girlfriend," "boyfriend," "wife," and "husband" unless the patient uses these terms |
| Do not make assumptions about relationships | Do not say, "and is this your sister [brother/mother/father]?" <br> Say, "and who has joined you today?" and allow the companion to identify themselves and their relationship to the patient |

patients may still be in the process of aligning their legal name with their gender identity. It is therefore important that until the patient's preferred gender pronoun or preferred name is known, they should be addressed by their preferred full name, not as "Mr. Smith" or "Ms. Smith." Secondly, never presume to know the relationship of anyone accompanying the patient; too often are significant others mistaken for "brother" "sister" or "friend." Making an assumption, no matter how benign and unintentional, can signal to the patient that the health care provider is at best not trained to manage LGBT patients and at worst intolerant or hostile. If the provider unintentionally makes an assumption, providing an immediate apology often corrects the *faux pas* and can allow the provider and the patient to set the encounter on the right path.

After greetings, introductions, and establishing rapport, the clinical encounter can transition to eliciting the chief concern of the patient. Providing undivided attention and exhibiting interest with non-verbal cues will signal engagement, and maintaining an appropriate level of eye contact will allow the patient to feel more welcome; too often have LGBT patients been dismissed by providers who looked at the patient with a degree of disgust or judgment or never looked them in the eye.

## Completing a Thorough and Competent History

As with any clinical encounter for the seasoned health care provider, determining the patient's agenda will allow both provider and patient to

efficiently direct the visit and ensure the explicit needs of the patient are addressed. As always, open-ended questioning is paramount and allowing adequate time for patients to answer questions will foster a more trusting relationship; interrupting a patient, especially one who may have experienced dismissive behavior from a health care provider in the past, will damage a budding patient–provider relationship. Table 6.2 shows a sample flow of questions you might consider using when interviewing patients.

After expertly eliciting the patient's chief concern and elaborating on the history of present illness, it is important to collect a thorough history, especially with first-time patients; this will build rapport and lay the groundwork for a productive patient–provider relationship for future visits. As is already explained in other texts and during the typical health care provider training, it is important to collect data regarding the past medical and surgical history, mental health history, current medications, allergies, family medical history, and social history including data about education, employment, family structure, substance use/abuse, sexual history, and other items as may be relevant to patient care and/or building rapport.

## Past Medical and Surgical History

Though LGBT patients have many of the same health concerns as the general population, there are particular issues of medical and surgical health that are distinct and should be considered when collecting the past medical and surgical history. Here, we will specifically make mention of issues related to cardiovascular disease, cancer,

**Table 6.2** Completing a thorough and competent history

---

**STEP 1: PUT PATIENT AT EASE**

"I am going to ask you a few questions about your sexual health and sexual practices. I understand that these questions are very personal, but they are important for your overall health."

"Just so you know, I ask these questions to all of my adult patients, regardless of age, gender, or marital status. These questions are as important as the questions about other areas of your physical and mental health. Like the rest of our visits, this information is kept in strict confidence. Do you have any questions before we get started?"

**PART 2: PARTNERS**

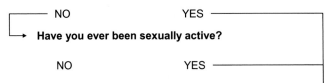

**Are you currently sexually active?**

NO            YES

**Have you ever been sexually active?**

NO            YES

**How many sexual partners have you had in the past 6 months?**

**When you have sex, do you do so with men, women, or both?**

**If both, how many male/female sexual partners have you had in the past 6 months?**

**Has anyone ever forced themselves on you sexually, or touched sexually you in an unwanted way?**

**PART 3: IDENTITY**

**Are you attracted to men, women, or both?**

**How do you identify your sexual orientation?**

**Are there any concerns you would like to discuss related to your sexuality, sexual orientation, or gender?**

**PART 4: PRACTICES / PROTECTION**

**When having sex, do you have vaginal, anal, and/or oral sex?**

**Do you use condoms/latex dams when having vaginal, anal, and/or oral sex? How often?**

NO or YES, SOMETIMES            YES, ALWAYS

**Do you and your partner(s) use any other protection against STI's?**

NO, or YES, SOMETIMES            YES, ALWAYS

**Could you tell me the reason why not?**            **What kind of protection do you use? How often?**

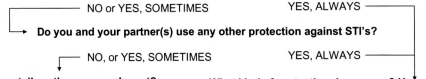

| For MSM, assess: | For WSW, assess: |
|---|---|
| - history and vaccination against Hep A and B | - use, frequency, sharing, and cleaning of sex toys |
| - history and results of anal pap smear | - frequency and protection with digital/vaginal sex |
| - use of alcohol/drugs during sex | - history of sex with men |

---

(continued)

**Table 6.2**   (continued)

---

PART 5: PAST HISTORY OF STIs

**Have you ever been diagnosed with an STI?**

NO                                              YES

**When were you diagnosed?**

**How were you treated?**

**Have you ever been tested for HIV or other STIs?**

**Would you like to be tested?**

**Has your current or any former partners ever been diagnosed or treated for an STI?**

NO                                    YES

**Were you tested for the same STI?**

PART 6: PREGNANCY PREVENTION

**Are you currently trying to conceive / father a child?**

NO                                     YES

**Are you concerned about getting pregnant or getting your partner pregnant?**

NO                                     YES

**Are you using contraception or practicing any form of birth control?**

**Do you need any information on birth control?**

PART 7: SEXUAL FUNCTION

**Do you have any concerns about sexual function?**

**Do you have pain with intercourse? Problems with erection, ejaculation, or orgasm?**

PART 8: COMPLETING HISTORY

"What other concerns or questions regarding your sexual health or sexual practices would you like to discuss?"

Thank the patient for being open and honest and praise any protective practices.

Express concern regarding high-risk practices, if necessary.

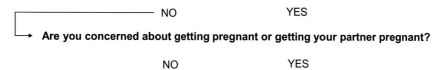

| Risk Reduction for MSM: | Risk Reduction for WSW: |
|---|---|
| - consistent use of condoms with oral/anal sex | - latex barriers minimize transfer of bodily fluids |
| - avoid excessive substance use | - lubricants to reduce tearing, abrasions |
| - counseling on HIV post-exposure prophylaxis | - clean sex toys with 1/10th bleach/water solution |

**Table 6.3** Cardiovascular risk factors in LGBT populations

| Tobacco use |
| --- |
| Alcohol abuse |
| Diabetes |
| Hypertension |
| Hyperlipidemia |
| Obesity |
| Sedentary lifestyle |
| Testosterone replacement/therapy |
| Bilateral oophorectomy |
| Anti-retroviral therapy |

**Table 6.4** Risk factors associated with breast cancer

| Tobacco use |
| --- |
| Alcohol abuse |
| Obesity |
| Nulliparity |

obesity, and surgical interventions as they are pertinent to the medical history, while Chap. 8 will discuss screening and preventive health related to these concerns.

## Cardiovascular Disease (Table 6.3)

There continues to be a significant burden of cardiovascular disease within the general population, but limited research has demonstrated that patients infected with HIV, lesbian women, and transgender patients taking masculinizing hormones are at increased risk. One prospective observational study of male and female participants noted a possible association between antiretroviral treatment and cardiovascular events such as myocardial infarction [12]. A review of cardiovascular health within the Los Angeles County Health Survey demonstrated a higher rate of heart disease diagnosis among lesbian women as compared to heterosexual women; bisexual women also had an elevated risk of heart disease compared to heterosexual women [13]. For transgender men, research suggests increased risks following bilateral oophorectomy [14, 15] and, several studies have found that transgender patients receiving hormone treatment had positive and negative changes in certain risk factors for cardiovascular disease [16]. However, the quality of the data has limited meta-analyses attempting to draw more robust conclusions from the data [17].

It is therefore important to consider these issues when collecting information from your patients.

## Cancer (Table 6.4)

LGBT patients have multiple risk factors that potentially place them at higher risk of having cancer at some point in their life time. There has been a long standing debate as to the possible increased risk for breast cancer among lesbian women as compared to heterosexual women, but the data remains limiting. While the relative risk for breast cancer is still being determined, there is enough evidence to suggest that lesbian women have a higher prevalence of risk factors associated with breast cancer, including nulliparity, alcohol use/abuse, tobacco use/abuse, and obesity [18–20]. This limited data stresses the importance of asking about these risk factors as well as sexual orientation when collecting the social history during the patient interview.

Similar to risk for cervical cancer, HPV infection in men who practice receptive anal intercourse has long been known to cause anal cancer [21–23]. There is research to suggest that a majority, as high as three-quarters, of men who have sex with men are positive for HPV [24–26]. Unlike cervical cancer prevalence, which peaks during the third decade of life in women, anal HPV infection is steady throughout the life of men who have sex with men [26]. This data highlights the need for anal cancer screening, which can be performed with cytology [25]; guidelines for routine screening and testing do not exist but study recommendations suggest screening HIV-negative men every 2–3 years and HIV-positive men annually [27, 28]. As men who have sex with men are at higher risk for infection with HPV types 6, 11, 16, and 18 and associated conditions, including genital warts and anal cancer, the US Advisory Committee on Immunization Practices (ACIP) recommends routine vaccination against HPV with the quadrivalent vaccine (HPV4) and vaccination for patients through the age of 26 years who have not been vaccinated

**Table 6.5** Patients who should be vaccinated against HPV

| Patients ≤26 years of age regardless of GI/SO |
| --- |

previously or who have not completed the three-dose series [29]; regardless of gender identity and/or sexual orientation, vaccination against HPV should be offered to patients 9–26 years of age (Table 6.5).

Unfortunately, data is limited on cancer among the transgender population. Case-reports do make note of breast cancer among transgender women receiving feminizing hormones [30–32] and transgender men receiving masculinizing hormones and undergone chest surgery [33, 34], ovarian cancer in transgender men on testosterone [35, 36], prostate cancer among transgender women receiving feminizing hormones [37, 38], and prolactinomas in transgender women receiving estrogen replacement therapy [39].[4] These reports stresses the importance of collecting information on prior medical and surgical treatments to more fully assess potential risks experienced by transgender patients.

It is worth stressing that the Surveillance Epidemiology and End Results database of the National Cancer Institute, the most comprehensive source of cancer statistics in the US, does not include sexual orientation or gender identity in the demographics data; this is another missed opportunity to estimate the incidence and prevalence of cancer in the LGBT population.

## Obesity

The American Medical Association (AMA) officially recognizes obesity as a disease entity that should be addressed as such [40]. There is an obesity endemic in the US and the Western world that does not leave LGBT populations unaffected. The most research available relates to obesity in lesbian women and bisexual women, demonstrating that lesbian women and

bisexual women are more likely to be overweight or obese when compared to heterosexual women [41–43]. Causation for this association remains unclear, but theories include minority stress, family rejection, and a rejection of societal standards of beauty [44].

There is also evidence that obese individuals may have worse HIV outcomes [45, 46]. Research has found that obese versus normal weight patients (based on BMI < 25 kg/m$^2$) had smaller increases in CD4 counts after initiating HAART; lower CD4 counts may now be another adverse consequence of obesity.

By recognizing obesity as a disease to be addressed during a patient visit, it is possible to reduce the risk of developing chronic diseases associated with being overweight or obese, including cardiovascular disease, diabetes mellitus type II, colon cancer, and sleep disorders.

## Surgical Interventions

The anatomy of the patient presenting to the clinic can direct the interview and influence the eventual physical exam and guide risk-reduction screening (see Chap. 8). For those reasons, it is important to enquire, when appropriate, about any prior surgeries, from mundane fractures to gender-affirming procedures such as colpectomy, vaginoplasty, phalloplasty, mastectomy, and other procedures to feminize or masculinize a patient. The interview should always be non-judgmental and the provider should aim to educate the patient as to the need for such information to be gathered.

For transgender patients who have undergone gender-affirming procedures, there are specific issues primary care providers and gynecologists should understand. According to WPATH, male-to-female patients who have had vaginoplasty should be counseled on the need for vaginal dilation or penetrative intercourse to maintain vaginal depth and width [47]. Further, due to the surgical shortening of the urethra, male-to-female patients experience urinary tract infections more frequently, and may suffer from function disorders as a result of damage to the autonomic nerve supply of the bladder floor during surgery [48, 49]. As most female-to-male patients do not undergo

---

[4] Causality should not be inferred from these case reports and there is a significant need to perform studies that determine prevalence of these conditions and risk/protection associated with these therapies.

colpectomy, preventive care must be tailored to anatomy and not gender. Similarly, patients receiving masculinizing hormones can experience atrophic changes of the vaginal lining which can lead to pruritus; such issues require sensitivity on the part of the health care provider as patients with a male gender identity and masculine gender expression may experience emotional discomfort or pain regarding their female genitals [50]. It is worth noting that despite surgical complications, patients rarely regret having undergone gender affirming procedures; the best predictor of overall outcomes of gender affirming procedures is the quality of surgical results [51].

For a more complete discussion of hormone treatment and gender affirming procedures and complications, please see section "5", Chaps. 18–21.

## Mental Health History

Research continues to find an increased risk for depression, anxiety, and suicide/suicidal behavior among LGBT patients [52–56]. Much of this is a result of the stigma, or minority stress, experienced every day by LGBT individuals in family, work, school, and social environments; explicit discrimination and harassment based on gender identity and/or sexual orientation have been demonstrated to be factors in stress, anxiety, depression, and mental illness [9, 57, 58].

As with all patients, the primary care provider should screen for mental illness. Depression remains a common affliction, and providers should ask about persistent depressed mood, anhedonia, and suicidal ideation, and treat or refer those with clinical depression. Referral for mental illness should be to a mental health provider with an understanding of LGBT care issues.

For further details on mental health in the LGBT population, please see Chap. 13.

## Current Medications

Enquiring about prescription medications, over-the-counter medications, supplements, and home remedies is a standard part of care. However, it is important to ask specifically about medications, hormones, and injectables (e.g. silicone) not obtained from a health care provider. Transgender patients may obtain hormone therapies and/or injectables either from other providers, internet pharmacies, or street vendors. Understanding the substances patients have used will guide prescription practices and recommendations.

Some transgender patients may already have been using hormones; they may have had them prescribed by a physician (and may be seeking a new physician for whatever reason), or they may have obtained hormones through overseas, "street," or internet sources, without any prior physician evaluation [59, 60]. In this latter instance, the WPATH provides recommendations for health care providers to continue the medical treatment of patients who have independently initiated hormone therapy, regardless of the patient's ability or desire to receive recommended gender-related psychiatric/psychological evaluation. Health care providers may provide treatment based upon the principle of harm reduction; when patients have demonstrated their determination to continue using medications without oversight, then it is usually advisable to assume their medical care and prescribe appropriate hormones. Denying them care will only result in their continued independent treatment, possibly to their detriment.

Electronic medical records are facilitating more rapid medication reconciliation across regional health systems [61].

## Allergies

Obtaining information about a patient's allergic and adverse reactions to medications, common environmental allergens (e.g. pet dander, mold, tobaccos smoke, et cetera), and other allergens (e.g. components of vaccines and other injectables) is standard of care. Understanding the allergy profiles of patients, particularly transgender patients, can alter the selection of hormones and other injectable therapies (e.g. cosmetic fillers such as silicone) [62]. Details regarding cosmesis can be found in Chaps. 15, 20, and 21.

## Family Medical History

To fully understand the potential risk factors of a patient, it is necessary to outline or diagram the age and health, or age and cause of death, of each immediate relative including parents, grandparents, siblings, children, and grandchildren; if there is a particular pattern either on the maternal or paternal side, it is worth enquiring about aunts and uncles and cousins as well. Collecting the family medical history is standard of care. However, as more governments, local and national, recognize the rights of same-sex couples to adopt, it will become increasingly important to educate adoptive parents of the need to obtain the medical records of their children's biological parents [63].

## Social History

What has typically been described as the "Social History" during the clinic encounter includes a range of information such as behavioral risk factors, environmental and societal factors that affect health, and support systems available to a patient. The order in and depth to which this information is collected can be left to provider preference but here we address *Substance Use/ Abuse*, *Socioeconomic Status*, *Support Systems*, *Sexual History*, and *Violence/Abuse*.

### Substance Use/Abuse

Enquiring about tobacco use, alcohol consumption, and the use of other illicit substances is standard of care as there is substantial data highlighting the health risks associated with each.

While there is a growing body of research that has focused on substance use among LGB patients (T to a lesser extent), an even larger body of research comparing heterosexual and non-heterosexual populations suggests that substance use is a problem for LGBT patients [10]. Numerous studies have shown that lesbian women and bisexual women have higher rates of past and current tobacco use [41, 64, 65]; the same has been found to be true of gay and bisexual men [65–67]. Overall, LGBT individuals in

the US are over 60 % more likely to smoke tobacco products as compared to the rest of the population [68]. Similarly, LGBT individuals are more likely to consume alcohol and more likely to become dependent [42, 64, 69, 70]. Not surprisingly, recreational drugs were used at higher rates among LGBT patients [70–73]. Given the unique stressors that factor into substance use and abuse, interventions have been tailored specifically for lesbian and gay communities [74].

See the webpage of the National LGBT Tobacco Control Network for a list of smoking cessation programs, referrals, and research.

### Socioeconomic Status: Education, Employment, Income

Socioeconomic factors are becoming recognized as significant determinants of health and health care outcomes. Arguably the more significant factors include education, employment, and income as each factor contributes to a patient's location within society, access to resources, and ability to overcome adverse situations. A complete social history will include information about a patient's level of education, employment status, and source(s) of income allowing the health professional to better understand the resources available to their patient and where they may need additional support.

The level of education, or educational attainment, of a patient can be a fair surrogate of the resources available to a patient as well as their support systems and possibilities for employment. Though the world economy no longer can guarantee employment for those furthering their education, it remains that those with high school/ secondary school degrees are generally better off than those without, those with college/university degrees are generally better off than those without, and so forth. However, LGBT individuals are less likely to have high school diplomas, bachelor's degrees, and advanced degrees compared to their heterosexual peers [79]. Knowing a patient's educational attainment and aspirations of such can allow the health provider to provide encouragement and possibly offer connections to resources (e.g. GED programs, skills training) [75].

Employment often provides many benefits including a support network, income, and health insurance. As a result, employment status greatly affects patient health outcomes as a result of access to economic and social resources. However, it is worth noting that lesbian, gay, bisexual and especially transgender patients face significant workplace and employment discrimination, making it important to enquire about employment status and appropriate to ask about workplace stressors as they relate to the visit presentation [76–78].

In addition to gainful employment, it important to ask about other sources of income (e.g. disability benefits, commercial sex work, bartering). Understanding the full extent of patients' economic resources can encourage an already prudent health provider to choose wisely to limit the burden of health care costs upon the patient as well as be mindful of possible social/institutional resources available to the patient [79, 80].

### Support Systems

The social network of a patient can be the source of significant frustrations as well as support. When thinking of social networks, many immediately look to biological family members to be the most significant sources of support. While this may be true for many patients, it is important to recognize that due to homophobia, transphobia, and intolerance of gender non-conforming identities or non-heteronormative social roles, many LGBT individuals have been rejected by their families [81]. Consequently, recognizing that a patient may not be closely connected to their family of birth can provide opportunities to enquire about other social networks (e.g. friends, work colleagues, et cetera) who serve as surrogate family or family of choice.

It is important to determine the support systems available to a patient in order to recommend the best therapies and treatment options available; research has demonstrated that patients with robust support systems have better healthcare outcomes [82]. This could not be truer than when it comes to elder care. Due to the high prevalence of rejection by family, many elder LGBT patients find themselves isolated as their other social net-

**Table 6.6** The 6 P's of a complete sexual health history

| Partners |
| --- |
| Practices |
| Protection from STIs |
| Past history of STIs |
| Prevention of/planning for pregnancy |
| Pleasure |

works age and pass away. Further, as they age and require higher levels of care, LGBT individuals have, in order to protect themselves, been forced to go back into the closet when they enter rehabilitation, long-term care, or nursing home facilities [83–87]. It is therefore important to recognize the anxiety many LGBT individuals may have when discussing any therapy plans that involve these services.

### Sexual Health History (Table 6.6)

When caring for LGBT patients, it is important to separate identity from behavior. As Chap. 1 clearly delineate's, a patient's sexual identity and/or gender identity cannot be used to assume their sexual behaviors and the disease risks they may encounter when engaging in sexual behavior. Therefore, taking the time to complete a thorough and non-judgmental sexual health history has the potential to both build the patient–provider relationship as the provider demonstrates a willingness to better understand the patient and be a powerful risk-reduction method as various behaviors are uncovered that could lead to pregnancy, sexually transmitted illnesses, or trauma while pursuing sexual satisfaction and intimacy.

While there are many entrées to the sexual health history, it is paramount to remain non-judgmental when opening the topic and exploring a patient's history. Establishing the purpose of this line of inquiry will go far in building rapport with the patient and making them, and the provider, comfortable in discussing sensitive information.

The CDC provides some of the more concise recommendations for completing the sexual health history and focuses on 5Ps: partners, practices, protection from STIs, past history of STIs, and prevention of/planning for pregnancy.

It is important to add a 6th P, Pleasure, to have a complete sexual health history. These are just guidelines, and the interview should be tailored to each patient's specific presentation and needs. However, these are a good starting point to the sexual health history.

> **Helpful Hint**
>
> An asexual individual is someone who does not experience sexual attraction, and, unlike celibacy, which people choose, asexuality is an intrinsic part of who asexual individuals are; just as it is important to understand the sexuality of some individuals as an intrinsic quality, it is important to recognize asexuality is an intrinsic quality for others. And just as sexually active individuals have emotional needs, so do asexual individuals; a person who is asexual may experience attraction to others, but they don't feel they need to act that attraction out sexually.

1. Partners

    To begin to assess the risk of contracting an STI, it is important to determine the number and gender of the patient's sex partners. As a recurring theme through this text, never make assumptions about the patient's sexual orientation. If only one sex partner is reported over the last 12 months, be certain to inquire about the length of the relationship. Also, ask about the partner's risk factors, such as current or past sex partners or drug use; it is not uncommon for the patient to not know their sexual partner's risks, but remains important to ask as this can direct prevention and treatment. If more than one sex partner is reported in the last 12 months, again be certain to explore for more specific risk factors, such as condom use/non-use, prophylaxis (e.g. PrEP), and partner risk factors.

> **Helpful Hint**
>
> If a patient has been sexually active in the past, but is not currently active, it is still important to take a sexual history as this may be an opportunity to explore the reasons why they are no longer sexually active (e.g. prior trauma, fear of transmitting or receiving STIs, et cetera).

2. Practices

    If a patient has had more than one sex partner in the past 12 months or has had sex with a partner who has other sex partners, you may want to explore further his or her sexual practices and methods of protection (e.g. condoms, barriers, PrEP). This is where it is critically important to enquire about behavior and to not make any assumptions based on identity. Asking about other sex practices will guide the assessment of patient risk, risk-reduction strategies, the determination of necessary testing, and the identification of anatomical sites from which to collect specimens for STI testing. Put bluntly, interview questions should aim to answer who is putting what, where, when, and how.

3. Protection from STIs

    It is necessary to determine the appropriate level of risk-reduction counseling for each patient; risk-reduction counseling for a patient in a monogamous relationship will be different from a patient who is a commercial sex worker or in an open-relationship. And even if a patient is in a monogamous relationship for over 12 months, it is still worth providing testing services if the patient is interested. However, in other situations, you may need to explore the subjects of abstinence, monogamy, condom use, the patient's perception of their own risk and their partner's risk, and the issue of testing for STIs.

4. Past history of STIs

A history of prior STIs can increase a patient's current risk for an STI. Therefore, it is essential to ask about prior diagnoses, when they occurred, how often, and courses of treatment.

5. Prevention of/planning for pregnancy

At this point in the interview, it should be possible to determine whether or not the patient is at risk of becoming pregnant or of fathering a child. If so, first determine if a pregnancy is desired. If not, then provide counseling on contraception methods for both the patient and their partner(s).

---

**Helpful Hint**

If biology allows and the patient is not planning to not have a child, they are planning to have a child.

---

6. Pleasure

Though this text is not intended to be an exhaustive review of sexual behavior and intimacy for LGBT individuals, it is important to recognize the importance of pleasure in sexual intimacy and well-being and the need to include it in a complete sexual health history [88, 89].

---

**Helpful Hint**

As often occurs, by the end of the interview, the patient may have come up with information or questions that they were not ready to discuss earlier. Allow the patient to circle back to prior topics if they feel comfortable doing so.

---

At this point, thank the patient for being open and honest as it is often difficult to discuss such culturally/socially sensitive information. Further, offer praise for any protective practices including those that offer a reduction of risk if not elimination of risk. After reinforcing positive behavior with praise, it is appropriate to specifically address concerns regarding high-risk practices. Expressing concern may help the patient accept a counseling referral, if one is recommended.

## Violence/Abuse

As with other areas of LGBT health, there is not much data on intimate partner violence. The CDC has recently begun to address this information gap with the National Intimate Partner and Sexual Violence Survey Overview of 2010 Findings on Victimization by Sexual Orientation [90]. The report indicates that individuals who self-identify as LGB have an equal or higher prevalence of experiencing intimate partner violence, sexual violence, and stalking as compared to self-identified heterosexuals. Bisexual women are disproportionately impacted; they experience a significantly higher lifetime prevalence of rape, physical violence, and/or stalking by an intimate partner, and rape and sexual violence other than rape by any abuser, when compared to both lesbian and heterosexual women.

Consequently, it is necessary to screen for intimate partner violence in order to provide referrals for individuals affected by abuse to culturally appropriate services. Consider initiating the interview with a question such as "Does your partner ever hit, kick, hurt, or threaten you?" or "Do you feel safe at home?" rather than asking if a patient has concerns about domestic violence or abuse. When providing referrals to other professionals, verify with the patient the level of disclosure of sexual orientation and/or gender identity that is appropriate. A detailed discussion of intimate partner violence can be found in Chap. 10.

## Laying the Groundwork for Future Encounters

Given the extensive history of discrimination and abuse by the health care community, ensuring a positive health care encounter will begin to address the health disparities experienced by the LGBT community. To that end, it is also important to be open to feedback from LGBT patients; often they are in a position to educate their providers and have had to do so in the past. Aside from offering a positive health care encounter, public advertising and community engagement will provide a positive impression for the community. It is important to note that LGBT patients have long been providing one another referrals to providers that have demonstrated culturally competent and compassionate care; the best referral comes from a satisfied patient. If the encounter has provided for at least the beginning of an open dialogue, LGBT patients will continue to seek care. The more positive encounters that occur between the health care professions and LGBT population, the sooner disparities in health care outcomes in LGBT patients will be understood and addressed.

## References

1. Lambda Legal. When health care isn't caring: lambda legal's survey of discrimination against LGBT people and people with HIV. New York: Lambda Legal; 2010. Available at www.lambdalegal.org/health-care-report.
2. Grant JM, Mottet LA, Tanis J, Harrison J, Herman JL, Keisling M. Injustice at every turn: a report of the national transgender discrimination survey, executive summary. Washington, DC: National Center for Transgender Equality and National Gay and Lesbian Task Force; 2011. Available at: http://www.transequality.org/PDFs/Executive_Summary.pdf.
3. Harrison AE, Silenzio VM. Comprehensive care of lesbian and gay patients and families. Prim Care. 1996;23(1):31–46.
4. Haas AP, Eliason M, Mays VM, Mathy RM, Cochran SD, D'Augelli AR, Silverman MM, Fisher PW, Hughes T, Rosario M, Russell ST, Malley E, Reed J, Litts DA, Haller E, Sell RL, Remafedi G, Bradford J, Beautrais AL, Brown GK, Diamond GM, Friedman MS, Garofalo R, Turner MS, Hollibaugh A, Clayton PJ. Suicide and suicide risk in lesbian, gay, bisexual, and transgender populations: review and recommendations. J Homosex. 2011;58(1):10–5.
5. Epstein S. Impure science: AIDS, activism, and the politics of knowledge. Berkeley, CA: University of California Press; 1996.
6. Crisp, C. Correlates of homophobia and gay affirmative practice in rural practitioners. J Rural Community Psychol. 2007;15:119–43.
7. Snowdon S. Equal and respectful care for LGBT patients. The importance of providing an inclusive environment cannot be underestimated. Healthc Exec. 2013;28(6):52, 54–5.
8. The Joint Commission. Advancing effective communication, cultural competences, and patient- and family-centered care for the lesbian, gay, bisexual, and transgender (LGBT) community: a field guide. Oak Brook, IL. Oct. 2011. Available at: http://www.jointcommission.org/assets/1/18/LGBTFieldGuide.pdf.
9. GLMA. Guidelines for lesbian, gay, bisexual, and transgender patients. GLMA. 2006. Available at: http://www.glma.org/_data/n_0001/resources/live/GLMA%20guidelines%202006%20FINAL.pdf.
10. IOM (Institute of Medicine). The health of lesbian, gay, bisexual, and transgender people: building a foundation for better understanding. Washington, DC: National Academies Press; 2011.
11. Bradford JB, Cahill S, Grasso C, Makadon HJ. Policy focus: how to gather data on sexual orientation and gender identity in clinical settings. Boston, MA: Fenway Institute; 2012. Available at http://www.fenwayhealth.org/site/DocServer/Policy_Brief_HowtoGather..._v3_01.09.12.pdf.
12. Friis-Moller N, Sabin CA, Weber R, d'Arminio Monforte A, El-Sadr WM, Reiss P, Thiebaut R, Morfeldt L, De Wit S, Pradier C, Calvo G, Law MG, Kirk O, Phillips AN, Lundgren JD. Combination anti-retroviral therapy and the risk of myocardial infarction. N Engl J Med. 2003;349(21):1993.
13. Diamant AL, Wold C. Sexual orientation and variation in physical and mental health status among women. J Womens Health. 2003;12(1):41.
14. Rivera CM, Grossardt BR, Rhodes DJ, Brown Jr RD, Roger VL, Melton 3rd LJ, Rocca WA. Increased cardiovascular mortality after early bilateral oophorectomy. Menopause. 2009;16:15–23.
15. Parker WH, Manson JE. Oophorectomy and cardiovascular mortality: is there a link? Menopause. 2009;16:1.
16. Gooren LJ, Giltay EJ, Bunck MC. Long-term treatment of transsexuals with cross-sex hormones: extensive personal experience. J Clin Endocrinol Metab. 2008;93(1):19.
17. Elamin MB, Garcia MZ, Murad MH, Erwin PJ, Montori VM. Effect of sex steroid use on cardiovascular risk in transsexual individuals: a systematic review and meta-analyses. Clin Endocrinol. 2010;72(1):1–10.
18. Diamant AL, Wold C, Spritzer K, Gelberg L. Health behaviors, health status, and access to and use of health care: a population-based study of lesbian, bisexual, and heterosexual women. Arch Fam Med. 2000;9(10):1043–51.
19. Tang H, Greenwood GL, Cowling DW, Lloyd JC, Roeseler AG, Bal DG. Cigarette smoking among lesbian women, gays, and bisexuals: how serious a problem? (United States). Cancer Causes Control. 2004;15(8):797–803.
20. Meads C, Moore D. Breast cancer in lesbian women and bisexual women: systematic review of incidence, prevalence and risk studies. BMC Public Health. 2013;13:1127. Available at: http://www.biomedcentral.com/1471-2458/13/1127.
21. Koblin BA, Hessol NA, Zauber AG, Taylor PE, Buchbinder SP, Katz MH, Stevens CE. Increased incidence of cancer among homosexual men, New York City and San Francisco, 1978–1999. Am J Epidemiol. 1996;144(10):916–23.

22. Ryan DP, Compton CC, Mayer RJ. Carcinoma of the anal canal. N Engl J Med. 2000;342(11):792.
23. Daling JR, Madeleine MM, Johnson LG, Schwartz SM, Shera KA, Wurscher MA, Carter JJ, Porter PL, Galloway DA, McDougall JK. Human papillomavirus, smoking, and sexual practices in the etiology of anal cancer. Cancer. 2004;101(2):270.
24. Friedman HB, Saah AJ, Sherman ME, Busseniers AE, Blackwelder WC, Kaslow RA, Ghaffari AM, Daniel RW, Shah KV. Human papillomavirus, anal squamous intraepithelial lesions, and human immunodeficiency virus in a cohort of gay men. J Infect Dis. 1998; 178(1):45–52.
25. Palefsky JM, Holly EA, Ralston ML, Jay N. Prevalence and risk factors for human papillomavirus infection of the anal canal in human immunodeficiency virus (HIV)-positive and HIV-negative homosexual men. J Infect Dis. 1998;177(2):361.
26. Chin-Hong PV, Vittinghoff E, Cranston RD, Buchbinder S, Cohen D, Colfax G, Da Costa M, Darragh T, Hess E, Judson F, Koblin B, Madison M, Palefsky JM. Age-specific prevalence of anal human papillomavirus infection in HIV-negative sexually active men who have sex with men: the EXPLORE study. J Infect Dis. 2004;190(12):2070.
27. Goldie SJ, Kuntz KM, Weinstein MC, Freedberg KA, Welton ML, Palefsky JM. The clinical effectiveness and cost-effectiveness of screening for anal squamous intraepithelial lesions in homosexual and bisexual HIV-positive men. J Am Med Assoc. 1999;281(19): 1822–9.
28. Goldie SJ, Kuntz KM, Weinstein MC, Freedberg KA, Palefsky JM. Cost effectiveness of screening for anal squamous intraepithelial lesions and anal cancer in human immunodeficiency virus-negative homosexual and bisexual men. Am J Med. 2000;108(8):634–41.
29. CDC. Recommendations on the use of quadrivalent human papillomavirus vaccine in males—advisory committee on immunization practices (ACIP). MMWR. 2011;60(50):1705–8.
30. Ganly I, Taylory EW. Breast cancer in a transsexual man receiving hormone replacement therapy. Br J Surg. 1995;82(3):341.
31. Pritchard TJ, Pankowsky DA, Crowe JP, Abdul-Karim FW. Breast cancer in a male-to-female transsexual: a case report. J Am Med Assoc. 1988;259(15):2278.
32. Symmers WS. Carcinoma of breast in trans-sexual individuals after surgical and hormonal interference with the primary and secondary sex characteristics. Br Med J. 1968;2(5597):83.
33. Burcombe RJ, Makris A, Pittam M, Finer N. Breast cancer after bilateral subcutaneous mastectomy in a female-to-male trans-sexual. Breast. 2003; 12(4):290.
34. Eyler AE, Whittle S. FTM breast cancer: community awareness and illustrative cases. Paper presented at XVII Harry Benjamin International Gender Dysphoria Association Symposium, Galveston, TX, 31 Oct–4 Nov 2001.
35. Hage JJ, Dekker JJ, Karim RB, Verheijen RH, Bloemena E. Ovarian cancer in female-to-male transsexuals: report of two cases. Gynecol Oncol. 2000; 76(3):413.
36. Pache TD, Chadha S, Gooren LJG, Hop WCJ, Jaarsma KW, Dommerholt HBR, Fauser BCJM. Ovarian morphology in long-term androgen-treated female to male transsexuals. A human model for the study of polycystic ovarian syndrome? Histopathology. 1991;19(5):445.
37. Markland C. Transexual surgery. Obstet Gynecol Annu. 1975;4:309.
38. van Haarst EP, Newling DW, Gooren LJ, Asscheman H, Prenger DM. Metastatic prostatic carcinoma in a male-to-female transsexual. Br J Urol. 1998;81(5):776.
39. Bunck MC, Debono M, Giltay EJ, Verheijen AT, Diamant M, Gooren LJ. Autonomous prolactin secretion in two male-to-female transgender patients using conventional oestrogen dosages. BMJ Case Rep. 2009;2009. pii: bcr02.2009.
40. AMA. H-150.953 obesity as a major public health problem. 2013. Available at: https://ssl3.ama-assn.org/apps/ecomm/PolicyFinderForm.pl?site=www.ama-assn.org&uri=%2fresources%2fhtml%2fPolicyFinder%2fpolicyfiles%2fHnE%2fH-150.953.HTM.
41. Case P, Austin SB, Hunter DJ, Manson JE, Malspeis S, Willett WC, Spiegelman D. Sexual orientation, health risk factors, and physical functioning in the nurses sexual orientation. J Womens Health. 2004; 13(9):1033.
42. Cochran SD, Mays VM. Relation between psychiatric syndromes and behaviorally defined sexual orientation in a sample of the US population. Am J Epidemiol. 2000;151(5):516–23.
43. Boehmer U, Bowen DJ, Bauer GR. Overweight and obesity in sexual-minority women: evidence from population-based data. Am J Public Health. 2007; 97(6):1134–40.
44. The Mautner Project. Lesbian overweight and obesity research: tackling the lesbian obesity epidemic. 2011. The National Lesbian Health Organization. Available at: http://www.whitman-walker.org/document.doc?id=289.
45. Crum-Cianflone NF, Roediger M, Eberly LE, Vyas K, Landrum ML, Ganesan A, Weintrob AC, Barthel RV, Agan BK. Infectious disease clinical research program HIV working group obesity among HIV-infected persons: impact of weight on CD4 cell count. AIDS. 2010;24(7):1069–72.
46. Crum-Cianflone NF, Roediger M, Eberly LE, Ganesan A, Weintrob A, Johnson E, Agan BK. Infectious disease clinical research program HIV working group. Impact of weight on immune cell counts among HIV-infected persons. Clin Vaccine Immunol. 2011;18(6): 940–6.
47. van Trotsenburg MAA. Gynecological aspects of transgender healthcare. Int J Transgend. 2009;11(4): 238–46.
48. Hoebeke P, Selvaggi G, Ceulemans P, De Cuypere GD, T'Sojoen G, Weyers S, Monstrey S. Impact of

sex reassignment surgery on lower urinary tract function. Eur Urol. 2005;47(3):398–402.

49. Kuhn A, Bodmer C, Stadlmayr W, Kuhn P, Mueller MD, Birkhauser M. Quality of life 15 years after sex reassignment surgery for transsexualism. Fertil Steril. 2009;92(5):1685–9.

50. Coleman E, et al. Standards of care for the health of transsexual, transgender, and gender-nonconforming people. 7th ed. Minneapolis, MN: WPATH; 2012.

51. Lawrence AA. Patient-reported complications and functional outcomes of male-to-female sex reassignment surgery. Arch Sex Behav. 2006;35(6):717–27.

52. Balsam KF, Beauchaine TP, Mickey RM, Rothblum ED. Mental health of lesbian, gay, bisexual, and heterosexual siblings: effects of gender, sexual orientation, and family. J Abnorm Psychol. 2005;114(3):471.

53. Bostwick WB, Boyd CJ, Hughes TL, McCabe SE. Dimensions of sexual orientation and the prevalence of mood and anxiety disorders in the United States. Am J Public Health. 2010;100(3):468.

54. Hatzenbuehler ML, Keyes KM, Hasin DS. State-level policies and psychiatric morbidity in lesbian, gay, and bisexual populations. Am J Public Health. 2009; 99(12):2275.

55. Bockting WO, Miner MH, Swinburne Romine RE, Hamilton A, Coleman E. Stigma, mental health, and resilience among an online sample of the U.S. transgender population. Am J Public Health. 2013; 103(5):943–51.

56. Budge SL, Adelson JL, Howard KH. Anxiety and depression in transgender individuals: the roles of transition status, loss, social support, and coping. J Consult Clin Psychol. 2013;81:545–57.

57. Meyer IH. Prejudice as stress: conceptual and measurement problems. Am J Public Health. 2003; 93(2):262f.

58. Berberet HM. San Diego lesbian, bisexual and transgender women needs assessment. 2005.

59. Anderson B. Deaths highlight illegal silicone use: trans pumping parties reportedly gaining popularity. Washington Blade. 2003.

60. Wallace P. Finding self: a qualitative study of transgender, transitioning, and adulterated silicone. Health Educ J. 2010;69(4):439–46. doi:10.1177/001789691 0384317.

61. Blumenthal D. The future of health care and electronic records. HealthIT Buzz. 2010. Available at: http://www.healthit.gov/buzz-blog/electronic-health-and-medical-records/the-future-of-health-care-and-electronic-records/.

62. Duffy DM. Liquid silicone for soft tissue augmentation. Dermatol Surg. 2005;31(11 Pt 2):1530–41.

63. Hill CM, Wheeler R, Merredew F, Lucassen A. Family history and adoption in the UK: conflicts of interest in medical disclosure. Arch Dis Child. 2010;95:7–11. doi:10.1136/adc.2009.164970.

64. Burgard SA, Cochran SD, Mays VM. Alcohol and tobacco use patterns among heterosexually and homosexually experienced California women. Drug Alcohol Depend. 2005;77(1):61.

65. Trocki KF, Drabble LA, Midanik LT. Tobacco, marijuana, and sensation seeking: comparisons across gay, lesbian, bisexual, and heterosexual groups. Psychol Addict Behav. 2009;23(4):620.

66. Gruskin EP, Greenwood GL, Matevia M, Pollack LM, Bye LL, Albright V. Cigar and smokeless tobacco use in the lesbian, gay, and bisexual population. Nicotine Tob Res. 2007;9(9):937.

67. Conron KJ, Mimiaga MJ, Landers SJ. A population-based study of sexual orientation identity and gender differences in adult health. Am J Public Health. 2010;100(10):1953.

68. King BA, Dube SR, Tynan MA. Current tobacco use among adults in the United States: findings from the National Adult Tobacco Survey. Am J Public Health. 2012;102(11):e93–100.

69. Gilman SE, Cochran SD, Mays VM, Hughes M, Ostrow D, Kessler RC. Risk of psychiatric disorders among individuals reporting same-sex sexual partners in the national comorbidity survey. Am J Public Health. 2001;91(6):933.

70. McCabe SE, Hughes TL, Bostwick WB, West BT, Boyd CJ. Sexual orientation, substance use behaviors and substance dependence in the United States. Addiction. 2009;104(8):1333.

71. Stall R, Paul JP, Greenwood G, Pollack LM, Bein E, Crosby GM, Mills TC, Binson D, Coates TJ, Catania JA. Alcohol use, drug use and alcohol-related problems among men who have sex with men. Addiction. 2001;96(11):1589.

72. King M, Semlyen J, Tai SS, Killaspy H, Osborn D, Popelyuk D, Nazareth I. A systematic review of mental disorder, suicide, and deliberate self harm in lesbian, gay and bisexual people. BMC Psychiatry. 2008;8:70.

73. Xavier JM, Bobbin M, Singer B, Budd E. A needs assessment of transgendered people of color living in Washington, DC. Int J Transgend. 2005;8(2/3):312.

74. American Lung Association. The LGBT community: a priority population for tobacco control. Available at: http://www.lung.org/stop-smoking/tobacco-control-advocacy/reports-resources/tobacco-policy-trend-reports/lgbt-issue-brief-update.pdf.

75. Wilkinson R, Marmot M, editors. Social determinants of health: the solid facts. 2nd ed. World Health Organization; 2003. http://www.euro.who.int/__data/assets/pdf_file/0005/98438/e81384.pdf.

76. Maguen S, Shipherd JC, Harris HN. Providing culturally sensitive care for transgender patients. Cogn Behav Pract. 2005;1(4):479–90.

77. Ash MA, Badgett MVL. Separate and unequal: the effect of unequal access to employment-based health insurance on same-sex and unmarried different-sex couples. Contemp Econ Policy. 2006;24(4):582.

78. Ponce NA, Cochran SD, Pizer JC, Mays VM. The effects of unequal access to health insurance for same-

sex couples in California. Health Aff. 2010;29(8):1539–48. doi:10.1377/hlthaff.2009.0583.

79. Albelda R, Badgett RVL, Schneebaum A, Gates GJ. Poverty in the lesbian, gay, and bisexual community. Los Angeles, CA: Williams Institute; 2009. March. http://williamsinstitute.law.ucla.edu/wp-content/uploads/Albelda-Badgett-Schneebaum-Gates-LGB-Poverty-Report-March-2009.pdf.

80. Badgett RVL, Durso LE, Schneebaum A. New patterns of poverty in the lesbian, gay, and bisexual community. Los Angeles, CA: Williams Institute; 2013. June. http://williamsinstitute.law.ucla.edu/wp-content/uploads/LGB-Poverty-Update-Jun-2013.pdf.

81. Ryan C, Huebner D, Diaz RM, Sanchez J. Family rejection as a predictor of negative health outcomes in White and Latino lesbian, gay, and bisexual young adults. Pediatrics. 2009;123(1):346–52.

82. Ryan C, Russell ST, Huebner D, Diaz R, Sanchez J. Family acceptance in adolescence and the health of LGBT young adults. J Child Adolesc Psychiatr Nurs. 2010;23(4):205–13.

83. Barker JC, Herdt G, de Vries B. Social support in the lives of lesbian women and gay men at midlife and later. Sex Res Soc Policy. 2006;3(2):1–23.

84. Blank TO, Asencio M, Descartes L, Griggs J. Intersection of older GLBT health issues: aging,

health, and GLBTQ family and community life. J GLBT Fam Stud. 2009;5(1):9–34.

85. Brotman S, Ryan B, Collins S, Chamberland L, Cormier R, Julien D, Meyer E, Peterkin A, Richard B. Coming out to care: caregivers of gay and lesbian seniors in Canada. Gerontologist. 2007;47(4):490.

86. Brotman S, Ryan B, Cormier R. The health and social service needs of gay and lesbian elders and their families in Canada. Gerontologist. 2003;43(2):192.

87. Cook-Daniels L, Munson M. Sexual violence, elder abuse, and sexuality of transgender adults, age 50+: results of three surveys. J GLBT Fam Stud. 2010;6(2):142.

88. Defining sexual health: report of a technical consultation on sexual health, 28–31 January 2002, Geneva: World Health Organization; 2006. http://www.who.int/reproductivehealth/topics/gender_rights/defining_sexual_health.pdf?ua=1.

89. Wolfe D. Men like us: the GMHC complete guide to gay men's sexual, physical, and emotional well-being. New York: Ballantine; 2000.

90. Walters ML, Chen J, Breiding MJ. The national intimate partner and sexual violence survey (NISVS): 2010 findings on victimization by sexual orientation. Atlanta, GA: National Center for Injury Prevention and Control, Centers for Disease Control and Prevention; 2013.

Edward J. Callahan, Catherine A. Henderson, Hendry Ton, and Scott MacDonald

## Learning Objectives

- Describe the role of electronic health records in providing care for LGBT patients (*ICS3, IPC1*).
- Discuss the importance of confidentiality for LGBT patients (*ICS2, Pr2*)
- Identify at least two strategies for effectively documenting sexual orientation and gender identity in electronic health records (*ICS3, Pr2*)

E.J. Callahan, Ph.D. (✉)
University of California, Davis School of Medicine,
Sherman Building, Suite 3900, 2300 Stockton Blvd,
Sacramento, CA 95817, USA
e-mail: callahan@ucdavis.edu

C.A. Henderson, B.A.
University of California, Davis, Davis, CA, USA
e-mail: chenderson1313@gmail.com

H. Ton, M.D.
Department of Psychiatry and Behavioral Sciences,
University of California, Davis School of Medicine,
2230 Stockton Blvd, Sacramento, CA 95817, USA
e-mail: hton@ucdavis.edu

S. MacDonald, M.D.
Department of Primary Care Network and
Information Technology, University of California,
Davis Health System, 2825 J St #300, Sacramento,
CA 95816, USA
e-mail: stmacdonald@ucdavis.edu

## Introduction

Electronic health records (EHRs) can provide an invaluable benefit to the provision of modern medical care. In order to ensure EHRs best accommodate lesbian, gay, bisexual, transgender, (LGBT) patients, often there must be a change in institutional culture. To date, a handful of medical centers have implemented fully inclusive EHR workflows. In this chapter, we will first address who must be invited into the challenge of changing institutional culture, describe the use of key informant interviews for inviting institutional leaders to become allies, and the determination of educational needs not only for providers but for all levels of personnel in the institution. We will further describe the process of developing support for all LGBT learners, staff, and faculty, while working to make it safe for LGBT patients to self-identity in clinical care. We will describe our process for caring for the sexual minority patient by identifying non-heterosexual and non-cis gender patients through discussion or demographic sexual orientation and gender identity (SO/GI) questions, and creating additional protections for those who self-disclose minority SO/GI status, while identifying key early targets for improving care of LGBT patients. This chapter describes how the University of California, Davis Health System became the first academic health center in the nation to introduce SO/GI in the EHR [1], while keeping a clear eye on the work

© Springer International Publishing Switzerland 2016
K.L. Eckstrand, J.M. Ehrenfeld (eds.), *Lesbian, Gay, Bisexual, and Transgender Healthcare*,
DOI 10.1007/978-3-319-19752-4_7

that still remains to ensure improvement of quality of care for LGBT patients.

In our institution, cultural change to enhance quality of care for LGBT patients is becoming more widely, if not universally, accepted. Such cultural change challenges entrenched unconscious bias, which makes change difficult. For that reason, it is highly unlikely that an institution can push hard for change during a set period of time and fully accomplish it; the more likely scenario is one of ongoing consciousness raising and skill development in a continuous quality improvement effort. Dealing with all these concerns is critical if we are to ask our patients to share their SO/GI demographics in the EHR.

## Creating Institutional Change in the Face of Unconscious Bias

The Institute of Medicine (IOM) acknowledged in 2003 that "Indirect evidence indicates that bias, stereotyping, prejudice, and clinical uncertainty on the part of healthcare providers may be contributory factors to racial and ethnic healthcare disparities. Prejudice may stem from conscious bias, while stereotyping and biases may be conscious or unconscious, even among the well intentioned." This 2002 IOM report "Inequality in Medicine" [2] fails to mention health disparities associated with sexual orientation or gender identity, reminding us how recently awareness of LGBT health disparities has emerged. The underlying mechanisms for LGBT health disparities are virtually identical to those underlying racial or ethnic minority health disparities: cultural stigma around the minority population resulting in development of conscious and unconscious bias, which in turn influences the process and quality of life for the population as well as the quality and process of care. Recognizing cultural stigma is critically important if we seek to understand the roots of health disparities and redesign and improve quality of clinical care delivery. Social stigma accurately predicts which groups will experience health disparities. In order to understand how those stigmas impact health and healthcare delivery, it is critical to acknowledge two related phenomena: unconscious bias [3, 4] and the influence of unconscious bias on clinical decision making [5, 6].

Unconscious bias or implicit bias is documented by the presence of behavioral indices of bias despite the individual's stated belief that they hold little or no bias in the area [3]. To even begin to deal with unconscious bias against LGBT populations on the institutional level, it is first necessary that leaders of the institution recognize that the IOM report [7] identifies unnecessary and unfair health disparities which in turn indicate personal and social ethical obligations to reduce those health disparities [8].

## Catalyzing Change at the University of California, Davis Heath System (UCDHS)

To begin to prepare UCDHS for the change of collecting SO/GI in the EHR, we selected several overlapping engagement/communication strategies. Examples of different messaging strategies are presented below to illustrate the array of communication efforts employed: elevator talking points, key informant interviews, senior leadership meetings and internal public relations. These efforts were preparatory to roll out of extensive provider training which was developed concurrently.

*Elevator Talking Points* The initial announcement of the charge of the Task Force for Inclusion of Sexual Orientation and Gender Identity in the Electronic Health Record triggered concerns from both clinicians and administrators that they were neither trained in how to discuss SO/GI, nor comfortable in doing so [2]. For the Task Force, this response was a systemic invitation to educate members of the healthcare delivery system and administration that serious LGBT health disparities exist, that gathering these sensitive demographic data from patients was feasible, and that systematically gathering SO/GI demographics

**Table 7.1** Elevator talking points on collecting sexual orientation and gender identity demographics in the electronic health record

| | |
|---|---|
| (I) | After going unnoticed for many years, staggering health disparities have been identified for people who have non-heterosexual sexual orientation (individuals who are lesbian, gay, and bisexual) or different gender identities (individuals who are transgender). Henceforth we refer to them collectively with the acronym LGBT |
| (II) | These health disparities appear to be rooted in multiple interacting factors, including stigma and efforts to avoid that stigma by hiding one's sexual orientation from others |
| (a) | Members of these populations have learned to avoid rejection and mistreatment by hiding their identity and becoming invisible. During encounters with healthcare professionals they often withhold information (e.g., risky same-sex sexual activity) or change aspects of their personal lives (e.g., discuss their same-sex partners as if they were opposite-sex partners) |
| (b) | Healthcare professionals and systems that hold negative attitudes or stereotypes regarding sexual minorities provide care that is ineffective, insensitive, discriminatory or even abusive. As a result, many patients who have experienced this kind of treatment or know others who have experienced it postpone seeking medical care, especially for nonurgent conditions |
| (c) | Nondisclosure of sexual orientation or gender identity and postponement of care reinforces the perceptions held by some healthcare providers that sexual minorities are too infrequently encountered in clinical practice to be worth learning about or accommodating their unique needs |
| (d) | Sexual minority individuals are at increased risk of stigmatization, discrimination and violence throughout their lifespan. These experiences, especially when they occur early in life, lead to the adoption of maladaptive coping behaviors (e.g., smoking, substance misuse, or early engagement in sexual behavior) that reduce stress immediately but which are ultimately associated with increased morbidity and mortality |
| (III) | Since the Stonewall riots in 1969, LGBT people in the US and industrialized western countries, but increasingly around the world as well, have rejected hiding their identity as a way to cope, discovering the power of claiming their identities instead |
| (IV) | With the onset of the internet and emergence of role models, LGBT children are discovering and announcing or questioning their sexual orientation and gender identity earlier. Nevertheless, discrimination and bullying for being different are still strong and families are not well prepared to support and nurture their children as they come out |
| (a) | There is a need to prepare healthcare providers to work with families through these developmental challenges |
| (b) | For LGBT children and youth whose families are unsupportive, healthcare providers need skills and attitudes to provide care to children and families that is supportive of both their confidentiality needs yet supportive of their developmental stage |
| (V) | LGBT people who are health providers have also been largely invisible and unaccounted for. Many federal and institutional surveys (for example, the American Association of Medical Colleges) do not yet acknowledge sexual minority identities: there is only very recent AAMC documentation of the existence of LGBT people in medicine as medical students, and not yet as applicants, residents or as faculty. We do not know whether LGBT people are admitted to medical schools at rates commensurate with their credentials, and we are only recently getting a sense of what their experience is like during medical school, while remaining largely unaware of their experience in residency, in practice or on faculty |
| (VI) | If we are to reduce health disparities for LGBT populations, we need their healthcare providers to know who they are. We can start that with building these demographics into the electronic health record (EHR) |
| (VII) | This also means that medical schools need to teach how sexual orientation and gender identity impact a person's development and life course, not just to which sexually transmitted infections they are vulnerable |

could facilitate improvement of quality of care for LGBT patients. To work toward this outcome, the Task Force developed Elevator Talking Points to use when appropriate to "sell" the need for SO/GI in the EHR (see Table 7.1).

*Key Informant Interviews* In order to prepare for the rollout of LGBT health disparity information, we felt it was critical that Health System leadership be systematically educated on the importance of reducing LGBT health disparities and invited to participate as allies in the process of changing the institutional culture. In order to invite leadership to participate in this cultural shift, we began conducting key informant interviews (Table 7.2), modeled on such interviews conducted to support implementation of the National Culturally and Linguistically Appropriate Services Standards [9]. In the key informant interview, we began by presenting the rationale for the discussion, "I would like to explore the potential of providing training to help our health system provide quality care to lesbian, gay, bisexual, transgender, those with differences of sex development, and queer or questioning patients. As a key leader in the Health System, we would like to speak to you to understand what you know about LGBT health disparities, and whether you are aware of any problems your unit may have experienced in providing care for LGBT patients. We would like to hear about your observations on how we might best educate our providers and staff. In order to develop our training as well as possible to meet the training needs and interests of your department, I would like to ask you some questions." Table 7.2 provides the questions we developed for this effort. Members of the Task Force then met with over 30 individual leaders to discuss these questions and experiences of LGBT patients in the care of their department. Each interview resulted in gathering data from the organizational leader as well as sharing LGBT patient experiences. After these discussions, each leader was invited to consider having a talk presented to their staff about care for LGBT patients. Virtually

**Table 7.2**  Key informant interview for SO/GI inclusion in EHR taskforce

| **Introduction** |
| --- |
| Please introduce yourself, thank the participant for spending time to speak with you, and describe the purpose of the interview to the participant |
| **Example introduction script:** "I would like to explore the potential of providing a training to help our health system provide quality care to patients who are lesbian, gay, bisexual, or transgender. You were identified as an important person to speak with because [please describe reason why participant was chosen]. In order to customize the training as much as possible to the needs and interests of your particular department, I would like to ask you some questions" |
| **Interview questions** |
| 1. Do you know what LGBT stands for? |
| 2. What is your opinion of the quality of care given to LGBT patients? |
| 3. Please describe what you think your department needs to enhance service to this community? |
| 4. Do you see a role for training in your department in improving LGBT health care? Please elaborate |
| 5. Do you recall past trainings on LGBT issues? What was the quality and how was it received? |
| 6. Have there been times when an LGBT patient has been uncomfortable in the way they or a family member was treated? |
| 7. It has been our experience that some providers are very open and engaged with the topic and others are very resistant. How might the current people in your department respond to an LGBT training? |
| 8. What challenges might we encounter in scheduling and conducting a training of this sort? Do you have thoughts on how we might address these challenges? |
| 9. Are there approaches or strategies that we should include in order to make the training as effective as possible while also conveying respect for the people in your department? |
| 10. Getting more to the nuts and bolts: Do you have suggestions on when and in what forum the training should be held? What types of formats—e.g., discussion, small groups, lectures—would be well received in your department? |
| 11. Before we end, is there anyone else that I should speak with or involve in this effort? |
| 12. Would you support our doing this training in your department? |
| 13. Would you be comfortable in collaborating in this training? |

**Fig. 7.1** Three staff show their ID badges with rainbow decals signaling their provision of a safe space for LGBT people. Photo credit: Kevin Ulrich, UC Davis Health System, copyright 2014 UC Regents. Used with permission

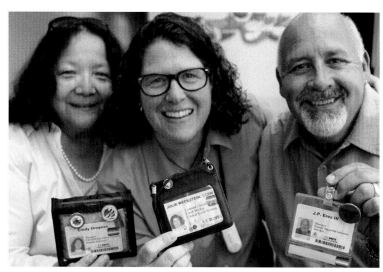

all who were interviewed were willing to step forward as collaborators to help make this process successful.

*Senior Leadership Meetings* LGBT health issues were also raised at upper level leadership meetings to further promote systemic awareness. Initial discussions about the project and its purpose were met primarily with silence, particularly among male leaders. Presenting the information in the context of humor helped people become more comfortable with the issue. For example, an LGBT staff support group was formed in May 2011, choosing to name itself GLEE (Gay and Lesbian Employees and Everyone who cares). Talking about GLEE was a welcome addition. GLEE members joked that they could not sing or dance and no one needed to fear that they would be subjected to that. Humor helped break the traditional silence around sexual orientation and gender identity, opening the way for increased comfort discussing LGBT health and the need to improve quality of care for LGBT patients.

*Internal Public Relations* A strategy was developed early to announce the efforts of the Task Force using *The Insider*, an intranet leadership column that appears whenever an employee logs onto a Health System computer. The Task Force

was introduced and its progress and plans were announced at different points using that medium. Announcements of National Coming Out Day and other celebrations of diversity appeared there as well. A recent *Insider* pictured faculty and staff with rainbow stickers placed on their Health System identification badges, signaling their commitment to providing a safe space for LGBT patients, learners and colleagues (Fig. 7.1). The stickers are worn not just by LGBT faculty and staff, but by all who care to signal their support for LGBT people; in fact, the majority of flag decal wearers to date are heterosexual and cis gender. As efforts began to generate changes in climate, the Task Force focused on developing and providing education about LGBT health disparities in preparation for asking SO/GI questions in the EHR.

## Using Education to Prepare for Culture Change

Multiple levels of education are needed to prepare a Health System to seriously commit to reducing health disparities. Since the IOM report [7] was published so recently, many people are not aware of the serious nature of the health disparities facing LGBT populations. Education is necessary for leadership, faculty, staff, medical students, as well as other health provider trainees within the health system. Two types of education are important: factual information on the existence of LGBT health disparities and consciousness raising efforts aimed at overcoming stigma associated with minority SO/GI. Significant efforts to raise awareness of LGBT health disparities, and the importance of collecting this information, were implemented over a course of several years. The disparities discussed are equivalent to those discussed elsewhere in this book. Central in the conversations, were concerns about interfacing with patients around these topics.

## Will Patients Accept Being Asked?

One challenge the Task Force faced was how to best ask the SO/GI questions: Which words ought to be used? How should questions be sequenced? Which populations were critical to capture? While the IOM report [7] delineated serious demonstrated health disparities for lesbian, gay and bisexual populations, data sources on transgender health were weaker in terms of sample sizes, yet the health problems of trans patients appeared even more profound. Also problematic is the virtual absence of systematic data on those with differences of sex development (intersex) and queer and questioning populations in the IOM report [1]. This de facto exclusion occurred because data exploring the health of these patients are not robust; while their existence as subpopulations is often not clear to researchers, it is very clear to those with these other identities that face a health workforce not skilled in their care. Health information on these populations is unclear because data is not ordinarily gathered on them and their health status as populations remain unknown.

Providers are also challenged with how to understand and value the terms the patient uses to self-describe their sexual orientation and/or gender identity. To aid our providers in understanding some of these less common terms, we developed a set of definitions for these terms that pop-up when a user allows the computer cursor to hover

over the terms (See Table 7.3). While genderqueer and pansexual are unusual terms for the medical community, they are terms that many younger patients use to identify themselves [10]. The provider needs to be comfortable exploring these and other terms used by patients. With definitions of populations of diverse sexual orientations and gender identities, it is critical to explore strategies to further educate leadership and clinicians about common health disparities experienced by LGBT populations. This became particularly clear with the 2011 publication of the results of a survey of Medical Education Deans in JAMA which revealed that most medical schools had poor to non-existent curricula on LGBT health [11].

## Patient Survey

After 3 years of atmosphere and curriculum building, we felt ready to launch the questionnaire in the electronic health record in the fourth year. To better inform our planning and decision making, we sought consultation from LGBT patients as well as heterosexual and cis gender patients about how they would feel about being asked their SO/GI. This survey effort was done as a quality improvement effort rather than as a research project. Responses of 200 heterosexual and cis gender patients were compared with responses from 100 lesbian, gay and bisexual (LGB) patients (no transgender, queer or intersex patients responded to this survey). All participants were adults aged 21–68 who received medical care in Northern California settings and identified their own SO/GI as part of the survey. Fewer than 20 % of LGB patients felt that they should not be asked their SO/GI. Similar percentages of heterosexual patients concurred stating, "It is no one's business what our sexual orientation is" and "I don't like anything about this idea, I think this is a private matter" At the other end of the spectrum, the plurality of patients in both heterosexual and LGB groups were positive about this discussion taking place. A bisexual person stated: "A person's sexual identity is an important part of their lifestyle and health; sharing it might be helpful for their health". A gay man added, "A doctor should have the most information possible to offer proper care and preventive strategies." Heterosexuals concurred, "Your personal doctor should know all about you as a patient, to be able to serve your needs as best possible." Another heterosexual patient stated, "Doctors may be more sensitive to a patient's feelings and concerns having this information." Among heterosexual patients, the largest group was neutral on the idea. For gay and lesbian patients, virtually half were positive about this information being collected.

Although not scientifically determined, there was some indication that people would prefer to have this information gathered in person by their physician but also found it acceptable to fill out a form at the physician's office or online in their own time. Very few, either heterosexual or LGB, were supportive of having this information discussed over the phone.

A bisexual individual added depth to the conversation by stating, "Only once the political and social environment has become more educated and homosexual fears have been lifted, would I ever admit my sexual orientation." Both heterosexual and LGB patients supported the idea of a physician directory in which providers declared themselves to be LGBT-supportive, although one gay man said that he would distrust such a self-description. Two thirds of LGB people stated a preference for a label for providers saying that they were LGBT-friendly or LGBT-welcoming, while less than half of heterosexual patients wanted physicians to make such statements. The bulk of respondents were supportive of trying to improve LGBT healthcare, with one heterosexual saying, "Everyone deserves the best care possible. Opening up a secure dialogue channel will encourage those with a specific orientation to come forward and share their information without fear." A lesbian added, "I think it's absolutely crucial that all human beings and all communities get the health care they need." A bisexual patient added, "I hope new developments occur such as this one proposed; they are desperately needed."

## Asking the Question in the Electronic Health Record

Institutional support, such as training in cultural awareness and education in LGBT health disparities, can improve patient experience. At present, however, few health providers are well versed in discussing issues around sexual orientation, while even fewer are prepared to meet the unique healthcare needs of transgender patients [12]. Until recently, many LGBT people lacked basic access to healthcare. For transgender patients, there has been little awareness of the need for pap smears and breast exams for trans men or prostate exams for trans women. The lack of capacity to track healthcare delivery and outcomes for LGBT patients has prevented programmatic efforts to improve quality of care to date. The ability to track health interventions undertaken and their results is necessary to improve quality of care for all populations.

That inability to identify and track LGBT patients can be addressed with the incorporation of SO/GI demographics in the EHR. Gathering that information requires conversations between patients and providers which in turn requires creating an environment in which patients feel safe disclosing their SO/GI. Coming "out" to LGBT-welcoming providers can reduce anxiety and allow for more honest, direct conversations about health. Patients are more likely to seek care when they need it if the environment is made safe for them.

Knowing patients' SO/GI is crucial for understanding where health disparities are occurring and learning how to prevent or intervene around those disparities. SO/GI EHR data can allow the systematic comparison of the epidemiology of health problems and health outcomes of LGBT patients with the outcomes of heterosexual, cis gender patients, giving us a measure of how well providers are meeting standards of care for LGBT patients. Health disparities will be made more visible, and harder to ignore, so that we can work to reduce them. EHR data can prove invaluable when researching better care utilization for LGBT populations, giving us direct feedback about the effectiveness of interventions. Having SO/GI data in the EHR can unlock the information we need to start providing high quality LGBT healthcare.

## Launching SO/GI in the Electronic Health Record

With reassurance that most patients could appreciate why these questions were being asked, and an overall favorable response toward launching the gathering of SO/GI data, the Task Force moved into the final build. To complete the build, the Task Force needed to address what questions should be asked and in what order. A literature review was done to explore what common terms had been used in prior research. We sought consultation from clinical settings such as Fenway Health [13] and the University of California, San Francisco Center for Excellence in Transgender Health [14]. These explorations led to both consensus on questions to use in determining SO/GI as well as recognition that it was critical to allow patients to use their own terms to describe themselves. For example, it is common in some African American male circles to use the term same gender loving to self-describe. While this was not included as a prompt, the questions may be revised in the future to include such a prompt. In addition, the youngest Task Force members (both LGBT and allies) were consulted carefully, asking that they share their preferred terms.

The younger Task Force members reported that it was critical that we capture self-descriptors such as pansexual (someone who is attracted to other people regardless of their gender identity or gender expression) and genderqueer [10]. The term genderqueer is often used by younger individuals. It sometimes indicates a person not subscribing to a male–female gender binary, and sometimes indicates that the person does not see her/himself as heterosexual. This lack of specificity in meaning requires providers to ask follow up questions to understand what their patient means by the term. The terms selected are presented in Table 7.3.

In the electronic record, definitions of terms are provided. These prompts provide a definition when a provider lets their cursor hover over a particular term. For example, differences of sex development is defined as having genetic, hormonal or anatomic development outside traditional bounds of male or female. If one selects differences of sex development, under comments they are asked to identify any associated medical condition.

## Options on Where and How One Provides Data

While members of the Task Force were immediately drawn to the idea of physicians gathering SO/GI as we launched this effort, it became clear that building in flexibility to the data collection would be a valuable strategy. First, one cannot mandate that all patients share their SO/GI demographics. Some have had such negative experiences with healthcare providers in the past that they will withhold that information. Second, among those who share their SO/GI data, some will not be comfortable with that information in the EHR. Employees can still be fired for their sexual orientation in 29 states and for their gender identity or expression in 31 states [15]. Individuals who anticipate moving to such states may not be willing to have that data shared in the future. Third, some individuals will only be comfortable sharing this information with their provider. This needs to be respected, but to optimize care delivery for LGBT patients it is critical to use that information to prompt prevention efforts and to monitor the timely delivery of early diagnostic tests, i.e. residual breast tissue examination and pap smear for female to male (FTM) trans patients who retain a cervix, and digital examination of the prostate for all male to female (MTF) patients. Fourth, we built a mechanism for declaring SO/GI from home by way of the patient portal into the EHR (called MyChart). Thus, the patient can provide these data from home, or the provider can enter the information after a discussion with the patient. If a patient declares SO/GI from home, we recommend that the provider review that data at the next visit to personalize the sharing. Our demographics allow sharing of marital status for LGBT individuals as well as identifying a partner if not married, both for advance directives and sharing health information.

**Table 7.3**  Cursor hover popups of SO/GI definitions

| Cursor hover popups for provider's Smartform | |
| --- | --- |
| **Gender identity** | How a person experiences/describes their own gender |
| Intersex | Having genetic, hormonal, or anatomic development outside traditional bounds of male or female; under comments, identify any associated medical condition(s). May be selected along with M or F |
| Trans FtM | Assigned female sex at birth, now identifies as male |
| Trans MtF | Assigned male sex at birth, now identifies as female |
| **Sexual orientation** | Categories describe exclusive or predominant attraction |
| Straight/heterosexual | A man attracted to women, or a woman attracted to men |
| Gay/homosexual | A man attracted to men |
| Gay/lesbian | A woman attracted to women |
| Bisexual | A man or woman attracted to both men and women |
| Questioning | A person unsure of, questioning, or testing sexual orientation or gender identity |
| Queer | A person identifying as non-heterosexual or as outside the male–female gender binary; younger generation claiming previously derogatory word/identity as positive |
| Other | A person experiencing an alternate sexual orientation; please ask for further specification |
| Pansexual | A person attracted to others regardless of their gender or gender expression |
| **Cursor hover popups for MyChart questionnaire** | |
| **Gender identity** | How you experience/describe your own gender |
| Intersex | At birth, you had genetic, hormonal or anatomic development outside traditional bounds of male or female; under comments, please describe any associated medical condition(s). This may be selected along with M or F |
| Trans FtM | You were assigned female sex at birth; now identify as a man |
| Trans MtF | You were assigned male sex at birth; now identify as a woman |
| **Sexual orientation** | Select term which best describes your exclusive or predominant attraction |
| Straight/heterosexual | As a man, you are attracted to women, or as a woman, you are attracted to men |
| Gay/homosexual | As a man, you are attracted to other men |
| Gay/lesbian | As a woman, you are attracted to other women |
| Bisexual | You are attracted to others of your gender as well as others of a different gender |
| Questioning | You are exploring, unsure of, or testing your sexual orientation or gender identity |
| Queer | You identify as non-heterosexual or as being outside the male–female gender identity binary |
| Other | You experience a sexual orientation outside those already described; please specify your sexual attraction further |
| Pansexual | You are attracted to others regardless of their gender or gender expression |

## Health Information Technology

Our EHR is built on an Epic base which has been incorporated since 2004. The revenue cycle has gone live in Spring, 2014. UCDHS has been selected for the Health Information and Management Systems Step 7 status (HIMSS 7), reflecting a high level of security and capacity for data analytics and clinical intervention. It is possible to provide a high level of monitoring of patient records for inappropriate access and use. The monitoring system is set to follow all those who declare sexual orientation or gender identity minority status closely to ensure there is no misuse of their data. Unauthorized access or sharing of information can lead to termination of employment.

Two final protections have been implemented for LGBT patients who declare SO/GI in the EHR. First, patient complaint service personnel were given special training in how to deal with complaints from heterosexual and cis gender patients offended at being asked about SO/GI, as well as how to respond to LGBT patient concerns about the security of the data. These service personnel shared that they were frequently asked to identify LGBT-welcoming primary care and specialty providers by patients new to the system. To accomplish this, in the 7 months leading to the launch of the EHR SO/GI demographic capacity, we began surveying providers seeking self-identification of LGBT-welcoming providers. We currently have nearly had over 300 individuals identify as LGBT-welcoming but many are not primary care providers. We need to continue to identify such providers in our system because many of these providers are at full capacity for patients. We invite LGBT residents to self-declare to enhance support services for them and to enhance the number of welcoming providers. Secondly, we have developed a website for all providers with helpful articles and links to videos which is also available on the web at https://myhs.ucdmc.ucdavis.edu/web/LGBTI/home [16].

We continue to add useful information to this website which is both internally accessible within the EHR and externally available through web search engines and the URL posted above.

## Conclusion: The Necessary Next Steps

Our SO/GI questionnaire is now on each of over 85,000 outpatient MyChart portals. Its presence is a key element in our institutional adoption of improvement in quality of care for LGBT patients. We are now undertaking comparisons of strategies for pushing these questionnaires out effectively to patients to encourage their sharing of data on the EHR portal. We are committed to learning how to do this most effectively. Considerable work remains if we are to optimize this tool to improve healthcare delivery for LGBT patients. That work will continue in different venues, since the Task Force for Inclusion of Sexual Orientation and Gender Identity in the Electronic Health Record has officially completed its charge with the launch of SO/GI demographics in the EHR. The Task Force has

been broken into subcommittees that now report to the Vice Chancellor's LGBT Advisory Council. There are multiple levels of effort ongoing and planned under this new Council.

These efforts include:

1. A committee to create comprehensive and effective policies to ensure respectful and quality care for trans patients.
2. Development of a mechanism to ensure staff is prompted to use the patient's preferred name for those who are transitioning.
3. A committee planning and overseeing patient centered outcomes research to explore mechanisms for enhancing quality of care for LGBT patients further. While we celebrate the adoption of LGBT Quality Improvement as a UCDHS initiative, accomplishing those improvements will take considerable effort and commitment.
4. An initiative to survey LGBT experiences of mistreatment at UCDHS and make recommendations to the Chancellor on how to improve experiences such as use of restorative justice [17] in conflict management.
5. Development of an anatomy checklist to determine what organs are present for transitioning patients.
6. Development of gay, lesbian, transgender, differences of sex development and other registries to assure that prevention and interventions can be launched and evaluated effectively.
7. Work with Press Ganey to assure that we seek SO/GI data in exploring our patient satisfaction responses.
8. Work within the Association of American Medical Colleges (AAMC) Faculty Forward program to assure that LGBT voices are heard in our next assessment of our faculty engagement as a School of Medicine.
9. Inclusion of sexual orientation and gender identity demographics for all faculty and staff hires at UCDHS.
10. Increasing cultural awareness through roll-out of Unconscious Bias training efforts.

11. Development of ongoing patient satisfaction and patient engagement measures to ensure that we are sensitive to patient wants and needs in the development of improved care.
12. Development of an LGBT patient advisory committee to use to oversee, comment on and recommend enhancements of care at UCDHS.

## References

1. Callahan EJ, Sitkin N, Ton H, Eidson-Ton WS, Latimore JP (2015) Introducing sexual orientation and gender identity into the electronic health record: one academic health center's experience. Acad Med 90(2):154–60. doi:10.1097/ACM.0000000000000467
2. Institute of Medicine (2002) Unequal treatment: what health care system administrators need to know about racial and ethnic disparities in healthcare. Washington, DC: National Academy Press
3. Greenwald AG, McGhee DE, Schwartz JL (1998) Measuring individual differences in implicit cognition: the implicit association test. J Pers Soc Psychol 74(6):1464–80. doi:10.1037/0022-3514.74.6.1464
4. Sabin J, Nosek BA, Greenwald A, Rivara FP (2009) Physicians' implicit and explicit attitudes about race by MD race, ethnicity, and gender. J Health Care Poor Underserved 20(3):896–913. doi:10.1353/hpu.0.0185
5. Dovidio JF, Fiske ST (2012) Under the radar: how unexamined biases in decision-making processes in clinical interactions can contribute to health care disparities. Am J Public Health 102(5):945–52. doi:10.2105/AJPH.2011.300601
6. Chapman EN, Kaatz A, Carnes M (2013) Physicians and implicit bias: how doctors may unwittingly perpetuate health care disparities. J Gen Intern Med 28(11):1504–10. doi:10.1007/s11606-013-2441-1
7. Institute of Medicine (2011) The health of lesbian, gay, bisexual, and transgender people: building a foundation for better understanding. Washington, DC: National Academies Press
8. Callahan EJ, Hazarian S, Yarborough M, Sanchez JP (2014) Eliminating LGBTIQQ health disparities: the associated roles of electronic health records and institutional culture. Hastings Cent Rep 44 Suppl 4:S48-S52. doi:10.1002/hast.371
9. Ton H, Steinhart D, Yang MS, Sala M, Aguilar-Gaxiola S, Hardcastle L, Bodick D (2011) Providing quality health care with CLAS: a curriculum for developing culturally & linguistically appropriate services. Facilitator's manual. Sacramento, CA: Office of Multicultural Health CDoPH and Department of Health Care Services
10. Wilchins R, Howell C, Nestle J (2002) Genderqueer: voices from beyond the sexual binary. Los Angeles, CA: Alyson
11. Obedin-Maliver J, Goldsmith ES, Stewart L, White W, Tran E, Brenman S, et al (2011) Lesbian, gay, bisexual, and transgender-related content in undergraduate medical education. JAMA 306(9):971–7. doi:10.1001/jama.2011.1255
12. Lambda Legal (2010) When health care isn't caring: Lambda Legal's survey on discrimination against LGBT people and people living with HIV.
13. Cahill S, Makadon H (2014) Sexual orientation and gender identity data collection in clinical settings and in electronic health records: a key to ending LGBT health disparities. LGBT Health 1(1):34–41. doi:10.1089/lgbt.2013.0001
14. Website for UCSF Center for Excellence for Transgender Health [12 June 2014]. Available from: http://www.transhealth.ucsf.edu/.
15. Human Rights Campaign. Employment Non-Discrimination Act [20 June 2014]. Available from: http://www.hrc.org/laws-and-legislation/federal-legislation/employment-non-discrimination-act.
16. UC Davis Health System. LGBTI health care [20 June 2014]. Available from: https://myhs.ucdmc.ucdavis.edu/web/LGBTI/home.
17. Zehr H (2002) The little book of restorative justice. Intercourse, PA: Good Books

# Part III

# LGBT Preventive Health and Screening

Keisa Fallin-Bennett, Shelly L. Henderson,
Giang T. Nguyen, and Abbas Hyderi

## Purpose

The purpose of this chapter is to provide an overview of the primary care needs of lesbian, gay, bisexual, and transgender (LGBT) patients including appropriate preventive and screening services and coordination of care.

K. Fallin-Bennett, M.D., M.P.H. (✉)
Department of Family and Community Medicine, University of Kentucky 2195 Harrodsburg Road, Ste 125, Lexington, KY 40504, USA
e-mail: keisa.bennett@uky.edu

S.L. Henderson, Ph.D.
Department of Family and Community Medicine, University of California Davis, 4860 Y Street, Suite 2300, Sacramento, CA 95817, USA
e-mail: shelly.henderson@ucdmc.ucdavis.edu

G.T. Nguyen, M.D., M.P.H., M.S.C.E.
Department of Family Medicine & Community Health and Student Health Service, University of Pennsylvania, 3535 Market Street, Suite 100, Philadelphia, PA 19104, USA
e-mail: GNguyen@upenn.edu

A. Hyderi, M.D., M.P.H.
Department of Family Medicine, University of Illinois at Chicago, M/C 785, 1819 Polk Street, Chicago, IL 60657, USA
e-mail: ahyder2@uic.edu

## Learning Objectives

- Identify at least three strategies for communicating effectively with LGBT patients using verbal and written communication and documentation strategies that respect the potentially sensitive nature of clinical information pertaining to patients' sexual orientation and gender identity (*ICS2, ICS3*)
- Describe screening tests, preventive interventions, and health care maintenance for LGBT patients (*PC3, PC4, PC5, PC6*)
- Discuss the importance of primary care providers recognizing patient autonomy in self-identification of sexual orientation and gender identity (*Pr2*)
- Identify at least three strategies for improving patient care within the health system by partnering and collaborating with LGBT community resources (*SBP4*)

## Overview of Primary Care

### Importance of Primary Care and the Patient-Centered Medical Home

In the modern-day urban America, many people have never experienced having a traditional "family doctor." Primary care, however, remains the backbone of healthcare, and is crucial for reducing the escalation of costs while maintaining high quality care. Sharma et al. demonstrate that the majority of care for the highest-cost chronic conditions is performed by primary care physicians [1]. With their focus on preventive care, primary care providers (PCPs) are also more cost-effective. Numerous studies worldwide demonstrate that health systems in which primary care is central and family physicians are the dominant specialty have better population health outcomes at a lower cost than sub-specialty dominated systems [2]. Many LGBT persons may be reluctant to access health care due to fear of stigmatization or discrimination, previous negative experiences, or concerns about provider knowledge and appropriate care [3]. Those concerns make it especially important for LGBT people to have a trusted PCP. The role of the PCP is to provide long-term, personalized care, and to coordinate care for a patient within the health care system as they build trust with the patient that facilitates health improvement.

Many decades after being proposed by the American Academy of Pediatrics, the modern movement to provide each patient with a Patient Centered Medical Home (PCMH) has gained momentum as the problems of an expensive and fragmented U.S. health care system have come to light. The purpose of a PCMH is for family physicians, general internists, pediatricians or nurse practitioners in primary care to establish systems that promote longitudinal, personalized, and yet, holistic care [4, 5]. The American Academy of Family Physicians describes the principles of the PCMH as access to a personal physician who leads the care team within a medical practice, a whole-person orientation to providing patient care, integrated and coordinated care, and focus on quality and safety [6]. The National Committee on Quality Assurance (NCQA) has devised detailed standards and guidelines for practices to be recognized at various stages on the way to being designated a full PCMH by the NCQA [7]. This recognition process is rigorous, involving establishment of electronic health records (EHR), flexible scheduling with after-hours and weekend access, integration of primary care and mental

health care, and continuous quality improvement involving patients and families. The movement toward medical homes was strengthened by the passage of the Affordable Care Act (ACA) in 2011. The law not only required health insurance coverage for almost every individual, but also incentivized elements of care already incorporated into the PCMH, such as meaningful use of electronic health records to facilitate quality improvement. If implemented fully, the law also creates incentives in terms of Medicare and Medicaid reimbursements as well as grant programs, to promote realignment toward primary care and prevention and more appropriate use of specialty and technical care [8].

## Preventive Health

### Patient–Provider Relationship

The patient–provider relationship is a keystone of primary care. The bond of trust between the patient and the provider (physician, nurse practitioner, or physician assistant) is vital to the diagnostic and therapeutic process. In order for the provider to make accurate diagnoses and provide optimal treatment recommendations, the patient must be able to communicate all relevant information about an illness or injury. Health outcomes can be improved when providers truly know their patients [9]. Knowing a patient's sexual orientation does more than just provide information about his or her sexual history. When providers truly know their patients, including salient identities, patients are more able to engage in their own care. From the perspective of whole person care, it is essential that patients feel comfortable disclosing aspects of their lives that may impact their ability to adhere to treatments. Patients filter provider instructions through their existing belief system; they decide whether the recommended actions are possible or desirable in the context of their everyday lives [10].

Providers can create an environment that is conducive to candid communication. Patients assess the office environment for signs of affirmation. Posters and patient education materials with relevant information in the waiting room help set a tone of acceptance. Using inclusive language on intake forms and training office staff to use inclusive language also may increase patients' comfort [3, 11]. In the examination room, it is important to ask patients open-ended questions that elicit who this patient is as a person. For example, a provider might ask whom a person lives with, who should be informed about health care issues, and how a patient prefers to be addressed. Phrasing these questions in a way that demonstrates openness to a variety of answers allows a trusting therapeutic relationship to develop [11].

---

**Helpful Hint**

To create a truly patient-centered environment for all patients, procedures and a culture of acceptance and awareness must be planned. Use the many available resources to facilitate patient-centeredness among LGBT patients.

---

## Health Promotion

Health promotion is an important function of primary care and the patient-centered medical home. Primary care physicians and providers also can and should play a role in promoting health in the community, considering the large contribution that social determinants of health have on population and individual health outcomes [12, 13]. LGBT patients deserve the same level of attention to health promotion as all patients, as well as the same level of investment in the health of their community. As is emphasized throughout this text, LGBT persons should be allowed and encouraged to self-define what community means to them.

### Nutrition and Physical Activity

Healthy lifestyles are critical elements in health promotion and have acquired added importance in the modern era in which obesity and health issues related to sedentary lifestyle and poor diet have become epidemics. In the LGBT community,

self-identified lesbians (and possibly bisexual women) are at an increased risk of overweight and obesity compared to heterosexual women [14, 15], while gay men tend to have lower BMI than their straight counterparts but express higher body dissatisfaction and may be at higher risk for eating disorders [16, 17]. Trends in physical activity for LGBT patients are difficult to ascertain and studies tend to be small and conflicting [18–21]. Primary care providers should be aware that body image ideals in the LGBT community may be different from typical cultural ideals, though those theorized differences seem to be minimal in recent, population-based studies [16, 17, 22–24]. Nevertheless, such cultural factors as lesbian women's greater idealization of muscularity [17] and gay men's greater internalization of media image ideals [25] could affect patient motivations to lose weight or adopt specific exercise plans. For some within the "bear" subculture of gay-identified men, obesity might even be normalized, and "excess" body weight can be a celebrated part of one's identity [26]. Motivational interviewing is a patient-centered approach that can help elicit a patient's values and assist in achieving culturally appropriate behavior change [27, 28].

### Mental and Emotional Health

LGBT people have an increased risk of mental health and substance use conditions; however, even those without a history of such conditions or any clear symptoms deserve the same attention to screening for depression, anxiety, violence victimization, and substance use as employed for all patients. Counseling on prevention of such conditions is also appropriate.

### Sexual Health

Sexual health is discussed in detail below and in other chapters. It is important to note here that LGBT patients should be asked the same details of sexual history and that assumptions about their behavior based on identity or past history should be avoided [3]. Prevention of sexually transmitted infections (STI's) and family planning are important discussions to have with all patients. It is important to recognize that lesbian-identified women and women who have sex with women (WSW) can transmit or receive any STI from a female partner and should not be dismissed as not-at-risk [29, 30]. In contrast, gay-identified men or men who have sex with men (MSM) should not be assumed to be at high risk simply based on identity or history, as some may be abstinent or monogamous [3]. It is also important to note that many LGBT patients are interested in pregnancy, surrogacy, or adoption, and that there are options to achieve parenthood for all patients and primary care providers should be ready to counsel or refer these patients appropriately [31]. Several articles and websites are helpful for primary care providers who wish to counsel patients more specifically [32–34]. It is also pertinent to remember that many WSW also have sex with men or will in the future and do need counseling concerning contraception [11, 29]. Transmen (transgender FTM) also often retain a uterus and ovaries, and testosterone therapy is not a reliable form of contraception; therefore they also require an exploration of their desires for fertility versus contraception, whether relevant to a current male partner or for future planning [35, 36].

---

**Helpful Hint**

Use a sensitive and comprehensive sexual history rather than assumptions about behavior to determine appropriate screening and diagnostic tests.

---

## Immunizations

Immunizations for LGBT persons generally follow accepted guidelines for children and adults, with the exception that the CDC does recommend full hepatitis A and B immunization for all MSM. Human papilloma virus (HPV) vaccination, which is recommended by the Centers for Disease Control (CDC) and the Advisory Committee on Immunization Practices (ACIP) for both females and males age 9–26, is also prudent to recommend to LGBT youth and young adults [37, 38]. Even lesbian-identified WSW

can benefit from HPV vaccination because HPV can be transmitted between women and the majority of such women also have sex with men in their lifetime [29]. Men benefit from HPV prevention in terms of both genital warts and anal cancer, as well as the reduction in transmission of HPV to male or female partners [37].

## Screening

### Cardiovascular Health

LGBT persons may be at higher risk of cardiovascular disease owing to their increased prevalence of risk factors such as smoking, depression, and (in women and some gay men), obesity [39, 40]. Nevertheless, there is no evidence supporting screening based on identity or sexual behavior alone. Screening for obesity, elevated blood pressure, cholesterol, lipids, and blood sugar are consistent with that of the general population and decisions for more or additional screening should be based on individual risk factors. The US Preventive Services Task Force (USPSTF) and the AAFP issue recommendations separately for each of the CV risk factors listed [41].

The Center of Excellence for Transgender Care at the University of California, San Francisco, recommends screening cholesterol/lipids and blood pressure for all patients planning to start hormone therapy within the coming year. They recommend a target systolic blood pressure at or below 130 and LDL at or below 135 prior to initiation of hormones [35]. Monitoring and treatment goals on hormones are covered in Chap. 19.

### Cancer

**Cervical Cancer** Cervical cancer incidence and prevalence have decreased dramatically in the last half-century thanks to widespread and frequent screening with Papanicolaou (Pap) tests and office-based colposcopy and treatment. Consequently, the vast majority of patients diagnosed with cervical cancer are those who have not undergone screening in over 10 years, including those who have never had a Pap test [29].

Most studies that include them find that WSW or lesbian-identified women are disproportionately represented among that group of infrequent or never screeners [42–44]. It is widely accepted that development of cervical neoplasia is highly associated with persistence of high-risk strains of HPV in the cervix. It is likely, therefore, that failure to screen is most commonly caused by a failure of the patient or the provider to recognize that WSW are at risk for HPV infection [29, 30]. In truth, WSW or lesbian identified women are at risk from multiple sources:

• The majority of WSW/lesbians also have a lifetime history of intercourse with men,
• Transmission of HPV between female partners is possible and has been documented,
• There exists a higher proportion of current or former smokers among sexual minority (SM) women, a known risk factor for cervical cancer [29].

In addition, many studies suggest that SM adolescents exhibit earlier sexual debut and higher risk sexual behavior (with partners of either or both sexes) than heterosexual teens [45–47]. Some research also demonstrates that women who have sex with both women and men are more likely to exhibit increased sexual risk-taking [45, 48]. Some WSW may therefore actually have higher risk for HPV acquisition than heterosexual women [30]. As with all patients, a detailed sexual history, including lifetime partners and measures taken toward safer sex, can help determine risk. (Please refer to Appendix A, Chaps. 2, 5, and 6 for suggested sexual history questions and more information on gathering history in a sensitive and patient-centered manner.) Nonetheless, all persons with a cervix and any history of sexual activity should be assumed to be susceptible to HPV, and recommended for screening with a Pap test according to usual guidelines [11, 49]. Those without a cervix due to hysterectomy should also be screened according to usual guidelines (See Table 8.1 for screening guidelines; note that those who have received the HPV vaccine series should continue to be screened per their age category.) [50]. At present, experts are considering the option of cervical cancer screening through HPV testing without cytology [52]; such recommendations are not currently in effect, however, and if HPV testing without cytology becomes an accepted screening option, it is unlikely that guidelines will advise an approach for screening SM women that differs from screening for the general population.

It is important to recognize that reduction in screening can also result from SM women's

**Table 8.1** Recommended cervical cancer screening for all persons with a cervix

| Age group/clinical feature | Screening method | Frequency | Other considerations |
| --- | --- | --- | --- |
| Under age 21 | Not recommended | | |
| Age 21–29 | Cytology alone | Every 3 years | Currently HPV testing alone not recommended; however, there is an FDA-approved HPV test (without Pap cytology), and ongoing studies are promising and likely to change practice[a] |
| Age 30–65 | HPV and cytology co-testing (preferred) | Every 5 years | |
| | Cytology alone (acceptable) | Every 3 years | |
| Age over 65 | Discontinue screening after adequate negative prior screenings | | Those with history of CIN 2–3 or CIS should continue screening per age 30–65 guidelines through 20 years after diagnosis |
| Status post total hysterectomy | Not recommended | | Applies to those without a cervix and without a history of CIN 2–3, CIS, or overt cancer in last 20 years |

*CIN* cervical intra-epithelial neoplasia, *CIS* carcinoma-in-situ
Adapted from *Table 1: Joint Recommendations of the American Cancer Society, the American Society for Colposcopy and Cervical Pathology, and the American Society for Clinical Pathology* appearing in the 2012 ACOG Practice Bulletin on Cervical Cancer Screening [50]; other than [a]references Ronco et al. [51] and U.S. FDA [52]

discomfort with the examiner and/or the exam itself. Anecdotally, many WSW find themselves subject to assumptions from the provider that their sexual activity is heterosexual and they may be chided for not using birth control [29, 30, 53]. This assumption reveals inadequate history-taking from the provider and does not engender confidence in the provider or the health care system. In addition, WSW may also experience more discomfort with the exam itself, especially those who are nulliparous and have not experienced significant vaginal penetration [29]. As is true with all patients, the WSW patient should be approached in a sensitive manner, the smallest speculum necessary for the patient's anatomy should be used, and the patient's reports of discomfort should be honored. Performing the bimanual exam prior to the speculum exam in order to assess pelvic landmarks and ease the patient into the exam is a reasonable option [54]. Williams and Williams [55] provides an excellent resource on using woman-centered language during a pelvic exam for female-identified patients.

Transgender patients should likewise be screened according to the organs and tissues present at any given time. Because the majority of FTM patients have not had genital reassignment surgery, most also require regular Pap screening as detailed in Table 8.1 [35]. As usual, a detailed sexual history helps the provider discuss the level of risk and benefit with the patient as necessary. Because FTM patients identify as men (and transspectrum natal born females in general do not identify completely as women), they may have particular difficulty managing emotions and physical sensations associated with pelvic exams. It is therefore important to employ extra sensitivity in using terminology that is comfortable for the patient and performing the exam efficiently. The Canadian organization "Check It Out, Guys" has a number of helpful recommendations for providers [56]. In addition, FTM patients have high prevalence of unsatisfactory pap smears compared to non-transgender patients possibly secondary to testosterone therapy causing growth in the clitoris and dryness of tissues, meaning that sensitivity to expected changes and more liberal use of lubrication within the limits of Pap test

sensitivity are important [57]. It is also critical to note the use of testosterone on the pathology order [36, 56]. An FTM who has had a hysterectomy or sexual reassignment surgery (SRS) with no history of cervical dysplasia can discontinue Pap screening. MTF individuals who have had SRS do not need Pap tests because they do not have a cervix and the neovagina consists of epithelial rather than mucosal tissue. They may of course need pelvic exams as indicated by symptoms or patient questions [35] (Note that rarely, especially in the past, neovaginas were constructed using tissue from the glans penis. If a patient knows of this surgical history, consensus guidelines are to use age-appropriate vaginal pap screening [58]). Not all patients broadly categorized as transgender identify as FTM or MTF, as described in Chap. 16, and it is the presence of a cervix rather than the gender identity, that determines the need for screening. In summary, cervical cancer screening should follow the same guidelines for all patients who have a cervix or had the cervix removed due to dysplasia or cancer [58].

**Helpful Hint**
The presence of a cervix rather than gender identity determines the need for cervical cancer screening.

**Breast Cancer** Evidence is mixed concerning whether lesbian women have a higher incidence of breast cancer than heterosexual or bisexual women. Some research, however, supports that risk factors such as lower parity and lactation, less use of hormonal contraception, higher rates of obesity, and lower rates of screening are more common in lesbian-identified women and might contribute to breast cancer risk [59]. With attention to the risk factors of the individual woman, breast cancer screening is recommended according to standard guidelines, either those of the United States Preventive Services Task Force (USPSTF), American College of Obstetricians and Gynecologists (ACOG), American Cancer Society (ACS), or others. The USPSTF, for example, recommends mammography screening every 1–2 years from age 50 to 74, with screening from age 40 to 50 and over 74 dependent on patient risk factors, values, and comorbidities [60]. In making shared decisions on mammography screening, the PCP and health care team should carefully consider the lesbian or bisexual-identified woman's risk factors concerning unopposed estrogen exposure over the lifetime and screening history, as well as family history.

Breast cancer screening in transgender persons on hormone therapy or after surgery is more complex. At this time there is no existing research on the incidence or natural history of breast cancer in these groups. Based on expert opinion, the UCSF Center for Transgender Health's primary care protocols recommend beginning mammography in MTF patients when patients are age 50 or over and have been on estrogen hormone therapy for 5 or more years (or age 50 with other risk factors such as body mass index (BMI) over 35 or strong family history) [35]. There is not a specific recommendation on stopping screening for MTF, though the USPSTF guideline of age 75 appears reasonable [60]. Many FTM undergo mastectomy (top surgery), and level of remaining risk may differ depending on whether the top surgery is a simple reduction versus a chest reconstruction. Those with a reconstruction are not thought to need mammograms in the absence of other major risk factors (e.g. strong family history/brca mutation), whereas a patient with only a reduction should be considered for screening as per natal females beginning at age 50. Similarly, FTM without top surgery should undergo screening every 1–2 years starting at age 50, as there is currently no evidence that testosterone therapy alone reduces breast cancer risk or the effectiveness of mammography. Due to lack of research in this area, the UCSF Center of Excellence for Transgender Health recommends annual chest wall and axillary node exam for all patients [35]. Given the low level of evidence that clinical breast exams are effective in reducing mortality from breast cancer in the general population, the benefit of annual chest wall exam is unclear.

**Colorectal Cancer (CRC)** Because sexual orientation and gender identity are not typically recorded in cancer registry data, national studies are unable to provide definitive evidence regarding the rates of colon cancer in LGBT populations. However, a recent analysis of Surveillance, Epidemiology, and End Results (SEER) data by Boehmer et al. showed that, independent of race and socioeconomic status, there is a significant positive association between CRC incidence and a higher geographic density of sexual minority persons. A similar association with regard to CRC mortality was also noted for sexual minority men [61]. Some data suggest that CRC screening may actually be higher for sexual minorities than for heterosexual persons. Data from the California Health Interview Survey showed that gay/bisexual men had 6–10 % greater screening than heterosexual men. However, vigilance is necessary, especially for some racial and ethnic minorities. For example, Asian/Pacific Islander men were much less likely to be up-to-date on CRC screening (41.0 % for gay/bisexual men, 43.8 % for heterosexual men) compared to gay/bisexual and heterosexual white men (59.8 % and 58.2 %, respectively) [62].

CRC screening can be accomplished through a number of methods (fecal occult blood testing/fecal immunochemical testing, sigmoidoscopy, or colonoscopy). The USPSTF recommends screening beginning at age 50 years and continuing until age 75 years [63]. This recommendation is no different for patients who identify as in sexual minority categories. Also, there does not appear to be an increased level of CRC risk for HIV-infected persons [64].

**Anal Cancer** Anal cancer is fairly uncommon in the general population, but the risk is about 30-fold higher for HIV-infected persons, and HIV+ MSM appear to be at highest risk [64]. Like cervical cancer, anal cancer is largely attributable to HPV. A multi-city trial reported anal HPV in 57 % of a large sample of HIV-negative MSM; this study also indicated that HPV infection risk was highest among men who practiced receptive anal intercourse and who had over five male partners in past 6 months [65]. Unlike cervical cancer, however, anal cancer is much less common (only about 5200 new cases per year in the U.S.), and guidelines for anal cancer screening are not as clear. Screening for anal cancer and its precursor, anal intraepithelial neoplasia (AIN), is accomplished through the use of anal cytology ("Anal Pap"). The sensitivity of anal cytology for detection of AIN is much better for HIV+ MSM than for HIV− MSM [66].

Cost-effectiveness models suggest that in the U.S. anal cytology done annually for HIV+ and biannually for HIV− MSM would be cost effective [67, 68]. The role of co-testing for high-risk HPV is unclear, and commercially available HPV detection methods are not yet FDA approved for anal samples. Abnormal anal cytology should prompt further investigation through high-resolution anoscopy (HRA). Techniques associated with this procedure are similar to those for colposcopy and include visualization under magnification, application of acetic acid, assessment of aceto-whitening and vascular changes (punctuation, mosaicism), and evaluation of Lugol's staining patterns. Biopsy of suspicious areas provides definitive diagnosis [69].

It has been recommended that biopsies showing high-grade anal intra-epithelial neoplasia (HG AIN; grade II or III) should be treated, while AIN grade 1 can be followed-up in 6 months, or treated if doing so would have minimal potential for morbidity. MSM with normal HRA may resume usual screening (annually if HIV+ and every 2–3 years if HIV−). Treatment of AIN may include cryotherapy, electrocautery, laser treatment, infrared coagulation, or topical therapies such as imiquimod, trichloroacetic acid, and 5-fluorouracil. It is important to note, however, in many cases, there may be limited availability of experienced cytopathologists who are able to accurately interpret anal cytology samples, as well as few clinicians capable of doing HRA or experienced in treating AIN. The process of screening should only be instituted if appropriate resources exist for evaluation and treatment of abnormal results [66, 69]. Because infection with HPV types 16 and 18 can be prevented by available vaccines, MSM should be offered immunization, hopefully before they become exposed to these strains of virus [38].

**Helpful Hint**
Screen HIV positive MSM annually with an anal Pap if resources are available for appropriate follow-up. Consider screening HIV negative MSM biannually.

**Prostate Cancer** Epidemiologic data on prostate cancer incidence is unavailable for gay/bisexual men, but there is no reason to believe that their risk would be lower than that of other populations. Given the lack of strong evidence to the contrary, screening considerations should follow the standard recommendations for non-LGBT populations. The USPSTF currently recommends against PSA-based screening, and does not make a recommendation considering other modalities [70]. Other organizations offer different recommendations [71]. MTF women are still at risk, and cases of prostate cancer have been reported among MTF transgender women on feminizing hormone therapy [72], though PSA levels are reduced by estrogen therapy and may not be adequate testing for prostate cancer when used alone [73]. Given that orchiectomy is a component of prostate cancer treatment [74], it is theoretically likely that removal of the testes as part of "bottom" surgery can reduce the chances that a trans woman might develop prostate cancer in the future.

**Testicular Cancer** The U.S. Preventive Services Task Force recommends against screening for testicular cancer [75] Recommendations are no different for men who have sex with men. While testicular cancer should be included in the differential diagnosis of testicular pain or masses in MSM, screening should not be part of routine screening for asymptomatic MSM.

**Lung Cancer** Although epidemiologic studies documenting lung cancer diagnoses by sexual orientation or gender identity are lacking, the disproportionately high prevalence of smoking among SGM portends a higher risk of lung cancer. One study suggests a higher incidence of and mortality from lung cancer in sexual minority men, though not women [76]. Lung cancer screening for those at high risk is controversial but currently recommended by the USPSTF. Criteria for screening with low-dose contrast computerized tomography (CT) scan include age 50–64 with over 30 pack year history and currently smoke or quit smoking less than or equal to 15 years prior [77]. Screening should be based on these elements of a patient's history, with awareness that SGM are more likely to meet these criteria than the general population [78]. Of course, SGM who use tobacco also have heightened risks for the effects of smoking other than lung cancer, such as chronic obstructive pulmonary disease, cardiovascular disease, and other non-lung cancers.

## Bone Density

Bone density screening is somewhat controversial even in the general population. Four organizations have somewhat different recommendations, but generally converge on dual-energy X-ray absorptiometry (DXA) screening at least once for all women age 65 and older or those under age 65 with risk factors for osteoporosis (smoking, history of significant corticosteroid exposure, low weight, strong family history) [79]. There is not yet agreement on the frequency or duration of screening, nor whether to screen routinely in men. Transgender patients present a challenge, as the effects of cross-sex hormones on bone density are not well understood. In particular, the effects of testosterone on bone density for FTM are unknown. The UCSF primary care protocols recommend starting screening at age 50–60 based on presence or absence of ovaries and duration of testosterone therapy [35] (see also "Part V", Chaps. 18–21). Note than some FTM, however, chose to taper to lower doses or off testosterone after surgical or natural menopause and should also be considered for DXA screening at that time. Estrogen's effect on bones that have also had prior exposure to testosterone is thought to protect MTF patients from osteoporosis. The primary care protocols recommend calcium, vitamin D and weight bearing exercise without

DXA screening in most MTF patients, with DXA recommended only in those patients who are post-orchiectomy/post-SRS, over 60, and off hormone therapy at least 5 years [35].

## Interpersonal Violence and Personal Safety

The USPSTF now recommends screening for IPV (more commonly known as intimate partner violence but recognized that violence can occur in a broader context) for women of child-bearing age, and finds insufficient evidence for screening the rest of the general primary care population [80]. Numerous studies demonstrate that LGBT people are at higher risk of intimate partner violence and overall violence victimization than the general population, likely associated with additional stressors such as experiences of stigma and discrimination, internalized homophobia, and the threat of being "outed" [81]. Helpful screening tools to use in primary care are listed and included in the CDC's guide [82]. PCPs should also be aware of community resources or hotlines to which to refer victimized patients as safely as possible. Attention to mental health consequences and specific state laws regarding reporting of violence are also important roles of PCPs. For more specific information on violence and LGBT health, see Chap. 10.

## Substance Use and Abuse

**Tobacco**  Tobacco use is up to two times more common in LGB versus heterosexuals [78, 83–86]. Although LGB tobacco use studies consistently demonstrate this risk behavior disparity, transgender persons have only recently been included in tobacco research. In a 2009–2010 nationally representative survey, 32.8 % of transgender-inclusive LGBT individuals reported current smoking, versus 19.5 % of heterosexuals [87]. In the National Transgender Discrimination Survey, the proportion of current smokers (29 % of transwomen and 33 % of transmen) were higher than the percentage in the general population and similar to that of other LGB/LGBT studies [88].

Measures of smoking initiation, daily versus non-daily smoking, and nicotine dependence are all important elements of tobacco use related to health outcomes. These aspects of use are still seldom studied in minority populations, but emerging data suggest that at least in some sub-groups of LGBT adults and adolescents, LGB persons are more likely to start smoking younger, smoke socially rather than not at all, and among regular smokers, to smoke more heavily than heterosexuals [84, 89]. Sexual minority adolescents also have higher nicotine dependence scores than their peers [89, 90]. Research on desire to quit and quit attempts among sexual minority groups is similarly limited mainly to young adult populations or is local in scope, but generally demonstrates lower odds of wanting to stop smoking and reduced quit ratios [86, 91].

Evidence supports the role of minority stress, social norms, social isolation, and targeting of sexual and gender minority (SGM) people by tobacco companies as contributing factors to this disparity. The tobacco industry actively and effectively targets advertising and promotion to LGB groups [92–95]. Minority stress theory [96] is reflected in studies showing that sexual minorities experience risk factors for cigarette smoking (e.g. stress, depression, alcohol use) at higher rates than the general population, while also experiencing factors unique to sexual minority groups such as discrimination, stigmatization, and victimization [97]. Stress among sexual minorities is also associated with mental health measures conditions such as distress, depression, and anxiety, which are in turn related to health risk behaviors including smoking and substance use [96–102]. Fortunately, there are some promising results from cessation programs focused on LGBT patients [103, 104].

**Helpful Hint**
Tobacco use may be the single largest contribution to mortality among the LGBT community. Screen every patient for tobacco use of all types and provide resources for motivational and behavioral change.

**Alcohol and Drug Use** Compared to heterosexual women, lesbian and bisexual women report heavier alcohol use and more alcohol related problems [105], and greater lifetime use rates of marijuana, cocaine and other illicit drugs [106]. Compared to heterosexual men, gay and bisexual men report greater lifetime use rates of cocaine, marijuana, MDMA, and methamphetamine [106]. Transgender MTF women report higher rates of intravenous drug use [107]. Alcohol and drug use are associated with higher sexual risk-taking among gay and bisexual men and MTF transgender women [108]. Methamphetamine, ecstasy (MDMA), ketamine, LSD and similar drugs are often referred to as "club drugs" and may be particularly associated with LGBT-oriented bars and clubs [109]. "Poppers" (amyl nitrite) are inhaled drugs used commonly by MSM to enhance sexual sensation and relax the anal sphincter [110]. Even at low frequencies, any illicit drug or excessive alcohol use increases risk of HIV and STI acquisition [111], and risk increases in a dose-dependent manner [112]. Alcohol and drugs may be used by LGBT people for a myriad of reasons similar to those associated with tobacco use above. Often LGBT people are marginalized within communities and historically have congregated at bars and clubs for socializing. Mental health comorbidities or using alcohol and drugs to escape feelings of loneliness and depression can complicate the diagnosis and treatment [98].

**Screening Tools** A number of tools, such as the SBIRT approach, CAGE, and AUDIT are available to screen for substance use and abuse in primary care settings. A convenient source of multiple online tools is the SAMHSA-HRSA Center for Integrated Health Solutions [113].

## Sexual Health

**STI Screening—MSM** According to CDC reports of multicenter studies, MSM had a prevalence of 14.9 % for gonorrhea and 11.2 % for Chlamydia. Moreover, MSM accounted for 62 % of all primary and secondary syphilis cases in the U.S. between 2005 and 2009, the syphilis

**Table 8.2** Primary care STI screening for MSM

| STI | Source/type | Indications | Timing |
| --- | --- | --- | --- |
| HIV | Serum or oral swab | All MSM | At least annually |
| Syphilis | Serology | All MSM | At least annually |
| Gonorrhea | Urine NAAT | Was anal insertive partner in last year | At least annually |
| | Rectal swab NAAT | Was anal receptive partner in last year | At least annually |
| | Oral swab NAAT | Was oral receptive partner in last year | At least annually |
| Chlamydia | Urine NAAT | Was anal insertive partner in last year | At least annually |
| | Rectal swab NAAT | Was anal receptive partner in last year | At least annually |
| Hepatitis B | HBsAg serology | All MSM | At least once and periodically until effective vaccination confirmed |
| HSV-2 HSV-1 | Serology | Consider if status unknown | Periodic for those with negative last status |

*NAAT* nucleic acid amplification testing
Source: US Public Health Service. Pre-exposure prophylaxis for the prevention of HIV infection in the United States—2014: A clinical practice guideline. Atlanta: CDC; 2014 [115]

seroreactivity rate for MSM was 11 % in 2008, and there has been a resurgence of syphilis with incidence in 2013 double what it was in 2000 (for which there was the lowest ever incidence) in which MSM are the sub-population with the greatest increase [114]. Many cases of STI are asymptomatic, so screening should be offered even if patients deny symptoms [72]. Consensus guidelines for STI screening among MSM from the CDC are summarized in Table 8.2 [116]. Screening at 3–6 month intervals are indicated for those with multiple partners, anonymous partners, or those who have sex along with illicit drug use or whose partners do so. Appropriate patient-centered care would also dictate that MSM in long-term monogamous relationships in which both partners have negative STI initial testing could reasonably forego or space out STI screening. It is always important to re-assess specific sexual history prior to testing. Note that testing for anal or oral HPV and its effects remains controversial. See the section on anal cancer above for more information. Additionally, some experts would recommend screening for both HSV-1 and HSV-2, given increasing rates of HSV-1 in genital samples [117, 118], though there is insufficient evidence for an official recommendation.

> **Helpful Hint**
> Utilize the Centers for Disease Control and Prevention (CDC) Sexually Transmitted Diseases Treatment Guidelines guidelines for guidance on screening MSM for STDs.

**STI Screening in WSW**  As with HPV infection, there is evidence of transmission of most STI's between female partners, though transmission is likely less efficient for most infections. HIV in particular is rare, with only one documented case considered to be confirmed as sexually transmitted [119] and a handful of others in which transmission was probable but less clear [30]. Conversely, bacterial vaginosis, though not an STI in the traditional sense, is more common in WSW with consistent strains documented in couples [30, 120]. Because HSV is transmitted similarly in various forms of sexual practices, transmission may be more common than most STIs in WSW. Evidence supports increased prevalence of HSV-1 with increasing female partners, possibly related to more frequent oral sex [30, 121]. As with all patients, a detailed sexual history, including lifetime partners and measures taken toward safer sex, can help determine risk.

(Please refer to Appendix A and Chaps. 5 and 6 for suggested sexual history questions.) Because of unclear risk of transmission, there are no established STI screening guidelines other than Pap screening under the same guidelines as for all women, and the recommendation to screen according to sexual history risk factors [116].

**STI Screening in Transgender Patients** In general, transgender persons should be screened commensurate with the body parts they have and their type of sexual activity. A transwoman who has oral or anal sex with men would therefore be screened according to guidelines for MSM, while a transman who has oral or vaginal sex with women would be screened according to guidelines for WSW. In practice, many trans persons may not identify in a specific category and may be in different stages of hormonal or surgical transition. As with all patients, trans persons may also have both male and female (or transgender) partners, as well. STI screening in this group must be customized in a patient-centered manner. For more information, please see Chaps. 16 and 17.

**Pre-exposure Prophylaxis Against HIV (PrEP)** In 2014, the US Public Health Service issued recommendations for the use of antiviral therapy to prevent HIV infection among individuals who are at high risk [115]. These recommendations apply to HIV-negative individuals who are at substantial risk of acquiring HIV infection. This includes anyone who is in an ongoing sexual relationship with an HIV-positive partner. It also includes anyone who is not in a mutually monogamous relationship with a partner who recently tested HIV-negative and who also meets any of the following criteria: (a) MSM who has had anal sex without a condom in the past 6 months, (b) MSM who has been diagnosed with an STI in the past 6 months, (c) heterosexual man or woman who does not regularly use condoms during sex with partners of unknown HIV status who are at substantial risk of HIV infection (e.g., people who inject drugs or have bisexual male partners). PrEP consists of one daily dose of tenofovir and emtricitabine, and it is generally well tolerated. Patients who are candidates for PrEP should be counseled about HIV transmission and prevention, as well as the risks and benefits of PrEP. Patients receiving PrEP should be screened for HIV every 3 months, and renal function should be assessed every 6 months.

**Mental and Emotional Health**
The majority of outpatient treatment for mental health disorders is delivered by PCPs rather than psychiatrists, psychologists, or social workers. Behavioral and emotional disorders are among the most frequent diagnoses seen in the primary care setting [122, 123]. The mental health of some LGBT patients is particularly influenced by constant concealment of true identity, victimization or fear of verbal or physical attack, problems with self-acceptance, and social isolation or lack of social support. Lastly, transgender and bisexual identified people can feel isolated from the gay and lesbian community [124].

The U.S. Preventive Services Task Force (USPSTF) recommends screening adults for depression in clinical practices that have systems in place to assure accurate diagnosis, effective treatment, and follow-up [125]. The same screening tools can be used for LGBT populations [113]. Further details on mental and emotional health appear in the section below and in Chap. 10.

A meta-analysis highlighted the prevalence of mental disorders in lesbians, gay men, and bisexuals (LGBs) and shows that people who identify as lesbian, gay, or bisexual have a higher prevalence of mental disorders than heterosexuals [96]. One framework for understanding this excess in prevalence of disorders is the concept of minority stress, which helps to explain that stigma, prejudice, and discrimination create a hostile and stressful social environment that causes mental health problems [126]. In the LGBT community, self-identified lesbians (and possibly bisexual women) are at an increased risk of overweight and obesity compared to heterosexual women [12, 14], while gay men tend to have lower BMI than their straight counterparts but express higher body dissatisfaction and may be at higher risk for eating disorders [16, 17]. PCPs should be aware that body image ideals in the LGBT community may be different from typical cultural ideals, though those theorized differences seem to be minimal in recent, population-based studies [16, 17, 22–24]. PCPs can increase their detection and understanding of mental health problems in their LGBT patients by knowing the stress processes that underlie prejudice events and internalized homophobia.

The health disparities experienced by LGBT populations derive from a complex network of cultural and institutional factors. In part, these disparities appear to stem from culturally sanctioned stigmatization of sexual and gender minorities, beginning early in childhood. Bullying at school or in the home is associated with elevated levels of anxiety and depression in LGBT youth, triggering maladaptive coping behaviors such as early experimentation with cigarettes, alcohol, drugs, sexual activity, and altered eating patterns. LGBT youth are significantly at higher risk for suicidal ideation and attempted suicide [99, 124]. LGBT people are also more likely to experience family rejection and adolescent homelessness. Running away to escape mistreatment or abuse drastically increases sexual and substance abuse risk and disrupts educational and employment opportunities. These factors in turn contribute to lifelong health disparities experienced by LGBT people [99].

## Family Models in LGBT Health

Recent groundbreaking publications have raised awareness of previously unrecognized health disparities experienced by LGBT populations [127]. PCPs can improve the health care of LGBT men and women and their families by maintaining a non-homophobic attitude, being sure to distinguish sexual behavior from sexual identity, communicating clearly and sensitively by using gender-neutral terms, and being aware of how their own attitudes affect clinical judgment.

The American Academy of Family Physicians defines family as, "a group of individuals with a continuing legal, genetic, and/or emotional relationship" [128]. PCPs play a special role in addressing patients' health from a holistic perspective that acknowledges and honors this broad definition of family. LGBT families include couples without children, couples with children and/or stepchildren, single parents with children, multiple parents raising children together, "families of choice" (close friends), and multiple adults in a committed relationship. PCPs can learn about their patient's family structure by asking patients who lives at home with them, who helps them make important health care decisions and inquiring further about the quality of relationships. When talking with children, physicians should initially use neutral language such as "parent(s)" rather than "mom" or "dad."

**Helpful Hint**
LGBT patients often define 'family' very broadly.

Related to emotional wellbeing and relationship health, LGBT couples are particularly vulnerable to the internalization of societal stigma. This can hamper the ability to form safe, strong, nurturing relationships. Lack of family and peer acceptance undermines LGBT relationship and contributes to psychological stress. Recent landmark decisions regarding legal marital status for lesbian and gay couples have improved financial and legal protections. However, in many states, the benefits of marriage remain unavailable, or at best, in flux for lesbian and gay couples [129]. PCPs can encourage LGBT families to protect themselves and their loved ones with legal documentation such as, living wills, medical power of attorney/health care proxy, durable power of attorney, second parent or joint adoption (where available), and sperm donor agreement.

## Brief Counseling within the Clinical Visit

Primary care providers are in a unique position to identify patients with potential mental health problems and intervene when appropriate. In the primary care setting, the mental health assessment includes asking patients about their most pressing mental health concern and assessing social factors and coping styles. Evidence supports brief interventions in primary care and brief interventions are especially relevant to the healthcare needs of LGBT patients, particularly in addressing substance abuse and patient activation [130–132].

As with any effective counseling modality, effective brief interventions begin with an active and empathic therapeutic style that respects patient autonomy and places responsibility for change on the patient. The focus of the intervention is on a specific problem with the intention of finding a solution that can be objectively measured. The provider incorporates patient values and beliefs into clearly defined goals related to specific behavior change and enhances patient self-efficacy so that patients can move toward change [133].

Counseling patients to change their behavior in an effort to support mental health (e.g., quitting smoking, decreasing alcohol use, exercising, medication adherence) can be a challenge for clinicians, particularly in a short amount of time. Evidence suggests that simply telling patients to change their behavior (e.g., eat less, exercise more) is not as effective as using a patient-centered approach, where the physician attempts to meet the patient "where he or she is at" in terms of internal motivation to change. For example, if the patient is resistant to change, then he or she will likely ignore any recommendations or guidelines. But if the patient is already taking steps to make a change, then one can take the opportunity to further motivate the patient, and to make further suggestions for taking action and committing to change. Therefore, prior to educating the patient about what changes to make, it is recommended that the PCP first assess the patient's readiness for making a change. This can be accomplished by asking how important the change seems to the patient, and then assessing how confident the patient feels in making the change [28].

The "transtheoretical model of change" proposes that people go through six predictable stages in their process of change. Progress through the stages can be slow, and many people regress to earlier stages during the process.

Once it is established which stage of change the patient is in, brief counseling techniques can be tailored to be more effective [134]. Motivational Interviewing is one patient-centered approach that can be used to increase motivation to change, and has been found to be successful in treating addiction. Many health professionals believe it can be easily adopted for other forms of behavioral change relevant to health promotion in the primary care setting [28].

## Coordination of Care

## Finding Appropriate Consultants

Although health care providers practice under codes of ethics that insist upon professionalism and respect for the patient, patients continue to report experiences of discrimination and insensitive communication or treatment in health care settings [88, 135, 136]. Studies as late as the early 2000s reveal significant bias of health care providers against LGBT patients [137–140], which have potential to affect patient experiences. How do PCPs protect their patients from discriminatory experiences or direct their patients to consultants more culturally competent in LGBT health? Unfortunately there are no standards or certifications demonstrating competence or sensitivity to which to refer. The GLMA directory is a national database open to providers of all specialties and can therefore be a resource in terms of screening consultants for sensitivity [141]. Some institutions, such as Vanderbilt University [142], and organizations such as Out, Proud, and Healthy in Missouri [143] have also established their own provider directories. Many areas of the country, however, have few to no listings in the GLMA directory and no local directory. In these areas, selecting more sensitive consultants to which to refer the patient, when possible, will be through personal networks and word-of-mouth. Of course, personal networks are not only the most effective way to refer in a patient-centered manner in all settings, but they also serve to reinforce sensitive and competent care through repeated referrals and personal feedback.

## Communication and Confidentiality

Documentation of sexual orientation and gender identity can be challenging, especially in settings in which registration forms and electronic health records (EHR) limit patients to hetero-normative and gender-normative designations. Evidence exists that patients still have concerns about confidentiality, especially the uncertainty induced by the EHR era [144.] There is no standard of care to guide documentation; however, national guidelines emphasize the need for transparency with patients about what information is recorded and the language used, and who has access to it. Of course it is appropriate to defer to the patient's preferences when necessary as befits patient-centered care [3, 145].

## Resources Most Relevant to Primary Care

The National LGBT Health Education Center—
Home
http://www.lgbthealtheducation.org/
The National LGBT Health Education Center—
Suggested Resources and Readings
http://www.lgbthealtheducation.org/publications/
lgbt-health-resources/
GLMA Guidelines for Care of Lesbian, Gay, Bisexual, and Transgender Patients
http://glma.org/_data/n_0001/resources/live/
GLMA%20guidelines%202006%20FINAL.
pdf
UCSF Center of Excellence for Transgender Health: Primary Care Protocol for Transgender Patient Care
http://transhealth.ucsf.edu/trans?page=
protocol-00-00
Mravcak SA. Primary care for lesbians and bisexual women. Am Fam Physician. 2006; 74(2):279–86.
http://www.aafp.org/afp/2006/0715/p279.html

## References

1. MA S, Cheng N, Moore M, Coffman M, Bazemore AW. Patients with high-cost chronic conditions rely heavily on primary care physicians. J Am Board Fam Med. 2014;27(1):11–2.
2. Starfield B, Shi L, Macinko J. Contribution of primary care to health systems and health. Milbank Q. 2005;83(3):457–502.
3. GLMA. Guidelines for care of lesbian, gay, bisexual and transgender patients. San Francisco, CA: GLMA; 2006.
4. Patient-Centered Primary Care Collaborative. Defining the medical home. 2013 [11 Mar 2014]. Available from: http://www.pcpcc.org/about/medical-home.
5. Rosenthal TC. The medical home: growing evidence to support a new approach to primary care. J Am Board Fam Med. 2008;21(5):427–40.
6. American Academy of Family Physicians. PCMH overview. 2014 [11 Mar 2014]. Available from: http://www.aafp.org/practice-management/pcmh/overview.html.
7. National Committee for Quality Assurance. Patient centered medical home recognition. [11 Mar 2014]. Available from: http://www.ncqa.org/Programs/Recognition/PatientCenteredMedicalHomePCMH.aspx.
8. Davis K, Abrams M, Stremikis K. How the affordable care act will strengthen the nation's primary care foundation. J Gen Intern Med. 2011;26(10):1201–3.
9. White JC, Dull VT. Health risk factors and health-seeking behavior in lesbians. J Womens Health. 1997;6(1):103–12.
10. Brock DW, Wartman SA. When competent patients make irrational choices. N Engl J Med. 1990; 322(22):1595–9.
11. Mravcak SA. Primary care for lesbians and bisexual women. Am Fam Physician. 2006;74(2):279–86.
12. Dysart-Gale D. Social justice and social determinants of health: lesbian, gay, bisexual, transgendered, intersexed, and queer youth in Canada. J Child Adolesc Psychiatr Nurs. 2010;23(1):23–8.
13. Hatzenbuehler ML, Bellatorre A, Lee Y, Finch BK, Muennig P, Fiscella K. Structural stigma and all-cause mortality in sexual minority populations. Soc Sci Med. 2014;103:33–41.
14. Boehmer U, Bowen DJ, Bauer GR. Overweight and obesity in sexual-minority women: evidence from population-based data. Am J Public Health. 2007; 97(6):1134–40.
15. Bowen DJ, Balsam KF, Ender SR. A review of obesity issues in sexual minority women. Obesity. 2008;16(2):221–8.
16. Peplau LA, Frederick DA, Yee C, Maisel N, Lever J, Ghavami N. Body image satisfaction in heterosex-

ual, gay, and lesbian adults. Arch Sex Behav. 2009;38(5):713–25.
17. Yean C, Benau EM, Dakanalis A, Hormes JM, Perone J, Timko CA. The relationship of sex and sexual orientation to self-esteem, body shape satisfaction, and eating disorder symptomatology. Front Psychol. 2013;4:887.
18. Aaron DJ, Markovic N, Danielson ME, Honnold JA, Janosky JE, Schmidt NJ. Behavioral risk factors for disease and preventive health practices among lesbians. Am J Public Health. 2001;91(6):972–5.
19. Boehmer U, Bowen DJ. Examining factors linked to overweight and obesity in women of different sexual orientations. Prev Med. 2009;48(4):357–61.
20. Deputy NP, Boehmer U. Determinants of body weight among men of different sexual orientation. Prev Med. 2010;51(2):129–31.
21. Yancey AK, Cochran SD, Corliss HL, Mays VM. Correlates of overweight and obesity among lesbian and bisexual women. Prev Med. 2003;36(6):676–83.
22. Austin SB, Ziyadeh N, Kahn JA, Camargo Jr CA, Colditz GA, Field AE. Sexual orientation, weight concerns, and eating-disordered behaviors in adolescent girls and boys. J Am Acad Child Adolesc Psychiatry. 2004;43(9):1115–23.
23. French SA, Story M, Remafedi G, Resnick MD, Blum RW. Sexual orientation and prevalence of body dissatisfaction and eating disordered behaviors: a population-based study of adolescents. Int J Eat Disord. 1996;19(2):119–26.
24. Polimeni AM, Austin SB, Kavanagh AM. Sexual orientation and weight, body image, and weight control practices among young Australian women. J Womens Health. 2009;18(3):355–62.
25. Blashill AJ. Gender roles, eating pathology, and body dissatisfaction in men: a meta-analysis. Body Image. 2011;8(1):1–11.
26. Gough B, Flanders G. Celebrating "obese" bodies: gay "bears" talk about weight, body image and health. Int J Mens Health. 2009;8(3):235–53.
27. Miller B. Motivational interviewing basics. [31 Mar 2014]. Available from: http://www.motivationalinterview.org/quick_links/about_mi.html.
28. Miller WR, Rollnick S. Motivational interviewing: preparing people for change. 2nd ed. New York: Guilford; 2002.
29. Fish J. Cervical screening in lesbian and bisexual women: a review of the worldwide literature using systematic methods. Leicester: De Montfort University; 2009.
30. Marrazzo JM. Barriers to infectious disease care among lesbians. Emerg Infect Dis. 2004;10(11):1974–8.
31. Ross LE, Tarasoff LA, Anderson S, Green D, Epstein R, Marvel S, et al. Sexual and gender minority peoples' recommendations for assisted human reproduction services. J Obstet Gynaecol Can. 2014; 36(2):146–53.
32. It's conceivable. It's conceivable: the path to parenting isn't always straight. [1 Apr 2014]. Available from: http://itsconceivablenow.com/.
33. Norton W, Hudson N, Culley L. Gay men seeking surrogacy to achieve parenthood. Reprod Biomed Online. 2013;27(3):271–9.
34. Steele LS, Stratmann H. Counseling lesbian patients about getting pregnant. Can Fam Physician. 2006; 52:605–11.
35. Center of Excellence for Transgender Health. Primary care protocol for transgender patient care. University of California, San Francisco; 2014 [28 Mar 2014]. Available from: http://transhealth.ucsf.edu/trans?page=protocol-00-00.
36. Check it out guys. Check it out guys: about the Pap test. Sherbourne: Sherbourne Health Centre; 2010 [28 Mar 2014]. Available from: http://www.checkitoutguys.ca/?q=about-the-pap-test.
37. Centers for Disease Control and Prevention. HPV vaccines. 2013 [1 Apr 2014]. Available from: http://www.cdc.gov/hpv/vaccine.html.
38. Centers for Disease Control and Prevention. Vaccines that might be indicated for adults based on medial and other indications. 2014 [1 Apr 2014]. Available from: http://www.cdc.gov/vaccines/schedules/hcp/imz/adult-conditions-shell.html.
39. Hatzenbuehler ML, McLaughlin KA, Slopen N. Sexual orientation disparities in cardiovascular biomarkers among young adults. Am J Prev Med. 2013;44(6):612–21.
40. Roberts SA, Dibble SL, Nussey B, Casey K. Cardiovascular disease risk in lesbian women. Womens Health Issues. 2003;13(4):167–74.
41. American Academy of Family Physicians. Summary of recommendations for clinical preventive services. Leawood, KS; 2014.
42. Frisch M, Smith E, Grulich A, Johansen C. Cancer in a population-based cohort of men and women in registered homosexual partnerships. Am J Epidemiol. 2003;157(11):966–72.
43. Marrazzo JM, Koutsky LA, Kiviat NB, Kuypers JM, Stine K. Papanicolaou test screening and prevalence of genital human papillomavirus among women who have sex with women. Am J Public Health. 2001; 91(6):947–52.
44. Tracy JK, Schluterman NH, Greenberg DR. Understanding cervical cancer screening among lesbians: a national survey. BMC Public Health. 2013;13:442.
45. Busseri MA, Willoughby T, Chalmers H, Bogaert AF. On the association between sexual attraction and adolescent risk behavior involvement: examining mediation and moderation. Dev Psychol. 2008;44(1):69–80.
46. Robinson JP, Espelage DL. Peer victimization and sexual risk differences between lesbian, gay, bisexual, transgender, or questioning and nontransgender heterosexual youths in grades 7–12. Am J Public Health. 2013;103(10):1810–9.
47. Saewyc EM, Bearinger LH, Blum RW, Resnick MD. Sexual intercourse, abuse and pregnancy among adolescent women: does sexual orientation make a difference? Fam Plan Perspect. 1999;31(3):127–31.

48. Tornello SL, Riskind RG, Patterson CJ. Sexual orientation and sexual and reproductive health among adolescent young women in the United States. J Adolesc Health. 2014;21:160–8.

49. American College of Obstetricians and Gynecologists. ACOG committee opinion no. 525: health care for lesbians and bisexual women. Obstet Gynecol. 2012;119:1077–80.

50. Committee on Practice Bulletins—Gynecology. ACOG practice bulletin number 131: screening for cervical cancer. Obstet Gynecol. 2012;120(5): 1222–38.

51. Ronco G, Dillner J, Elfström KM, Tunesi S, Snijders PJF, Arbyn M, et al. Efficacy of HPV-based screening for prevention of invasive cervical cancer: follow-up of four European randomised controlled trials. Lancet. 2014;383(9916):524–32.

52. HPV test recommended as primary screening tool. Cancer Discov. 2014;4(6):OF6.

53. Phillips-Angeles E, Wolfe P, Myers R, Dawson P, Marrazzo J, Soltner S, et al. Lesbian health matters: a Pap test education campaign nearly thwarted by discrimination. Health Promot Pract. 2004;5(3):314–25.

54. Carter S, Rad M, Schwarz B, Sell S, Marshall D. Creating a more positive patient experience of pelvic examination. J Am Assoc Nurse Pract. 2013;25(11):611–8.

55. Williams AA, Williams M. A Guide to performing pelvic speculum exams: a patient-centered approach to reducing iatrogenic effects. Teach Learn Med. 2013;25(4):383–91.

56. Check it out guys. Tips for providing paps to trans men. Sherbourne: Sherbourne Health Centre; 2010 [28 Mar 2014]. Available from: http://checkitoutguys. ca/sites/default/files/Tips_Paps_TransMen_0.pdf.

57. Peitzmeier SM, Reisner SL, Harigopal P, Potter J. Female-to-male patients have high prevalence of unsatisfactory Paps compared to non-transgender females: implications for cervical cancer screening. J Gen Intern Med. 2014;29(5):778–84.

58. Committee on Health Care for Underserved Women. Committee opinion no. 512: health care for transgender individuals. Obstet Gynecol. 2011;118(6):1454–8.

59. Brown JP, Tracy JK. Lesbians and cancer: an overlooked health disparity. Cancer Causes Control. 2008;19(10):1009–20.

60. U.S. Preventive Services Task Force. Screening for breast cancer. United States Preventive Services Task Force; 2009 [24 Apr 2014]. Available from: http://www.uspreventiveservicestaskforce.org/ uspstf/uspsbrca.htm.

61. Boehmer U, Ozonoff A, Miao XP. An ecological analysis of colorectal cancer incidence and mortality: differences by sexual orientation. BMC Cancer. 2011;11:8.

62. Heslin KC, Gore JL, King WD, Fox SA. Sexual orientation and testing for prostate and colorectal cancers among men in California. Med Care. 2008;46(12):1240–8.

63. U.S. Preventive Services Task Force. Screening for colorectal cancer. 2008 [21 Apr 2014]. Available from: http://www.uspreventiveservicestaskforce. org/uspstf/uspscolo.htm.

64. Sigel K, Dubrow R, Silverberg M, Crothers K, Braithwaite S, Justice A. Cancer screening in patients infected with HIV. Curr HIV/AIDS Rep. 2011;8(3):142–52.

65. Chin-Hong PV, Vittinghoff E, Cranston RD, Buchbinder S, Cohen D, Colfax G, et al. Age-specific prevalence of anal human papillomavirus infection in HIV-negative sexually active men who have sex with men: the EXPLORE study. J Infect Dis. 2004;190(12):2070–6.

66. Park IU, Palefsky JM. Evaluation and management of anal intraepithelial neoplasia in HIV-negative and HIV-positive men who have sex with men. Curr Infect Dis Rep. 2010;12(2):126–33.

67. Goldie SJ, Kuntz KM, Weinstein MC, Freedberg KA, Palefsky JM. Cost-effectiveness of screening for anal squamous intraepithelial lesions and anal cancer in human immunodeficiency virus-negative homosexual and bisexual men. Am J Med. 2000;108(8):634–41.

68. Goldie SJ, Kuntz KM, Weinstein MC, Freedberg KA, Welton ML, Palefsky JM. The clinical effectiveness and cost-effectiveness of screening for anal squamous intraepithelial lesions in homosexual and bisexual HIV-positive men. JAMA. 1999;281(19): 1822–9.

69. Darragh TM, Winkler B. Anal cancer and cervical cancer screening: key differences. Cancer Cytopathol. 2011;119(1):5–19.

70. U.S. Preventive Services Task Force. Screening for prostate cancer. United States Preventive Services Task Force; 2012 [24 Apr 2014]. Available from: http://www.uspreventiveservicestaskforce.org/ prostatecancerscreening.htm.

71. American Cancer Society. American Cancer Society recommendations for prostate cancer early detection. 2013. Updated 25 Feb 2014 [24 Apr 2014]. Available from: http://www.cancer.org/cancer/prostatecancer/ moreinformation/prostatecancerearlydetection/ prostate-cancer-early-detection-acs-recommendations.

72. IOM (Institute of Medicine). The health of lesbian, gay, bisexual, and transgender people: building a foundation for better understanding. Washington, DC: National Academies Press; 2011.

73. Gooren L, Morgentaler A. Prostate cancer incidence in orchidectomised male-to-female transsexual persons treated with oestrogens. Andrologia. 2014;46(10):1156–60.

74. Scherr D, Swindle PW, Scardino PT. National Comprehensive Cancer Network guidelines for the management of prostate cancer. Urology. 2003;61(2 Suppl 1):14–24.

75. U.S. Preventive Services Task Force. Screening for testicular cancer. 2011 [21 Apr 2014]. Available from: http://www.uspreventiveservicestaskforce.org/ uspstf/uspstest.htm.

76. Boehmer U, Ozonoff A, Miao X. An ecological approach to examine lung cancer disparities due to sexual orientation. Public Health. 2012;126(7): 605–12.

77. U.S. Preventive Services Task Force. Screening for lung cancer. United States Preventive Services Task Force; 2013 [24 Apr 2014]. Available from: http://www.uspreventiveservicestaskforce.org/uspstf/uspslung.htm.

78. Lee JGL, Griffin GK, Melvin CL. Tobacco use among sexual minorities in the USA, 1987 to May 2007: a systematic review. Tob Control. 2009;18(4):275–82.

79. National Guideline Clearinghouse. Guideline synthesis: screening and risk assessment for osteoporosis. Agency for Healthcare Research and Quality; 2008. Updated November 2012 [21 Apr 2014]. Available from: http://www.guideline.gov/syntheses/synthesis.aspx?id=38658&search=bone+density.

80. U.S. Preventive Services Task Force. Screening for intimate partner violence and abuse of elderly and vulnerable adults. 2013 [24 Apr 2014]. Available from: http://www.uspreventiveservicestaskforce.org/uspstf/uspsipv.htm.

81. Ard KL, Makadon HJ. Addressing intimate partner violence in lesbian, gay, bisexual, and transgender patients. J Gen Intern Med. 2011;26(8):930–3.

82. Basile KC, Hertz MF, Back SE. Intimate partner violence and sexual violence victimization assessment instruments for use in health care settings: version 1. In: Prevention CfDCa, editor. Atlanta, GA: National Center for Injury Prevention and Control; 2007.

83. Conron KJ, Mimiaga MJ, Landers SJ. A population-based study of sexual orientation identity and gender differences in adult health. Am J Public Health. 2010;100(10):1953–60.

84. Gruskin EP, Greenwood GL, Matevia M, Pollack LM, Bye LL. Disparities in smoking between the lesbian, gay, and bisexual population and the general population in California. Am J Public Health. 2007;97(8):1496–502.

85. McElroy JA, Everett KD, Zaniletti I. An examination of smoking behavior and opinions about smoke-free environments in a large sample of sexual and gender minority community members. Nicotine Tob Res. 2011;13(6):440–8.

86. Pizacani BA, Rohde K, Bushore C, Stark MJ, Maher JE, Dilley JA, et al. Smoking-related knowledge, attitudes and behaviors in the lesbian, gay and bisexual community: a population-based study from the US Pacific Northwest. Prev Med. 2009;48(6):555–61.

87. King BA, Dube SR, Tynan MA. Current tobacco use among adults in the United States: findings from the National Adult Tobacco Survey. Am J Public Health. 2012;102(11):e93–100.

88. Grant JM, Mottet LA, Tanis J. National transgender discrimination survey report on health and health care. Washington, DC: National Center for Transgender Equality; 2010.

89. Corliss HL, Wadler BM, Jun HJ, Rosario M, Wypij D, Frazier AL, et al. Sexual-orientation disparities in cigarette smoking in a longitudinal cohort study of adolescents. Nicotine Tob Res. 2013;15(1):213–22.

90. Austin SB, Ziyadeh N, Fisher LB, Kahn JA, Colditz GA, Frazier AL. Sexual orientation and tobacco use in a cohort study of US adolescent girls and boys. Arch Pediatr Adolesc Med. 2004;158(4):317–22.

91. Remafedi G, Jurek AM, Oakes JM. Sexual identity and tobacco use in a venue-based sample of adolescents and young adults. Am J Prev Med. 2008; 35(6):S463–70.

92. Dilley JA, Spigner C, Boysun MJ, Dent CW, Pizacani BA. Does tobacco industry marketing excessively impact lesbian, gay and bisexual communities? Tob Control. 2008;17(6):385–90.

93. Ling PM, Neilands TB, Glantz SA. Young adult smoking behavior: a national survey. Am J Prev Med. 2009;36(5):389–94.e2.

94. Smith EA, Thomson K, Offen N, Malone RE. "If you know you exist it's just marketing poison": meanings of tobacco industry targeting in the lesbian, gay, bisexual, and transgender community. Am J Public Health. 2008;98(6):996–1003.

95. Stevens P, Carlson LM, Hinman JM. An analysis of tobacco industry marketing to lesbian, gay, bisexual, and transgender (LGBT) populations: strategies for mainstream tobacco control and prevention. Health Promot Pract. 2004;5(3 suppl):129S–34.

96. Meyer IH. Prejudice, social stress, and mental health in lesbian, gay, and bisexual populations: conceptual issues and research evidence. Psychol Bull. 2003;129(5):674–97.

97. Blosnich J, Lee JG, Horn K. A systematic review of the aetiology of tobacco disparities for sexual minorities. Tob Control. 2013;22(2):66–73.

98. Amadio DM. Internalized heterosexism, alcohol use, and alcohol-related problems among lesbians and gay men. Addict Behav. 2006;31(7):1153–62.

99. Bontempo DE, D'Augelli AR. Effects of at-school victimization and sexual orientation on lesbian, gay, or bisexual youths' health risk behavior. J Adolesc Health. 2002;30(5):364–74.

100. Hatzenbuehler ML. How does sexual minority stigma "get under the skin"? A psychological mediation framework. Psychol Bull. 2009;135(5):707–30.

101. McCabe SE, Bostwick WB, Hughes TL, West BT, Boyd CJ. The relationship between discrimination and substance use disorders among lesbian, gay, and bisexual adults in the United States. Am J Public Health. 2010;100(10):1946–52.

102. Meyer IH. Minority stress and mental health in gay men. J Health Soc Behav. 1995;36(1):38–56.

103. Eliason MJ, Dibble SL, Gordon R, Soliz GB. The last drag: an evaluation of an LGBT-specific smoking intervention. J Homosex. 2012;59(6):864–78.

104. Matthews AK, Li CC, Kuhns LM, Tasker TB, Cesario JA. Results from a community-based smoking cessation treatment program for LGBT smokers. J Environ Public Health. 2013;2013:984508.

105. Wilsnack SC, Hughes TL, Johnson TP, Bostwick WB, Szalacha LA, Benson P, et al. Drinking and drinking-related problems among heterosexual and

sexual minority women. J Stud Alcohol Drugs. 2008;69(1):129–39.

106. Cochran SD, Ackerman D, Mays VM, Ross MW. Prevalence of non-medical drug use and dependence among homosexually active men and women in the US population. Addiction. 2004;99(8):989–98.

107. Herbst JH, Jacobs ED, Finlayson TJ, McKleroy VS, Neumann MS, Crepaz N. Estimating HIV prevalence and risk behaviors of transgender persons in the United States: a systematic review. AIDS Behav. 2008;12(1):1–17.

108. Wong W, Chaw JK, Kent CK, Klausner JD. Risk factors for early syphilis among gay and bisexual men seen in an STD clinic: San Francisco, 2002–2003. Sex Transm Dis. 2005;32(7):458–63.

109. Lea T, Reynolds R, de Wit J. Alcohol and club drug use among same-sex attracted young people: associations with frequenting the lesbian and gay scene and other bars and nightclubs. Subst Use Misuse. 2013;48(1–2):129–36.

110. Pebody R. Making it count briefing sheet 7: poppers. In: Aidsmap N, editor. Sigma Research; 2011. http://sigmaresearch.org.uk/files/MiC-briefing-7-Poppers.pdf

111. Colfax G, Coates TJ, Husnik MJ, Huang Y, Buchbinder S, Koblin B, et al. Longitudinal patterns of methamphetamine, popper (amyl nitrite), and cocaine use and high-risk sexual behavior among a cohort of San Francisco men who have sex with men. J Urban Health. 2005;82(1 Suppl 1):i62–70.

112. Santos GM, Coffin PO, Das M, Matheson T, DeMicco E, Raiford JL, et al. Dose-response associations between number and frequency of substance use and high-risk sexual behaviors among HIV-negative substance-using men who have sex with men (SUMSM) in San Francisco. J Acquir Immune Defic Syndr. 2013;63(4):540–4.

113. SAMHSA-HRSA Center for Integrated Health Solutions. Screening tools. Health Resources and Services Administration [24 Apr 2014]. Available from: http://www.integration.samhsa.gov/clinical-practice/screening-tools.

114. Patton ME, Su JR, Nelson R, Weinstock H. Primary and secondary syphilis—United States, 2005–2013. MMWR Morb Mortal Wkly Rep. 2014;63(18):402–6.

115. United States Public Health Service. Pre-exposure prophylaxis for the prevention of HIV infection in the United States—2014: a clinical practice guideline. 2014.

116. Centers for Disease Control and Prevention. Sexually transmitted disease treatment guidelines, 2010: special populations. Centers for Disease Control and Prevention; 2010 [21 Apr 2014]. Available from: http://www.cdc.gov/STD/treatment/2010/specialpops.htm.

117. Bernstein DI, Bellamy AR, Hook 3rd EW, Levin MJ, Wald A, Ewell MG, et al. Epidemiology, clinical presentation, and antibody response to primary infection with herpes simplex virus type 1 and type 2 in young women. Clin Infect Dis. 2013; 56(3):344–51.

118. Wald A. Genital HSV-1 infections. Sex Transm Infect. 2006;82(3):189–90.

119. Chan SK, Thornton LR, Chronister KJ, Meyer J, Wolverton M, Johnson CK, et al. Likely female-to-female sexual transmission of HIV—Texas, 2012. MMWR Morb Mortal Wkly Rep. 2014;63(10): 209–12.

120. Marrazzo JM, Koutsky LA, Eschenbach DA, Agnew K, Stine K, Hillier SL. Characterization of vaginal flora and bacterial vaginosis in women who have sex with women. J Infect Dis. 2002;185(9):1307–13.

121. Marrazzo JM, Stine K, Wald A. Prevalence and risk factors for infection with herpes simplex virus type-1 and -2 among lesbians. Sex Transm Dis. 2003;30(12): 890–5.

122. Gonzalez J, Williams Jr JW, Noel PH, Lee S. Adherence to mental health treatment in a primary care clinic. J Am Board Fam Pract. 2005;18(2): 87–96.

123. Roca M, Gili M, Garcia-Garcia M, Salva J, Vives M, Garcia Campayo J, et al. Prevalence and comorbidity of common mental disorders in primary care. J Affect Disord. 2009;119(1–3):52–8.

124. Savin-Williams RC. Verbal and physical abuse as stressors in the lives of lesbian, gay male, and bisexual youths: associations with school problems, running away, substance abuse, prostitution, and suicide. J Consult Clin Psychol. 1994;62(2): 261–9.

125. U.S. Preventive Services Task Force. Depression in Adults: Screening. United States Preventive Services Task Force; 2009 [29 Oct 2015]. Available from: http://www.uspreventiveservicestaskforce.org/Page/Document/RecommendationStatementFinal/depression-inadults-screening.

126. Frost DM, Lehavot K, Meyer IH. Minority stress and physical health among sexual minority individuals. J Behav Med. 2015;38:1–8.

127. Krehely J. How to close the LGBT health disparities gap: disparities by race and ethnicity. Center for American Progress; 2009 [21 Apr 2014]. Available from: http://www.americanprogress.org/issues/2009/12/lgbt_health_disparities.html.

128. American Academy of Family Physicians. Policies & recommendations: family, definition of. 2014 [21 Apr 2014]. Available from: http://www.aafp.org/about/policies/all/family-definition.html.

129. Movement Advancement Project. All children matter: how legal and social inequalities hurt LGBT families (Full Report). 2011.

130. Harrison AE, Silenzio VM. Comprehensive care of lesbian and gay patients and families. Prim Care. 1996;23(1):31–46.

131. Lang AJ. Brief intervention for co-occurring anxiety and depression in primary care: a pilot study. Int J Psychiatry Med. 2003;33(2):141–54.

132. Roy-Byrne P, Veitengruber JP, Bystritsky A, Edlund MJ, Sullivan G, Craske MG, et al. Brief intervention for anxiety in primary care patients. J Am Board Fam Med. 2009;22(2):175–86.

133. Center for Substance Abuse Treatment. Brief interventions and brief therapies for substance abuse. Rockville, MD; 1999. Contract no: 34.

134. Prochaska JO, DiClemente CC, Norcross JC. In search of how people change. Applications to addictive behaviors. Am Psychol. 1992;47(9): 1102–14.

135. Saulnier CF. Deciding who to see: lesbians discuss their preferences in health and mental health care providers. Soc Work. 2002;47(4):355–65.

136. Sinding C, Barnoff L, Grassau P. Homophobia and heterosexism in cancer care: the experiences of lesbians. Can J Nurs Res. 2004;36(4):170–88.

137. East JA, El Rayess F. Pediatricians' approach to the health care of lesbian, gay, and bisexual youth. J Adolesc Health. 1998;23(4):191–3.

138. Eliason MJ, Hughes T. Treatment counselor's attitudes about lesbian, gay, bisexual, and transgendered clients: urban vs. rural settings. Subst Use Misuse. 2004;39(4):625–44.

139. Lena SM, Wiebe T, Ingram S, Jabbour M. Pediatricians' knowledge, perceptions, and attitudes towards providing health care for lesbian, gay, and bisexual adolescents. Ann R Coll Physicians Surg Can. 2002;35(7):406–10.

140. Sanchez NF, Rabatin J, Sanchez JP, Hubbard S, Kalet A. Medical students' ability to care for lesbian, gay, bisexual, and transgendered patients. Fam Med. 2006;38(1):21–7.

141. GLMA. Find a provider. [25 Apr 2014]. Available from: http://www.glma.org/index.cfm?fuseaction=Page.viewPage&pageId=939&grandparentID=534&parentID=938&nodeID=1.

142. Vanderbilt University School of Medicine. Program for LGBTI health. Nashville, TN: Vanderbilt University; 2014 [25 Apr 2014]. Available from: https://medschool.vanderbilt.edu/lgbti/.

143. Out Proud and Healthy in Missouri. LGBT Tobacco Project. [12 Sept 2013]. Available from: http://www.outproudandhealthy.org/research-2/tobacco/.

144. Stablein T, Hall JL, Nissenbaum H, Anthony TD. Gay males and electronic health records: privacy perceptions, age, and negotiating stigma. Paper presented at the annual meeting of the American Sociological Association Annual Meeting, Colorado Convention Center and Hyatt Regency, Denver, CO; 2012.

145. Bradford J, Cahill S, Grasso C, Makadon HJ. Policy focus: how to gather data on sexual orientation and gender identity in clinical settings. Boston, MA: Fenway Health; 2012.147.

# LGBT Parenting

Christopher E. Harris

## Learning Objectives

- Identify at least three unique parenting challenges faced by LGBT couples and at least three opportunities to overcome these challenges (*KP4*, *PC5*, *SBP1*)
- Describe outcomes of children raised by LGBT parents (*KP3*)
- List the current recommendations from national medical societies regarding LGBT parenting (*PC6*, *PBL13*)

As the struggle for LGBT rights has progressed over the past half century, parenting issues have also received increasing attention. In part, this is due to LGBT people acknowledging sexual orientation and gender identity throughout the life span. This may include coming out after marriage to an opposite sex partner and having children. This then leads to the stories that abound of parents coming out to children at all ages. Unfortunately, this often occurs with dissolution of a marriage and the consequent heartbreak for all parties involved. However, as LGBT people have established relationships earlier in life, many have sought to bring children into the family in a purposeful and well considered fashion. This is a profound change and represents part of broader social acceptance. As proof, in 2013, a nationwide survey estimated that 28 % of male same sex couples were raising children, which had grown considerably from the 5 % estimate in 1990 [1, 2]. It can be said that growth in gay male parenting is proof of establishing this as part of their life course trajectory, fulfilling the developmental task of adulthood proposed by Erikson—generativity (creating contributions that will last beyond the present) [3]. In addition, lesbian parenting has also grown over the recent decades, but not nearly as much. Data show that 22–28 % of lesbian households in 1990 had children compared to 35 % in 2010 [2]. Research from the 2011 National Transgender Discrimination Survey demonstrates that 38 % of transgender individuals are parents [4]. Overall, many LGBT people are parenting with substantial growth over the past decade.

However, in spite of this growth, controversy continues to exist about LGBT parenting. In particular, as society discusses same-sex marriage, the key question is almost always about the effect upon the children. This affects families on a deeply personal and emotional level as these concerns are often used in custody battles to prevent LGBT people from obtaining custody or, perhaps, even having any access to their children.

C.E. Harris, M.D. (✉)
Department of Pediatrics, Cedars Sinai Medical Center, 8700 Beverly Blvd., NT-4230, Los Angeles, CA 90048, USA
e-mail: christopher.harris@cshs.org

© Springer International Publishing Switzerland 2016
K.L. Eckstrand, J.M. Ehrenfeld (eds.), *Lesbian, Gay, Bisexual, and Transgender Healthcare*,
DOI 10.1007/978-3-319-19752-4_9

In recent years, the study by Mark Regnerus attempted to show, using a population based approach, negative outcomes for children who had one parent in a "same-sex romantic relationship" at some point during childhood [5]. However, his study used improper sampling technique and the results have been called into question. More important, the ethics of the study itself has been found wanting as the funders of the study directed the methods and the results of the research [6]. However, in spite of this, these results has been used to justify animus toward LGBT people throughout the world. Because of concern 'for the children', it is important that physicians and other healthcare providers be conversant in the issues discussed in this chapter.

As LGBT people come out and establish relationships, children arrive by various means. Surrogacy is the process of carrying a pregnancy for intended parents. This may involve transfer of an embryo created by *in vitro* fertilization such that the child is not related to the surrogate. In traditional surrogacy, the fertilization may occur naturally or artificially with the baby being related to the woman carrying the fetus to delivery. Gestational surrogacy involves fertilization of an egg from a donor with sperm that may or may not belong to the father. Surrogacy is performed with the assistance of an agency that can assist with both medical and legal issues. Much case law has been established over the years that clearly delineate the rights and responsibilities for all parties concerned.

Adoption has been known as a way to create families and can also take place through various forms. Agency adoptions employ the services of a state licensed organization that will interview and assess the prospective parent for the demands of childrearing. A home study is also done to ensure that child safety measures are in place in the domicile. Often, health and financial assessments may be needed along with letters of recommendation. Once completed, a family may be deemed suitable to adopt. Some agencies also work within the foster care system to assist children who have been brought into the care of the state. Once parental rights have been terminated, these children are then made available for adoption.

## Demographics of LGBT Parenting

Data provided by the Williams Institute estimate that 37 % of LGBT identified individuals have had a child at some time in their lives. It is estimated that three million LGBT Americans have a child; conversely as many as six million American children or adults have had an LGBT parent. Same sex couples are four times more likely than their different sex counterparts to be raising an adopted child. In addition, LGBT couples are six times more likely to be raising foster children. Nearly 40 % of persons in same-sex couples raising children are persons of color. Children of lesbian or gay couples are also more likely to be members of racial or ethnic minorities. Among non-white individuals in same sex couples, one-third are raising a child compared to 18 % of their white counterparts [1].

With regard to geography of LGBT parents, it is found that these families are most common in the South, Mountain West and Midwest areas of the US. In particular, the states with the highest proportions of same sex couples with children are Mississippi, Wyoming, Alaska, Idaho and Montana. LGBT families are found in 96 % of US counties [1].

Economic factors must also be considered for LGBT families. Analysis of data gathered in the Gallup Daily Tracking Survey in 2012 show that there are some characteristics of LGBT families that are associated with a greater likelihood of being in poverty. Based on this national data set, LGBT families are more likely to be female, younger and be a member of a racial or ethnic minority. In particular, single and married LGBT adults raising children were more likely to report incomes less than the poverty threshold [1]. In addition, certain governmental programs established to assist families under financial stress may not provide services to LGBT families due to the official definition of 'family'. For example, Temporary Assistance for Needy Families only recognizes **legal** parents of a child or children when considering the 'assistance unit'. Given the variety of state laws on gay marriage, obviously, this can create major hardship for parents and children alike [7].

## Legal Issues for LGBT Families

Most regulation of parenting rights and responsibilities is codified in state law. This then leads to wide variation for LGBT families. For example, depending upon the state, dissolution of a relationship may be impossible if parents have gotten married in a state that recognizes same sex marriage, but wish to divorce in the home state which does not. In this instance, simple access to the court is denied, contrary to the ideals of due process and equal access embodied in the Constitution. Further, there are many states that outlaw two parent adoptions by LGBT couples. The same is true for families that wish to provide foster care where prohibitions may be absolute.

In the case of surrogacy, some states provide legal recognition as a parent to the person who donated either egg or sperm; certainly this is contrary to the wishes of the parents involved. There is also case law where the legality of a surrogacy contract is questioned, leading to the potential of children being removed from the home of the intended parent. The best known case occurred in New Jersey, Robinson vs. Hollingsworth [8]. This case lasted for years in the New Jersey Superior Court. The eventual finding was that contracts for surrogacy were invalid in New Jersey. Fortunately, however, the court found that, in order to preserve the stability of the home for the girls, it was best for them to remain with the same-sex parents. See Fig. 9.1.

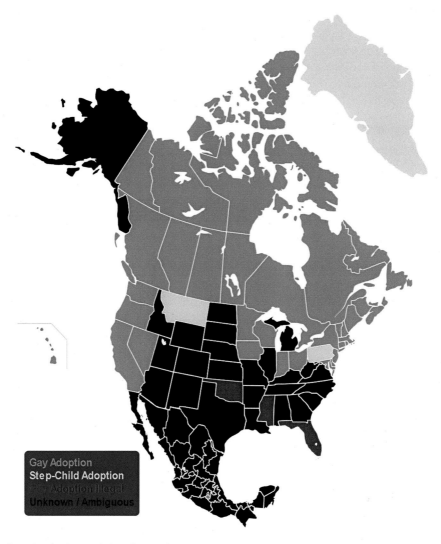

**Fig. 9.1**   Gay adoption in North America as of December 2013 (image courtesy, J. Ehrenfeld)

Also, in situations involving end of life and survivorship, Social Security benefits and veterans' survivor benefits may not automatically be transferred to the surviving spouse. This, obviously, may have major implications for the financial well-being of a family after a tragic loss. In particular, this may leave children without health insurance benefits or even access to the surviving spouse if the couple lived in a state without legal recognition of the relationship. Other benefits that automatically accrue to a married spouse include the ability to provide consent for medical care on a routine or emergent basis. In addition, many couples have reported that travel as a same-sex couple involves the constant need to provide documentation of the relationships in the family. Sometimes, even with proof of birth certificates and legal orders, various officials may still harbor suspicion about the family makeup.

Many families with significant immigration challenges are parenting. Data analyzed over the past decade show that nearly 80,000 binational families, dual non-citizen families and dual citizen families are raising 40,700 children [9]. Due to current US immigration policy, opposite sex married couples are treated differently than same-sex couples. Couples with one citizen or permanent resident would benefit from procedures that expedite application for the non-citizen partner. Legislation has been proposed (Uniting American Families Act) in both the US House and Senate that would change immigration regulations to make a same sex partner equivalent to spouse. Hopefully, as more states grant LGBT couples equivalent legal status in marriage, the tide will shift and this legislation will pass.

In summary, there are a multitude of laws that deny same sex couples equality when compared to opposite sex couples. Ranging from healthcare to taxation, the impact of this unequal treatment is especially marked on those who have no access to petition for proper protection. Indeed, by their very nature, these rules denigrate and demean LGBT families. Much effort must go toward ensuring the children in these families that their family constellation is just as valid and stable as other families in society. Like all children, they must rely on parents for assistance in

all things; parents will feel tremendous stress by not being able to ensure a safe and secure family environment.

## Outcomes for Children

Given that children exist within LGBT families, it is indeed reasonable to ask how children fare in this environment. As clinicians, our goal is to ensure that children have optimal physical, emotional and social health. Obviously, we would want to base our assessment on rigorous investigation using the best scientific methods. Fortunately, several researchers have accepted this challenge and provide valuable insight into the key question: How do the children do?

Dr. Nanette Gartrell has provided valuable insight into this question with the National Longitudinal Lesbian Family Study. This study began in 1986 by selecting a cohort of families comprised of lesbian mothers with children conceived by artificial insemination. All mothers identified as lesbian at the time of enrollment. Studied as toddlers, 5 year olds, 10 year olds and as adolescents, these young people have provided remarkable data in areas such as health, division of household labor, relationship satisfaction, parenting style and experience of discrimination. As toddlers, mothers had children who were, in general, very healthy. They found that relationships with extended family had improved once the children were born; conversely, career became less important as children were added [10]. As 5 year olds, the mothers again reported that the children were healthy and developing normally. The stress of parenting was acknowledged by many mothers with some of the families having divorced in the 3 year interval. Children had experienced some homophobic attitudes and mothers had been deliberate in providing children with tools to handle this discrimination. They also had sought out schools that were diverse in many ways; indeed, children had diverse groups of friends as a result [11]. When the children had reached 10 years of age, individual personal interviews were performed using a standard psychological instrument. In addition, the Child Behavior Checklist was given to the children's mother and used to assess competencies and behavioral/emotional problems. Domains analyzed include school functioning and extracurricular activities, such as sports and hobbies. Based on the mothers' report, the children in the study were developmentally normal. The only difference noted was that the girls in the study group had lower scores on the Externalizing behavior scale, indicating fewer problems in this area. More than 40 % of the children had experienced homophobic attitudes about their family; they were very well prepared with responses to insults made. The mothers also reported that they also spoke up when racist or sexist remarks were uttered in their presence [12]. In summary, the youngsters were resilient and thriving after the first decade of life.

The next time point for assessment of the children occurred at 17 years; again the Child Behavior Checklist was used to assess social functioning as well as potential emotional or behavioral problems. Interviews with the mothers and an online questionnaire of the adolescents themselves showed that there was higher rating on social, academic and total competences areas and less social, rule-breaking, aggressive and problem behavior than an age matched control group of American teenagers [13]. The research team has also investigated the sexual behaviors and sexual orientation of the teens, using the Kinsey scale [14]. None of the teens had been sexually abused. When assessing the age of first sexual contact, the researchers found that, compared to the national sample, the children of the lesbian couples were significantly older at first sexual contact. None of the girls of lesbian parents had become pregnant as late teens, though the difference from the representative sample was not statistically significant. Overall, this research is vitally important in show that the children of lesbian mothers are well adjusted emotionally and have normal maturation in matters of sexual development.

Other researchers have looked at the well being of adults reared by lesbian, gay and bisexual parents. Dr. Patterson and colleagues have evaluated how social climate of a given locale affects levels of stress in the offspring of gay and bisexual people. Studying 91 adults raised by non-heterosexual parents, it was found that this group predominantly was reared by coupled lesbian mothers. The sexual orientation of the parent became known early in life (~7 years). The educational attainment of the subjects was high with approximately two-thirds having a college degree. Positive psychological adjustment was routinely noted in the subjects; in particular, average to high life satisfaction was found. Results showed that two particular factors correlated with social climate. First, voting patterns reflecting a majority Democratic zip code, favorable local policies regarding LGB adoption, hate crimes and employment non-discrimination showed a positive correlation. Second, the demographic components of the local population (size of the overall population along with number and percentage of households headed by same-sex couples) combined to create a second factor that correlated with a favorable social climate. These findings certainly correlate with those suggested by theories regarding minority stress—members of minority groups living in more tolerant areas are subjected to less stress compared to those living in areas with negative social climate [15].

Another study using the National Longitudinal Study of Adolescent Health data set evaluated the adjustment of teens growing up in a lesbian-headed household. They were compared to a matched group living with opposite sex parents. There were no significant differences in psychological well-being (self-esteem, anxiety), measures of school outcome (grades, difficulties in school), or measures of family relationships [13]. Regarding the developmental tasks of adolescents, the teens raised by lesbian women were as likely to have been in a romantic relationship over the prior 18 months. There were no significant differences in peer relationships, self-reported use of substances or peer victimization between the two groups of teens [14]. In summary, this investigation, using a large sample representative sample of adolescents from across the US, shows that having same-sex parents is associated with normal developmental outcomes.

The considered conclusion of much research all confirm the fact that children of LGBT parents do very well in multiple spheres of life. No behavioral problems are found. Academically, the children are as intelligent as peers. In particular, regarding sexual orientation and gender identity, the great concern that the children will be somehow harmed by their parents is proven patently false. In addition, the sexual orientation and gender identity conforms to statistical norms. These data should ensure that all who must make decisions about child welfare will consider factors other than the sexual orientation of the parents involved.

## Marriage and Health

In June 2013, the United States Supreme Court had a docket that would forever change the landscape of American culture. Hearing the cases of *Hollingsworth vs. Perry* and *United States vs. Windsor*, the court had to wander into the thicket of society's approval or approbation of same-sex marriage. The case of *United States vs. Windsor* decided that the Defense of Marriage Act violated the Due Process Clause of the Fifth Amendment of the Constitution [16]. Stating poetically,

> The differentiation (of marriages) demeans the couple…whose relationship the State has sought to dignify….it humiliates tens of thousands of children now being raised by same-sex couples. The law in question makes it even more difficult for the children to understand the integrity and closeness of their own family and its concord with other families in their community and in their daily lives…Under DOMA, same-sex married couples have their lives burdened, by reason of government decree, in visible and public ways. By its great reach, DOMA touches many aspects of married and family life, from the mundane to the profound.

The effect of this ruling has been a rapid and steady progression of rulings declaring that same-sex marriages are proper for state recognition. The speed with which these rulings have occurred is nearly dizzying. Also, it has been associated with major changes in how society views same-sex marriage. Multiple polls by various public opinion organizations confirm that the majority of Americans now approve of same-sex marriage. But does this have any bearing on health?

In a commentary for the American Journal of Public Health, Dr. Buffie delineates how unequal treatment leads to adverse health outcomes and why marriage is important in ameliorating those outcomes [17]. The continuous stress of dealing with one's minority status in our society leads persons to devalue themselves as one's stature in society is continually questioned. Often the invisibility of lesbian and gay people compounds this stress. Internalizing this stress can then lead to behaviors that are self-destructive. Conversely, in a very concrete fashion, marriage improves health by increasing access to health insurance. Many companies and municipalities reserve spousal insurance benefits for those who are civilly married. Perhaps, even more importantly, the psychology of marriage is vital, also. In reviewing data collected by Massachusetts, the first state to recognize same-sex marriage, members of married same sex couples stated that they felt more committed to their partners after having been accorded official state recognition. Children in these families overwhelmingly felt happier and better off after receiving society's approval. Other data show that married same-sex couples are more connected to families of origin. Married couples, whether gay or straight, are less depressed and show less anxiety. Couples who have wed are less likely to engage in behavior that is associated with sexually transmitted infection. This then shows the multiple ways that marriage improves society—the couple is strengthened, the children are happier, families are more connected and, in general, health is improved.

## Healthcare Organization Statements on LGBT Parenting

Many different healthcare organizations have made statements regarding same-sex parenting.

### American Medical Association
Health Care Disparities in Same Sex Partner Households Our American Medical Association: (1) recognizes that denying civil marriage based on sexual orientation is discriminatory and

imposes harmful stigma on gay and lesbian individuals and couples and their families; (2) recognizes that exclusion from civil marriage contributes to health care disparities affecting same-sex households; (3) will work to reduce health care disparities among members of same-sex households including minor children; and (4) will support measures providing same-sex households with the same rights and privileges to health care, health insurance, and survivor benefits, as afforded opposite-sex households [18].

Health Disparities Among Gay, Lesbian, Bisexual and Transgender Families Our AMA will work to reduce the health disparities suffered because of unequal treatment of minor children and same sex parents in same sex households by supporting equality in laws affecting health care of members in same sex partner households and their dependent children [19].

Partner Co-adoption Our AMA will support legislative and other efforts to allow the adoption of a child by the same-sex partner, or opposite sex non-married partner, who functions as a second parent or co-parent to that child [20].

## American Academy of Pediatrics

Coparent or Second-Parent Adoption by Same-Sex Parents …Children born or adopted into families headed by partners who are of the same sex usually have only 1 biologic or adoptive legal parent. The other partner in a parental role is called the "coparent" or "second parent." Because these families and children need the permanence and security that are provided by having 2 fully sanctioned and legally defined parents, the Academy supports the legal adoption of children by coparents or second parents. Denying legal parent status through adoption to coparents or second parents prevents these children from enjoying the psychologic and legal security that comes from having 2 willing, capable, and loving parents… [21]

Promoting the Well-Being of Children Whose Parents Are Gay or Lesbian The AAP works to ensure that public policies help all parents, regardless of sexual orientation and other characteristics, to build and maintain strong, stable and healthy families that are able to meet the needs of their children. In particular, the AAP supports:

1. Marriage equality for all capable and consenting couples, including those who are of the same gender, as a means of guaranteeing all federal and state rights and benefits and long-term security for their children.
2. Adoption by single parents, coparents adopting together or a second parent when 1 parent is already a legal parent by birth or adoption, without regard to the sexual orientation of the adoptive parent(s).
3. Foster care placement for eligible children to qualified adults without regard to their sexual orientation [22].

## American Psychiatric Association

The American Psychiatric Association supports same-sex marriage as being advantageous to the mental health of same-sex couples and supports legal recognition of the right for same-sex couples to marry, adopt and co-parent. [23].

## American Psychological Association

Child Custody or Placement The sex, gender identity, or sexual orientation of natural, or prospective adoptive or foster parents should not be the sole or primary variable considered in custody or placement cases [24].

Sexual Orientation & Marriage …Therefore be it resolved that the APA believes that it is unfair and discriminatory to deny same-sex couples legal access to civil marriage and to all its attendant benefits, rights, and privileges;

Therefore be it further resolved that APA shall take a leadership role in opposing all discrimination in legal benefits, rights, and privileges against same-sex couples;

Therefore be it further resolved that APA encourages psychologists to act to eliminate all discrimination against same-sex couples in their practice, research, education and training (American Psychological Association, 2002);

Therefore be it further resolved that the APA shall provide scientific and educational resources that inform public discussion and public policy development regarding sexual orientation and marriage and that assist its members, divisions, and affiliated state, provincial, and territorial psychological associations [25].

Sexual Orientation, Parents, & Children Therefore be it resolved that the APA opposes any discrimination based on sexual orientation in matters of adoption, child custody and visitation, foster care, and reproductive health services;

> Therefore be it further resolved that the APA believes that children reared by a same-sex couple benefit from legal ties to each parent; Therefore be it further resolved that the APA supports the protection of parent-child relationships through the legalization of joint adoptions and second parent adoptions of children being reared by same-sex couples; Therefore be it further resolved that APA shall take a leadership role in opposing all discrimination based on sexual orientation in matters of adoption, child custody and visitation, foster care, and reproductive health services; Therefore be it further resolved that APA encourages psychologists to act to eliminate all discrimination based on sexual orientation in matters of adoption, child custody and visitation, foster care, and reproductive health services in their practice, research, education and training (American Psychological Association, 2002);
> Therefore be it further resolved that the APA shall provide scientific and educational resources that inform public discussion and public policy development regarding discrimination based on sexual orientation in matters of adoption, child custody and visitation, foster care, and reproductive health services and that assist its members, divisions, and affiliated state, provincial, and territorial psychological associations [25].

Resolution on Marriage Equality for Same-Sex CouplesTherefore be it resolved that the American Psychological Association supports full marriage equality for same-sex couples;

> Be it further resolved that the American Psychological Association reiterates its opposition to ballot measures, statutes, constitutional amendments, and other forms of discriminatory policy aimed at limiting lesbian, gay, and bisexual people's access to legal protections for their human rights, including such measures as those that deny same-sex couples the right to marry;
> Be it further resolved that the American Psychological Association calls on state governments to repeal all measures that deny same-sex couples the right to civil marriage and to enact laws to provide full marriage equality to same-sex couples;
> Be it further resolved that the American Psychological Association calls on the federal government to extend full recognition to legally married same-sex couples, and to accord them all of the rights, benefits, and responsibilities that it provides to legally married different-sex couples;
> Be it further resolved that the American Psychological Association encourages psychologists and other behavioral scientists to conduct

quality research that extends our understanding of the lesbian, gay, and bisexual population, including the role of close relationships and family formation on the health and well-being of lesbian, gay, and bisexual adults and youths;
Be it further resolved that the American Psychological Association encourages psychologists and other professionals with appropriate knowledge to take the lead in developing interventions and in educating the public to reduce prejudice and discrimination and to help ameliorate the negative effects of stigma;
Be it further resolved that the American Psychological Association will work with government and private funding agencies to promote such research and interventions to improve the health and well-being of lesbian, gay, and bisexual people [26].

## American Academy of Child and Adolescent Psychiatry

> **Gay, Lesbian, Bisexual, or Transgender Parents.** All decisions relating to custody and parental rights should rest on the interest of the child. There is no evidence to suggest or support that parents who are lesbian, gay, bisexual, or transgender are per se _**superior or inferior**_ from or deficient in parenting skills, child-centered concerns, and parent-child attachments when compared with heterosexual parents. There is no _**credible evidence that shows**_ that a parent's sexual orientation or gender identity will adversely affect the development of the child.
> Lesbian, gay, bisexual, or transgender individuals historically have faced more rigorous scrutiny than heterosexual people regarding their rights to be or become parents. The American Academy of Child & Adolescent Psychiatry opposes any discrimination based on sexual orientation or gender identity against individuals in regard to their rights as custodial, foster, or adoptive parents [27].

## Summary

LGBT people have experienced tremendous growth in visibility over the past generation. For many LGBT people, the dream of children seemed to vanish during the coming out process; time, however, has past, society has changed and, through concerted effort and expense, family has been created. For others, coming out after marriage and children was part of a particular life course. Nonetheless, for all of these variously constructed families, children of LGBT parents are a reality. Many social scientists have taken on the task of asking the question: Are the children ok? Overwhelmingly, the answer is affirmingly positive. They have normal peers. They do well in school. They aren't troubled emotionally or psychologically. Most importantly, they grow up to be accepting people who love their parents. We should wish this for ALL of our children.

## References

1. Gates GJ. LGBT parenting in the United States. Los Angeles, CA: Williams Institute at UCLA Law School; 2013. http://williamsinstitute.law.ucla.edu/wp-content/uploads/LGBT-Parenting.pdf.
2. Bradford J, Barrett K, Honnold JA. The 2000 census and same-sex households: a user's guide. New York: The National Gay and Lesbian Task Force Policy Institute, The Survey and Evaluation Research Laboratory, and The Fenway Institute; 2002. www.ngltf.org.
3. Erikson JM, Erikson EH. The Life Cycle Completed. New York, NY: WW Norton; 1997.
4. National Center for Transgender Equality and National Gay and Lesbian Task Force. Injustice at Every Turn: A Report of the National Transgender Discrimination Survey. http://www.thetaskforce.org/static_html/downloads/reports/reports/ntds_full.pdf. Published on February 4, 2011. Accessed December 3, 2013.
5. Regnerus, M. How different are the adult children of parents who have same-sex relationships? Findings from the New Family Structures Study. *Soc Sci Res* 2012; 41(4): 752–70.
6. The Regnerus Fallout. Human Rights Campaign. http://www.regnerusfallout.org/ Accessed November 15, 2015.
7. Movement Advancement Project, Family Equality Council and Center for American Progress, "All Children Matter: How Legal and Social Inequalities Hurt LGBT Families, " October 2011, (Condensed Version).
8. N.J. gay couple fight for custody of twin 5-year-old girls. NJ.com http://www.nj.com/news/index.ssf/2011/12/nj_gay_couple_fight_for_custod.html Accessed January 17, 2014.
9. Konnoth CJ, Gates GJ. Same-sex couples and immigration in the United States. Williams Institute, UCLA; May 2014. Retrieved from http://williamsinstitute.law.ucla.edu/wp-content/uploads/Gates-Konnoth-Binational-Report-Nov-2011.pdf.
10. Gartrell N, Banks A, Hamilton J, et al. The National Lesbian Family Study: 2. Interviews with mothers of toddlers. *Am J Orthopsychiatry* 1999;69(3): 362–369.
11. Gartrell N, Banks A, Reed N, et al. The National Lesbian Family Study: 3. Interviews with mothers of five-year-olds. *Am J Orthopsychiatry* 2000; 70(4):542–548.
12. Gartrell N, Rodas C, Deck A, et al. The USA National Lesbian Family Study: Interviews with Mothers of 10-Year-Olds. *Feminism & Psychology* 2006;16(2):175–192.
13. Gartrell N, Bos H. US National Longitudinal Lesbian Family Study: Psychological Adjustment of 17-Year-Old Adolescents. *Pediatrics* 2010; 126(1):28–36.
14. Gartrell NK, Bos HMW, Goldberg NG. Adolescents of the U.S. National Longitudinal Lesbian Family Study: sexual orientation, sexual behavior, and sexual risk exposure. *Arch Sex Behav* 2011;40(6): 1199–209.
15. Lick DJ, Tornello SL, Riskind RG, et al. Social Climate for Sexual Minorities Predicts Well-Being Among Heterosexual Offspring of Lesbian and Gay Parents. *Sex Res Soc Policy* 2012;9:99–112.
16. United States vs. Windsor, 570 U.S. ____(2013). (Docket NO. 12–307).
17. Buffie WC. Public Health Implications of Same-Sex Marriage. *Am J Public Health* 2011;101(6): 986–90.
18. Health Care Disparities in Same Sex Partner Households. American Medical Association. https://www.amaassn. org/ssl3/ecomm/PolicyFinderForm.pl?site=www.ama-assn.org&uri=/resources/html/PolicyFinder/policyfiles/HnE/H-65.973.HTM
19. Health Disparities Among Gay, Lesbian, Bisexual and Transgender Families. American Medical Association. https://www.amaassn.org/ssl3/ecomm/PolicyFinderForm.pl?site=www.ama-assn.org&uri=/resources/html/PolicyFinder/policyfiles/DIR/D-65.995.HTM
20. Partner Co-Adoption. American Medical Assocation. https://www.ama-assn.org/ssl3/ecomm/PolicyFinderForm.pl?site=www.amaassn.org&uri=%2fresources%2fhtml%2fPolicyFinder%2fpolicyfiles%2fHnE%2fH-60.940.HTM.
21. Coparent or Second-Parent Adoption by Same-Sex Parents. Pediatrics 2002;109(2):339–40.
22. Promoting the Well-being of Children whose Parents are Gay or Lesbian. Pediatrics 2013; 131(4):827–30
23. Position Statement on Issues Related to Homosexuality. American Psychiatric Association. http://www.psychiatry.org/File%20Library/Learn/Archives/Position-2013-Homosexuality.pdf. Retrieved November 23, 2015.
24. Conger, J.J. (1977). Proceedings of the American Psychological Association, Incorporated, for the year 1976: Minutes of the Annual Meeting of the Council of Representatives. *American Psychologist, 32*, 408–438.

25. Paige, R.U. (2005). Proceedings of the American Psychological Association, Incorporated, for the legislative year 2004. Minutes of the meeting of the Council of Representatives July 28 & 30, 2004, Honolulu, HI

26. Resolution on Marriage Equality for Same Sex Couples. American Psychological Association. http://www.apa.org/about/policy/samesex.aspx. Retrieved December 3, 2013.

27. Gay, Lesbian, Bisexual, or Transgender Parents. American Academy of Child & Adolescent Psychiatry. http://www.aacap.org/AACAP/Policy_Statements/2008/Gay_Lesbian_Bisexual_or_Transgender_Parents.aspx. Retrieved December 3, 2013.

# Intimate Partner Violence

## Tulsi Roy

## Purpose

The purpose of this chapter is to define intimate partner violence, explore the issues around this complex and sensitive topic, outline challenges unique to LGBT communities, and provide clinicians guidance to confront and address this public health challenge.

## Learning Objectives

After reading this chapter, learners will be able to:

- Discuss the risk factors, effects on health, and public health impact that intimate partner violence (IPV) has on LGBT communities (PC5)
- Identify at least three differences in individual and structural challenges in addressing IPV for same-sex relationships compared to opposite-sex relationships (KP4, SBP1)
- Discuss forms of abuse and social challenges exclusively faced by transgender individuals (KP3, PC3, SPB4)
- Discuss opportunities for healthcare providers to communicate with LGBT patients, address, and document concerns about IPV (ICS1, ICS2)

T. Roy, M.Sc., M.D. (✉)
University of Chicago Medical Center, Chicago, IL, USA
e-mail: Tulsi.roy@uchospitals.edu

## Introduction

Intimate partner violence (IPV) is defined as the physical, emotional, psychological, or sexual harm inflicted on an individual by a current or former partner or spouse. IPV describes patterns of abusive behavior used by one partner to gain or maintain control over the other, including physical and sexual violence or threats of violence, social isolation, psychological aggression, stalking, economic deprivation, neglect, and controlling a partner's sexual or reproductive health. According to the National Intimate Partner and Sexual Violence Survey (NIPSVS), more than one in three women (35.6 %) and more than one in four men (28.5 %) in the United States have experienced rape, physical violence, and/or stalking by an intimate partner in their lifetime [1]. It is estimated that the costs of intimate partner rape, physical assault, and stalking exceed $5.8 billion each year, nearly $4.1 billion of which is for direct medical and mental health care services. Many survivors of these forms of violence can experience physical injury, mental health consequences such as depression, anxiety, low self-esteem, and suicide attempts, and physical health consequences such as gastrointestinal disorders, substance abuse, sexually transmitted diseases, and gynecological or pregnancy complications [1]. These consequences can lead to hospitalization, homelessness, disability, or death.

© Springer International Publishing Switzerland 2016
K.L. Eckstrand, J.M. Ehrenfeld (eds.), *Lesbian, Gay, Bisexual, and Transgender Healthcare*,
DOI 10.1007/978-3-319-19752-4_10

The effects of IPV are wide reaching, affecting not just those abused, but also their families, friends, businesses, and economic productivity. The total costs of IPV include nearly $0.9 billion in lost productivity from paid work and household chores for those suffering from nonfatal IPV and $0.9 billion in lifetime earnings lost by victims of IPV homicide [2]. Though IPV has been a serious and preventable public health issue for decades, until a significant grassroots movement gained momentum in the late 1970s and 1980s, little in the way of research or policy addressed it, due in part to the lack of awareness and stigma surrounding IPV and abuse [3]. Furthermore, despite the significant burden of violence, only limited policies, procedures, and programs have been enacted to address this costly and preventable public health challenge.

The LGBT community in particular faces unique challenges regarding IPV. Research suggests that prevalence of IPV is at least as high for same-sex couples compared to their opposite-sex counterparts [4]. Same-sex IPV is more likely to go unacknowledged and less likely to be addressed adequately by healthcare providers, law and policy makers, educators, and social services.

Traditionally, addressing IPV was under the exclusive purview of the legal system and penal code, but as focus shifts towards a more holistic approach to IPV prevention and treatment of individuals suffering from abuse social workers and healthcare providers serve a critical role as first-line responders to survivors. History, however, reflects a failure on the part of physicians to adequately address IPV, particularly for the LGBT community, due to lack of cultural competency, paucity of resources, and incomplete or absent educational tools. This chapter will explore the issues around this complex and sensitive topic, outline challenges unique to LGBT communities, and provide clinicians guidance to confront and address this public health challenge.

## Defining Abuse

The lack of standardized definitions of abuse and violence contributes to a failure in cultural competency on the part of physicians and remains a major obstacle in addressing IPV in a systematic and effective way. This confusion stems from the development of terminology within multiple disparate domains: healthcare, social services, and the legal system. Lawmakers now face the task of consolidating different operative legal definitions from 50 states, which may differ from those definitions used by professionals in violence and abuse prevention [5].

In order for physicians to adequately respond to such sensitive issue, they must familiarize themselves with some basic terminology:

*Physical violence* and/or abuse is the intentional use of physical force or power, threatened or actual, against another person or against oneself or against a group of people, that results in or has a high likelihood of resulting in injury, death, psychological harm, or deprivation. Physical violence or abuse includes, but is not limited to scratching, pushing, shoving, throwing, grabbing, biting, choking, shaking, hair pulling, slapping, punching, hitting, burning, and use of restraints or one's body, size, or strength against another person. The unwarranted administration of drugs and physical restraints, force-feeding, and physical punishment of any kind are additional examples of physical abuse. Physical violence includes, but is not limited to, use of a weapon against a person [6].

*Sexual violence* and/or abuse is divided into three categories: (a) the use of physical force to compel a person to engage in a sexual act against his or her will, whether or not the act is completed; (b) an attempted or completed sex act involving a person who is unable to consent to the act or understand the nature or condition of the act, to decline participation, or to communicate unwillingness to engage in a sexual act due to age, illness, disability, influence of alcohol or other drugs, intimidation or pressure; and/or (c) abusive sexual contact. Sexual contact includes, but is not limited to, unwanted touching, and sexually explicit photographing [6].

*Psychological/emotional abuse* encompasses a range of verbal and mental methods designed to emotionally wound, coerce, control, intimidate, harass, insult, and psychologically harm. Isolation and withholding of information from the target of said behaviors also falls under this title of psychological aggression and emotional abuse [6].

As with any complicated social dynamic, definitions of abuse and violence are informed in large part by their historical and cultural context and the evolving boundaries and challenges of relationships and commitments. The complexity and depth of social and romantic interaction may make it especially difficult at times to clearly delineate abuse or violence from poor conflict management skills, especially in conditions of psychological aggression and emotional abuse. For this reason, it is necessary to examine the intent or function of the violence in each couple. Domination, intimidation, degradation, and control may also be elements of abusive intimate partner violence, wherein a partner seeks to control the thoughts, beliefs or conduct of the other or to punish the other partner [7].

## Etiologies and Epidemiology

Violence is a preventable outcome of a series of learned behaviors in which aggressors try to maintain control of their partners. While there is no singular etiology for violence, abuser tend to blame life stressors or unfulfilled expectations for their outbursts, and often individuals suffering from abuse are held responsible for exacerbating pre-existing stress or resisting control or punishment. Typically, IPV occurs in a controlling cycle, in which an assault is followed by a period wherein the abuser is remorseful, apologetic, or even loving, before tensions and abuser-perceived "transgressions" build to precipitate another episode of violence. Over time, these cycles generally become more frequent and more severe.

One of the most common myths of intimate partner violence is that it is an action perpetrated by cis-gender men against cis-gender women. The reality is that IPV affects men and women at all levels and demographics of society, regardless of race, religion, or economic status. While no one knows what exactly what causes IPV, economic stress, history of mental illness, history of abuse, perceived disparate power differentials, and social dysfunction are all correlated with

violence in both same-sex and opposite-sex relationships [8]. In a cross-sectional study of MSM, depression and substance abuse were among the strongest correlates of intimate partner violence [9]. Risk markers and correlates of intimate violence in same-sex relationships are notably similar to those associated with heterosexual partner abuse. An extended list of factors can be viewed in Table 10.1.

**Table 10.1** Risk factors for perpetration of violence

| Multiple factors influence the risk of perpetrating IPV [13, 14]: |
| --- |
| • History of physical or psychological abuse |
| • Prior history of being physically abusive |
| • Low self-esteem |
| • Low income |
| • Low academic achievement |
| • Young age |
| • Involvement in aggressive or delinquent behavior as a youth |
| • Heavy alcohol and drug use |
| • Anger and hostility |
| • Personality disorders and mood disorders |
| • Unemployment |
| • Economic stress |
| • Emotional dependence and insecurity |
| • Belief in strict gender roles (e.g. male dominance and aggression in relationships) |
| • Desire for power and control in relationships |
| • History of experiencing neglect or poor parenting as a child |
| • History of experiencing physical discipline as a child |
| Relationship factors |
| • Marital conflict |
| • Marital instability |
| • Economic stress |
| • Unhealthy family relationships and interactions |
| Community factors |
| • Poverty and associated factors (e.g., overcrowding) |
| • Low social capital-lack of institutions, relationships, and norms that shape the quality and quantity of a community's social interactions |
| • Weak community sanctions against IPV (e.g., unwillingness of neighbors to intervene in situations where they witness violence) |
| • Patriarchal gender norms (especially those concerning female submission and male dominance) |

Until the 1990s, few studies had examined the prevalence of IPV in same-sex couples. More robust research has since developed to address the major disparities in research and policy. Meta-analyses of the research to date suggest that LGBT individuals are at least as likely—if not more likely—to be abused by their partners as heterosexual men and women. According to the National Coalition of Anti-Violence Programs (NCAVP), LGBT and queer (LGBTQ) youth, people of color, gay men, and transgender women were more likely to suffer injuries, require medical attention, experience harassment, or face anti-LGBTQ bias as a result of IPV. Although it is unknown whether the severity of abuse is comparable between opposite-sex and same-sex couples, gay individuals suffering from IPV were almost twice likely to require medical attention as a result of violence [10]. In a 2009 study, males suffering from same-sex IPV reported more verbal abuse than males suffering from of opposite-sex IPV. Females suffering from (lesbian, bisexual, and straight), by contrast, did not report differences by type of IPV [11]. In an analysis of the California Health Interview Survey, 1250 of the 31,623 respondents who identified as LGB or WSW/MSM reported higher rates of physical and sexual violence than their heterosexual counterparts, though this figure was significant only for bisexual women and gay men. Notably, for bisexual women, 95 % of violent incidents were perpetrated by a male partner [12].

The Gender, Violence and Resource Access Survey found that 50 % of transgender respondents reported assault or rape by a partner, while 31 % identified as an IPV survivor [10]. Transgender survivors, specifically, were twice as likely to face threats/intimidation, 1.8 times more likely to experience harassment, and over four times (4.4) more likely to face police violence as a result of IPV than people who did not identify as transgender. Moreover, transgender people of color and transgender women experienced this violence at even higher rates and were more likely to face these abuses as part of IPV [15]. It should also be noted that, although transgender people comprise approximately 8 % of the LGBT com-

munity, of the 21 LGBT IPV homicides reported in 2012, 3 (14 %) of the individuals suffering from IPV identified as transgender [10].

Despite considerable challenges in research, studies on intimate partner violence in LGBT youth relationships have yielded compelling results. Studies estimate that around 25–40 % of gay, bisexual and lesbian youth report at least one lifetime incident of emotional, physical, or sexual abuse by a same-sex partner, figures that are similar to or higher than lifetime reports of violence from heterosexual samples [16, 17]. Of note, male adolescents within exclusively same-sex relationships were less likely than females to report experiencing the violent behaviors. These results underscore the need for early screening and intervention in this population [18].

## Challenges in Reporting, Research, and Policy

Studies examining the prevalence and severity of IPV in LGBT relationships are limited by many of the same obstacles of research on heterosexual IPV, particularly small sample populations. Many individuals affected by IPV are reluctant to report IPV for many reasons: fear of retaliation by the abuser, fear of judgment by healthcare providers or law enforcement, fear of further isolation, fear of disrupting family and children, or a desire to protect the abuser by internally diminishing the severity of the violence. Additionally, many individuals suffering from IPV (and the general public at large) are often unaware of what constitutes IPV, either due to denial or lack of education [5]. To overcome this obstacle, many studies based on large samples typically have used nonrandom sampling methods, often with recruitment through gay and lesbian publications, organizations, and activities. The result is that same-sex intimate violence is often studied using nonrepresentative samples.

Setting aside methodological challenges, LGBT relationships face not only increased risk factors for violence, but LGBT survivors also experience identity-specific forms of abuse. The unique possibilities for extortion make it especially difficult for LGBT individuals to leave or report abusive relationships. These forms of IPV are summarized here:

*Internalized guilt* Many LGBT individuals choose not to disclose their abuse because they feel that their relationship must appear outwardly "perfect" either to compensate for the stigma of homosexuality/gender nonconformity or not to validate heterosexist bigotry that suggests that LGBT relationships are less valid or "serious" [7]. This is particularly true of younger individuals, who may harbor more conflicted feelings about their sexual identity [19].

*Homophobia/biphobia/transphobia* Societal oppression of LGBT people has allowed heterosexism to be used as another psychological weapon in the arsenal of a abuser keen on controlling and manipulating his or her partner. For instance, abusive partners of transgender survivors may tell their partners they are not "real" men or women, that no one else would want to be with him or her, or that they would be more unsafe "on the streets" outside the relationship. Other forms of heterosexist abuse may include shaming gender-nonconforming behaviors, telling a partner that the abuser is the only one who understands their sexual identity, or threatening to "out" a partner to his or her family, employer, or community. These behaviors ultimately exploit insecurities concerning the social ramifications of his or her sexual orientation. In addition to psychological trauma, outing may result in the loss of support systems, housing, jobs, or even child custody. Often, individuals affected by may be reluctant to report IPV based on fears of the negative consequences of revealing their true sexual orientation [20].

*Children* When same-gender couples have children, the abuser may threaten to take the children away. If the abuser is the biological or adoptive parent, this threat could easily be carried out because many states have adoption laws that do not permit same-gender parents to adopt each other's

children. In this situation, the non-biological parent has no legal rights to child custody if the couple separates. Similarly, if the abuser is a non-biological parent, he or she may threaten to "out" the biological parent in order to jeopardize the biological parent's custody and transfer the child to a heterosexual household [21].

*Lack of support from law enforcement* For those LGBT individuals affected by IPV that do seek help, they may encounter a lack of cultural competency from law enforcement that believe that IPV is perpetrated by straight men against straight women. There is often a concomitant misconception that LGBT IPV refers to conditions of mutual combat rather than victimization [22]. According to the 2012 NCAVP report, in nearly a third of the LGBTQ-specific IPV cases reported to the police, the survivor was arrested instead of the aggressor. LGBTQ IPV survivors also experienced other forms of police misconduct including verbal abuse, slurs or bias language, or physical violence. Particularly in the transgender community, half of individuals reported feeling discomfort in seeking assistance from police, and close to a quarter of individuals had experienced police harassment [10]. This mistrust in law enforcement serves to reinforce the degree of isolation transgender individuals experience.

*Access to social services* Since the reauthorization of the Violence Against Women Act (VAWA) of 2013—which included provisions for LBGT individuals—domestic violence or intimate partner violence is no longer legally defined as violence between straight male aggressors and females. That being said, LGBT individuals may encounter homophobic bias in court should they choose to press charges [21]. Should these individuals reveal their sexual orientation and decide to leave their partners, many have been denied access to social services and safety nets such as shelters. Shelters not only provide safe and stable housing, they also provide other social services such as counseling, legal and employment services, and child services. Domestic violence services that are LGBT-specific have been designed primarily for LGBT communities, with providers specializing in work with LGBT individuals and families. But despite LGBT individuals facing higher rates of social isolation, prejudice, and mental illness in daily life, LGBT-specific shelters are rare or nonexistent particularly in rural areas, only compounding the needs of an underserved community. Most domestic violence services have been designed primarily for the heterosexual community—with varying degrees of LGBT acceptance—and providers of these services may not have received training in LGBT domestic violence and usually receive variable amounts of training in LGBT issues. For those individuals who are able to access social services, lack of cultural competency often contributes to the already-present sense of isolation and may actually re-traumatize those affected by IPV, leading them to return to their aggressors or stop seeking support altogether [23]. In fact, many non-LGBT specific shelters that do exist have historically operated under the belief that IPV is a heterosexual phenomenon and did not accept men or trans women. For this reason, while women have the option of going to female-focused shelters, limited resources are available for male and transgender individuals affected by IPV. The recent reauthorization of VAWA, however, now contains a nondiscrimination clause that prohibits LGBT individuals from being turned away from shelters on the basis of sexual orientation or gender identity, so there is hope that more programs will rise to the challenge of providing culturally-competent care to future victims. Despite expanding access for LGBT individuals, however, it must be noted that VAWA came under considerable criticism for the relatively paltry provision of only $4 million to LGBT organizations of its larger $1.6 billion budget. While the reauthorization of VAWA should be applauded as a major step towards legal equality for the LGBT community, disparities in funding only underscore that more work must be done to address the issue of IPV within this vulnerable population.

## The Role of Clinicians

Clinicians serve an important role in identifying, supporting, treating, and intervening on behalf of individuals affected by IPV. However, one of the most difficult tasks is screening for IPV, since clinical manifestations of IPV are subtle in all but most obvious cases. Lack of knowledge or training, time limitations, inability to offer lasting solutions or external resources, and fear of offending the patient all contribute to provider-specific barriers that IPV victims face. Compounding the stigma of abuse and violence, classism, racism, homophobia, and transphobia also adds to a culture of inertia and victim-shaming within medicine. Providers must fix this culture through information, trust, empathy, and objectivity.

While signs of trauma (e.g. bruises, burns, scratches to the face, abdomen, and genitals) are thought to be most consistent with IPV, in most cases, abused patients present with either no symptoms at all or may present with non-traumatic diagnoses such as IBS, depression, abdominal pain, anxiety, substance abuse, or STIs. Given this vague constellation of symptoms, it is important for providers to consider IPV as an etiology or even lower thresholds for IPV screening, particularly for gay and transgender patients. Careful history and physical exam skills are essential so that the subtle signs of IPV can be screened for and recognized.

Given that many in the LGBT community feel stigmatized, marginalized, and judged for their sexual orientation, many individuals do not reveal their sexual orientations or gender identity in the clinical setting, complicating the already challenging task of addressing a patient's unique needs and obstacles. As previously mentioned, disclosing one's sexual identity—especially in a setting where trust and rapport have not been established—is a major deterrent for many LGBT victims in seeking help and breaking a cycle of abuse. Establishing rapport with patients tactfully and professionally in a nonjudgmental way is key with any survivor of IPV but is especially paramount in LGBT communities. The first step is to interview the patient alone in a quiet room and verbally assure them of confidentiality. Then, rather than running through a formal IPV screening questionnaire, it may be more prudent for the provider to open a dialogue with the patient when taking a sexual history ("Are you sexually active?", "Are you in a relationship?", "Do you have sex with men, women, or both?"). Such questions are respectful, relevant, and set up a professional conversation for inquiry about all aspects of sexual and emotional health without appearing voyeuristic or judgmental.

> **Helpful Hint**
> After establishing rapport, ask about specific behaviors (hitting, punching, nonconsensual sexual activity, etc.) and try to explore the patient's feelings of fear in the relationship.

By asking pertinent follow-up questions using inclusive, non-heteronormative language, a provider can establish trust with a patient before delving into more sensitive IPV-history questions, such as "Do you feel unsafe in your relationship?" or "Have you been hit, punched, kicked, or physically threatened by your partner or previous partner?". If affirmative, asking "In what context, did these events happen?" and "How have these events affected you?" are good follow-up questions. If a patient discloses how they feel about the violence, it is important to validate and affirm their feelings, particularly given the challenge of discussing IPV with a provider.

Inquiring about specific IPV experiences rather than asking about a more general "history of domestic violence" is beneficial for two reasons: First, IPV often goes unacknowledged not only on an institutional level, but also on a cultural level, even within the LGBT community [24]. Many individuals affected by IPV do not have the knowledge to label their experiences as abusive or violent—particularly in cases of sexual assault or emotional/psychological abuse—so inquiring and correctly identifying IPV fulfills a much-needed educational role for these patients.

Second, identifying specific violent or abusive experiences may aid in furthering dialogue, educating the patient, guiding the physical exam, and developing a treatment plan that suits a patient's specific needs. Once providers are able to obtain a proper history of IPV and trauma, they can then extend their screening and physical exam to include physical injury, substance abuse, depression, anxiety, HIV and other STIs, the prevalence of which is much higher in individuals affected by IPV.

> **Helpful Hint**
> Remember to validate and affirm a patients feelings and experiences to maintain rapport and trust.

## Physical Exam

Patterns of injury that might be suspicious for abuse include multiple injuries in various stages of healing, cuts, scratches, or bruises on the face, abdomen, and genitalia, or any acute injury that does not have a clear cause. The presence of STIs or signs of self-harm and substance abuse, while not direct signs of IPV, should prompt discussions about emotional health and relationship history. As previously mentioned, however, most individuals affected by IPV present without any overt signs of trauma.

## A Brief Note on Documentation

The role of clear and accurate medical records cannot be understated. Medical documentation is readily admissible in court as evidence that can substantiate a individual's assertion of harm, even when a victim is unable to testify against his or her aggressor. Correct documentation also enables providers to effectively communicate amongst each other about a patient's history of IPV, permitting more individualized patient care in the future. Whenever possible, the patient's own words should be documented in the chart, and the relationship of the aggressor and indivdual abused be stated along with supporting photographs and descriptions from the physical exam. Areas of tenderness or concern, even without visual evidence of trauma, should be documented on a body map, along with descriptions of the symptoms.

## IPV Intervention

After listening to the patient, affirming their experiences, and conducting a thorough history and physical exam, the next step in IPV intervention is ensuring patient safety. Patient safety can be addressed on several fronts. The first is to ask the patient if he or she subjectively feels safe going home at all, and, if not, if he or she has a safe place to stay. Another key step may be determining whether there are firearms in the household, or if the aggressor has access to firearms or other weapons. Not only will this allow one to make appropriate referrals to social services, it can also give the provider better insight into the volatility of the domestic situation. It is also crucial to note if children are present in the home and if their safety is also jeopardized. The physician should alert the patient of their legal protections, and that restraining orders and civil protection orders are available in the United States. These protections may even mandate temporary child custody and mandate rent or mortgage payments by the aggressor.

Creating a personalized safety plan is simple and powerful tool for patients who feel endangered. Patients should be advised to take measures to establish independence and security. Such activities may include ensuring that important phone numbers are available at all times, rehearsing realistic escape routes from their homes, workplaces, or anywhere partners may threaten them, developing outside contacts, seeking support regularly from friends, colleagues, or professionals, and keeping a list of secure places to seek refuge if their safety is imminently threatened. Keeping change for phone calls, opening separate bank accounts, and leaving extra money, car keys, clothes, or copies of important papers with a friend or in a safe place serves as a way for an individual affected by IPV to discreetly build their independence without a possibly dangerous confrontation with their abuser [25].

Different interventions may be appropriate if the patient is a minor. Almost half of LGBT youth and adolescents report feeling abused in at least one past relationship; therefore, screening and intervention is especially crucial in this vulnerable demographic [26]. More specifically, males reporting exclusively same-sex relationships are less likely than females to report experiencing violence [18]. If the patient's safety is imminently jeopardized, it may be advisable to discuss the situation with the patient's parents. In the pediatric population, referring to social work may also provide an important role in managing complex social dynamics in the home or at school.

A host of health risks are associated with IPV and have been outlined in Table 10.2. Chronic pain, gastrointestinal distress, and frank physical injuries are all physical findings important to document and address with the appropriate medical management and pharmacotherapy. Sexually transmitted infections and psychiatric illness such as depression, anxiety, and post-traumatic stress disorder are far more prevalent in abusive relationships, and individuals affected by IPV are often not empowered to seek treatment. Therefore, the clinical encounter should also include STD screening, depression and anxiety screening (including assessing risk of suicidal ideation), and discussion of safe sex practices [23]. Particularly

**Table 10.2** The impact of IPV on health

Intimate partner violence in heterosexual and LGBT all victims of IPV is associated with increased health risks of the following:

- Substance use disorders
- Trauma and stress related disorders (ex. PTSD)
- Depression, suicidal ideation and attempts
- Sexually transmitted diseases
- Unplanned or early pregnancy and pregnancy complications
- Eating disorders
- Gastrointestinal disorders
- Chronic pain disorders
- Psychosomatic symptoms

in pediatric and adolescent populations, physicians should initiate frank discussions about safe sex, STDs, and consent. Substance abuse in particular has been found consistently to correlate with IPV in both heterosexual and LGBT populations, so the clinician should explore the patient's coping mechanisms and evaluate the patient for substance dependence [27].

Many individuals affected by IPV remain in abusive relationships for a number of reasons, be they emotional, physical, or financial, and the process of extricating themselves from the relationship often takes a long time. Even so, many individuals who have been abused may refuse help altogether. Particularly in these situations, the most essential advice for the clinician is to patiently listen, providing accessibility, support, and frequent and regular follow-up both during the abusive relationship and after the relationship has been terminated [23]. Identifying IPV allows the provider to educate his or her patients and advocate for their wellbeing. Physicians should reaffirm that intimate partner violence is a crime and inform their patients that there is help available should he or she be willing to receive it.

Below is a list of domestic violence resources organized by region, reproduced from the 2007 National Resource Center on Domestic Violence Information & Resource Guide [28].

Gay Men's Domestic Violence Project
  (GMDVP)
955 Massachusetts Avenue, PMB 131
Cambridge, MA 02139
Telephone: 800-832-1901
Email: Support@gmdvp.org
Web: http://www.gmdvp.org/
Founded as a non-profit organization by a survivor of domestic violence in 1994, The Gay Men's Domestic Violence Project (GMDVP) provides community education and direct services to gay, bisexual, and transgender male victims and survivors of domestic violence. It now has a growing pool of volunteers and speakers, and four staff members. GMDVP relies on the grassroots support of survivors, its volunteer base, the LGBT community, and other allies.

Lambda GLBT Community Services
216 South Ochoa Street
El Paso, TX 79901
Telephone: 208-246-2292
Fax: 208-246-2292
Email: admin@lambda.org
Web: http://www.lambda.org/
LAMBDA has led the effort to create an awareness of homophobia and its effects, becoming a major source of information for decision makers and news media. LAMBDA has also worked to protect gays and lesbians from discrimination and violence in homes, businesses, and schools through educational campaigns, non-discrimination leadership, and anti-violence efforts. LAMBDA's Anti-Violence Project (AVP) provides victim services to survivors of hate crimes, domestic violence, sexual assault, and other crimes. AVP's services include crime prevention and education, a 24-h bilingual (English-Spanish) hotline, peer-to-peer support groups, and accompaniment to and advocacy with police, the courts, and other service providers.

The National Coalition of Anti-Violence
  Programs (NCAVP)
240 West 35th Street, Suite 200
New York, NY 10001
Telephone: 212-714-1184
TTY: 212-714-1134
Web: http://www.ncavp.org
The National Coalition of Anti-Violence Programs (NCAVP) is a coalition of over 20 lesbian, gay, bisexual, and transgender victim advocacy and documentation programs located throughout the United States. Before officially forming in 1995, NCAVP members collaborated with one another and with the National Gay and Lesbian Task Force (NGLTF) for over a decade to create a coordinated response to violence against LGBT communities. NCAVP member organizations have increasingly adapted their missions and their services to respond to violence within the community. The first annual domestic violence report was released in October of 1997.

**Arizona**

Wingspan Anti-Violence Project

300 East Sixth Street

Tucson, AZ 85705

Telephone: 520-624-1779

Fax: 520-624-0364

TDD: 520-884-0450

Email: wingspan@wingspan.org

Web: http://www.wingspanaz.org/content/WAVP.php

The Wingspan Anti-Violence Project is a social change and social service program that works to address and end violence in the lives of lesbian, gay, bisexual, and transgender (LGBT) people. WAVP provides free and confidential 24-h crisis intervention, information, support, referrals, emergency shelter, and advocacy to LGBT victim/survivors of violence. Additionally, the project offers extensive outreach and education programs.

**California**

Community United Against Violence (CUAV)

60 14th Street

San Francisco, CA 94103

Business Telephone: 415-777-5500

24-h Support Line: 415-333-HELP

Fax: 415-777-5565

Web: http://www.cuav.org/

Community United Against Violence (CUAV) is a 20-year old multicultural organization working to end violence against and within lesbian, gay, bisexual, transgender and queer/questioning (LGBTQ) communities. Believing that in order for homophobia and heterosexism to end, CUAV must fight all forms of oppression, including racism, sexism, ageism, classism and ableism. CUAV offers a 24-h confidential, multilingual support line, free counseling, legal advocacy, and emergency assistance (hotel, food, and transportation vouchers) to survivors of domestic violence, hate violence, and sexual assault. CUAV uses education as a violence prevention tool through the speakers bureau, the youth program, and the domestic violence prevention program.

Los Angeles Gay & Lesbian Center/STOP Partner Abuse/Domestic Violence Program

1625 North Schrader Boulevard

Los Angeles, CA 90028

Telephone: 323-860-5806 (clients)

Fax: 323-993-7699

E-mail: domesticviolence@laglc.org

Website: http://www.laglc.org/domesticviolence

The L.A. Gay & Lesbian Center's STOP Partner Abuse/Domestic Violence Program provides a comprehensive continuum of partner abuse and domestic violence services designed to address the specific and unique needs of the lesbian, gay, bisexual and transgender communities.

San Diego Lesbian, Gay, Bisexual, Transgender Community Center

3909 Centre Street

San Diego, CA 92103

Telephone: 619-692-2077

Fax: 619-260-3092

Web: http://www.thecentersd.org/

Group and individual counseling offered to both victims and offenders struggling with relationship violence. This program is also probation/court-certified for court-ordered clients. Lesbian, gay, bisexual and transgender youth are also served. [The Relationship Violence Treatment & Intervention Program] is targeted towards victims and offenders of same-sex relationships.

**Colorado**

Colorado Anti-Violence Program

P.O. Box 181085

Denver, CO 80218

Telephone: 303-852-5094; or 303-839-5204 Crisis Line: 888-557-4441

Fax: 303-839-5205

E-mail: coavp@hotmail.com

Web: www.coavp.org

The Colorado Anti-Violence Program is dedicated to eliminating violence within and against the lesbian, gay, bisexual, and transgender (LGBT) communities in Colorado. CAVP provides direct client services including crisis intervention, information, and referrals for LGBT victims of violence 24 h a day and also provides technical assistance, training, and education for community organizations, law enforcement, and mainstream service providers on violence issues affecting the LGBT community.

**Illinois**

Center on Halsted Horizons Anti-Violence
    Project
961 W. Montana, 2nd Floor
Chicago, IL 60614
Telephone: 773-472-6469
Fax: 773-472-6643
TTY: 773-472-1277
E-mail: mail@centeronhalsted.org
Web: http://www.centeronhalsted.org/coh/calen-
    dar/home.cfm
The Center on Halsted Anti-Violence Project
    (AVP) has assisted thousands of victims of
    anti-lesbian, gay, bisexual, or transgender
    (LGBT) hate crimes, domestic violence, sex-
    ual assault, discrimination, and police miscon-
    duct. Staff and trained volunteers counsel,
    support, and advocate for all victims and sur-
    vivors of such violence. All AVP victim ser-
    vices are free and confidential.

**Massachusetts**

Fenway Community Health Violence Recovery
    Program
7 Haviland Street
Boston, MA 02115
Telephone: 617-267-0900
Toll-free: 888-242-0900
Spanish information: 617-927-6460
TTY: 617-859-1256
Web: http://www.fenwayhealth.org/services/vio-
    lence.htm
The Violence Recovery Program (VRP) at
    Fenway Community Health provides counsel-
    ing, support groups, advocacy, and referral ser-
    vices to Gay, Lesbian, Bisexual and
    Transgender (GLBT) victims of bias crime,
    domestic violence, sexual assault and police
    misconduct. VRP staff members frequently
    present at trainings for police, court personnel
    and human service providers on GLBT crime
    survivor issues. Other services include a sup-
    port group for GLBT domestic violence survi-
    vors, the region's only support group for male
    survivors of rape and sexual assault, advocacy
    with the courts and police, and assistance with
    victim compensation. VRP provides short-
    term counseling to survivors and their families,
    and referrals to longer-term counseling through
    their mental health department.

The Network/La Red
P.O. Box 6011
Boston, MA 02114
Telephone (V/TTY): 617-695-0877
Fax: 617-423-5651
E-mail: info@thenetworklared.org
Web: http://www.biresource.org
The Network/La Red was formed to address batter-
    ing in lesbian, bisexual women's, and transgen-
    der communities. Through (a) the formation of
    a community-based multi-cultural organization
    in which battered/formerly battered lesbians,
    bisexual women, and transgender folks hold
    leadership roles; (b) community organizing,
    education, and the provision of support services;
    and (c) coalition-building with other move-
    ments for social change and social justice, the
    Network/LaRed seeks to create a culture in
    which domination, coercion, and control are no
    longer accepted and operative social norms.
    Agency services include a Hotline, Safe Home
    program, Advocacy program, and Organizing/
    Outreach program. All services are bilingual
    and wheelchair and TTY-accessible. ASL inter-
    preters, air filters, and reimbursement for child-
    care are available as needed.

**Michigan**

Triangle Foundation
19641 West Seven Mile Road
Detroit, MI 48219-2721
Telephone: 313-537-7000
Fax: 313-537-3379
Web: http://www.tri.org/ Triangle Foundation is
    Michigan's leading organization serving the gay,
    lesbian, bisexual, transgender (GLBT) and allied
    communities. The Triangle Foundation Anti-
    Violence Program is a social change and social
    service program that works to address and end
    violence in the lives of GLBT people. We pro-
    vide free and confidential intervention, informa-
    tion, support, attorney referrals, emergency
    shelter referrals, and advocacy to GLBT victim/
    survivors of violence. Additionally, we offer
    extensive outreach and education programs.

**Minnesota**

OutFront Minnesota
310 East 38th Street, Suite 204 Minneapolis, MN
    55409

Telephone: 612-824-8434 [Hotline]
Telephone: 612-822-0127
Toll-free: 800-800-0350
E-mail: info@outfront.org
Web: http://www.outfront.org
OutFront Minnesota offers direct services to victims of domestic violence and offers training concerning same-sex domestic abuse to DV service providers.

**Missouri**

Anti-Violence Advocacy Project of the St. Louis region
P.O. Box 63255
St. Louis, MO 63163
Telephone: 314-503-2050
Web: http://www.avap-stl.org/
The mission of the Anti-Violence Advocacy Project (AVAP) of the St. Louis Region is to provide education and advocacy that addresses intimate violence and sociopolitical oppression based on sexual orientation and/or gender identity. This project addresses all forms of violence that affect the lesbian, gay, bisexual, transgender, queer community, including (but not limited to) domestic violence, sexual violence, anti-gay harassment and hate crimes.

Kansas City Anti-Violence Project
PO Box 411211
Kansas City, MO 64141-1211
Telephone: 816-561-0550
Email: info@kcavp.org Web: http://www.kcavp. org
KCAVP was created to provide information, support, referrals, advocacy and other services to LGBT survivors of violence including domestic violence, sexual assault, and bias crimes, focusing these services within the Kansas City metropolitan area. KCAVP also educates the community at large through training and outreach programs.

**New York**

Gay Alliance of the Genesee Valley
Rochester, NY 14605
Telephone: 585-244-8640
Fax: 585-244-8246

Web: http://www.gayalliance.org/ The Gay Alliance of the Genesee Valley is dedicated to cultivating a healthy, inclusive environment where individuals of all sexual orientations and gender expressions are safe, thriving, and enjoy full civil rights.

In Our Own Voices
245 Lark Street
Albany, NY 12210
Telephone: 518-432-4188
Fax: 518-432-4123
Email: info@inourownvoices.org
Web: http://www.inourownvoices.org
In Our Own Voices is an autonomous organization dedicated to addressing the many needs of the LGBT community. The purpose of [the Capital District LGBT Anti-Violence Project] is to improve domestic violence services for lesbian, gay, bisexual and transgender people, particularly people of color, in the Capital District.

Long Island Gay and Lesbian Youth
34 Park Avenue
Bay Shore, NY 11706-7309
Telephone: 361-655-2300
Fax: 631-655-7874
Web: http://www.ligaly.org
Long Island Gay and Lesbian Youth (LIGALY) is a not-for-profit organization providing education, advocacy, and social support services to Long Island's gay, lesbian, bisexual, and transgender (GLBT) youth and young adults, and all youth, young adults, and their families for whom sexuality, sexual identity, gender identity, and HIV/AIDS are an issue. Our goals are to empower GLBT youth, advocate for their diverse interests, and to educate society about them. [The Long Island Gay and Lesbian Youth Anti-Violence Project] will serve GLBT and HIV-positive victims of violence, and others affected by violence, by providing free and confidential services enabling them to regain their sense of control, identify and evaluate their options and assert their rights. In particular, the Project will assist survivors of hate-motivated violence, domestic violence and sexual assault.

The New York City Gay & Lesbian Anti-Violence
   Project
240 West 35th Street, Suite 200
New York, NY 10001
Telephone: 212-714-1141 [Hotline]
Telephone : 212-714-1184 TTY: 212-714-1134
   [Hotline]
Fax: 212-714-2627
E-mail: clientservices@avp.org
Web: http://www.avp.org
The New York City Gay & Lesbian Anti-Violence
   Project serves lesbian, gay, transgender, bisexual and HIV-positive victims of violence, and
   others affected by violence, by providing free
   and confidential services. The Project assists
   survivors of hate-motivated violence (including HIV-motivated violence), domestic violence, and sexual assault, by providing
   therapeutic counseling and advocacy within
   the criminal justice system and victim support
   agencies, information for self-help, referrals
   to practicing professionals, and other sources
   of assistance. The larger community is also
   served through public education about violence directed at or within LGBT communities and through action to reform government
   policies and practices affecting lesbian, gay,
   transgender, bisexual, HIV-positive and other
   survivors of violence.

**North Carolina**
North Carolina Coalition Against Domestic
   Violence (NCCADV)
115 Market Street, Suite 400
Durham, NC 27701
Telephone: 919-956-9124
Fax: 919-682-1449
Web: http://www.nccadv.org
Project Rainbow Net, an initiative of the North
   Carolina Coalition Against Domestic Violence
   (NCCADV) addresses issues related to
   domestic violence in lesbian, gay, bisexual
   and transgender relationships. The initiative is
   a grassroots effort based on the insight of an
   advisory council made up of lesbian, gay,
   bisexual and transgender people who have an
   understanding of domestic violence in LGBT
   relationships and a desire to end it. Project

Rainbow Net provides training to LGBT community groups and domestic violence service
   providers in North Carolina, in an effort to
   improve the state's response to LGBT survivors of domestic violence. This website, as
   well as the NCCADV website (www.nccadv.
   org) contains information about domestic violence in LGBT relationships, tools for domestic violence service providers, tips on helping
   a friend experiencing domestic violence, and
   links to other online resources.

**Ohio**
Buckeye   Region   Anti-Violence   Program
   (BRAVO)
PO Box 82068
Columbus, OH 43202
Telephone: 614-268-9622
E-mail: bravoavp@earthlink.net
Toll-free: 866-86-BRAVO [Hotline]
Web: http://www.bravo-ohio.org
BRAVO works to eliminate violence perpetrated
   on the basis of sexual orientation and/or gender
   identification, domestic violence and sexual
   assault through prevention, education, advo-
   cacy, violence documentation and survivor ser-
   vices, both within and on behalf of the Lesbian,
   Gay, Bisexual and Transgender communities.

The Lesbian Gay Community Center of Greater
   Cleveland
6600 Detroit Avenue
Cleveland, OH 44102
Telephone: 216-651-LGBT (651-5428)
Toll-free: 888-GAY-8761 (429-8761)
E-mail: info@lgcsc.org
Web: http://www.lgcsc.org/
The Center works toward a society free of
   homophobia and gender oppression by advancing the respect, human rights and dignity of the
   lesbian, gay male, bisexual and transgender
   communities. The Center is a non-profit organization that provides direct service, social
   support, community-building and programs to
   empower lesbian, gay, bisexual, transgender
   and intersex people. Core program areas are
   Education, Health and Wellness and Youth
   Services.

**Ontario**

The 519 Anti-Violence Programme
519 Church Street
Toronto, ON M4Y 2C9
Canada
Telephone: 416-392-6877 [Hotline]
E-mail: avp@the519.org
Web: http://www.the519.org
The 519 Anti-Violence Programme provides support to and advocacy for people who have experienced same-sex partner abuse or hate motivated violence or harassment, works with the LGBTQ Communities in Toronto to provide education on responding to and preventing violence, works with other service providers to ensure that their services are accessible and appropriate for LGBTQ people and works with other agencies to develop new services to address service gaps.

**Oregon**

Survivor Project
P.O. Box 40664
Portland, OR 97240
Telephone: 503-288-3191
Email: info@survivorproject.org
Web: http://www.survivorproject.org/defbarresp.html
Survivor Project is a non-profit organization dedicated to addressing the needs of intersex and trans survivors of domestic and sexual violence through caring action, education and expanding access to resources and to opportunities for action. Since 1997, Survivor Project has provided presentations, workshops, consultation, materials, information and referrals to many anti-violence organizations and universities across the country, as well as gathered information about issues faced by intersex and trans survivors of domestic and sexual violence.

**Pennsylvania**

Equality Advocates
1211 Chestnut Street, Suite 605
Philadelphia, PA 19107
Telephone: 215-731-1447
Toll Free: 866-LGBT-LAW (866-542-8529) [Hotline, available within PA only.]
Email: info@equalitypa.org
Web: http://www.equalitypa.org
Equality Advocates' mission is to advocate equality for lesbian, gay, bisexual, and transgender individuals in Pennsylvania through direct legal services, education, and policy reform.

**Texas**

Montrose Counseling Center, Inc. (MCC)
701 Richmond Avenue
Houston, TX 77006-5511
Telephone: 713-529-3211 [Hotline]
Toll Free: 800-699-0504 [Hotline: Regional Toll-Free]
Telephone: 713-529-3590 [Youth Line]
Telephone: 713-529-0037
Fax: 713-526-4367
E-mail: avp@montrosecounselingcenter.org Web: http://www.montrosecounselingcenter.org
MCC, a Joint Commission on Accreditation of Healthcare Organizations facility, provides comprehensive behavioral health and social services for the Gay, Lesbian, Bisexual, Transgender and Questioning communities in and around metropolitan Houston. Anti-violence services include 24-h hotline, advocacy/case management, safety planning, medical, legal and court accompaniment, professional and peer counseling, assistance with Crime Victim's Compensation applications, Victim Impact Statements and protective orders, and legal advocacy for bias/hate crimes, domestic violence and sexual assault. Emergency shelter and transitional housing is also available for domestic violence survivors. Other services available include licensed outpatient substance abuse treatment and GLBTQ youth enrichment programs.

Resource Center of Dallas
P.O. Box 190869
Dallas, TX 75219-0869
Telephone: 214-528-0144
Fax: 214-522-4604
The Resource Center's Family Violence Program promotes self-autonomy, safety and long-term independence for gay, lesbian, bisexual and transgender individuals involved in family violence.

**Vermont**
Safespace
PO Box 158
Burlington, VT 05402
Telephone: 802-863-0003
Toll-free hotline: 866-869-7341
E-mail: Info@SafeSpaceVT.org
Web: http://www.SafeSpaceVT.org
SafeSpace is a social change and social service
organization working to end physical, sexual,
and emotional violence in the lives of lesbian,
gay, bisexual, transgender, queer and questioning (LGBTQQ) people. SafeSpace provides direct services to survivors of violence
through its Support Line, and provides educa-
tion/outreach to the community about issues
of violence in the LGBTQQ community. The
organization provides information, support,
referrals, and advocacy to LGBTQQ survivors
of domestic, sexual and hate violence/dis-
crimination. Advocates work with survivors,
helping them access legal, medical, financial,
housing, and other community resources.
Finally, SafeSpace provides education, training and professional consultation to
individuals, groups, schools, and organizations about the issues of violence in the
LGBTQQ community.

**Virginia**
Equality Virginia
403 North Robinson Street
Richmond, VA 23220
Telephone: 804-643-4816
Fax: 804-643-1554
E-mail: va4justice@aol.com
Web: http://www.equalityvirginia.org/
Equality Virginia is a statewide, non-partisan,
lobbying, education and support network for
the gay, lesbian, bisexual, transgender, and
straight allied (GLBT) communities in
Virginia. The Anti-Violence Project is an
Equality Virginia Education Fund-based pro-
gram that works to address and end violence
in the lives of lesbian, gay, bisexual, transgen-
der, queer and HIV-affected people across the
Commonwealth.

**Washington**
The Northwest Network of Bi, Trans, Lesbian
and Gay Survivors of Abuse
PO Box 20398
Seattle, WA 98102
Telephone: 206-568-7777
TTY message: 206- 517-9670
E-mail: info@nwnetwork.org
Web: http://www.nwnetwork.org/about.html
The Northwest Network acts to increase its communities' ability to support the self-determination
and safety of bisexual, transgender, lesbian, and
gay survivors of abuse through education, organizing and advocacy. The Northwest Network
works within a broad liberation movement dedicated to social and economic justice, equality
and respect for all people and the creation of loving, inclusive and accountable communities.
Services are free and confidential and include
support groups, individual counseling, legal
advocacy, shelter referrals, safety planning, basic
needs assistance, community education and
community organizing.

**Wisconsin**
Milwaukee LGBT Community Center
315 West Court Street
Milwaukee, WI 53212
Telephone: 414-271-2656 [For AVP program,
dial extension 111]
Fax: 414-271-2161
Web: http://www.mkelgbt.org
The Milwaukee LGBT Community Center's mission is to improve the quality of life for people
in the Metro Milwaukee area who identify as
LGBT by providing a home for the birth, nur-
ture and celebration of LGBT organizations,
culture and diversity; initiating, implementing
and advocating for programs and services that
meet the needs of LGBT communities; educating the public and LGBT communities to
encourage positive changes in systems affecting
the lives of people identifying as LGBT;
empowering individuals and groups, who identify as LGBT to achieve their fullest potential;
and cultivating a culture of diversity and inclusion in all phases of the project.

# References

1. Black MC, Basile KC, Breiding MJ, Smith SG, Walters ML, Merrick MT, Chen J, Stevens MR. The National Intimate Partner and Sexual Violence Survey (NISVS): 2010 Summary Report. Atlanta, GA: National Center for Injury Prevention and Control, Centers for Disease Control and Prevention; 2011.
2. National Center for Injury Prevention and Control. Costs of intimate partner violence against women in the United States. Atlanta, GA: Centers for Disease Control and Prevention; 2003.
3. Burke LK, Follingstad DR. Violence in lesbian and gay relationships: theory, prevalence, and correlational factors. Clin Psychol Rev. 1999;19(5):487–512.
4. McClennen JC. Domestic violence between same-gender partners: recent findings and future research. J Interpers Violence. 2005;20(2):149–54.
5. Gay and Lesbian Medical Association and LGBT Health Experts. Healthy people 2010 companion document for lesbian, gay, bisexual, and transgender (LGBT) health. San Francisco, CA: Gay and Lesbian Medical Association; 2010.
6. Saltzman LE, Fanslow JL, McMahon PM, Shelley GA. Intimate partner violence surveillance: uniform definitions and recommended data elements, version 1.0. Atlanta, GA: National Center for Injury Prevention and Control, Centers for Disease Control and Prevention; 1999.
7. Rohrbaugh JB. Domestic violence in same-gender relationships. Fam Court Rev. 2006;44(2):287–99.
8. Jewkes R. Intimate partner violence: causes and prevention. Lancet. 2002;359:1423–9.
9. Houston E, McKirnan D. Intimate partner abuse among gay and bisexual men: risk correlates and health outcomes. J Urban Health. 2007;84(5):681–90.
10. National Coalition of Anti-Violence Programs (NCAVP). A report from the National Coalition of Anti-Violence Programs (NCAVP): lesbian, gay, bisexual, transgender, queer, and HIV-affected intimate partner violence in 2012. New York City Gay and Lesbian Anti-Violence Project; 2013.
11. Blosnich JR, Bossarte RM. Comparisons of intimate partner violence among partners in same-sex and opposite-sex relationships in the United States. Am J Public Health. 2009;99(12):2182–4.
12. Goldberg NG, Meyer IH. Sexual orientation disparities in history of intimate partner violence: results from the California Health Interview Survey. J Interpers Violence. 2013;28(5):1109–18.
13. Garcia-Moreno C, Heise L. Violence by intimate partners. In: Krug EG, Dahlberg LL, Mercy JA, Zwi AB, Lozano R, editors. World report on violence and health. Geneva: World Health Organization [WHO]; 2002. p. 87–121.
14. Tjaden P, Thoennes N. National Institute of Justice and the Centers of Disease Control and Prevention, "Extent, nature and consequences of intimate partner violence: findings from the National Violence Against Women Survey". 2000.
15. Greenberg K. Still hidden in the closet: trans women and domestic violence. Berkeley J Gend Law Justice. 2012;27(2):199–224.
16. Freedner N, Freed LH, Yang YW, Austin SB. Dating violence among gay, lesbian, and bisexual adolescents: results from a community survey. J Adolesc Health. 2002;31:469–74.
17. Hipwell AE, et al. Examining links between sexual risk behaviors and dating violence involvement as a function of sexual orientation. J Pediatr Adolesc Gynecol. 2013;26(4):212–8.
18. Halpern CT, Young ML, Waller MW, Martin SL, Kupper LL. Prevalence of partner violence in same-sex romantic and sexual relationships in a national sample of adolescents. J Adolesc Health. 2004;35(2):124–31.
19. Edwards KM, Sylaska KM. The perpetration of intimate partner violence among LGBTQ college youth: the role of minority stress. J Youth Adolesc. 2013;42(11):1721–31.
20. Ristock JL. Relationship violence in lesbian/gay/bisexual/transgender/queer communities: moving beyond a gender-based framework. 2005. Violence Against Women Online Resources, Office for Violence Against Women. Available at http://www.mincava.umn.edu/documents/lgbtqviolence/lgbtqviolence.html.
21. Aulivola M. Outing domestic violence: affording appropriate protections to gay and lesbian victims. Fam Court Rev. 2004;42(I):162–77.
22. Finneran C, Stephenson R. Gay and bisexual men's perceptions of police helpfulness in response to male-male intimate partner violence. West J Emerg Med. 2013;14(4):354–62.
23. Ard KL, Makadon HJ. Addressing intimate partner violence in lesbian, gay, bisexual, and transgender patients. J Gen Intern Med. 2011;26(8):930–3.
24. Island D, Letellier P. Men who beat the men who love them: battered gay men and domestic violence. New York: Routledge; 1991.
25. Holt S, Couchman D. The L.A. Gay & Lesbian Center's STOP Partner Abuse/Domestic Violence Program. LA Gay & Lesbian Center. 2011. http://laglc.convio.net/site/DocServer/Info_Bookletcv__2_.pdf?docID=14323. Accessed 11 June 2014.
26. Tham K, et al. Queer youth relationship violence. Community United Against Violence and Lavender Youth Recreation & Information Center, California State Department of Health Services. 2000.
27. Klostermann K, Kelley ML, Milletich RJ, Mignone T. Alcoholism and partner aggression among gay and lesbian couples. Aggression Violent Behav. 2011;16:115–9.
28. Allen M, Brancom PL, Burnett D, Hernandez A, List-Warrilow J. LGBT communities domestic violence information & resources. 2007. http://nwnetwork.org/wp-content/uploads/2011/11/National-Resource-Center_LGBTDV-Full.pdf. Accessed 11 June 2014.

# Part IV

# LGBT Health in Specialty Medicine

# Pediatric and Adolescent LGBT Health

# 11

## Henry H. Ng and Gregory S. Blaschke

## Purpose

The purpose of this chapter is to describe the socioecologic factors influencing the health of LGBT youth, identify the challenges LGBT youth face in their experience of adolescence, learn strategies to interact with LGBT youth and meet them where they are, apply best practices in caring for LGBT youth, and provide clinicians resources to better care for sexual minority youth.

## Learning Objectives

After reading this chapter, learners will be able to:

H.H. Ng, M.D., M.P.H. (✉)
Center for Internal Medicine-Pediatrics,
The MetroHealth System/Case Western Reserve
University School of Medicine,
2500 MetroHealth Dr., H574, Cleveland,
OH 44109, USA
e-mail: hng@metrohealth.org

G.S. Blaschke, M.D., M.P.H.
Department of Pediatrics, Oregon Health and Science
University, Doembecher Children's Hospital,
707 SW Gaines St, CDRC-P, Portland,
OR 97239-2998, USA
e-mail: Blaschke@ohsu.edu

- Describe the development of sexuality, sexual orientation, gender identity, and gender expression *(KP3)*
- Discuss how the challenges faced by LGBT youth impact risk behaviors and health *(PC5, KP4, KP5, SPB4)*
- Discuss the importance of confidentiality in healthcare for LGBT youth *(ICS2, Pr2)*
  - Identify at least three protective factors that can promote resilience among LGBT youth *(KP3, PC5, PC6)*

## Introduction

### Introductory Case Presentation [1, 2]

Imagine you are a nurse, medical student, resident or physician working in the Emergency Department of a middle-sized city. Your next patient is LH. You walk into the room and begin to obtain the following information:

LH is a 21-year-old male to female (MTF) transgender individual presenting to the Emergency Department with a complaint of increasing diffuse abdominal pain for 2–3 days. She reported that the pain did not radiate to other parts of her abdomen. She denied any vomiting, blood in the stool, dark tarry stools or any changes in her bowel habits. She denied any fevers or weight loss, changes in diet or blunt force trauma to the abdomen.

© Springer International Publishing Switzerland 2016
K.L. Eckstrand, J.M. Ehrenfeld (eds.), *Lesbian, Gay, Bisexual, and Transgender Healthcare*,
DOI 10.1007/978-3-319-19752-4_11

**Past medical history**: None

**Past surgical history**: None

**Medications**: Premarin (a form of conjugated estrogen) as prescribed by her endocrinologist for hormonal transitioning

**Allergies**: No known drug allergies

**Social history**: LH denied using tobacco. She reported social alcohol use. She denied illicit drugs or intravenous drug use. She reported working as a female impersonator at a local night club.

**Family history**: Negative for gastrointestinal disease

You proceed to perform a focused physical exam/assessment:

**General appearance**: LH was in no apparent distress. She was androgynous appearing.

**Vital signs**: Afebrile, vital signs stable.

**Abdominal exam**: Except for slight diffuse abdominal tenderness to light palpation, the exam was normal.

LH declined genital and rectal exams. The patient's exam was otherwise unremarkable.

At this time, what additional information would you like to obtain from LH?

You obtain the additional information:

**Sexual history**: LH is currently single and partners with males. She reports using barrier methods (condoms) inconsistently. She has not had sexual reassignment surgery. She denied any penile or rectal symptoms.

**Medication history**: Although LH had been prescribed Premarin to take BID (twice daily), she had been taking 5–10 pills daily for the last 2 weeks. The patient reported desiring the effect of the hormonal treatment to occur more rapidly and believed that greater doses of the medication would achieve that goal.

**Additional social history**: Moreover, LH is a silicone injection user who just attended a "pump party" where she received non-medical augmentation services to enhance her physical attributes. LH paid $500 for a local "beautician" (non-licensed, non-medically trained personnel) to inject industrial grade quality silicone into her breasts.

## Introductory Case Wrap-Up and Questions to Consider

The common causes of abdominal pain, including appendicitis, colitis, gallbladder disease, infectious hepatitis and pancreatitis, were ruled out based on physical exam and history findings for LH. Her abdominal pain was attributed to the supratherapeutic overdose of the Premarin. Premarin is metabolized by the liver and excessive amounts can cause some degree of drug-induced hepatitis. She was discharged from the emergency department with instructions to decrease her intake of Premarin to the dose prescribed. A follow-up note was sent to her endocrinologist informing him of her evaluation.

Health care providers reviewing this introductory case may also want to consider the following questions:

1. How does one decide what pronoun is appropriate to use in addressing LH?
2. How does one ask about sexual behaviors, gender identity and sexual orientation in a culturally competent manner?
3. With the information you have obtained from LH, what additional measures, if any, should be or could be taken to address her presenting problem of abdominal pain?
4. What is this patient's anticipatory guidance or aftercare education?
5. How would you counsel her to prevent this from occurring again?
6. What other health conditions is she at risk?
7. What health resources are available to her to reduce risks of illness and promote health?

LH was not a fictitious character, but an actual patient. The health concerns and problems illustrated in her case are not uncommon for members of the Lesbian, Gay, Bisexual and Transgender (LGBT) community.

The goal is that, after reading this chapter, the reader will be more comfortable and familiar with best practices and culturally sensitive approaches to the care of sexual minority youth. To that end and to better address health issues of sexual minority youth, this chapter also will provide a framework for understanding LGBT-related health disparities, an overview of adolescent sexuality development and a brief review of the epidemiology of pertinent adolescent health-focused issues.

## Health Disparities among LGBT Youth

The overarching framework for understanding LGBT health disparities is found in the Institute of Medicine Report: *The Health of Lesbian, Gay, Bisexual, and Transgender People: Building a Foundation for Better Understanding* [3]. The report posits that four perspectives guide the discussion on LGBT Health (see Chap. 1 for more details):

1. The minority stress model: calls attention to the chronic stress that sexual and gender minorities may experience as a result of their stigmatization;
2. Life course perspective: looks at how events at each stage of life influence subsequent stages;
3. Intersectionality perspective: examines an individual's multiple identities and the ways in which they interact; and
4. Social ecology perspective: emphasizes that individuals are surrounded by spheres of influence, including families, communities, and society.

The net effect of such discrimination based on sexual orientation and gender identity/expression culminates in negative physical and emotional health outcomes. Combined with other forms of inequality (i.e. racism, sexism, ageism, ableism, heterosexism), LGBT youth are subject to macro- and micro-inequalities in their day-to-day navigation of local and geographic social groups as well as society at large.

Concepts of "gay-related stress" [4] and "minority stress" [5, 6] describe a range of stressors resulting from individual and institutional discrimination against people with sexual minority identities. The impact of these stressors on mental health was described in the MacArthur Foundation's National Survey of Midlife Development in

the United States (MIDUS) Study [7] in which respondents reported measures of discrimination in four domains:

- Lifetime discriminatory experiences
- Frequency of day-to-day discrimination
- Reasons for discrimination
- General effects of discrimination

Respondents were asked about mental health indicators of five stress-sensitive psychiatric disorders and drug and alcohol dependence. Homosexual and bisexual individuals reported lifetime and day to day experiences with discrimination more frequently than heterosexuals and over 40 % of respondents attributed this in part, or in total, to their sexual orientation.

## Gender and Sexuality Development

Gender and sexuality development for children and adolescents is complex, dynamic, and a multifactorial process. Gender identity awareness can begin early in life, and, by age three, some children can become conscious of physical differences between males and females. Gender is learned by children very early and Kohlberg in 1996 [8] described a sequence from gender identification, gender stability and gender constancy confirmed by the research of others [9–13]. Most 2-year olds know their gender and can identify the gender of strangers. Three year olds consistently apply gender labels although preschoolers are not certain that gender is a permanent attribute, most 4–5 year olds apply many learned social stereotypes.

By middle childhood, children's interest in same-gender peer play and behavior reflect the ongoing process of gender identity formation. Some children may exhibit gender variant or gender incongruent behavior, more than a lack of interest in culturally defined gender roles or behavior. For example, some girls may prefer to play with trucks, cars and other stereotypically "masculine" toys while some boys may prefer to play with dolls, dresses or other stereotypically "feminine" toys. Some of these children with gender variant behaviors may experience gender conflict or dysphoria. Though some children and youth resolve their dysphoria by the end of adolescence, a proportion of youth will persist with these feelings of gender dysphoria and seek gender transition care [14].

In the face of uncertainty about ultimate outcomes, a clinically practical approach is to consider that gender dysphoria would occur at the extreme end of the continuum. Perrin identified three clear principles for parents of children with gender dysphoria: "It is legitimate (1) to help children feel more secure about their gender identity as boys or girls, perhaps preventing adult transgenderism; (2) to diminish as much as possible peer ostracism and social isolation; and (3) to treat evidence of associated behavioral/emotional stress" [15].

The variation in expression of gender and sexuality is certainly a developmental process impacted by many biologic, psychological and contextual factors in society and culture. The extensive literature looking at genetic, neuro-anatomic and psycho-endocrine factors will not be reviewed here; nor a discussion of family, social or the impact of fear, bias and stigma on development of complex sexual behaviors. Instead, many have described mature stages in lesbian and gay identity formation [16–19].

Ultimately sexual orientation also has a developmental trajectory across childhood and adolescence. Data from Youth Risk Behavior Surveys have demonstrated that a proportion of youth identify their sexual orientation as other than heterosexual and that this number has been stable over time. "…The prevalence of homosexuality among adolescents is unknown because gender roles and sexual identity may take years to evolve and be acknowledged. Although only 1 % of 12th-grade males and less than 1 % of 12th-grade females viewed themselves as mostly or completely homosexual, 10 % were unsure of their sexual orientation" [20]. Historically, sexual minority youth were more likely to select same sex attraction than to select a self-identifying label. "Students were most likely to endorse same-sex attractions, followed by fantasies and experiences, and then were least likely to describe themselves as homosexual" [21].

However, sexual minority youth are coming out younger and identifying their sexual orientation earlier. A 2011 report on LGBT Youth Risk Behavior Surveillance found that, across the nine sites that assessed sexual identity, students identified themselves as:

- Heterosexual: 90.3–93.6 % (median: 93.0 %)
- Gay or lesbian: 1.0–2.6 % (median: 1.3 %)
- Bisexual: 2.9–5.2 % (median: 3.7 %)

The percentage of students who were unsure of their sexual identity ranged from 1.3 to 4.7 % (median 2.5 %) [22].

Coming out may be specifically challenging in various cultural environments and communities as sexuality holds different meaning within different cultures and ethnicities [23]. Specific challenges for LGBT Youth of Color beyond identity development, for example, include integration of sexual and gender identity, consolidation with race and ethnicity, racism and bias within larger LGBT community as well as homophobia, biphobia, and/or transphobia within their own ethnic communities [23]. Despite the need for culturally competent interventions and best practices to support LGBT Youth of Color, however, research is lacking in this area. Of the 168 publications and articles published between 1972 and 1999 on health and mental health concerns of LGBT youth, only 16 were on LGBT youth of color including 3 book chapters, 4 empirical studies and 9 additional articles on social service/provider training needs of transgender youth [24].

## Health Vulnerabilities among LGBT Youth: A Review of the Literature

It is clear from the literature that a number of physical and mental health concerns may challenge sexual minority youth as they journey toward adulthood. Health professionals caring for LGBT youth need to become sensitive to the psychological, medical and social issues that impact the well-being of LGBT youth and become proficient in discussing these health issues with their patients.

## Mental Health

Poor mental health and suicide are among the most important and concerning health issues LGBT youth face. In 2010, suicide was the second leading cause of death among young people ages 10–24, accounting for 4867 deaths [25]. In general, the incidence and prevalence of suicide among LGBT populations is largely unknown as death records do not include a deceased person's sexual orientation or gender identity. Across many different countries, however, a strong and consistent relationship between sexual orientation and nonfatal suicidal behavior has been observed. A meta-analysis of 25 international population-based studies found the lifetime prevalence of suicide attempts in gay and bisexual male adolescents and adults was four times that of comparable heterosexual males. Among lesbian and bisexual females, lifetime suicide attempt rates were almost twice those of heterosexual females. Lesbian, gay, and bisexual (LGB) adolescents and adults were also found to be almost twice as likely as heterosexuals to report a suicide attempt in the past year [26]. Research also indicates that nearly half of young transgender people have seriously considered suicide, with nearly 25 % reporting a previous suicide attempt [27]. A different study finds that LGB youth are four times more likely, and questioning youth are three times more likely, to attempt suicide compared to heterosexual youth [28].

In addition, sexual orientation seems to be a stronger indicator of suicide attempts in males than in females [29]. And, compared to heterosexual youth, suicide attempts by LGB youth and questioning youth are 4–6 times more likely to result in injury, poisoning, or overdose requiring treatment from a medical professional [29]. One non-random sample of LGB adolescents and young adults reported over half of the youth who attempted suicide used methods classified as moderate to lethal [30].

In addition to suicide, other mental health disparities among LBGT youth and their psychosocial antecedents have been described in the literature, including social isolation, running away, substance abuse, compromised mental health, damaged self-esteem, depression and anxiety [31]. A 2009 survey of more than 7000 LGBT middle and high school students aged 13–21 years found that in the past year, because of their sexual orientation:

- Eight of ten students had been verbally harassed at school
- Four of ten had been physically harassed at school
- Six of ten felt unsafe at school
- One of five had been the victim of a physical assault at school [32]

In 2014, Blashill and Safran identified increased use of anabolic steroids among sexual minority boys [33]. The authors found that sexual minority adolescent boys were at an increased odds of 5.8 (95 % confidence interval 4.1–8.2) to report a lifetime prevalence of anabolic steroid use (21 % vs. 4 %) compared with their heterosexual counterparts.

Analysis of data from the Growing Up Today Study (GUTS) has identified differences in patterns of tobacco use, alcohol use and eating disorders in sexual minority youth. GUTS is a longitudinal cohort study of United States adolescent boys and girls who are children of women who participated in the Nurses' Health Study II. Findings include that youth of minority sexual orientation reported earlier initiation of alcohol use and that there is greater risk of alcohol use among heterosexual males and bisexual females. These disparities in alcohol use among youth with a minority sexual orientation emerge in early adolescence and persist into young adulthood [34]. With respect to tobacco use, youth who identified as mostly heterosexual girls or bisexual and lesbian were more likely to smoke, whereas Gay/Bisexual self-identified boys were no more likely to smoke than heterosexual boys. The findings persisted even when controlling for multiple socio-demographic and psychosocial covariates [35].

Findings from Austin et al. in 2009 revealed that mostly heterosexual girls and boys had greater concerns with weight and appearance and were less happy with their bodies compared with same-gender heterosexuals. Specifically, mostly heterosexual girls were more likely to vomit and/or use laxatives to control weight and more likely to binge eat in the past year. However, the researchers also found gay/bisexual boys were more concerned with trying to look like men in the media and more likely to binge compared to heterosexual boys. In this study, lesbian/bisexual girls reported feeling generally happier with their bodies than mostly heterosexual girls and were less concerned with trying to look like women in the media [36].

## Physical and Sexual Health

LGBT youth also face challenges in navigating healthy sexuality compared to heterosexual youth. Studies show that LGBT youth are more likely than heterosexual teens to have had sexual intercourse, to have had more partners, and to have experienced sexual intercourse against their will [37]. Substance use before sex, high-risk sexual behaviors and issues surrounding personal safety including prostitution have been reported more often by lesbian, gay, and bisexual youth than heterosexual youth [31, 38]. In addition, Lane found in 2002 that young men who partner with both sexes have reduced odds of condom use and increased odds of having had multiple sexual partners [39].

Research studies also identify that lesbian and bisexual teens are twice as likely as their heterosexual peers to experience unintended pregnancy. Moreover, some lesbian youth may use intentional pregnancy as a strategy or coping mechanism in an attempt to hide their sexual identity [40, 41].

As compared to their heterosexual peers LGBT teens also are at an increased risk of STIs, including HIV [38]. Although the number of incident cases of HIV in the United States has plateaued, new HIV infections in LGBT youth, especially in communities of young men who have sex with men (MSM) continue to rise. According to CDC HIV surveillance data, youth aged 13–24 accounted for approximately 26 % of all incident HIV infections in the United States in 2010, with

most new HIV infections among youth occurring among gay and bisexual males. Young bisexual and gay males experienced a 22 % increase in incident HIV infections between 2008 and 2010, with young Hispanic/Latino and African American/Black MSM especially affected. Nearly 60 % of youth with HIV living in the United States are unaware that they are HIV positive [42]. Factors which potentially contribute to the spread of HIV in young LGBT people include youth low perception of risk, low rates of HIV testing, low rates of condom use, high rates of sexually transmitted infections, older sexual partners some of whom are likely to be infected with HIV, substance use, homelessness, inadequate HIV education and feelings of social isolation [42].

## Risk and Protective Factors for Mental and Physical Health

LGBT adolescents face the same concerns of all adolescents; however, they have additional challenges primarily due to stigmatization, isolation, discrimination and barriers than those experienced by heterosexual teens (see Fig. 11.1). Their dynamic, complex and often changing understanding of their own gender identity, sexual orientation, attraction and behaviors lead to many needs outlined in the position paper of the Society for Adolescent Health and Medicine [43]. While health disparities will require health care providers to assess and address risk, followed by prioritized risk reduction strategies, the majority of LGBT youth are healthy and well adjusted.

The high risk behaviors of LGBT youth are often a result of reactions to social stigma and non-acceptance by peers, family and society, including our health care systems. These may in turn lead to internalized homophobia, isolation, bullying and other forms of victimization. As with all adolescents, an LGBT teen's family member, peer, or others of importance to them (like teacher, coach, physician) response to their disclosure of identity may serve to build resiliency or compound risk.

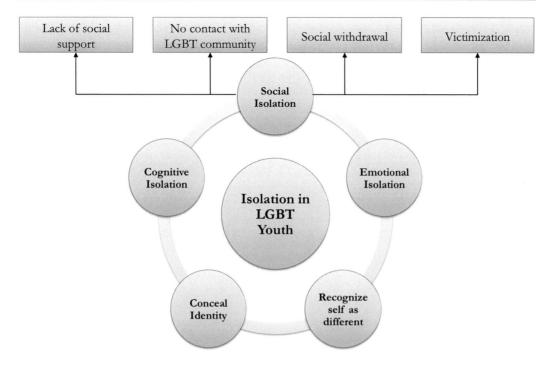

**Fig. 11.1**  Dimensions of isolation for LGBT youth (adapted from Johnson MJ, et al. Isolation of lesbian, gay, bisexual and transgender youth: a dimensional concept analysis. J Adv Nurs. Mar 2014)

## Family Response

Family connectedness is an important factor in response to adversity in adolescence. Family relationships do improve as parents when families become more aware of the challenges teens face. When compared to their peers, LGBT teens with high levels of family rejection lead to significant increased risk of suicide, depression, illegal drug use and unprotected sexual intercourse [44]. Those who report family acceptance show better overall health outcomes and well-being [45].

Research by Ryan [44] published in the journal *Pediatrics* reported significantly higher rates of mental and physical health problems among LGB young adults who experienced high levels of rejection from their parents while they were adolescents. Specifically, LGB adolescents who reported higher levels of rejection were:

- 8.4 times more likely to have attempted suicide;
- 5.9 times more likely to report high levels of depression;
- 3.4 times more likely to use illegal drugs; and
- 3.4 times more likely to have engaged in unprotected intercourse

## Individual and Community Consideration

Peer rejection, bullying including social media have resulted in teen and young adult suicides that have raised community awareness via the media. Unfortunately this can happen even based on perceived sexual orientation and/or gender expressions. School aged LGBT teens have reported being victims of verbal (85 %) or physical (40 %) harassment and nearly 20 % physical assault [46]. Victimization in turn correlates with suicide attempts [47] and sexual risk and substance abuse [48]. Policy implications for LGBT youth are paramount within systems where they are disproportionately represented, as in foster care, homelessness, and juvenile justice systems [49, 50].

## School Policy

As a place where children and youth spend significant time, schools matter! Significant bullying occurs within schools which have short and long term implications [51]. Even modest reductions in school based victimization would result in significant improvement for LGBT youth health. Four key policy recommendations were published in 2011 by Russel et al. [52].

1. Enforce clear and inclusive antidiscrimination/anti-harassment policies inclusive of LGBT identity and gender expression
2. Make clear where students should go for LGBT information and support
3. Regular intervention by staff when bias-motivated harassment happens
4. Support gay-straight alliances and other student sponsored diversity clubs
5. Integrate LGBT topics into curriculum

## Societal Stigma

A growing understanding of trauma-informed care, cumulative life stress as a result of adverse childhood events (ACE), and increased understanding of neuro-biologic changes as a result of early brain development, leads one to also postulate a growing emergence of awareness that health disparities are not only prevalent in racial and ethnic groups, but are also common in sexual and gender minority populations. LGBT children, youth and LGBT headed families are all vulnerable populations.

## Internalized Homophobia

The society stigma from potential family, peer, and role model rejection often leads to internalized homophobia compounded by isolation and discrimination that may occur. Health professionals must first recognize how their own (or their systems) response may also lead to injury or re-injury. The high level of stress may manifest as anxiety, depression, and exaggerated risk taking behavior of adolescents. Shame, guilt and denial are all potential cofounders. Adolescents are also not likely equipped with skills and neurodevelopmental maturation including reasoning, limit setting, impulsiveness etc. Familial, societal

reaction also likely contributes to truancy, homelessness, self-medication via substance abuse or counterintuitively, attempts to reduce of feelings of isolation through risky sexual behaviors.

## Isolation

In 2002, Hazler and Denham conceptualized teen isolation as resulting from peer on peer abuse including bullying, teasing and harassment [53]. Johnson and Amella expanded on this in 2013, identifying several forms of isolation contributing to risk and therefore potentially amenable via supports. They describe isolation of LGBT youth as a complex interaction between social isolation, emotional isolation, recognition of a "different" self-identity, leading perhaps to identity concealment and further cognitive isolation of the teen, These are postulated to be enhanced by lack of traditional supports (rejection by family, friends), lack of contact with LGBT community and role models, leading to social withdrawal and often victimization.

Cognitive isolation may include inaccurate information and lack of role models, or others to discuss self-identity, gender and sexual attraction or orientation [54].

## Resiliency

Despite these risks, the majority of LGBT youth do remarkably well suggesting resiliency, skill acquisition, and perhaps rapidly changing social acceptance. Mayer et al. suggested many helpful strategies for clinicians and systems including a public health approach [55]. Clinicians must be prepared to deliver nonjudgmental education, advice and services to this vulnerable population. Many children may need assistance in planning for coming out, considering potential reactions of friends, family and others with whom they rely. They require accurate information and community resources. Risk assessment and risk reduction using preventive medicine and clinical tools like screening instruments, motivational interviewing and brief intervention and referral to therapy are imperative for all adolescents including LGBT youth. As the majority of LGBT youth are already seeing providers, becoming comfortable with adolescent discussions regarding sexuality is important. While adolescent health clinics and clinics specific to

LGBT communities are sometimes available in urban centers, the majority of teens will not have ability to access such centers. Recognizing this is only one of many populations that primary care providers in particular must develop knowledge, attitudes and skills a list of resources, policy statements, and educational materials are included in Appendix 1.

## Supporting Parents of Sexual Minority Youth

While culture, religion, tradition and prior status of family relationships will all impact the parents' reaction and response to the news of a child's sexual and gender identity, every family is really a unit unto itself. Culture, religion, tradition and relationships are all highly individualized by individuals and families. Many parents may 'already know' the 'secret' that their child reveals. Parents may also experience stages of grief. Their own personal experience or knowledge of bias, discrimination, victimization and protecting their child are all items that parents will need to process. Doing so with others is often necessary. Health care providers for children also have a relationship with parents. While their primary duty is to protection of the child, pediatricians and others providers caring for children, can assist parents as their response or reaction may evolve over time. Providing factual data about risks, risk reduction and/or gender transitions will be needed. Providers of children and youth will need to educate themselves about community agencies that can assist with more in depth information and/or support groups for their children and/or themselves. Again using techniques like motivational interviewing, readiness for change and focusing on long term outcomes for their children may be beneficial. Self-affirming assistance to the youth while simultaneously guiding parents in their supportive role may require separate sessions and/or providers. The American Medical Association, the American Psychological Association, the American Academy of Pediatrics, the Society of Adolescent Health and Medicine, all have policies/positions that reject consideration of conversion therapy (therapies which have a goal to change sexual orientation) as unsubstantiated and harmful.

## LGBT Youth in the Context of Their Development, Family and Community

Adolescence is often a difficult stage developmentally (and psychosocially) for everyone involved in some way. Parents, family members, friends and trusted adult role models may struggle with any adolescent's behavior. Adding sexual minority status may compound the difficulty. This can be explained in part by understanding some basic principles of neurodevelopmental differences in children and adolescents, and recalling how normal neural maturation affects coping mechanisms of children and youth.

Young children, for example, respond to stickers to change behavior more than expected in part because of how developing brains respond to rewards at that stage. A small reward (sticker) can result in much jubilation and pays off in achieving behavioral change. Adolescents, on the other hand, would say "*lame*" or "*whatever*" to any care provider who attempt to change behavior through the use of stickers. Instead their 'reward pathways' respond to more dramatic behaviors that often involve risk, including "sex, drugs (alcohol), and rock and roll." In general, a child's brain also develops from 'inside out' (brain stem to fine motor skills) and from 'back to front' (caudal to cephalic development.) Executive functions, decision making, and working through anticipated and unanticipated consequences are examples of frontal lobe functions that gain strength in late adolescence and young adulthood. Children with anatomic or physiologic (organic) changes in these areas and individuals with variable expression of these incompletely understood functions may never develop strengths in these domains. The timing of the development of these skills is also individualistic and subject to both genetics and environment.

Parents (or parent equivalent figures) when present may struggle in guiding their youth in many areas since peer influence and role models play such an important role in this age group. When LGBT orientation and sexual behaviors are added to this mix, one can realize additional stressors these youth (and families) may face as described in Chap. "epidemiology".

In caring for LGBT youth, many clinicians will encounter parents, families and other trusted adults who are struggling with their child's sexuality. This presents an opportunity for physicians and health professionals to provide messages of acceptance and support which are central to improving health outcomes for sexual minority youth. An example of such an accepting message is:

> As your child's health care provider, I recognize it must be difficult for you to grapple with your child's emerging sexuality. What we know is that youth who receive supportive messages about themselves tend to do better and have better health outcomes. I know you must care about your child, and that is why you came to see me. How can I help you offer your child a parental message of support and acceptance?

In the effort to better understand the experience of LGBT youth within the context of their development, family and community, it is important to acknowledge how little is known from population based research versus high-risk sampling of the gay community. These facts make it imperative to follow the IOM report recommendations to expand knowledge in the many subgroups of the LGBT population.

## Reaching LGBT Youth in the Clinical Setting

Research indicates that the majority of youth do value their physician's advice about sexuality. Factors contributing to greater youth comfort when discussing such matters with their own regular health provider included addressing issues of general sexual health and the adolescent's own high self-esteem [56].

In addition, Ginsberg et al. assessed LGBT Youth Comfort and Safety in Health Settings in 2002 and found that LGBT youth value the same clinic characteristics desired by all adolescents: privacy, cleanliness, honesty, respect, competency and a non-judgmental stance [57]. Less but somewhat important factors included having a LGBT provider, a site that focuses on LGBT youth, having magazines for LGBT people in waiting rooms, and having health information

offered in a private place. Actions that were perceived as offensive included an assumption of heterosexuality, a negative reaction to revealing sexuality, an assumption of greater risk of disease (as orientation does not equal behavior) and delivery of health care information from a judgmental point of view.

One way health professionals can improve health outcomes for LGBT youth is to exhibit both cultural and clinical competency when working with sexual minority youth. Start the interview in a manner that elicits the patient's preferred name, pronoun and any gender-referent terms used in self-identification. (Refer to terms and vocabulary covered in previous chapters for a more in depth review of terminology used for self-identification.) It is important to remember, that for some youth, the terms used for self-identification are fluid and may change over time. Additionally, some may use words like "Queer" or "Genderqueer" as an all-encompassing term if self-identification.

When obtaining a sexual history, it is important to be aware that youth commonly perceive providers as authority figures. Always preface any inquiry into behavior or risk-based screening in the framework of confidentiality, consent and normalization. Confidentiality is important to gain an adolescent's honest response and trust in a provider's guidance. Not all revelations can be maintained in confidence, however, and a provider should always explain the limits of confidentiality, which vary by state. Such limits generally include a break in confidentiality when the adolescent's behaviors or answers to questions place him/her (or others) in danger. Providers also are generally mandated reporters for child abuse, variably for intimate partner violence reporting, and age differences between sexual partners as defined by state law. State specific laws often address age difference between intimate partners where one is below 18. Homicidal and suicidal ideation also obligates action by providers. Discussion of consent for treatment of mental health, alcohol and drugs, options regarding pregnancy, contraception and sexually transmitted infections can vary somewhat by state. In addition, the same definitions may not apply from a legal, ethical or moral framework.

Parents or other adult figures involved may also need to understand the limits of disclosure for youth. Provide reassurance, however, that a provider will inform authorities/parents or other responsible adults, if something arises that can or must be shared such as danger to self/others. Involving a trusted parent, adult family member or friend may be indicated and lead to better outcomes for many domains, but it's important to remember that breaking confidentiality when necessary does not necessarily mean telling them all the details. Alternatively, seeking permission from the involved youth and negotiating the details of what can be shared with parents is possible. (Examples include: SADD Contract for Life; substance abuse treatment; making decisions about unwanted and/or unplanned pregnancy.)

Be careful to realize providers are in a powerful position compared to youth, and one's own moral, ethical and religious beliefs can influence this interaction, either consciously or unconsciously. Unconscious or systematic racism in medicine as demonstrated in health care is an example of how this may also occur in the setting of sexual minority youth. Many organized medicine and specialty organizations, including the American Medical Association and the American Academy of Pediatrics, also suggest that providers refer patients to other care providers when there are significant conflicts that may interfere with providing care in such situations.

Also keep in mind safety for adolescents and LGBT youth specifically. As noted previously, suicide, homelessness (often by familial rejection), intimate partner violence, substance misuse, bullying, and potential trafficking are examples of significant risk factors within this population. While encouraging 'coming out' and self-acceptance is important, doing so in a safe environment and keeping safety in mind is important. Negotiating and facilitating this process maybe one role where providers can assist youth. It is not the provider's job to "out" the child to anyone; on the other hand, facilitating difficult conversations

with the permission of the child may be an important role entrusted to the provider by the involved LGBT youth.

Prior to asking a patient about sexual attraction or behaviors, generally preface the discussion by normalizing the questions themselves. For example, begin by stating "*I ask all my patients these questions, and in this way.*" Generic open-ended questions may also facilitate open and honest communication. Opening the conversation with "*Tell me about your partner*" could be one way to begin. Others may be more comfortable asking "*What type of person are you attracted to? Who are you sexually active with?*" Remember that adolescents may not understand generic terms like sexual activity until they are significantly mature. As one example, the provider may need to specifically ask about each behavior as adolescents often do not consider oral sex to be sexual activity. By normalizing this discussion, you are relieving anxiety that adolescents sometimes feel that adults '*can tell they had sex by just looking at them.*' You do not want any adolescent to feel that you are singling them out by asking them the 'gay questions' because they look, sound or act in a gender non-conforming way.

Stereotypes are generally only partially true, and cultural assumptions made by many can be off putting if overly applied. Every family and individual is a 'culture' unto themselves. Everyone owns their own religious, ethnic, racial, cultural and social norms. Stated another way, no two African American, Roman Catholics, or North Westerners share the exact same characteristics. Similarly, no two Master's degrees, in the same field and even from the same university are ever exactly the same.

As discussed in a prior chapter, common terminology used by LGBT adolescents may vary by many factors, including generation, slang, geography, culture, etc. Providers should demonstrate fluidity of language and use of Queer/Genderqueer as a potentially all-encompassing identity term. Utilize active listening skills, defined as listening for meaning. Strength of conviction, concern or terminology may be crucial.

Listening for affirming or dis-congruent language or meaning, affect, or descriptions of family acceptance can be crucial when interacting with LGBT adolescents. Prefacing a conversation with *"I care for you, no matter what you say"* is one way to express a non-judgmental stance.

Providing generic examples of how others have responded may sometimes assist in breaking the ice. Just as addressing suicide does not increase the individual rate/risk of suicide, providers should not fear asking questions and taking a comprehensive history. If nothing else, even if a teen does not respond or disclose at the time of initial questioning, it will prompt them to know that you and/or your clinic is a place to come in the future with any of their LGBT concerns.

Remember that adolescents and youth will be actively listening to your response to their questions and are likely to over-interpret a facial expression, unintended attitude, or some other form of non-verbal communication. Sexual minority youth, like most adolescents, are savvy and can sense negative emotional reactions from a health provider. Thus, assessing the youth's understanding may allow clarification of any unintended non-verbal communication cue or comment. Avoiding a negative response is important. Likewise, acknowledging and/or apologizing for a misstatement if one should occur in a heartfelt way is important to gain, sustain and maintain trust.

Mnemonics such as HEADDSS, SHADDES or HEADSFIRST can help a provider organize an adolescent or young adult visit. These clinical tools, originally developed by Goldenring [58], have been adapted as foundational questions to discuss in an adolescent's social history and essentially complete 'developmental and risk based' surveillance. The HEADSFIRST mnemonic below, for example, can provide a framework to explore how adolescent sexuality and/or gender identify may impact different aspects of an adolescent's life and health.

- **H**ome: Separation, support, "space to grow"
- **E**ducation: Expectations, study habits, achievement
- **A**buse: Emotional, verbal, physical, sexual

- **D**rugs: Tobacco, alcohol, marijuana, cocaine, others
- **S**afety: Hazardous activities, seatbelts, helmets
- **F**riends: Confidant, peer pressure, interaction
- **I**mage: Self-esteem, looks, appearance
- **R**ecreation: Exercise, relaxation, TV, media games
- **S**exuality: Changes, feelings, experiences, identity
- **T**hreats: Depressed or upset easily, harm to self or others

These methods, however, have not been validated as a method for population or risk-based screening of youth. Screening tools for mental health and substance use that can be used at the population or risk-based, individual level, include PHQ2, PHQ 9A, CRAFFT, AUDIT, POSSIT, SCARED, Vanderbilt ADHD, etc. Universal and risk-based medical screening based on age, sexual and other behaviors, and pertinent anatomic organs in the Trans person can be completed as indicated per national guidelines (mammogram, vaginal and/or rectal pap, etc.).

Some authors advocate for a strength-based approach to adolescents [59]; questioning and responding toward an adolescent's strengths in each of these areas (and in general) rather than a risk-based approach. By developmental definition, adolescents and youth are more oriented to peers and environment, but this must also be placed in the context of the individual person, the family (biologic or by choice), and the community where they reside (peers, culture, religion/ spirituality, school, etc.)

Finally, a provider must also address their entire system and practice of care where LGBT youth are seen. It is difficult for any provider to overcome a negative experience sometimes inadvertently initiated further up-stream by other care team members, or by culturally incompetent forms, handouts or other 'hidden' messages delivered that indicate less openness by the practice or facility where these youth may be seen. Indeed, much of the research we have on a variety of subgroups in this population actually comes from alternative locations where care may be sought. Many youth are seen in settings other than a medical home (pediatric, family medicine or internal medicine settings.) School based health centers, urgent care, sports medicine clinics, homeless or at-risk centers, and juvenile justice programs are just some examples where LGBT youth may be seen.

## Guidelines and Best Practices for Care of Sexual Minority Youth

The LGBT Advisory Committee to the AMA Board of Trustees helped create a "Compendium of Health Profession Association LGBT Policy and Position Statements." This includes 101 policy or position statements by 10 major health professional associations. This list was last updated in 2013 and is available on line at the GLMA website.

The most recent American Academy of Pediatrics (AAP), *Bright Futures: Guidelines for Health Supervision of Infants, Children and Adolescents, 3rd Edition* [60] was funded by the US Department of Health and Human Services, Health Resources and Services Administration, and the Maternal Child Health Bureau. These specific guidelines contain a theme chapter on promoting healthy sexual development and sexuality. The AAP also recently published specific guidelines on providing LGBT care in office settings.

One of the more comprehensive lists of resources available for a variety of audiences was published by Perrin et al. [61] The AMA also convened and published proceedings from an adolescent educational forum addressing youth bullying [62]. The Trevor Project™ founded in 1998 by the creators of Academy Award® winning short film TREVOR is a LGBT youth crisis intervention and suicide prevention program. The film addresses adolescent angst of coming out [63]. The It Gets Better Project™ was created by Dan Savage to bring messages of hope to LGBT youth around the world [64].

For medical educators, the videos from the Adolescent Reproductive and Sexual Health Education Project http://prh.org/teen-reproductive-health/arshep-explained/ can be extremely useful in practicing discussions for learners in medicine.

A list of references, tools, resources and organizations that support efforts to ameliorate health disparities for LGBT individuals and to improve the climate for LGBT health professionals (including allies) is listed in Appendix 1 for general LGBT topics and Appendix 2 for transgender topics. Appendix 3 includes some simple measures practices may take to improve LGBT friendliness. Appendix 4 reviews some anticipatory guidance regarding sexuality applicable to all adolescents.

## Guidelines and Best Practices for Care of Gender Non-conforming Youth

There are limited guidelines for assisting the transgender population. The World Professional Association for Transgender Health's Standards of Care (WPATH) were published in 2001 and updated in 2011 [65]. In addition the Endocrine Society published "Endocrine Treatment of Trans-sexual Persons: An Endocrine Society Clinical Practice Guideline" in 2009 [66]. These guidelines focus on proper diagnosis and treatment of gender dysphoria and any comorbidity if present. The experienced therapist will focus on self-affirming therapy. Classification for the process is based on reversible, partially reversible and irreversible treatment. In conjunction with guidance from therapists, reversible pubertal suppression using GnRH analogs is advised no earlier than Tanner stage 2 or 3. This allows the adolescent to achieve best desired results with hormonal therapy after age 16. Often Trans teens present too late to start suppressive therapy, necessitating further interventions at later stages of pubertal development. Partially reversible cross gender hormonal therapy should be monitored for desired and adverse medical complications (see Table 11.1). Recommendations are that irreversible surgical therapy should occur after age 18. Many more details are available via the American Academy of Pediatrics Committee on Adolescence 2013 statement and technical report

**Table 11.1** Side effects of cross-sex hormones

| MTF patients | FTM patients |
|---|---|
| **Estrogen** | **Testosterone** |
| Deep venous thrombosis | Hyperlipidemia |
| Prolactinomas | Polycythemia |
| Hypertension (BP) | Male pattern baldness |
| Liver disease (LFTs) | Acne |
| Decreased libido | |
| Increased breast cancer | |
| **Spironolactone** | |
| Hyperkalemia | |
| Hypotension | |

on the Office-Based Care for Lesbian, Gay, Bisexual, Transgender and Questioning Youth [67, 68].

In conclusion, LGBT youth have many challenges, barriers and disparities in comprehensive health care including physical, sexual and mental health. While facing the same concerns of all adolescents, they have additional challenges due to stigmatization, isolation, discrimination when compared to heterosexual teens. These combine to place LGBT youth and increased risk for many items that will require providers to focus motivational interviewing and risk reduction strategies. Family response, provider supportiveness and social support at the school and community level all help mitigate negative outcomes. While the vast majority of LGBT youth do quite well many helpful strategies for the providers, clinics and communities of care have been shared. Ongoing efforts and research into resiliency and supports, understanding risks, risk reduction and prevention and treatment of HIV in particular, remain paramount to the health of this community.

## Supplement 1: Resources

### Useful Books for Youth, Counselors, and Family

#### Books
*Losing generations: adolescents* in *high-risk settings:* panel on high-risk youth. Commission on Behavioral and Social Sciences and Education, National Research Council. 1993.

Males M. *Framing youth: 10 myths about the next generation.* Common Courage Press. 1999.

### Books for Children
Heron, *How would you feel if your dad was gay?*—Examines the concerns of three children with gay parents.

Newman, *Heather has two mommies*—Illustrates the loving and supportive family of 5-yearold Heather and her two lesbian mothers. So lovingly done, you'll wonder what all the fuss was about in the NYC School Board.

Willhoite, *Daddy's roommate*—Illustrates many family situations with this non-traditional family.

Willhoite, *Families, a coloring book*—Appreciating diverse (racial, generational, cultural, sexual) families, Ages 2–6.

### Books for Adolescents Self Help
Bass and Kaufman, *Free your mind: The Book for Gay, Lesbian, and Bisexual Youth and Their Allies.* Harper Perennial.

*Be yourself: Questions and answers for gay, lesbian and bisexual youth*—Factual, nononsense, homo-positive 22-page pamphlet available from PFLAG.

Due, *Joining the tribe: Growing up Gay and Lesbian in the 90's.* Doubleday.

Marcus, *Is It a Choice? Answers to 300 of the Most Frequently Asked Questions about Gays and Lesbians.* Harper Collins.

McNaught, *On being gay: Thoughts on family, faith, and love*—Gay-positive essays on family, faith, and love, and what it means to be gay.

Rench, Understanding *sexual identity: A book for gay teens and their friends*—Discusses coming out, healthy sexuality, homophobia, religious views, and resources.

### Novels and Autobiographies
Due, *Joining the tribe: Growing up gay and lesbian in the 90's*—Interviews with several teens of varied backgrounds.

## Books and Articles for Counselors

Bergstrom and Cruz, *Counseling lesbian and gay male youth: Their special lives/special needs.* Increases counselors' awareness of the issues.

Berzon, *Positively gay: New approaches to gay and lesbian life*—Valuable anthology on living a fulfilling lesbian or gay life.

Shiman, *The prejudice book: Activities for the classroom*—Although the book does not explicitly mention lesbians and gays, the discussion can certainly address these groups. Excellent vehicle for exploring prejudice, stereotypes, and discrimination.

## Coming-Out and Parental Acceptance Handbooks

Bernstein, *Straight parents/gay children*—Addresses parental fear and helps parents appreciate their child. Told through the vehicle of author accepting his lesbian daughter.

Borhek, *Coming out to parents: A two-way survival guide for lesbians and gay men and their parents*—Good resource for lesbians and gay men, counselors, and parents. Chapter on religious issues.

Borhek, *My son Erik*—Acceptance after initial difficulty relative to fundamentalist religious beliefs. Good for parents with religious issues.

Fairchild and Hayward, *Now that you know: What every parent should know about homosexuality.* Harcourt Brace Jovanivich.

## Reference and Office Books to Consider

Mastoon, Adam. *The Shared Heart-Portraits and Stories Celebrating Lesbian, Gay, and Bisexual young people.* Harper Collins Press 1997

Lathom, Bob. *The invisible minority: GLBTQ Youth at Risk.* Point Richmond Press 2000

Owens, Robert. *Queer Kids: The Challenges and promises for Lesbian, Gay and Bisexual Youth* Harrington Park Press 1998. (State by State reference list of resources included.)

Boykin, K. *One More River to Cross: Black and Gay in America.* New York: Anchor Books, 1996.

Brown, L. S. Lesbian Identities: Concepts and Issues. In A. R. D'Augelli and C. J. Patterson (eds.), *Lesbian, Gay and Bisexual Identities over the Lifespan.* New York: Oxford University Press, 1995.

Butler, J. *Gender Trouble: Feminism and the Subversion of Identity.* New York: Routledge, 1990.

Butler, J. *Bodies That Matter: On the Discursive Limits of Sex.* New York: Routledge, 1993.

Catallozzi M, Rudy B. Lesbian, gay, bisexual, transgendered, and questioning youth: The importance of a sensitive and confidential sexual history in identifying the risk and implementing treatment for sexually transmitted infections. Adolescent Medicine Clinics, Volume 15, Number 2—June 2004.

Clare, E. *Exile and Pride: Disability, Queerness, and Liberation.* Boston: South End Press, 1999.

Creed, B. Lesbian Bodies: Tribades, Tomboys, and Tarts. In E. Grosz and E. Probyn (eds.), *Sexy Bodies: The Strange Carnalities of Feminism.* New York: Routledge, 1995.

D'Augelli, A. R. Identity Development and Sexual Orientation: Toward a Model of Lesbian, Gay, and Bisexual Development. In E. J. Trickett, R. J. Watts and D. Birman (eds.), *Human Diversity: Perspectives on People in Context.* San Francisco: Jossey-Bass, 1994.

Diaz, R. Latino Gay Men and Psycho-Cultural Barriers to AIDS Prevention. In M. Levine, J. Gagnon and P. Nardi (eds.), *In Changing Times: Gay Men and Lesbians Encounter HIVIAIDS.* Chicago: University of Chicago Press, 1997.

Fassinger, R. E. The Hidden Minority: Issues and Challenges in Working with Lesbian Women and Gay Men. *Counseling Psychologist,* 1991, 19(2),157–176.

Feinberg, L. *Transgender Warriors: Making History from Joan of Arc to Dennis Rodman.* Boston: Beacon Press, 1996.

Feinberg, L. *Trans Liberation: Beyond Pink or Blue.* Boston: Beacon Press, 1998.

Fox, R. Bisexual Identities. In A. R. D'Augelli and C. J. Patterson (eds.), *Lesbian, Gay, and Bisexual Identities over the Lifespan: Psychological Perspectives.* New York: Oxford University Press, 1995.

Halberstam, J. *Female Masculinity.* Durham: Duke University Press, 1998.

Harry Benjamin International Gender Dysphoria Association. The HBIGDA Standards of Care for Gender Identity Disorders, Sixth Version. 2001. http://www.wpath.org/documents2/socv6.pdf

Klein, F. The Need to View Sexual Orientation as Multivariable Dynamic Process: A Theoretical Perspective. In D.P. McWhirter, S. A. Sanders and J. M. Reinisch (eds.), *Homosexuality/Heterosexuality: Concepts of Sexual Orientation.* New York: Oxford University Press, 1990.

Klein, F. *The Bisexual Option.* (2nd ed.) New York: Haworth Press, 1993.

Raffo, S. Introduction. In S. Raffo (ed.), *Queerly Classed.* Boston: South End Press, 1997.

Renn, K. A., and Bilodeau, B. Analysis of LGBT Identity Development Models and Implications for Practice. In R. Sanlo (ed.), *Gender Identity and Sexual Orientation Research, Policy and Personal Perspectives.* San Francisco: Jossey-Bass, 2005.

Rhoads, R. A. *Coming Out in College: The Struggle for a Queer Identity.* Westport, Conn.: Bergin and Garvey, 1994.

Savin-Williams R. The New Gay Teenager. Harvard University Press, Cambridge, MA, 2005.

Wilchins, R. A. *Read My Lips: Sexual Subversion and the End of Gender.* New York: Firebrand Books, 1997.

Wilchins, R. A. Queerer Bodies. In J. Nestle, C. Howell and R. A. Wilchins (eds.), *Genderqueer: Voices from Beyond the Sexual Binary.* Los Angeles: Alyson, 2002.

Wilson, A. How We Find Ourselves: Identity Development in Two-Spirit People. *Harvard Educational Review,* 1996, 66(2), 303–317.

## Videos

*It's elementary: Talking about gay issues in school*—Explores the teaching of tolerance in six different classrooms (available from Women's Educational Media, San Francisco, 415-641-4632).

*Pride and prejudice: The life and times of gay and lesbian youth*—Focuses on a Toronto weekly youth group showing the significance of this service for teens (available at 416-924-21 00).

*Safe schools: Making schools safe for gay and lesbian students* (available from Donna Brathwaite, Safe Schools Program, Massachusetts Department of Education, 617-388-3300, ext. 409. Plan to send blank tape).

*Teaching respect*—Produced by the Gay, Lesbian, and Straight Teachers Network. This video explains why educators should be concerned about homophobia and abuse in school (available at 212-727-0135).

*Both My Moms' Names Are Judy* is a provocative 10-min video that shows elementary school children who have gay or lesbian parents talking about their experiences at school. The video is available from Lesbian & Gay Parents Association, 519 Castro St., Box 52, San Francisco, CA 94114-2577, Phone: 415-522-8773, e-mail: LGPASF@aol.com (10 min, $25 individual/$50 institution).

*Gay Youth.* This powerful video is extremely effective in showing why sexual orientation education is important. A variety of young people are interviewed, and the effect of family support is revealed. The results range from suicide to having a same-sex date for the senior prom. I have used this video for faculty at all grade levels as well as for high school students. Audiences always gave it high marks on the evaluation form (40 min, $59.95).

*Out of the Past* traces the emergence of gay men and lesbians in American history through the eyes of a young woman coming to terms with herself. This film by Jeff Dupre won the Sundance Film Festival Audience Award for Best Documentary as well as a Bronze Apple from National Educational Media Foundation in 1998 (65 min, $25 individual/$99 institution).

The Trevor Project: www.trevorproject.org
It Gets Better: www.itgetsbetter.org
PRCH: Adolescent Reproductive and Sexual Health Education Project
http://prh.org/teen-reproductive-health/arshep-explained/

www.prch.org email: info@prch.org, phone: 646-366-1890

Physicians for Reproductive Choice and Health

55 West 39th St, suite 1001, New York, NY, 10018-3889

Fax 646-366-1890

## National Organizations

- Coalition for Lesbian and Gay Student Groups (214) 621-6705
- *Gay, Lesbian, Straight Education network*: http://www.glsen.org
- *National Coalition for LGBT Youth*: http://www.outproud.org
- *Sexuality information for Teens, by Teens*: http://www.sxect.org
- The UCSF Center for AIDS Prevention Studies: http://hivinsite.ucsd.edu
- An AIDS and HIV information resource: http://thebody.com
- *National AIDS Advocacy Organization*: http://aidsaction.org/
- Information on AIDS and HIV in Spanish: http://www.ctv.ed/USERS/fpardo/home.html
- *The HIV/AIDS Treatment Information Service* (ATIS): http://hivatis.org
- The American Academy of Child and Adolescent Psychiatry—Facts for Families: http://www.aacap.org/publications/factsfam/index.htm (AIDS #30 GL Adol #63)
- National Gay and Lesbian Hotline: 1-800-SOSGAYS
- National Runaway Switchboard and Adolescent Suicide Hotline: 1-800-621-4000
- National Youth Advocacy Coalition (NYAC): http://www.nyacyouth.org
- The Trevor Project: http://www.trevorproject.org 866-4-U-TREVOR
- Transfamily: http://transfamily.org
- Transkids Purple Rainbow: http://www.transkidspurplerainbow.org
- Family Acceptance Project: http://familyproject.sfsu.org
- It Gets Better: http://www.itgetsbetter.org

- National Federation of Parents, Family and Friends of Lesbians and Gays (PFLAG): http://www.community.pflag.org
- Youth Resource: http://www.amplifyyourvoice.org/youthresource

## Medical Professional Organizations

GLMA: Health Professionals Advancing LGBT Equality: http://www.glma.org

AMA LGBT Advisory Committee: https://www.ama-assn.org/ama/pub/about-ama/our-people/member-groups-sections/glbt-advisory-committee.page

The World Professional Association for Transgender Health, Inc (WPATH): http://wpath.org

Adolescent Reproductive and Sexual Health Education Project: http://www.prh.org/ARSHEP

## Talk Lines/Hotlines/Crisis Lines

| | |
|---|---|
| AIDS Foundation Hotline (English and Spanish) | (800) for AIDS |
| GLBT Peer Youth Hotline | (800) 399-PEER |
| Gay, Lesbian, and Bisexual Youth Line | (800) 347-TEEN |
| Gay Men's Health Crisis (GMHC)—HIV/AIDS | (212) 807-6655 |
| LYRIC Gay Youth Talk Line and Info Line | (800) 246-PRIDE |
| Lesbian AIDS Project HIV/AIDS info and referral | (212) 337-3532 |
| National Center for Lesbian Rights | (800) 528-6257 |
| National HIV/AIDS Hotline | (800) 342-AIDS |
| National Lesbian and Gay Crisis Line | (800) 221-7044 |
| National Native American AIDS Prevention Center | (800) 283-AIDS |
| National Runaway Hotline | (800) 843-5200 |
| National Suicide and Runaway Switchboard | (800) 621-4000 |
| National Suicide Hotline | (800) 882-3386 |
| Out Youth Hotline | (800) 96-YOUTH |
| Parents and Friends of Lesbians and Gays | (415) 921-8850 |
| | (202) 638-4200 |
| Project Inform Hotline—HIV/AIDS Information | (800) 822-7422 |

## Supplement 2: Transgender

### Medical

Bilodeau, Brent. *Genderism: Transgender Students, Binary Systems and Higher Education.* Saarbriicken, Germany: VDM Verlag Dr. Muller Aktiengesellshaft, 2009.

Bockting, Walter, and Eric Avery. *Transgender Health And HIV Prevention: Needs Assessment Studies from Transgender Communities Across the United States.* Binghamton, NY: The Haworth Medical Press, 2005

Bockting, Walter, and Joshua Goldberg (eds). *Guidelines for Transgender Care.* Binghamton, NY: The Haworth Press, 2007.

Coleman, Edmond J., Walter 0. Bockting, and Sheila Kirk. *Transgender And HIV: Risks, Prevention, and Care.* Binghamton, NY: Haworth Press, 2001.

Denny, Dallas, ed. *Current Concepts in Transgender Identity.* Garland Reference Library of Social Science, 1998.

Drescher, Jack, and Ubaldo Leli, eds. *Transgender Subjectivities: A Clinician's Guide (Journal of Gay & Lesbian Psychotherapy Monographic Separates).* Binghamton, NY: Haworth Medical Press, 2004.

Ellis, Alan L., Melissa White, and Kevin Schaub. *The Harvey Milk Institute Guide to Lesbian, Gay, Bisexual, Transgender, and Queer Internet Research (Haworth Gay & Lesbian Studies).* Harrington Park Press, impt of Haworth Press, Binghamton, NY, 2002

Ettner, Randi, Stan Monstrey, and Even Eyler. *Principles of Transgender Medicine and Surgery (Human Sexuality).* Binghamton, NY: Haworth Press, 2007.

Gottlieb, Andrew. *Interventions With Families of Gay, Lesbian, Bisexual, And Transgender People: From the Inside Out.* Binghamton, NY: Haworth Press, 2006.

Harcourt III, John P. *Current Issues in Lesbian, Gay, Bisexual, And Transgender Health.* Binghamton, NY: Harrington Press (impt of Haworth Press), 2006.

Hines, Sally. *TransForming Gender: Transgender Practices of Identity, Intimacy and Care.* Bristol, UK: Policy Press, Univ of Bristol, 2007.

Kirk, Sheila. *Hormones for the Female to Male.* Available from www.ifge.com.

Lev, Arlene. *Transgender Emergence: Therapeutic Guidelines for Working With Gender Variant People and Their Families (Haworth Marriage and the Family).* The Haworth Clinical Practice Press, impt of Haworth Press, Binghamton, NY, 2004.

MacGillivray, Ian K. *Gay-straight Alliances: A Handbook for Students, Educators, and Parents (Haworth Series on GLBT Youth &Adolescence).* Binghamton, NY: Harrington Park Press, 2007

Makadon, Harvey J., et al. *Fenway Guide to Lesbian, Gay, Bisexual & Transgender Health.* American College of Physicians, 2008.

Mallon, Gerald P. *Social Work Practice with Transgender and Gender Variant Youth.* New York: Routledge, 2009.

Meezan, William, and James I. Martin, eds. *Research Methods With Gay, Lesbian, Bisexual, and Transgender Populations (Journal of Gay & Lesbian Social Services, 3/4)*

Nunter, Nan D., Courtney G. Joslin, and Sharon M. McGowan. *The Rights of Lesbians, Gay Men, Bisexuals, and Transgender People (American Civil Liberties Union Handbook).* Southern Illinois UP, ACLU, 2004

Meyer, Ilan H., and Mary E. Northridge, eds. *The Health of Sexual Minorities: Public Health Perspectives on Lesbian, Gay, Bisexual and Transgender Populations.* New York: Columbia UP, 2006.

O'Keefe, Tracie, and Katrina Fox, eds. *Finding the Real Me: True Tales of Sex and Gender Diversity.* San Francisco: Jossey Bass, 2003.

Sanlo, Ronni L., ed. *Working with Lesbian, Gay, Bisexual, and Transgender College Students: A Handbook for Faculty and Administrators (The Greenwood Educators' Reference Collection).* Westport, CT: Greenwood Press, 1998.

Sears, James T. *Gay, Lesbian, And Transgender Issues In Education: Programs, Policies, And Practice (Haworth Series in GLBT Community and Youth Studies).* Binghamton, NY: Harrington Park Press, 2005.

Valentine, David. *Imagining Transgender: An Ethnography of a Category*. Durham, NC: Duke University, 2007.

Whittle, Stephen, and Susan Stryker. *The Transgender Reader*. Binghamton, NY: Haworth Park Press, 2005; New York: Routledge, 2006.

Winters, Kelley. *Gender Madness* in *American Psychiatry: Essays from the Struggle for Dignity*. ISBN 1-4392-2388-2, GID Reform Advocates

## Medical Journals

Gagne, Patricia, Richard Tewksbury and Deanna McGaughey, Coming out and Crossing over: Identity Formation and Proclamation in a Transgender Community. *Gender and Society*, Vol. 11, No.4 (Aug., 1997), pp. 478–508. http://www.jstor.org/stable/190483

P Lee, C Houk—The Diagnosis and Care of Transsexual Children and Adolescents: A Pediatric Endocrinologists' Perspective. J Ped Endocrin Metab, 2006, vol. 19 (no. 2)

Rosenberg, Miriam, M.D., Ph.D. Recognizing Gay, Lesbian, and Transgender Teens in a Child and Adolescent Psychiatry Practice. J Am Acad Child Adolesc Psychiatry. 2003 Dec; 42(12): 1522–3.

Stoller, R.J. (1979). Fathers of Transsexual Children. J. Amer. Psychoanal. Assn., 27:837–866.

## General Adult and Professionals

Beam, Cris. *Transparent: Love, Family, and Living the T with Transgender Teenagers*. Orlando, FL: Harcourt Brace, 2007.

Boenke, Mary, ed. *TransForming Families: Real Stories about Transgendered Loved Ones*, 3rd ed. New York: PFLAG, 2003.

Boyd, Helen. *She's Not the Man I Married: My Life with a Transgender Husband*. Emeryville, CA: Seal Press, 2007.

Brill, Stephanie A. and Rachel Pepper. *The Transgender Child: A Handbook for Families and Professionals*. San Francisco: Cleis Press, 2008.

Brown, Mildred, and Chloe Rounsley. *True Selves: Understanding Transsexualism: For Families, Friends, Coworkers and Helping Professionals*. San Francisco: Jossey-Bass, 2003.

Cascio, J., Catherine Brown, and Beatrice Gordon. *Dragonfly Stories: Stories Celebrating the LGBTQ Community*, (vol. 1). Kearney, MI: Rainbow Legends, LLC, 2007. Published in the *Journal of GLBT Family Studies*, Volume 4, Issue 4 September 2008, pages 543–545.

Feinberg, Leslie. *Trans Liberation: Beyond Pink or Blue*. Boston: Beacon Press, 1998. Gold, Mitchell, with Mindy Drucker. Crisis: Growing Up Gay in America. Greenleaf Book Club Press, 2008.

Green, Jamison. *Becoming a Visible Man*. Nashville: Vanderbilt UP, 2004.

Heman, Joanne. *Transgender Explained For Those Who Are Not*. Bloomington, IN, AuthorHouse, 2009.

Howard, Kim, and Steven Drukman. *Out & About Campus: Personal Accounts by Lesbian, Gay, Bisexual & Transgender College Students*. Los Angeles: Alyson Publications, 2000.

Huegel, Kelly. *GLBTQ: The Survival Guide for Queer and Questioning Teens*. Minneapolis, MN: Free Spirit, 2003.

Israel, Gianna E., Donald E. Tarver and Diane Shaffer. *Transgender Care: Recommended Guidelines, Practical Information, and Personal Accounts*. Philadelphia: Temple UP, 1997.

Jennings, Kevin, and Pat Shapiro. *Always My Child: A Parent's Guide to Understanding Your Gay, Lesbian, Bisexual, Transgendered or Questioning Son or Daughter*. New York: Fireside, 2003.

"Just Evelyn." *Mom, I Need to be a Girl*. Imperial Beach, CA: Walter Trook Publishing, 1998. [276 Date St. Imperial Beach, *CA* 91932]

Kane-Kanedemaios, J. Ari, and Vern L. Bullough, eds. *Crossing Sexual Boundaries: Transgender Journeys, Uncharted Paths*. New York: Prometheus, 2006.

Kerry, Stephen. *Are You a Boy or a Girl? Intersex and Genders: Contesting the Uncontested: A Comparative Analysis between the Status of Intersex in Australia and the United States of*

*America.* Saarbriicken, Germany: VDM Verlag, 2008

Kotnla, Dean. *The Phallus Palace: Female to Male Transsexuals.* Los Angeles, Alyson Press, 2002.

Lundschien, Randy P. *Queering Creole Spiritual Traditions: Lesbian, Gay, Bisexual, and Transgender Participation in African Inspired Traditions in the Americas.* Binghamton, NY: Haworth Press, 2004.

Matzner, Andrew. *0 Au No Keia: Voices From Hawai'i's Mahu and Transgender Communities.* 2001 (out of print)

O'Keefe, Tracie, and Katrina Fox. *Trans People in Love.* New York: Routledge, 2008. Rose, Lannie. *How To Change Your Sex: A Lighthearted Look at the Hardest Thing You'll Ever Do.* Lulu Press, 2004.

Rudacille, Deborah. *The Riddle of Gender: Science, Activism, and Transgender Rights.* New York: Pantheon Books, 2005.

Stryker, Susan. *Transgender History (Seal Studies).* Berkeley: Seal Press, 2008

## Books for Children

Dyer, Wayne, Kristina Tracy, and Melanie Siegel. *Incredible You: 10 Ways to Let your Greatness Shine Through.* Carlsbad, CA: May Mouse, 2005.

Ewert, Marcus, and Rex Ray. *10,000 Dresses.* New York: Seven Stories Press, 2008.

Jimenez, Karleen Pendelton. *Are You a Boy or a Girl?* Toronto, Canada: Green Dragon Press, 2000.

Kates, Bobbi. *We're Different, We're the Same.* New York: Random House, 1992.

Parr, Todd. *It's OK to be Dif.forent.* Little, Brown, 2001.

Perel, Ronnie. *Fluffy the Bunny.* Available at www.IFGE.org

Wanzer, C. Kevin. *Choose To Love: A Poem About Life, Love & Choices.* Bloomington, IN: AuthorHouse, 2006.

## Books for Children (Spanish)

Dyer, Wayne. *Eres increible!: 10 formas de permitir que tu GRANDEZA brille a traves de ti,* Carlsbad, CA: May House, 2006.

## Books for Teens

Anders, Charlie. *Choir Boy.* [available on Amazon.com]

St. James, James. *Freak Show.* New York: Penguin, 2007.

Saint Clair, C.C. *Morgan in the Mirror.* ISBN-10: 0980334438 ISBN-13: 978-0980334432. POD.

Bomstein, Kate. *Hello Cruel World: 1OJ Alternatives to Suicide for Teens, Freaks and Outlaws.* Kindle Edition, 2006.

Sardella, Rebecca. *My Brother Beth* (out of print)

Bomstein, Kate. *My Gender Workbook: How to Become a Real Man, a Real Woman, the Real You, or Something Else Entirely.* New York: Routledge, 1998.

Peters, Julie Anne. *Luna.* New York: Little Brown, 2006. Wittlinger, Ellen. *Parrotfish.* New York: Simon & Schuster, 2007.

## References for Gender Dysphoria

Brown, M.L., and Rounsley, A.C. (1996). *True Selves: Understanding Transsexualism for Families, Friends, Coworkers, and Helping Professionals.* San Francisco, CA: Jossey-Bass.

Brill, S.A. & Pepper, R. (2008). *The Transgendered Child: A Handbook for Families and Professionals.* San Francisco, CA: Cleis Press Inc.

Cohen- Kettenis, P.T. and Pfafflin, F. (2003). *Transgenderism and intersexuality in childhood and adolescents: Making choices.* Thousand Oaks, Sage Publications.

Cohen-Kettenis, P.T., Delemarre-van de Waal, H.A., and Gooren, L.J. The treatment of transsexual adolescents: Changing insights. *Journal of Sexual Medicine*, 2008, 5, 8, 1892–1897.

Delemarre-van de Waal, H.A. and Cohen-Kettenis, P.T. Clinical management of gender identity disorder in adolescents; A protocol on psychological and pediatric endocrinology aspects. *European Journal of Endocrinology*, 2006, Nov 155, Suppl 1: 131–137.

Drummond, K.D., Bradley, S.J., Peterson-Badali, M., and Zucker, K.J. A follow-up study of girls with gender identity disorder. *Developmental Psychology*, 2008, 44, 34–45.

Hembree, W., Cohen-Kettenis, P.T., Delemarre-van de Waal, H., Gooren, L.J., Meyer III, W. Spack, N., et al. Endocrine treatment of transsexual persons: an endocrine society clinical practice guideline. *Journal of Clinical Endocrinology and Metabolism*, 2009, 94, 3132–3154.

Spack NP. Transgenderism, *Lahey Clinic Medical Ethics*, 2005, 12(3). Fall issue.

Speigal, A. (May 2008). "All Things Considered:" An Interview with Dr. Norman P. Spack on Pubertal Suppression in Transgender Adolescents. National Public Radio "Driveway Moments" 2009 Series;

http://www.npr.org/templates/story/story.php/?storyId=90247842 (part 1)

http://www.npr.org/templeates/story/storyId=90273278 (part 2)

Wren, B. (2000). Early physical intervention for young people with atypical gender identity development. *Clinical Child Psychology and Psychiatry*, 5, 220–231.

Zucker, K.J. "I'm half-boy, half-girl": Play psychotherapy and parent counseling for gender identity disorder. In R.L. Spitzer, M.B. First, J.B. W. Williams, and M. Gibbons (Eds.), *DSM-IV-TR' casebook, Volume 2. Experts tell how they treated their own patients.* Washington, DC: American Psychiatric Publishing, 2006, pp. 321–334

Zucker, K.J. On the "natural history" of gender identity disorder in children [Editorial]. *Journal of the American Academy of Child and Adolescent Psychiatry*, 2008, 47, 1361–1363

Zucker, K.J. Children with gender identity disorders: Is there a best practice? [Enfants avec troubles de l'identite sexuee: y-a-t-il une pratique la meilleure?] *Neuropsychiatric de l'Enfance et de l'Adolescence*, 2008, 56, 358–364.

Zucker, K.J. The DSM diagnostic criteria for gender identity disorder in children. *Archives of Sexual Behavior*, 2010, 39, 477–498.

## Supplement 3: Making Your Health Care Setting Safer for LGBTQ Youth

(A) Conduct training for staff around homophobia, cultural competency, confidentiality and privacy for GLBTQ Youth.

(B) Use broad inclusive language for human sexual behavior and relationships that is gender neutral.

(C) Insure understanding of consent, confidentiality and legal/policies that govern your practice.

(D) Address anti-gay behavior and language in clear and consistent manner and according to same rules that apply to other groups/cultures.

(E) Designate a resource person (and/or provider) who is knowledgeable in existing resources and community contacts/programs.

(F) Books, magazines, posters, hotline numbers, handouts and brochures specific or inclusive of LGBTQ should be available. These should be visible and accessible (perhaps in a private manner.)

(G) Connect with LGBTQ and/or allies to assist with family navigation, and/or with health promotion and prevention programs.

(H) Be prepared to help children, youth and families, as well as other family members, and refer them to services they may need.

(I) Items like rainbow stickers, upside down pink triangle located in exam rooms or at front desk can be a subtle way to communicate the LGBT friendly practice.

## Supplement 4: Adolescent Anticipatory Guidance for Sexuality

### Early Adolescence: 11–14 Years

Abstinence for those who have not had sex, and as an option to those who are sexually experiences, is the best protection from pregnancy, STIs and the emotional distress of disrupted relationships. Knowing how to protect oneself and one's partner is critical for those sexually active. Delaying sexual debut, is beneficial for children.

### Sample Questions

**Parent**: How do you plan to help your child deal with pressures to have sex? How does your culture help you do this?

**Youth**: Have you had sex? Was it wanted or unwanted? Have you ever been force or pressured to do something sexual that you haven't wanted to do? How many partners have you had in past year? Were your partners male or female or have you had both male and female partners? Were your partners young, older or your age? Did you use a condom and other contraception?

### Anticipatory Guidance

**For parent:**
- Encourage abstinence or a return to abstinence
- Help your child make a plan to resist pressures. Be there when support is needed
- Support safe activities
- If uncomfortable talking about these topics, learn more from reliable sources
- Talk about relationships and sex when issues arise on television, at school or with friends. Be open, nonjudgmental, but honest about your views

**For youth:**
- Abstaining from sexual intercourse, including oral sex, is the safest way to prevent pregnancy and STIs

- Figure out ways to make sure you can carry through on your decisions. Plan how to avoid risky places and relationships
- If you are sexually active, protect yourself and your partners from STIs and pregnancy

### Middle Adolescence: 15–17 Years

Sexuality and relationships are an important issue in middle adolescence. Parents and adolescents need accurate information and support to help them communicate with each other.

### Sample Questions

**For youth**: Have you talked with your parents about crushes you've had, about dating and relationships, and about sex? Are you attracted to males, females or both, or are you undecided? Do you have any questions or concerns about who your gender identity or who you are attracted to? Have you had sex?

**For parent**: Do you monitor or supervise your adolescent's activities and friends? Do you enjoy talking with your adolescent and her friends? Have you established house rules about curfews, parties, dating and friends? How do you plan to help your adolescent deal with pressures to have sex? Does he have any special relationships or someone he dates steadily?

### Anticipatory Guidance

**Youth:**
- It's important for you to have accurate information about sexuality, your physical development, and your sexual feelings. Please ask me if you have any questions.

**Parent:**
- Communicate frequently and share expectations clearly.
- Help your adolescent make a plan to resist pressures to have sex.
- Be there for her when she needs support or assistance.

## Late Adolescence: 18–21 Years

For the young adult, the issue of sexuality is central. Some young adults still may have questions or concerns about their sexual orientation, gender identity, or sexual maturity. For some the decision to have and intimate relationship and become sexually active may be relevant. For thoughts about emotional intensity of a romantic relationships, or protection from STIs and pregnancy may be uppermost in their minds.

### Sample Questions

**For young adult**: What are your values about dating and relationships? Are you attracted to males, females, or both? Do you have any questions or concerns about your gender identity (as a male or female)? Have you had sex? What are your plans and values about relationships, sex, and future family or marriage? have you talked with your parents/family about stable relationships or marriage?

**For parent**: Your teen in now a young adult. Are you comfortable with her development?

### Anticipatory Guidance

- Sexuality is an important part of your normal development as a young adult.
- If you have any question s or concerns about sexuality, or your development, I hope you will consider me one of the people with whom you can discuss these issues.

Hagan JF, Shaw JS, Duncan PM, eds. 2008. *Bright futures: Guidelines for Health Supervision of Infants, Children and Adolescents,* Third addition. Elk Grove Village, IL: American Academy of Pediatrics.

Access for free at:

http://brightfutures.aap.org/
http://brightfutures.aap.org/3rd_edition_guidelines_and_pocket_guide.html

## References

1. Ng H. Clinical cases: LGBTQ youth. Medscape case #1, 3 Dec 2010. http://www.medscape.com/viewarticle/733052_1.
2. Alternative case from www.pedicases.org; *Michael's Disclosure* by Maurice Melchiono; Case advisors: S. Jean Emans and Cathryn Samples. Harvard Medical School and Children's Hospital, Boston. http://pedicases.org/wp-content/uploads/2011/07/sexuality4.pdf.
3. IOM (Institute of Medicine). The health of lesbian, gay, bisexual, and transgender people: building a foundation for better understanding. Washington, DC: National Academies Press; 2011.
4. Rosario M, Schrimshaw EW, Hunter J, Gwadz M. Gay-related stress and emotional distress among gay, lesbian and bisexual youths: a longitudinal examination. J Consult Clin Psychol. 2002;70(4):967–75. doi:10.1037/0022-006X.70.4.967.
5. Meyer IH. Minority stress and mental health in gay men. J Health Soc Behav. 1995;36(1):38–56.
6. Meyer IH. Prejudice, social stress, and mental health in lesbian, gay and bisexual populations: conceptual issues and research evidence. Psychol Bull. 2003;129:674–97. doi:10.1037/0033-2909.129.5.674.
7. Mays VM, Cochran SD. Mental health correlates of perceived discrimination among lesbian, gay, and bisexual adults in the United States. Am J Public Health. 2001;91(11):1869–76. doi:10.2105/AJPH.91.11.1869.
8. Kohlberg L. A cognitive-developmental analysis of children's sex-role concepts and attitudes. In: Maccoby E, editor. The development of sex differences. Stanford, CA: Stanford University Press; 1996. p. 82–173.
9. Fagot BI. Sex differences in toddlers' behavior and parental reaction. Dev Psychol. 1974;10:554–8.
10. Fagot BI. Consequences of moderate cross-gender behavior in preschool children. Child Dev. 1977;48:902–7.
11. Fagot BI. Changes in thinking about early sex role development. Dev Rev. 1985;5:83–9.
12. Fagot BI. Review: The "sissy boy syndrome" and the development of homosexuality. Arch Sex Behav. 1992;21:327–32.
13. Marcus D, Overton WF. The development of cognitive gender constancy and sex role preferences. Child Dev. 1978;49:434–44.
14. Perrin EC, Siegel BS, Committee on Psychosocial Aspects of Child and Family Health of the American Academy of Pediatrics. Promoting the well-being of children whose parents are gay or lesbian. Pediatrics. 2013;131(4):e1374–83. Available at: www.pediatrics.org/cgi/content/full/131/4/e1374 pmid:23519940.
15. Perrin EC. Sexual orientation in child and adolescent health care. New York: Springer; 2002.

16. Savin-Williams RC. Theoretical perspectives accounting for adolescent homosexuality. J Adolesc Health Care. 1988;9:95–104.
17. Troiden RR. Becoming homosexual: a model of gay identity acquisition. Psychiatry. 1988;42:362–73.
18. Troiden RR. Homosexual identity development. J Adolesc Health Care. 1988;9:105–13.
19. Cass VC. Homosexual identity formation: a theoretical model. J Homosex. 1979;4:19.
20. Emans SJ, Brown RT, Davis A, Felice M, Hein K. Society for adolescent medicine position paper on reproductive health care for adolescents. J Adolesc Health. 1991;12:649–61.
21. Remafedi G, Resnick M, Blum R, Harris L. Demography of sexual orientation in adolescents. Pediatrics. 1992;89(4):714–21.
22. Centers for Disease Control and Prevention. MMWR Early Release. 2011;60(7). Accessed 11 May 2014.
23. Ryan C. Lesbian, gay, bisexual, and transgender youth: health concerns, services, and care. Clin Res Regul Aff. 2003;20(2):137–58.
24. Ryan C. A review of the professional literature & research needs for LGBT youth of color. Washington, DC: National Youth Advocacy Coalition; 2002.
25. CDC Injury Center: Violence Prevention. Youth Violence: National Statistics. Five leading causes of death among persons 10-24 years of age, United States, 2010. http://www.cdc.gov/violenceprevention/youthviolence/stats_at-a_glance/lcd_10-24.html.
26. U.S. Department of Health and Human Services (HHS) Office of the Surgeon General and National Action Alliance for Suicide Prevention. 2012 National strategy for suicide prevention: goals and objectives for action. Washington, DC: HHS; 2012.
27. Grossman AH, D'Augelli AR. Transgender youth and life-threatening behaviors. Suicide Life Threat Behav. 2007;37(5):527–37.
28. CDC. Sexual identity, sex of sexual contacts, and health-risk behaviors among students in grades 9-12: youth risk behavior surveillance. Atlanta, GA: U.S. Department of Health and Human Services; 2011.
29. Garofalo R, Wolf R, Wissow LS, Woods ER, Goodman E. Sexual orientation and risk of suicide attempts among a representative sample of youth. Arch Pediatr Adolesc Med. 1999;153(5):487–93. doi:10.1001/archpedi.153.5.487.
30. Remafedi G, Farrow JA, Deisher RW. Risk factors for attempted suicide in gay and bisexual youth. Pediatrics. 1991;87(6):869–75.
31. Remafedi GJ. Adolescent homosexuality issues for pediatricians. Clin Pediatr. 1985;24(9):481–5.
32. Kosciw JG, Greytak EA, Diaz EM, Bartkiewicz MJ. The 2009 National School Climate Survey: the experiences of lesbian, gay, bisexual and transgender youth in our nation's schools. New York: Gay, Lesbian Straight Education Network; 2010. Available at www.glsen.org/binary-data/GLSEN_ATTACHMENTS/file/000/001/1675-5.PDF.
33. Blashill AJ, Safren SA. Sexual orientation and anabolic-androgenic steroids in U.S. adolescent boys. Pediatrics. 2014;133(3):469–75. doi:10.1542/peds.2013-2768. Epub 2014 Feb 2.
34. Corliss HL, Rosario M, Wypij D, Fisher LB, Austin S. Sexual orientation disparities in longitudinal alcohol use patterns among adolescents: findings from the growing up today study. Arch Pediatr Adolesc Med. 2008;162(11):1071–8. doi:10.1001/archpedi.162.11.1071.
35. Austin S, Ziyadeh N, Fisher LB, Kahn JA, Colditz GA, Frazier A. Sexual orientation and tobacco use in a cohort study of US adolescent girls and boys. Arch Pediatr Adolesc Med. 2004;158(4):317–22. doi:10.1001/archpedi.158.4.317.
36. Austin SB, Ziyadeh NJ, Corliss HL, Rosario M, Wypij D, Haines J, Field AE. Sexual orientation disparities in purging and binge eating from early to late adolescence. J Adolesc Health. 2009;45(3):238–45.
37. Saewyc E, Bearinger L, Blum R, Resnick M. Sexual intercourse, abuse and pregnancy among adolescent women: does sexual orientation make a difference? Fam Plann Perspect. 1999;31(3):127–31.
38. Gibson P. Gay male and lesbian youth suicide. In: Feinleib M, editor. Report of the secretary's task force on youth suicide, vol. 3. Washington, DC: Department of Health and Human Services; 1989. p. 110–42.
39. Lane T. Among sexually experienced male adolescents, those with partners of both sexes exhibit riskiest behavior. Perspect Sex Reprod Health. 2002;34:3.
40. Blake SM, Ledsky R, Lehman T, Goodenow C, Sawyer R, Hack T. Preventing sexual risk behaviors among gay, lesbian, and bisexual adolescents: the benefits of gay-sensitive HIV instruction in schools. Am J Public Health. 2001;91(6):940–6.
41. Davis V. Lesbian health. Obstetrician Gynaecologist. 2005;7:98–102.
42. CDC. HIV among youth. Fast facts. 2014. www.cdc.gov/hiv/risk/age/youth/index.html.
43. Reitman DS, Austin B, Belkind U, et al. Recommendations for promoting health and well-being of lesbian, gay, bisexual, and transgender adolescents: a position paper of the Society for Adolescent Health and Medicine. J Adolesc Health. 2013;52:506–10.
44. Ryan C, Huebner D, Diaz RM, Sanchez J. Family rejection as a predictor of negative health outcomes in white and Latino lesbian, gay, and bisexual young adults. Pediatrics. 2009;123(1):346–52.
45. D'Augelli AR, Grossman A, Starks MT. Parent's awareness of lesbian, gay and bisexual youth's sexual orientation. J Marriage Fam. 2005;67:474.
46. Kosciw JG, Greytak EA, Diaz EM, et al. The 2009 National School Climate Survey: the experiences of

lesbian, gay, bisexual and transgender youth in our nation's schools. GLSEN. 2009. Available at: http://www.glsen.org/binary-data/GLSEN_attachments/file/000/001/1675-1.pdf.

47. Herschberger SL, Pilkington NW, D'Augelli AR. Predictors of suicide attempts among gay, lesbian, and bisexual youth. J Adolesc Res. 1997;12:477.

48. Garofalo R, Wolf RC, Kessel S, et al. The association between health risk behaviors and sexual orientation among a school-based sample of adolescents. Pediatrics. 1998;101:895.

49. Wilber S, Ryan C, Marksamer J. CWLA best practice guideline: serving LGBT youth in out-of-home-care. Washington, DC: Child Welfare League of America; 2006.

50. Leeuwen JM, Boyle S, Salomonsen-Sautel S, et al. Lesbian gay, and bisexual youth: an eight-city public health perspective. Child Welfare. 2006;85:181.

51. O'Malley Olson E, et al. School violence and bullying among sexual minority high school students, 2009-2011. J Adolesc Health. 2014;55(3):432–8.

52. Russell ST, et al. Lesbian, gay, bisexual, and transgender adolescent school victimization: implications for young adult health and adjustment. J Sch Health. 2011;81(5):223–30.

53. Hazler RJ, Denham SA. Social isolation of youth at risk: conceptualizations and practical implications. J Couns Dev. 2002;80(4):403–9.

54. Johnson MJ, et al. Isolation of lesbian, gay, bisexual and transgender youth: a dimensional concept analysis. J Adv Nurs. 2014;70(3):523–32.

55. Mayer KH, Garofalo R, Makadon HJ. Promoting the successful development of sexual and gender minority youths. Am J Public Health. 2014; 104(6):976–81.

56. Boekeloo BO, Schamus LA, Cheng TL, Simmens SJ. Young adolescents' comfort with discussion about sexual problems with their physician. Arch Pediatr Adolesc Med. 1996;150(11):1146–52.

57. Ginsburg K, Winn R, Rudy B, Crawford J, Zhao H, Schwarz D. How to reach sexual minority youth in the health care setting: the teens offer guidance. J Adolesc Health. 2002;31:407–16.

58. Goldenring MN, Cohen E. Getting into adolescent heads. Contemp Pediatr. 1998;5:75–90.

59. Ginsburg KR, Kinsman SB, editors. Reaching teens: strength-based communications strategies to build resilience and support healthy adolescent development. Elk Grove Village, IL: American Academy of Pediatrics; 2014.

60. Hagan JF, Shaw JS, Duncan PM. Bright futures: guidelines for health supervision of infants, children and adolescents. 3rd ed. Elk Grove Village, IL: American Academy of Pediatrics; 2008.

61. Perrin E, Cohen K, Gold M, Ryan C, Savins-Williams R, Schorzman C. Gay and lesbian issues in pediatric health care. Curr Probl Pediatr Adolesc Health Care. 2004;34:355–98.

62. Fleming M, Towey K, editors. Educational forum on adolescent health: youth bullying. Chicago, IL: American Medical Association; 2002. Copies available at www.ama-assn.org/go/adolescenthealth.

63. www.thetrevorproject.org

64. www.itgetsbetter.org

65. World Professional Association for Trans-gender Health. Standards of care for the health of transsexual, transgender, and gender nonconforming people. Minneapolis, MN: World Professional Association for Transgender Health; 2011. Available at: www.wpath.org.

66. Hembree WC, Cohen-Ketternis P, Delemarre-van de Waal HA, Endocrine Society, et al. Endocrine treatment of transsexual persons: an Endocrine Society clinical practice guideline. J Clin Endocrinol Metab. 2009;94(9):3132–54.

67. The Committee on Adolescence. Office-based care for lesbian, gay, bisexual, transgender, and questioning youth. Pediatrics. 2013;132(1): 198–203.

68. Levine DA, The Committee on Adolescence. Technical report: office-based care for lesbian, gay, bisexual, transgender, and questioning youth. Pediatrics. 2013;132:e297–313.

# Geriatric Care and the LGBT Older Adult

# 12

## Michael Clark, Heshie Zinman, and Edwin Bomba

## Purpose

The purpose of this chapter is to provide an overview of the health needs of LGBT older adults. The chapter assumes that clinicians who are interested in improving health outcomes for this population must be strong advocates in building an evidence-base as well as improving systems of care. Functional status, quality of life and the need for inter-professional collaboration with be emphasized.

## Learning Objectives

- Identify at least five ways in which LGBT older adults may express their needs based on their individual construction of their identity that includes intersecting aspects of sexual orientation and aging *(KP3, KP4)*
- Describe the demographics of the LGBT older adult population and identify emerging data

M. Clark, Dr.N.P., A.P.N.-B.C., D.C.C. (✉)
Rutgers School of Nursing-Camden,
Camden, NJ, USA
e-mail: mike.clark@rutgers.edu; maitrimike@outlook.com

H. Zinman, B.A., M.B.A. • E. Bomba, B.A., M.B.A.
LGBT Elder Initiative, Philadelphia, PA, USA
e-mail: hjzinman@lgbtei.org; ebomba@aol.com; ebomba@lgbtei.org

sources that may lead to a better understanding of this population *(KP3, PBLI3)*
- Discuss the health disparities faced by LGBT older adults, including support and caregiving needs, and effective interventions that may support optimal health for LGBT older adults *(PC5, Pr1, Pr2, SBP1)*
- Discuss ways in which current conceptual models of chronic care may relate to the unique needs of LGBT older adults *(PC5, Pr2, SBP1)*

## Key Concepts

- Community of practice: Healthcare professionals who interact in order to share knowledge and experiences as well as advocate for the needs of LGBT older adults (Adapted from Lave and Wenger) [1]
- Community of interest: A diverse range of people and groups who interact and collaborate to decrease disparities and improve health outcomes for LGBT older adults
- Informal support network: Caregivers and supportive others who are not paid for the services needed to support the care needs of LGBT older adults. This network may include family, significant others, friends as well as other community group members and volunteers
- Formal support network: Health professionals and other paid workers who provide supportive services for LGBT older adults.

© Springer International Publishing Switzerland 2016
K.L. Eckstrand, J.M. Ehrenfeld (eds.), *Lesbian, Gay, Bisexual, and Transgender Healthcare*,
DOI 10.1007/978-3-319-19752-4_12

## Chapter Overview

There are few evidence-based practice recommendations for the LGBT older adult population. In many ways, care of this population has to be built "from the ground up". Efforts to improve health outcomes will take the collaborative efforts of those within and outside of clinical practice in order to build effective delivery systems as well as a research base that informs best practices. This chapter will attempt to situate best practices in the care of LGBT older adults within a broad professional, social and political context.

This chapter begins with an overview of some of the data on health disparities in the LGBT older adult population as well as current and projected efforts to improve the quality of these data. Threaded throughout the chapter are the four dimensions of the conceptual framework as put forth by the IOM report "The Health of Lesbian, Gay, Bisexual, and Transgender People: Building a Better Understanding for Better Understanding" as outlined in Table 12.1.

This chapter also suggests how the clinician may partner with a group such as the Elder Initiative which is a grass roots organization with a mission to develop a community of interest that addresses issues related to the care of LGBT older adults in a comprehensive manner. We believe that robust communities of interest will play a vital role in improving health outcomes for LGBT older adults.

## The Institute of Medicine Conceptual Framework as Applied to LGBT Older Adults

Efforts to improve the healthcare of LGBT older adults requires a better understanding of issues related to healthcare access as well as medical and social factors that affect health outcomes. A summary report on the health of LGBT persons published by the Institute of Medicine provides excellent conceptual frameworks that may support efforts to build knowledge to improve the

**Table 12.1** Institute of Medicine conceptual frameworks related to the health of LGBT older adults [2]

- Life course framework: The experiences of individuals at every stage of their life affect subsequent experiences. Older adults can't be viewed in a "snapshot" manner. Their unique life course as a LGBT person influences their relationships, choices, and experiences as an older adult. Their lives must also be viewed within a historical context. Older LGBT adults "came out" in a very different social milieu compared to younger LGBT adults. Their options regarding relationships, choices and experiences have had a significant impact on their life course.

- Minority stress model: Sexual minorities experience chronic stress due to stigmatization. Although some older adults have developed a certain amount of resilience in the face of stigmatization, in general, the adaptive capacities of older adults decrease with age. As LGBT older adults become more frail they may be less able to cope with the stresses associated with stigmatization.

- Intersectionality: Socially constructed dimensions such as race, gender, sexual orientation and age interact in complex ways to contribute to experiences of marginalization. Social inequality is associated with patterns of unequal distribution of goods and resources and result in unequal treatment of marginalized individuals and groups. Marginalization is reinforced by societal views and expectations. LGBT older adults have multiple dimensions that may be viewed in a socio-historical context. They may experience marginalization due to being seen as belonging to more than one marginalized group. Ageism both from within and outside of the LGBT community is a dimension of marginalization that is unique to LGBT older adults.

- Social ecology model: Assumes that there is a complex interaction between individual and population-level determinants of health. Behaviors have an impact on the environment and, conversely, the environment have an impact on individual behavior. The model has multiple levels which include the individual, families, relationships, community and society. Health determinants for LGBT older adults are made more complex by the challenges of dealing with an increased number of co-morbid conditions and issues related to functional dependence.

healthcare of in all age groups. However, there are certain characteristic that are unique to LGBT older adults. These frameworks are revisited here with special considerations for understanding the healthcare needs of LGBT older adults.

## The LGBT Older Adult Population

### Defining and Describing the LGBT Older Adult Population

#### Demographics of the LGBT Older Adult Population

Efforts to decrease health disparities through an improvement in quality of health and social services require the development of a robust database on the LGBT older adult population. Basic demographic data on the LGBT population as a whole are lacking.

Current data suggests that 3.5 % of adults in the United States identify as LGBT. Among this group 1.7 % identify as lesbian/gay, 1.8 % as bisexual and 0.3 % identify as transgender [3]. An estimated 19 million Americans (8.2 %) report that they have engaged in same-sex sexual behavior [4].

The older adult population in the U.S. will grow rapidly over the next 30 years as the "baby boomers" reach old age. The proportion of the population over age 65 is expected to grow from 13.3 % in 2011 to 21 % of the population in 2040 [5]. A special Gallup poll on the LGBT population estimated that 1.9 % of those older than age 65 identified as LGBT. However, this age group also had the highest rates of identifying as neither LGBT nor heterosexual (6.9 %) [6]. This may reflect a reluctance on the part of LGBT older adults to be "out". The Gallup poll indicated that those in the 18–29 age group more than three times as likely to be out as those older than age 65 [7].

### Research on Health Disparities and LGBT Older Adults

Some research indicate that LGBT older adults may have higher rates of disability, substance use and mental health problems [8, 9]. However, research also suggests that in order to assess individual risk, one needs to consider certain contextual factors such as socio-economic status, relationship status, and factors that affect minority stress such as race, gender and gender identity. These contextual factors are associated with a great deal of variability in individual health status and health risk factors. They represent inter-dependent effects of factors related to life course, intersectionality, minority stress and social ecology.

Efforts to identify and decrease disparities in health outcomes for LGBT older adults face a number of challenges. There are limited data on health determinants and health outcomes for LGBT older adults. A review of the medical literature from 1950 to 2007 indicates that about one third of all of the published literature on LGBT populations related to HIV and sexually transmitted diseases. Approximately 1 % of any literature on LGBT health issues specifically addressed the needs of LGBT older adults [10].

Attempts to gather useful data are affected by intersectionality issues such as gender, race, socio-economic status and ageism. The need to synthesize data on specific smaller subpopulations with that of aggregate data on larger populations of LGBT individuals presents significant challenges for researchers. Newer research and sampling methods are needed to derive estimates of health disparities that are specific to individuals with unique clusters of defining characteristics [11].

### Important Research Studies on LGBT Older Adult Health (Table 12.2)

### Health Determinants in Older Adults (Table 12.3)

Research on the relationship between healthcare and health outcomes for all older adults is limited. Older adults, especially the very old are frequently excluded from clinical research studies. There are few randomized control trials to guide therapeutic decisions and screening. Also due to the diversity in this LGBT older adult population more longitudinal studies are needed in order to understand the effects of aging over time [12, 17].

Many of the studies that purport to study LGBT older adults include subjects as young as

**Table 12.2** Selected major studies on health issues for LGBT older adults

| Study | Sample population | Methodology | Main findings |
|---|---|---|---|
| Analysis of 2003–2010 Washington State Risk Factor Surveillance System (WA-BRFSS) [12] Examined health outcomes, chronic conditions, and access to care, behaviors and screening. The BRFSS (Behavioral Risk Factor Surveillance System) is a national survey conducted by each state, however, Washington State began including LGB identifiers in 2003. This study allows for comparison of LGB vs. heterosexual population. Transgender individuals were not included. | $N = 96{,}992$ LGB age range (50–98) Women aged 50 years and older ($n = 58{,}319$) Lesbian = 1.03 % ($n = 562$) Bisexual women = 0.54 % (291) Men age 50 years and older (37,820) Gay men = 1.28 % (463) Bisexual men = 0.51 % (215) 0.51 % ($n = 215$) | Random direct dial surveys Response rate 43–50 % Sample weights provided by WA-BRFSS Analysis of data aggregated from annual WA-BSS from 2003 to 2010 | LGB older adults had a higher risk of disability, poor mental health, smoking, and excessive drinking than did heterosexuals. Lesbian women and bisexual women had a higher risk of cardiovascular disease and obesity. Gay and bisexual men had higher risk of poor physical health and living alone than did heterosexuals. Lesbian women reported a higher rate of excessive drinking than did bisexual women. Bisexual men reported a higher incidence of diabetes and a lower testing rates than did gay men. |
| Caring and Aging with Pride (CAP) (2011) [12] Study to determine health disparities as well as risk and protective factors that affect health and well-being. | $N = 2560$ Age of subjects: 50–64 = 44 % 65–79 = 46 % 80+ = 10 % Sexual and gender identity Gay male (some respondents reported multiple identities) Gay male (60 %) Lesbian (33 %) Bisexual women (2 %) Bisexual men (3 %) Transgender (7 %) Within transgender population: Male to female (60 %) Female to male (26 %) Other (6 %) No response (7 %) Race Non-Hispanic White (87 %) Hispanic (4 %) African American (3 %) Asian-Pacific Islander (2 %) Native American/Alaskan Native (2 %) Other: 4+ years of college (73 %) Household incomes <200 % of the poverty level (31 %) Employed (44 %) Retired (43 %) Have children (25 %) Live with others (45 %) Live alone (55 %) | Survey Began with an analysis of the WA-BRFSS data to look for aggregate data on health disparities The study then conducted an in-depth analysis of survey data from 2560 LGBT individuals of to take a closer look at risks and protective factors related to health and well-being. These subjects were enrolled through 11 LGBT service agencies around the country. | Nearly one-half had a disability. Nearly one-third reported depression. Almost two-thirds have been victimized three or more times. Thirteen percent have been denied healthcare or received inferior care. More than 20 % do not disclose their sexual or gender identity to their physician. About one-third do not have a will or durable power of attorney for healthcare. Respondents identified that the most needed services included: senior housing, transportation, legal services, social events. |

(continued)

**Table 12.2** (continued)

| Study | Sample population | Methodology | Main findings |
|---|---|---|---|
| Met Life Study (2006) [13] To understand the specific needs and concerns of "baby boomers" to support planning efforts once they reach old age. | 1000 Self-identified LGBT individuals ages 40–61 Gender, sexual orientation and gender identity Male (56 %) Female (43 %) Transgender (1 %) Gay (52 %) Lesbian (33 %) Bisexual (15 %) Relationship status Civil unions (46 %) | On-line survey and interviews conducted by Zogby International | One in four provided care for adult friend or family member One in five is unsure about who would provide care for them should they, themselves, require it. 27 % expressed great concern about age discrimination. 12 % of lesbian women lack confidence that they will be treated respectfully by healthcare professionals. 40 % believe that being LGBT gives them resilience and helps them to prepare for aging. Two thirds would like to die at home. |
| Met Life Study (2010) [28] | 1201 Self-identified LGBT individuals ages 45–64 Demographics for LGBT populations Male (66 %) Female (34 %) Age 45–49 (28 %) Age 50–54 (23 %) Age 55–59 (37 %) Age 60–64 (12 %) Gay male (46 %) Lesbian (25 %) Bisexual (24 %) Transgender (5 %) High School + (84 %) 4 years College + (35 %) Own home (67 %) Rent (27 %) Health self rating: Excellent (9 %) Very good (30 %) Good (34 %) Fair (23 %) Poor (4 %) | Comparison of 1201 LGBT on-line survey responses with matched survey responses from 1206 individuals of the same age from the general population. | Comparison of findings for LGBT vs. general population Partnered 61 %/77 % Relying on friends for: Confiding 54 %/40 % Errands 32 %/20 % Emotional support 53 %/41 % Support in emergency 42 %/25 % Advice 53 %/43 % LGBT individual reporting being mostly or completely out/ having an accepting family Lesbian women 76 %/61 % Gay men: 74 %/57 % Bisexuals: 16 %/24 % Transgender: 39 %/42 % Being LGBT helps prepare for aging Yes 74 % no 26 % Being LGBT makes aging harder Yes 54 % no 46 % |

(continued)

**Table 12.2** (continued)

| Study | Sample population | Methodology | Main findings |
|---|---|---|---|
| Women's Health Initiative (1991–2005) [14] | Approximately 160,000 women ages 50–79 of these 93,311 participants were asked about their sexual orientation: Heterosexual (97.1 %) Lifetime lesbian women (0.3 %) Lesbian women after age 45 (0.3 %) Bisexuals (0.8 %) | 3 randomized clinical trials (cardiovascular disease, cancer, osteoporosis, cancer) and an observational study | Lesbian and bisexuals women [15] Higher socioeconomic status Used alcohol and cigarettes more often Scored lower on measures of mental health and social support Exhibited higher risk factors for reproductive cancer and cardiovascular disease |
| Health of Aging Lesbian, Gay and Bisexual Adults in California: Summary findings from the California Health Interview Surveys (analysis from 2003, 2005 and 2007 data) [16] | Self-identified LGB individuals age 50–70 Analysis included a sub-set of the total number surveyed that identified as lesbian, gay or bisexual, $N = 1052$ LGB/heterosexual: Male (61 %/47.7 %) Female (39 %/52.3 %) Age 65–70 (13.1 %/18.2 %)) Person of color (22.5 %/40.9 %) Low income (below 200 % Federal Poverty Level) (19.5 %/24.2 %) Any graduate level education (35.0 %/16.6 %) Men who live alone (50 %/13.4 %) | Random-dial ongoing telephone survey completed in 2 year cycles with 50,000 Californians surveyed in each cycle. Discriminant question: "Do you think of yourself as straight or heterosexual, as gay (lesbian) or homosexual, or bisexual?" Transgender individuals were not identified. | GB men reported higher rates of hypertension, diabetes, physical disability and fair/poor health status and psychological distress. LB women reported higher rates of psychological distress. GB men higher rates of doctor's visits. LB women with increased delay in seeking care. |

50 years of age. These populations are for the most part mobile and socially active. There are almost no studies that have significant numbers of subjects greater than 75 years of age. This bias in the research significantly limits our understanding of frail LGBT older adults.

## Geriatric Care of LGBT Older Adults

### General Considerations and Approaches in Caring for LGBT Older Adult (Table 12.4)

The LGBT older adult population is extremely diverse. In additions to sexual orientation and gender identity there is great variability in the health status of individuals based on age and the degree of frailty. Despite this complexity, recommendations are emerging that guide the clinician

in meeting the needs of this population. A large national study, *The aging and health report-disparities and resilience among lesbian, gay, bisexual and transgender older adults* [8] gathered data from 2500 LGBT individuals from age 50 to 95. Table 12.4 summarizes the recommendations derived from this study.

### Contextual Issues That Impact Geriatric Care

Providing effective care for LGBT older adults requires that providers be both clinically and culturally competent. Older patients, particularly those with complex medical problems and a high degree of frailty, require specialized geriatric care that employs effective care coordination to optimize functional status and quality of life outcomes. Experts in the field of geriatrics state their

**Table 12.3** Summary of the evidence for improving health outcomes in LGBT older adults

| Issues that impact the evidence | General considerations |
|---|---|
| 1. General lack of research on older adults<br>2. No uniform age criteria for defining the older adult population in survey and research data<br>3. Older adults are not sufficiently included in survey and research data that effect health services policy and funding.<br>4. Quality outcomes for health services provided to LGBT older adults is lacking | • Research on older adults in general is less robust than younger cohorts. This is particularly true with respect to longitudinal studies that assess the effects of health determinants over time.<br>• Criteria for including and describing older adults in the research literature ranges from age 50 to 90. This age range represents a very heterogeneous population in terms of financial resources, social support needs, frailty and other health issues such as comorbidities. This limits the ability to appropriately generalize and apply research findings.<br>• Policy and funding for health and social services is largely determined by an analysis of needs at the population level. Lack of quality data limits efforts to improve funding for services.<br>• There is a need for significant improvements in measuring quality outcomes for health services proved to LGBT older adults. These efforts should be addressed at the systems level within and among healthcare organizations. Significant improvements may occur if demographics on LGBT older adults are integrated in electronic health records. In addition, if older adults are identified as a "vulnerable population" social services that are funded through the Older American's Act will be encouraged to collect data related to quality metrics. |

**Table 12.4** National Resource Center on LGBT aging: data collecting guidelines in LGBT older adults [8]

| **Look for the effect of lifetime stigma, discrimination and violence and assess for:** |
|---|
| Social isolation |
| Depression and anxiety |
| Poverty |
| Chronic illness |
| Delayed care-seeking |
| Poor nutrition |
| **Address common misconceptions among providers:** |
| Assuming that there are no LGBT individuals being served |
| Assuming that LGBT individuals can be easily identified without asking |
| It is illegal to ask about sexual orientation |
| Older LGBT individuals will resist disclosing their sexual orientation or gender identity |
| **Integrate methods of collecting data on sexual orientation and gender identity into all aspects of providing care:** |
| Within the healthcare encounter |
| Within all processes related to demographic data collection |
| Ensure and negotiate issues related to confidentiality |
| Questions of sexual orientation, gender identity and the sexual behavior history should be addressed separately as these may intersect in ways that are not readily apparent to the clinician |
| Consider and explain how particular information contributes to quality of care |
| Documentation needs to support the best patient outcomes (for instance, it may be necessary to code transgender patients according to their assigned gender at birth to get insurance coverage for screening and other health services) |

LGBT older adults may suffer due to a "double effect" of being cared for by providers who may lack general geriatric clinical competencies along with a lack of cultural competence. Since older adults need integrated interprofessional care, it is important that these issues be addressed at the level of provider systems.

**Frailty and the Care of LGBT Older Adults**

Approaches to care of older adults is largely determined by the frailty of the patient. Frailty is primarily a condition of diminished ability to respond effectively to challenges or stressors.

concern over the lack of education and training in the knowledge and skills needed to effectively care for older adult patients [18]. There have been calls for reform of education in the health professions to close the current gap in clinical knowledge and skills [19].

It has physical, cognitive, emotional and social dimensions [20]. Frailty is loosely correlated with chronologic age. However, this correlation is not absolute. It correlates more closely with chronic co-morbid conditions that impact functional status and self-efficacy. It has been suggested that health outcomes, particularly for frail individuals, be measured in terms of quality of life which correlates most closely with an optimal functional status as well as high quality social relationships. There has been a shift toward measuring the cost effectiveness of care in terms of "quality life years".

## Frailty vs. Resilience

Older adults who exhibit characteristics of healthy aging demonstrate a high degree of resilience in adapting to the limitations and challenges associated with aging. Limited data suggests that some LGBT older adults demonstrate a high degree of resilience [21, 22]. These individuals attribute this resilience to the development of coping strengths in response to dealing with the effects of social stigma. There is a need for more research on the identification and support of resilience factors, particularly among LGBT people of color [23, 24].

## The Impact of Social Stigma on Health Outcomes

Utilization of health services by the current cohort of LGBT older adults has been limited by negative experiences associated with social stigma. As a result, certain LGBT older adults may have excess disease burden due to a lack of screening and early prevention and management of chronic health conditions. The extent of this problem is largely unknown [8].

## Factors That Impact Adaptive Capacity of LGBT Older Adults

## Financial Resources and Access to Healthcare

On average, LGBT older adults, particularly women and single individuals are poorer than the population as a whole. There are data to support

that poor lesbian women and bisexual women are less likely than heterosexual women to have health insurance and that this affects utilization of preventive and other health services [12]. An analysis of the Massachusetts Behavioral Risk Factor Surveillance System, found that transgender adults have lower household incomes and higher rates of unemployment compared cisgender individuals [25].

LGBT older adults may have a pattern of under-employment due to a need to "settle" for jobs for which they were overqualified due to issues of social stigma associated with gender, sexual orientation and gender identity. They were more likely to work in jobs with minimal or no health insurance benefits. The effects of under-employment has an impact on the financial stability of these individuals in old age since they have fewer assets and their Social Security benefits may be less due to decreased lifetime taxable incomes.

Research indicates that many Americans erroneously think that the "gay" population is more affluent than the general population. While this may be true for some individuals, many LGBT older adults are poorer than the general population. Some LGBT individuals, due to issues associated with stigma and discrimination, were marginally employed with a work history that was characterized by fragmentation of low pay. For these individuals, federal entitlement benefits are lower due to a history of lower wage tax contributions. For instance, in order to avoid extra premiums for Medicare benefits, an individual has to pay federal wage taxes for at least 10 years. Social Security benefits are also indexed to amount of federal wage taxes.

Many older adults, even those with Medicare, pay a significant amount of their healthcare costs out of pocket [26]. Costs of healthcare not covered by insurance disproportionately affects the poor as these costs consume a much higher percentage of their discretionary income health expenses. Poverty is frequently calculated only on estimations of factors such as food and housing. They do not include healthcare and medication costs which are increasing at a rate greater than that of inflation. These costs may be prohibitive for those who are poor. As a result poor LGBT older adults may have limited healthcare options.

The implementation of the Affordable Care Act (ACA) may improve access to care for LGBT older adults aged 50–65. Individuals who live in states that participate in the new Medicaid eligibility requirements may qualify with incomes up to 138 % of the federal poverty level. Previous eligibility required that individuals be at or below the poverty level and the individual had to have a "categorical determinant" such as a chronic or debilitating condition. The categorical determinant has been eliminated in the minority of states that are participating in the Medicaid federal/state partnership agreements put forth in the ACA. The near poor (income up to 400 % of the federal poverty level) qualify for federal subsidies to purchase insurance on exchanges. All health plans on the exchange can't deny enrollment based on pre-existing conditions [27]. These changes may dramatically increase health care access to a significant number of LGBT older adults 50–65 years of age who are poor or near-poor.

Older adults who are on Medicaid are faced with significantly fewer choices in seeking healthcare as many providers do not accept this insurance. This may have a significant impact on health maintenance and preventive services that are important in this population. Funding for needed services, supplies and medications are also limited.

## Social Networks and the Health of LGBT Older Adults

Social networks play a large role in the health of older adults. For heterosexual older adults the social network is comprised primarily of members of their "family of origin". The social network of LGBT older adults is more likely to consist of long term stable relationships with friends. The relationships that LGBT older adults have with their "family of origin" may be negatively affected by social stigma.

Relationship status for older adults in general and LGBT older adults in particular is affected by the presence or absence of a partnered relationship. Single LGBT older adults are particularly at risk for poverty, social isolation and poor health outcomes. A significant percentage of LGBT older adults, particularly in large urban areas, are single [28]. Some LGBT older adults may become single due to the death of a partner. This may be particularly true for gay men who have lost partners due to HIV disease. Single older lesbian women, are particularly at risk for poverty. There are very limited data on the relationship status of transgender older adults [29].

## Clinical Care of LGBT Older Adults

### LGBT Older Adults as Two Populations

In caring for older adults, clinicians and other service providers must address issues related to physical, social, emotional and spiritual health. Some gerontologists differentiate the health status of older adults based on frailty. Some make a dichotomous distinction and use the term "young-old" and "old-old" based on an estimation of frailty [30]. For the "young old" the goals of care are the identification and management of disease in order to achieve an optimal number of "quality life years". For frail older adults, the goal of disease management shifts toward the management of symptoms that impair self-efficacy and healthy social interactions.

The research literature that does address the needs of LGBT older adults focuses mostly on the "young-old" population or the later adult population age 50–65. This is reflected in the IOM report that attempted to synthesize the literature on LGBT older adults. They state that they were limited in finding data on LGBT older adults and chose to review the literature for all individuals greater than age 50 [9].

### Care of the LGBT "Young-Old"

The general approach to care for the young-old typically seeks to identify and manage specific clinical problems. Most of the health issues can be identified in standard history and screening methods. In order to provide culturally competent care, the clinician needs to establish an open and honest relationship in which the patient is comfortable disclosing important medical and social information that pertain to maintaining their health.

In one large study, LGBT older adults identified the core competencies that they thought were essential in providing high quality care. These include that the clinician reflect upon their own values and preferences; apply contemporary theories of aging and social gerontology; integrate contextual factors specific to LGBT older adults in conducting a health and social assessment and use culturally sensitive and age appropriate language to establish and build rapport [31].

The cultural competence of clinicians and healthcare workers who work in clinics and other outpatient settings is a key determinant of quality care for this population. LGBT older adults who have experienced discrimination from health care providers and services may be reluctant to share essential information that may be important for screening, prevention and disease management.

## Selected Health Problems in LGBT Older Adults

Certain health disparities are found in LGBT individuals who are entering later adulthood. Life course factors such as social stigmatization may play a role in these disparities. Some of these conditions such as depression, suicide and violence may be associated with minority stress. Other conditions such as obesity, alcohol intake and smoking may be associated with behavioral patterns enhanced by socialization patterns and group norms.

### Behavioral Health Issues

There are very limited data that describe behavioral health issues for transgender individuals. A systematic review of the epidemiology literature identified certain mental health problems that have a higher prevalence in LGB individuals. These problems should guide screening efforts in the LGB older adult population [33]. The findings indicate that LGB individuals are at higher risk for suicidal ideation and behaviors, mental disorder and substance misuse and dependence. There was

a twofold increase risk of suicide attempts in the year prior to the study and a fourfold excess lifetime risk for gay and bisexual men [33].

The relative risk for depression, anxiety, and alcohol and substance misuse were at least 1.5 more common compared to heterosexuals [33]. Lesbian and bisexual women were at particular risk for substance dependence. The review found few prospective studies. Therefore the data on risk factors are very limited. This study did not include transgender individuals [33].

A cross sectional study found that transgender individuals have an increased risk of smoking but little is known about other health related behaviors such as alcohol misuse, lack of exercise and obesity [34]. An online survey of transgender individuals indicated high levels of depression, anxiety and somatization [22].

## General Health Problems in Older LGBT Individuals

LGB older adults, compared to age matched heterosexuals, are at increased risk for disability, poor mental health, smoking and excessive drinking. Older lesbian women were more likely to engage in excessive drinking than bisexual women. Older lesbian and bisexual women are at increased risk for cardiovascular disease and obesity. Older gay men are at increased risk for poor physical health and they are more likely to live alone [12].

## Sexual Health in LGBT Older Adults

The care of all LGBT older adults should include taking a thorough and accurate sexual history. The guidelines for a culturally sensitive approach for obtaining a history are put forth elsewhere in this text. The only point worth noting is that there may be a need to distinguish current vs. past sexual practices for this population.

For LGBT older adults it may be particularly important to distinguish sexual orientation and gender identity from patterns of sexual activity. For instance, lesbian women and bisexual women may report a history of having sex with men. The sexual histories as well as the reproductive history of women have important implications for screening of a number of diseases. These include testing for risks associated with hepatitis, herpes simplex and human papilloma virus as well as the risk for HIV and sexually transmitted diseases such as syphilis.

Little is known about sexual practices and problems of older adults in the general population. One review of the literature found two thirds of those over age 50 were excluded from research trials on the prevention of sexually transmitted infections [35].

One large study indicate that the prevalence of sexual activity in the general population decreases with age from approximately 73 % in the 57–64 year age group to 26 % among respondents who were 75–85 years of age. About one half of both men and women reported at least one bothersome sexual problem [36]. In women these included low desire, difficulty with vaginal lubrication and inability to climax. In men erectile dysfunction was the most frequent problem (37 %) [36]. Only 38 % of men and 22 % of women over the age of 50 reported having discussed sex with a physician [36]. Having frank discussion about sexual practices, including higher risk sexual activity, may be particularly important for older gay men. Self-reported risk behavior among MSM over the age of 50 indicates that the number of sexual partners can remain quite high. In a 12 month telephone survey of MSM, 25 % of those age 60–69 reported nine or more partners in the previous year [37].

There is some evidence to suggest that older adults underestimate their risk for acquiring sexually transmitted infections [38]. This may be particularly true if individuals are coming out of long term monogamous relationships either due to separation or the death of a partner. Mental health issues, especially depression, and issues such as social isolation and loneliness may increase the potential for higher risk behaviors [39].

For older men, including gay men, the use of drugs for erectile dysfunction may increase the risk of sexually transmitted disease, although the data on this are mixed [38]. Although data are emerging in younger age cohorts, it is unclear as to the effects that the internet and social media may have on sexual activity patterns among LGBT older adults [40].

There is little research on the transmission of sexually transmitted infections in women who have sex with women. However, it is particularly important to assess behaviors that may include recent or remote sexual contact with men. Heterosexual contact is the predominant risk factor for women who acquire HIV infection [41]. The risk of transmission must be evaluated in the context of specific sexual practices (i.e. sharing of sex toys in vaginal or anal sex). There is some concern about increased transmission risk for older women due to a thinning and drying of the vaginal mucosa. This may place the woman at increased risk for small tears or abrasions that may increase the transmission risk.

**Clinical Tips:**

- Requests for and discussions about medications for erectile dysfunction provides an excellent opportunity for a broader discussion of sexuality and specific risks for sexually transmitted infections. In one study of the general older adult population, 17 % of men indicted that they used ED medication during their last sexual encounter [36].
- Condom use should be encouraged. In one study among older adults who were not in long term monogamous relationships, 20 % of men and 24 % of women used a condom in their last sexual encounter. This same group indicated that 5 % of their partners had a sexually transmitted infection at the time of their last sexual encounter [39].
- For men and women a discussion about the use of sex toys should be addressed as these may be a vector for transmission of infections. Women who have sex with women may underestimate thier risk of transmission of sexually transmitted diseases when using sex toys [42].

## HIV Disease and LGBT Older Adults

HIV disease is a significant problem for older adults, including LGBT older adults. There are two cohorts of interest in this group: Older gay men who contracted HIV earlier in life and those who are newly infected as older adults. Expert consensus opinion guidelines for older adults with HIV have recently been published by the American Academy of HIV Medicine and the AIDS Community Research Initiative of America [43].

The increased prevalence of HIV in the older adult population is due to an increase in survival of those infected earlier in life as well as an increase in the incidence of newly acquired infections. By 2015, half of all HIV positive individuals will be age 50 or older [41]. The largest cohort of HIV positive older adults in the general population are in the 50–54 age group [44]. Among those over the age of 50, 60 % of the infections are attributed to sexual behaviors in men who have sex with men [44]. The HIV rates for older African American men 12 times higher than those for whites [45]. Of particular concern is the fact that one in six of all newly acquired cases of HIV infection in the general population occur in men older than 50 years of age [41].

Older women typically contract HIV primarily through heterosexual contact. Lesbian and bisexual women may report significant rates of previous sexual activity with men. There are theoretical reasons as to why older women may be at increased risk for HIV infection, including a thinning, more friable vaginal mucosa due to postmenopausal changes [46].

## Care of the HIV Positive LGBT Older Adult

Care for HIV positive older adults can be characterized as consisting of three phases: early care (screening, diagnosis and initiation of treatment); managing the HIV disease; and, addressing emerging issues that may be specific to the aging process itself [47].

### Initiation of Therapy

It is recommended that the primary provider consult with a specialist who has expertise in managing HIV disease when initiating therapy. However, many of these specialist may have limited experience in managing this disease in older adults. This will likely change as the number of HIV infected older adults increases. Professional groups such as the American Academy of HIV Medicine and the AIDS Community Research Initiative of America have recently published recommended treatment strategies for HIV positive older adults [43]. Primary care providers will need to stay current on treatment guidelines and recommendations as these continue to evolve.

The response of older adults to antiretroviral therapy (ART) compares well to the responses found in younger individuals [48]. However, decreases in morbidity and mortality depend on early detection. Current guidelines suggest that treatment be offered to all HIV positive individuals regardless of age [49]. Researchers are only beginning to explore the safety and efficacy of ART in older individuals [49].

In general, older adults being treated for HIV have drug adherence rates approaching 95 % with fewer interruptions in therapy compared to younger cohorts [50]. Older adults treated with ART achieve acceptable decreases in viral load, however, some tend to have less favorable improvements in CD4 counts. This may be partially related to being diagnosed later and thus having lower CD4 counts at the initiation of therapy [51].

HIV positive older adults present special treatment challenges due to an increased number of co-morbid conditions and medications. Older adults with HIV have higher rates of drug-drug interactions due largely to the higher number of medications used to treat co-morbid conditions [52]. One study indicated that 76 % of participants were taking nine or more drugs. Among these drugs a significant number had unacceptable interaction profiles [52]. Little is known about the pharmacokinetic and pharmacodynamics of ART in older patients [51]. Medication simplification to decrease these interactions may have increased importance in this population.

**Clinical tips:**

• Incorporate screening for substance misuse disorder when initiating ART therapy

Patients who do not take their ART consistently have significantly worse health outcomes as a results of the effect of poorly controlled HIV disease on the immune system, cardiovascular system, neurologic system and the kidneys. Poor ART adherence correlates with rates of substance abuse. In one study 22 % of those with suboptimal ART adherence screened positive for unhealthy alcohol use. It is estimated that approximately 10 % of LGBT older adults drink excessively [8]. Standardized screening tools have been tested and validated in HIV positive patients [53].

## Maintenance of Therapy

HIV positive older adults are at increased risk for certain HIV-associated non-AIDS (HANA) conditions. These conditions include an increased risk for cardiovascular disease, malignancies and osteoporosis. Other factors related to health behaviors include diet, exercise, tobacco use and substance use as well as an adequate management of HIV and other chronic conditions. HANA conditions occur more frequently with lower CD4 counts and higher viral loads, but they can also occur in patients with well controlled HIV disease [54]. HANA conditions associated with cardiovascular events, non-AIDS malignancies, and end stage kidney and liver disease are responsible for as many as 60 % of deaths in HIV infected individuals [55].

Chronic hepatitis B and C infections pose a special risk for HIV infected older adults. Hepatitis C is responsible 90 % of liver related deaths in HIV infected individuals [56]. The United States Preventive Services Task Force recommends one time screening for all adults born between 1945 and 1965 [57]. This age group represents approximately 75 % of all patients who have chronic hepatitis C infection [58].

Most patients with Hepatitis C are unaware that they are infected. Many can't remember a specific risk factor. It is not known how the rates of Hepatitis C for LGBT individuals compares to the general population. Specific risk factors such as I.V. drug use and sex with IV drug users are considered behavioral risk factors. Although sexual transmission of hepatitis C in men who have sex with men is thought to be low; there is some increase in risk with unprotected receptive anal sex. Those within the LGBT community who currently use or have previously used IV drugs are at highest risk.

## Screening for Cancer in HIV Positive Individuals

Although cancer screening is not an issues specific to LGBT older adults, some patients may present for the first time in later years due to bad past experiences with healthcare providers or a lack of insurance. This delay in care may lead to worse outcomes.

HIV positive men who have sex with men are at increased risk for anal cancer. Detection of epithelial changes suggesting an increased risk of early cancer can be accomplished by performing and anal Pap test. A significant barrier to effective screening exists due to a lack of clinical expertise as well as equipment such as a high-resolution anoscope in most practice settings. In addition, many pathologists lack experience in interpreting pathology specimens from rectal samples and there is a concern about inter-rater reliability.

One author recommends that an anal Pap test should be performed at the time of the initial diagnosis of HIV. The Pap should be repeated at 6 month intervals until two normal cytology results are obtained. Abnormal cytology results should prompt follow up evaluation with high-resolution anoscopy and biopsy of suspicious lesions [59]. There is no evidence that early testing for prostate cancer in HIV positive patients is beneficial [59].

Cervical Pap testing should be performed twice within the first year after an HIV diagnosis and annually thereafter (provided that the cytology results are normal). There is very limited data on Pap testing rates for HIV positive lesbian and bisexual women. However, up to one fourth of all HIV positive women in the general population fail to get annual Pap tests [60]. Clinicians need to be vigilant in recommending Pap testing and provide appropriate referral.

## Clinical Issues in the Care of Older Transgender Patients

Transgender individuals experience significant difficulties in navigating the healthcare system. Transgender individuals report denial of care because of their gender identity (19 %); verbal harassment in the medical setting (28 %) and a postponement of care due to discrimination and disrespect (33 %) [61].

Older adults who are transgender are more likely to have increased morbidity as a result of a lack of appropriate screening and early intervention for a variety of conditions [61]. They may also have a history of problems related to the use of non-medical sources of hormones due to a lack of trust in or a lack of access to supportive health services [62]. A welcoming care environment and health insurance coverage may have a positive effect on care seeking behavior [63].

Recent trends in policy and healthcare funding hold forth the promise that increasing numbers of older transgender individuals will have healthcare coverage. Medicare covers routine care and hormonal therapy [64]. In addition, the department of Health and Human Services has determined that transgender individuals may no longer be automatically denied coverage for sex reassignment surgeries [65].

The transgender population is exceedingly complex. Transgender individuals may undergo various degrees of surgical and hormonal gender-confirming therapies. They may have undergone sex reassignment surgery or begun gender-confirming therapy at an early age or they may begin the process of gender transitioning later in life. Transgender individuals may develop gender dysphoria later in life. For these individuals, the transition can be particularly difficult since hormone therapy may produce less pronounced changes in physical characteristics.

Screening and preventive care of transgender older adults is based upon a consideration of the body organs of the individual as well as surgical and hormonal gender-confirming therapy. Currently there are no clear evidence-based guidelines that are specific to the care of transgender persons [66].

Little is known about the long terms risks of hormone therapy in transgender patients. Providers must pay attention to organs in place for a particular transgender patient. Transgender women need a consideration of prostate cancer risk. Transgender men who have not had total hysterectomies need to have their cancer risk assessed for reproductive organs that remain intact.

There is some evidence that transgender women have a higher risk for osteoporosis [67]. In one cross sectional study involving 100 transgender persons, 6 % of transgender women experienced a thrombotic event and 6 % experienced cardiovascular problems. The risk of thromboembolism may be greater with higher doses of estrogen, especially in late adult transgender women who are obese or who smoke. The average length of hormone use was 11.3 years [67]. There is also some concern about the health risks associated with breast implants [68].

Transgender men usually tolerate androgen therapy well. There are some concerns about the risk for osteoporosis; however, there are no current guidelines for bone density studies for transgender men. A few case studies of vaginal, cervical and endometrial cancer have been reported. A few cases of cancer of the breast in residual breast tissue has been reported [69].

Transgender individuals experience higher rates of depression. A review of the literature identified several factors that influence depression including a lack of social support, violence, sex work and challenges associated with gender identity [70]. In general, transgender persons have higher rates of drug use, HIV infection and sex work compared to the general population [70]. There is a concern that depression in transgender persons is associated with increased rates of substance use and high risk sexual behavior [71]. These interaction effects in older transgender persons has not been studied.

**Clinical consideration:**

- Transgender individuals typically sign an elaborate informed consent document before beginning care.
- The transgender person may benefit from periodic follow up regarding risk: benefit decisions regarding health risks associated with hormone therapy as they age.
- These interventions might allow for more informed choices regarding treatments and screening.

## Care of the Frail LGBT Older Adult

### Frailty as a Factor in Framing Care

The care of frail older adults is complex. These patients tend to have an increased number of co-morbid conditions and they are frequently taking a large number of drugs. Chronic disabling conditions or cognitive impairment impede their capacity for self-care. As a result of the complex and multi-dimensional challenges faced by these individuals, care must be provided by a team that includes professionals, as well as friends and family. Paid service providers are frequently called "formal caregivers" and unpaid or volunteer providers are called "informal caregivers".

Clinicians who work with frail individuals must become competent in the principles of geriatrics as well as develop systems and expertise that support high-quality care coordination. Competent coordination must incorporate inter-professional clinical care as well as a wide range of social services. The delivery of high quality care also requires that each clinician and service provider be culturally competent in caring for LGBT older adults.

Frail older adults have unique needs. The main factors that affect care include geriatric syndromes, polypharmacy, and recognition of atypical and non-specific presentation of disease. Geriatric syndromes such as falls, incontinence and acute changes in mental status are frequently manifestations of underlying disease. Clinicians must work closely with caregivers in order to identify and manage these issues.

## Factors That Promote Health Aging in Frail Individuals

### Aging in Place

Recently an emphasis has been placed on keeping frail older adults in the community and out of institutions. Policy initiatives are in place to frame services based on frailty vs. chronological age. For instance, the Administration on Aging which provides many of the federal and state programs for older adults are now part of the Administration for Community Living which is designed to coordinate service for all individuals with disabilities that place them at risk for needing institutional care. This includes those with intellectual, developmental and other disabilities [72]. Moving forward, programs and policies are likely to place increasing emphasis on providing and coordinating services based on the need for functional support outside of institutional settings [73].

The concept of "aging in place" is becoming a popular concept that describes efforts to keep frail individuals out of institutions. Central to the ability for older adults to remain in the community is the provision of care that supports functional status. Care provided by family and friends must be coordinated with community-based services such as senior centers and home health care. [74].

Innovative models that integrate the volunteer efforts of neighbors with formal healthcare and social services are evolving. There are several models that are emerging such as Naturally Occurring Retirement Communities (NORCs) [75] and the Village to Village Network [76]. These are local organizations that provide volunteer support by neighbors to frail older adults living in their community. These organizations typically partner with health and social service organizations. Although these organizations are not targeted specifically to LGBT older adults, they may become an important "aging in place" support in areas with higher concentrations of LGBT older adults.

Some cities have or are beginning to develop senior housing that primarily serve LGBT older adults. These projects are partnering with social and health services in the community that specialize in serving the LGBT community.

Gay senior housing projects have opened in a number of large cities in the U.S. These centers, such as the one in Philadelphia, are partnering with an LGBT health center and an LGBT social services organization. Models that integrate LGBT-friendly housing with LGBT-friendly social and medical services holds forth promise for supporting a high quality of health for its residents [77].

## Supporting Informal Caregiver Networks

Caregiver burden is a source of concern since maintaining the health of the caregiver is a crucial determinant as to whether the older adult can "age in place". Although there has been much speculation as to the negative health impacts of caregiving, research is needed to better understand this phenomenon [78]. The relationship between overall health and caregiver burden is a complex one. Some caregivers report that caregiving is a positive experience that provides a sense of accomplishment and increased self-esteem.

Although there is no centralized national-level surveillance system on informal caregivers of older disabled adults [79] it is estimated that approximately 80 % of the home care for severely disabled patients, such as those with Alzheimer Disease, is provided by family members such as spouses and adult children. These individual comprise the patient's "family of origin".

A significant challenge that will be faced by clinicians and social service providers is to identify and support informal networks of individuals who provide needed care for LGBT older adults who seek to "age in place". Among the general population of older adults 72 % of men and 41 % of women live with a spouse [80]. Among LGBT older adults approximately 40 % have a partner. Only 20–25 % of LGBT older adults report having one or more living children compared to 40 % for heterosexual older adults [81] The social networks of LGBT older adults are characterized as "families of choice" as opposed to the "families of origin" [82].

For LGBT older adults a significant amount of care support may be provided by a network of individuals that are part of a "family of choice". The capacity of these informal networks for providing supportive care for LGBT older adults is not known. Some research suggests that while friends may provide emotional support, they may be limited in their ability to provide the kind of constant functional support that is required for aging in place. There is concern that LGBT older adults are more at risk for requiring institutionalized care. Also, "family of choice" caregivers frequently do not receive the kinds of social supports that are afforded caregivers who are part of a "family of origin". For instance, LGBT partners and friends may not be considered eligible under the Federal Medical Leave Act (FMLA) which allows time for workers to take time off to care for sick and disabled family members.

The United States v. Windsor decision in which the U.S. Supreme Court struck down the federal Defense of Marriage Act, FMLA eligibility varied by state. In determining eligibility a distinction was made between the "place of domicile" (state in which the same-sex spouse lives) and the "place of celebration" (state in which they are married) [83]. The subsequent Supreme Court ruling that legalized same-sex marriage in all states eliminates this variability.

Some caregivers who are members of a "family of choice" may be unaware of services and resources to which they are entitled. The National Family Caregiver Support Act has broad language that can be interpreted to include LGBT caregivers. However, LGBT elders and caregiver support programs are often unaware of this more inclusive language [84]. Of the limited federal funds provided for caregiver support programs, almost no funds have been provided for programs specifically designed to meet the needs of LGBT elders [85].

## Assessment of Functional Status and Functional Supports

Although there are many functional status tools with good reported psychometrics, these have not been tested specifically with regard to LGBT individuals. In addition, there are no tools to assess the nature and quality of support networks for LGBT older adults. Care must be taken to avoid assumptions that caregiving will be provided by a heterosexual "wife" or "husband".

Suggested approaches include:

- Begin with open ended questions:
  - "Who helps you with your day to day activities?"
  - "If you had an emergency, who would you call?"
  - "Who would maintain your apartment or house if you became ill?" (This may include pet care)

Functional status tools must be modified to include the needs of the support network for LGBT older adults, which may be broader and more variable than that of the general population.

## Financial Issues That Impact the Health of LGBT Older Adults

The quality of life for all individuals depends upon adequate healthcare benefits, financial resources and economic stability. The financial status of older adults is determined by the assets at the time of retirement as well as retirement income. Single LGBT older adults, particularly females, often have fewer assets and lower incomes.

However, as the status of federal laws have recently evolved with the legalization of same sex marriage, a growing gap will continue to develop between married and single individuals. There are major differences in the economic status of partnered vs. single LGBT older adults. In general, single individuals tend to be poorer and either uninsured or underinsured. The majority of LGBT older adults are single. The changes in federal entitlement program benefits that are being afforded same sex couples do not always benefit single individuals.

Some poor LGBT older adults who have not yet reached 65 years of age may receive limited

healthcare benefits through the Medicaid Program. Eligibility is based on a having few assets as well as having an income near or below the federal poverty line [88].

## Support for Planning for Decreasing Capacity

### Financial Planning for Long Term Care

Paying for the cost of long term care is a major challenge for LGBT older adults. This is particularly true, but not limited to, paying for nursing home care. The average cost of nursing home care is $ 80,000 per year [89]. Costs for long term care provided in the home are substantial both in terms of direct and indirect costs.

Typically individuals pay out of pocket for nursing home care until their financial resources are depleted. At that time they apply for Medicaid as the source of funding for nursing home care. Since Medicaid is a program with "means testing" individuals must have little in the way of personal assets or income in order to qualify. Unmarried partners who share assets with an individual requiring long term care are at financial risk of losing their portion of any shared assets of investments. This is particularly problematic if an unmarried couple co-owns a home [84].

Issues related to financial planning for long term care are very complex and beyond the scope of this text. However, financial resources have a major impact on the health and healthcare options for LGBT older adults. Clinicians can assist LGBT older patients by providing referral to information sources that may assist in advance planning.

### Advance Directives

The proportion of Americans who have advance directives has been increasing. One study found that from the years 2000 to 2010 the percentage of Americans with advance directives increased from 47 to 72 % [90]. This same study found that in 2010, approximately 71 % of adults had at least one hospitalization in the last two years of their life. Approximately 35 % died in the hospital [90]. In the absence of an advance directive, hospitals and other healthcare organizations typically turn to family and friends to serve as surrogate decision-makers. These individuals are asked to consider treatment options based on their understanding of the patient's values, wishes and preferences. Research indicates that difference of opinion about a patient's preferences may cause significant conflict between members of the "family of origin" and the "family of choice" [81].

Clinicians should advise LGBT older adults on the important components of an advance directive as well as the importance of ensuring that the designated decision-maker will have the power to execute the patient's wishes and preferences [91]. Many patients erroneously assume that a living will document is sufficient in ensuring that their preferences for end of life care will be honored. They fail to realize that these documents need to be interpreted within the complex and often hectic context of the circumstances surrounding the execution of this document.

The MetLife study in 2006 found that just over half of 1000 LGBT participants had not prepared living wills and only about 44 % had designated a surrogate decision-maker in a formal document [13]. Single LGBT older adults are even less likely than partnered individuals to have completed this process.

This issue is complicated for LGBT individuals due to variability in the recognition of identified surrogate decision-maker who may be neither the patient's spouse nor a member of the "family of origin". It is unwise for LGBT individuals to assume that hospitals and healthcare providers will turn to a member of their "family of choice" for making decisions in the absence of a legally enacted advanced directive. In some states the designation of a surrogate decision maker may require complex legal consultation to create valid documents to ensure the legitimacy of a chosen surrogate decision-maker.

The Human Rights Campaign (HRC) has categorized states based on their recognition of LGBT surrogate decision-makers [92]. LGBT older adults should be strongly encouraged to become familiar with state laws regarding advance directives and surrogate decision-making.

## Long Term Care Issues Specific to LGBT Older Adults

Older adults with decreased functional status, cognitive impairment or complex chronic comorbidities require supportive long term care. This care may be provided in the community or in long term care settings. In general, LGBT older adults report significant concerns about these services. One community needs assessment found that slightly more than half of LGBT elders were dissatisfied with federal, state and local services [93]. In another study of 127 LGBT adults, 33 % thought that they would have to hide their sexual orientation or gender identity if they moved to a nursing home [94]. A health disparities study conducted with over 3500 LGBT people in New York found that 8.3 % reported being neglected by a caregiver and 8.9 % experienced financial exploitation [95].

Clinicians should be aware of the vulnerability that LGBT older adults perceive or experience in utilizing long term care services. One of the barriers to promoting culturally competent services and environments in nursing homes is that many of these institutions believe that they do not have LGBT residents. LGBT older adults worry that they will experience discrimination and poor care if they disclose their sexual or gender identity. The fear of disclosure creates a kind of "Catch 22". This lack of disclosure on the part of LGBT residents inhibits efforts to improve efforts to deliver culturally competent care. It remains to be seen whether the current cohort of gay baby boomers, will be more willing to disclose their sexual orientation or gender identity and advocate for higher quality care.

The federal Nursing Home Reform Act requires all nursing homes that receive Medicare or Medicaid funding (almost all nursing homes) to provide written policies to residents regarding their rights under this law. These "resident bill of rights" include the right to choose one's physician; the right to privacy; dignity and respect; the right to use one's clothing (allowing transgender individuals to dress according to their gender identity); the right to be free from abuse and restraints; and the right to voice grievances without retaliation [84]. However, there may be variation in the ways that nursing homes interpret these requirements when it comes to LGBT older adults.

Enactment of these rights for LGBT older adults is at best uneven. Residents may experience neglect and abuse from staff members as well as other residents. Staff may fail to identify and respond to the needs of LGBT-identified individuals in long-term care settings [96]. In general, staff are not trained to manage interactions between LGBT and heterosexual residents and families. This could result in problems that range from ostracism to hostility. Residents may have limitations set on their visitation rights that may restrict access to supportive spouses, partners and friends. Often LGBT residents are too frail to advocate for themselves.

Most of the paid personal care provided to older adults across settings is provided by poorly paid, unlicensed personal care assistants. It will be important to reach out to these workers in order to optimize the quality of the living environments of dependent LGBT older adults. Some potential targets for disseminating information on culturally competent care are Area Agencies on Aging as well as ombudsman programs and advocacy groups. Communities of interest that involve consumers, supportive others, medical providers, social workers, personal care workers and others can support efforts to improve the care of LGBT older adults.

The National Senior Citizen Law Center and 11 other advocacy groups have drafted comments that propose a number of changes to expand the rights of nursing home residents. These changes include: adding anti-discriminatory language to include sexual orientation, gender identity, as well as marital status and family status. In addition, it recommends allowing same sex partners to share a room and extend unlimited visiting hours to any "friendly visitor" (currently only family members are extended this privilege) [97].

## Retirement Community and Assisted Living Issues Specific to LGBT Older Adults

Some older adults choose to live in assisted living settings. Little is known about the experiences of LGBT older adults in this type of setting. There are variable, limited, anecdotal reports in the literature regarding a perception of the effects of stigma in these settings. Unlike nursing homes, assisted living facilities are not highly regulated. Recently, some LGBT friendly assisted living facilities have opened. One report indicates that LGBT residents felt acceptance and an ability to form expanded social networks in this setting [98].

## Future Directions: Building Capacity for Improving the Care of LGBT Older Adults

### Policy

Significant efforts are needed at the federal, state and local level to collect demographic data on LGBT older adults. One strategy that would promote these efforts is to have LGBT older adults identified as a vulnerable population [84]. The Older Americans Act (OAA) has provisions that require state and local aging services agencies funded by this act to engage in systematic efforts to identify vulnerable populations and their needs. If LGBT older adults are identified as a vulnerable population, Area Agencies on Aging (AAA) that provide a variety of community services at the state and county level, would be required to track outcomes related to the utilization and quality of services delivered to LGBT older adults.

### LGBT Older Adults and New Care Delivery Models

The federal and state governments are seeking innovative ways to decrease cost and improve the quality of chronic care. At the federal level, service delivery is being retooled to target support for people with disabilities regardless of age. One of the primary changes involves providing effective and integrated services that will allow frail older adults and others with disabilities to remain in the community.

In 2009, the Department of Human Services launched the Community Living Initiative to direct important changes in chronic care for people with disabilities. Many of the goals of this initiative could potentially improve the quality of care for LGBT older adults. Innovative new programs might promote flexibility and choice for LGBT older adults and their caregivers. Some options that might be considered include: Deciding where and with whom they live; having control over the services they receive and who provides those services; having the ability to work and earn money; choosing friends and family to help them participate in community life (and in some cases pay them for these services); and, receive information and services that take into account their cultural and linguistic needs.

The Agency on Aging (AoA) is now a part of the Administration for Community Living which in is in turn a part of the Department of Health and Human Services. Service domains for the Agency on Aging will include: Elder rights services; health prevention and wellness programs; national family caregiver support programs; and support services [72].

The Agency on Aging has begun to include LGBT older adults in its language on diversity. At present, the main funded effort has been to support the SAGE National Resource Center on LGBT Aging [99]. Advocacy will be needed to push for inclusive language and transparent inclusion of LGBT older adults within all appropriate Agency on Aging programs and initiatives.

Recently a Community Living Policy Center at the University of California has undertaken efforts to identify and study promising long term care practices that are being implemented at the state and federal level in order to make recommendations regarding the development of model state-level long term care services and support systems for LGBT older adults. Currently state-run systems are very uneven in the types of services provided. The CMS Center for Innovation and other funding sources are currently supporting a number of demonstration project to improve long term services in the community. LGBT older adults may benefit from specific aspects of potential improvements that are being discussed and tested [100]. A common theme in the planning and analysis of these programs is the development of consumer directed services. This includes mechanisms for community involvement in the planning and evaluation of services.

There are proposals to develop a registry of agencies that match the specific needs of consumers. Information provided by these registries might include LGBT friendly agencies. Proposals to allow for employing family members should include language that designate an LGBT older adult's "family of choice". Programs that give money directly to consumers to hire their own direct care workers should provide a list of direct care workers who are competent in caring for LGBT older adults [100].

## Clinician Involvement in Practice Improvement for LGBT Older Adults

As previously outlined, the main consideration for high quality direct care is the development of warm, welcoming, supportive, open and collaborative relationships with LGBT older adults. In addition, clinicians need to keep abreast of developments in emerging evidence-based research on health disparities and best practices that may specifically benefit LGBT older adults. In addition clinicians will need to explore ways to improve their practice settings in order to promote culturally competent care.

Currently, most arguments for inclusion of LGBT patients has been based on normative principles such as justice. Clinicians need to find ways to craft pragmatic arguments that seek to link improved care for LGBT patients with an improvement in established quality metrics that drive payment for services. To accomplish this, clinicians must explore ways to align LGBT care with evolving models of care delivery that will drive payment. These models place particular emphasis on behavioral determinants of chronic health problems. Examples include the Chronic Care Model, and the Patient-Centered Medical Home. These models reframe care to give the patient more control over choices regarding their care. They emphasize the need for an "activated patient" who is a collaborative partner in planning and executing care. The quality of the provider-patient relationship will be a key factor in the collaborative process. Process metrics are being designed to capture these characteristics of care. It is important that LGBT individuals be clearly identified in quality measurement processes.

Clinicians can advocate for change in existing statutes, policies and programs at the federal, state and local level. They must also seek to influence professional organizations to include LGBT care issues in their mission, policies and strategic plans.

## Resources for Clinicians Caring for LGBT Older Adults

A number of different types of resources are available for clinicians. Many of these resources are not directed specifically to the needs of LGBT older adults. Further work needs to be done to ensure that these groups specifically include the needs of the LGBT older population. References for these resources are listed below:

**General resources:**

– **The National Resource Center on LGBT Aging**: This is the most comprehensive source of practical information, guidelines as well as education and training programs for clinicians and consumers who seek to improve the lives of LGBT older adults. This site is continually updated with new resources. http://www. lgbtagingcenter.org/
– **AARP Website: Home and Family: LGBT**: Webpage designed to share information on issues related to LGBT older adults. http://www.aarp. org/relationships/friends-family/aarp-pride. html?intcmp=FTR-LINKS-WWA-LGBT
– **The Aging and Health Report: Disparities and Resilience among Lesbian, Gay, Bisexual, and Transgender Older Adults**: Aging and health issues facing lesbian, gay, bisexual and

transgender(LGBT) baby boomers. This report has many resources that support a better understanding of health needs of LGBT adults 50 years of and older. http://caringandaging.org/
– **LGBT Aging Issues Network (LAIN)**
LAIN, a constituent group of the American Society on Aging, works to raise awareness about the concerns of LGBT elders and about the unique barriers they encounter in gaining access to housing, healthcare, long-term care and other needed services. LAIN has an excellent website with a great deal of information including the LGBT Aging Resources Clearinghouse. http://www.asaging.org/lain
– **Outing Age 2010: Public Policy Issues Affecting Lesbian, Gay, Bisexual and Transgender (LGBT) Elders**
This report provides an in-depth look at public policy issues and challenges facing millions of lesbian, gay, bisexual and transgender people in the United States as they get older. http:// www.thetaskforce.org/reports_and_research/ outing_age_2010
– **LGBT Older Adults in Long Term Care Facilities: Stories from the Field**
This report, funded by the Arcus Foundation, was co-authored by six national organizations and reports on the results of a survey conducted to better understand the experiences of LGBT older adults in long-term care settings. http://www.lgbtlongtermcare.org/wp-content/ uploads/NSCLC_LGBT_report.pdf
– **Tools for Protecting Your Health Care Wishes**
A guide prepared by Lambda Legal to assist LGBT in protecting their rights in health care settings. http://www.lambdalegal.org/ publications/take-the-power/your-health-care-wishes.html

**Academic resources for clinical knowledge, research and policy:**

– **University of California Center of Excellence for Transgender Health**. The mission of this center is to increase access to comprehensive, effective and affirming health care services for transgender and gender-variant communities. One of its programs works

to develop evidence-based primary care protocols for the care of transgender patients. www.
transhealth.ucsf.edu
- **The Williams Institute**: national think tank
  organization at the University Of California
  Los Angeles School Of Law. The mission of
  the institute is to conduct rigorous, independent research on sexual orientation and gender
  identity law and public policy. http://william-
  sinstitute.law.ucla.edu/

**Professional society and specialty organiza-
tion resources:**

- **American Geriatrics Society Sections &
  Special Interest Groups: Needs of Older
  Gay and Lesbian, Bisexual and Transgender
  Persons**. www.americangeriatrics.org/about_
  us/who_we_are/sections_special_interest_
  groups/
- **American Medical Association: GLBT
  Health Resources: Treating Older GLBT
  Patients: Clinical resources and clinical
  research related to the care of LGBT older
  adults**.    http://www.ama-assn.org/ama/pub/
  about-ama/our-people/member-groups-sec-
  tions/glbt-advisory-committee/glbt-resources/
  lgbt-health-resources.page

## Communities of Interest and the Potential for Change: The Elder Initiative Experience

### Overview of the LGBT Elder Initiative

Founded in October 2010 as an outcome of the a
local LGBT Elder Initiative Summit, the LGBT
Elder Initiative (LGBTEI) is an all-volunteer,
advocacy organization dedicated to assuring that
LGBT older adults have every opportunity to age
successfully. The LGBTEI, which is based in
Philadelphia, PA, serves the geographic area
known as the Delaware Valley (Southeastern
Pennsylvania, Southern New Jersey and the State
of Delaware).

The Elder Initiative works to assure access to
information, resources, services, and institutions
that are culturally competent. The EI focuses on
building bridges between the Aging services network, LGBT service and community organizations such as the William Way LGBT Community
Center (WWCC), the local (SAGE), and LGBT
seniors. In addition, the LGBT Elder Initiative
seeks to align with the efforts other groups such
as the Human Rights Campaign (HRC), National
Gay and Lesbian Task Force (NGLTF), FORGE,
a transgender rights organization, and other advocates for the rights of LGBT people.

Rather than creating new organizations and
institutions, the EI is focused on assuring that the
services and resources currently available are
safe, welcoming and sensitive to the unique needs
of LGBT older adults in the Delaware Valley.
They work to accomplish this goal through advocacy, education, information dissemination,
referral, and training.

The work of the LGBT Elder Initiative
evolved out of the LGBT Rights Movement and
the AIDS epidemic. Also as a result of those
two historic forces, large numbers of LGBT
people "came out" of the closet over the past
half-century. Those people, members of the
baby boomer generation, are now reaching the
age of 65. The LGBT Elder Initiative recognized that attention needed to shift to these
older individuals, including those with new and
chronic HIV infections.

### Targeting Key Issues

The LGBT Elder Initiative recognizes certain key
problems and barriers for improving services. In
particular, these include the lack of cultural competency among service providers and a lack of
attention to the needs of LGBT older adults from
government and social service agencies.
Clinicians as well as federal, state and local agencies must become aware of the need for improved
services. The LGBT Elder Initiative seeks to create
a local community of interest in order to educate
and address these issues.

Congressional recognition of LGBT older
adults as a vulnerable population in the Older
Americans Act (OAA) has been stalled for years.

This lack of recognition in the OAA and by the aging services network, coupled with fear of social and institutional discrimination by consumers, has meant that the LGBT older adult population has not been counted. Without data—census numbers, health disparities studies, socio-economic analyses—development of targeted efforts to improve the health of this population have been weak. The opportunity for improved data collection, outreach efforts and development of targeted programs is limited by the lack of current data and the lack of a federal mandate in the OAA to designate LGBT older adults as a vulnerable population. This designation would require state and regional Agencies on Aging to track demographics and evaluate program outcomes for LGBT older adults.

## Growing Awareness

Despite the lack of government recognition and support, institutional awareness of the needs of the LGBT older adult population is emerging; a shift in consumer perspective is occurring simultaneously. Advocacy efforts by many organizations and individuals have effected significant policy changes that have helped spur these shifts. The end of Don't Ask; Don't Tell (DNDT), the policy excluding LGBT people from serving in the military, and the Supreme Court ruling granting legal recognition to same-sex marriage in all states have been major milestones in changing perceptions, laws and regulations.

## Collaborative Political and Social Action

Decades of lobbying and grassroots political organizing at the federal, state and local levels have slowly created an environment in which all of these efforts have begun to result in both policy and social change. Contributing to this change environment are openly LGBT people and allies at all levels of elected government and throughout government bureaucracies.

## The Service Provider Network

For large numbers of LGBT older adults, accessing the aging services network engenders fear of discrimination and mistreatment. These fears are based on past, negative experiences with health care and social service providers. The perception and the reality are that social service and other aging service providers are not LGBT culturally competent and sensitive regarding the LGBT older adult population. LGBT service providers and organizations, by and large youth-centric, are not aware of, nor sensitive to, the needs of older adults in the community. For the aging population, the issue of cultural competency has therefore become a top priority.

## Identifying Local Needs

Limited data is available regarding the needs of LGBT older adults. Given the lack of date, the LGBTEI's first step in beginning the local effort was to conduct a community needs assessment survey. This survey, circulated in summer 2010, received over 325 responses from LGBT-identified individuals over 55 years of age. From that survey, the priority needs of the community were identified to be physical and emotional health and well-being; safe, affordable and welcoming housing; social networking and engagement opportunities; and culturally competent social services and case management.

## Developing a Strategy

A regional aging summit was convened in October 2010 to review the survey data and develop recommendations for action. The summit included representatives from aging and LGBT organizations, academicians, government representatives, and community members. Modeled after community organizing efforts used during the AIDS crisis, this process of engagement resulted in constituent and provider buy-in.

The outcome of the summit was a directive to:

1. Empower LGBT older adults to advocate for their own health and well-being
2. Work to assure that the providers in the aging services network are culturally competent
3. Advocate for legislation and public policies that create a climate in which members of the LGBT communities can age successfully at every age

The broad outline of action for achieving these goals was modeled on HIV/AIDS community organizing with advocacy, education, information dissemination, referral, and training as the primary tactics.

## The HIV/AIDS Experience

For grassroots organizations, the process of community building is challenging. Identifying and impacting difficult to reach and at-risk populations, those who are deeply closeted, those in communities and cultures that are not accepting of LGBT people, is a daunting task. The AIDS crisis presented what was perceived as a dire threat and created an environment of urgency. Aging does not create the same sense of urgency and in this less "urgent" environment, organizing is a slower process.

## Existing Systems of Support

Unlike the early stages of the AIDS crisis, a community infrastructure for people with HIV disease is now in place. There are many organizations and systems of supports within the LGBT communities. These supports, however, are not necessarily attuned to the needs of older adults. Conversely, structures are in place to provide health care and social services for older adults as a whole. These services are not necessarily welcoming to, inclusive of, or viewed as safe by, LGBT older adults.

## Primary Goals

To overcome the ageism, homo- and transphobia, and discrimination that do exist and to take advantage of the community support structures built throughout the AIDS crisis, the Elder Initiative's strategy for action simultaneously targets consumers, providers and policy makers. An overriding goal of the effort is to avoid creation of an alternate, separate but equal system of services and supports. The existing structures of aging and LGBT services are vast. The goal is to make those providers and services culturally competent to meet the needs of the LGBT older adult population. The EI works with the community; the existing aging services network and LGBT service and community organizations to realize its goals. Collaboration involving as many community assets as possible is a key tactic along with advocacy, education, information dissemination, referral, and training.

## Implementation

In the original community needs assessment survey in 2010, issues of importance to the LGBT older adult community were identified. Today, those overarching issues are broken down into sub-topics and addressed in "campaigns." Each campaign is designed to raise community awareness and empower community members with information and resources that they can use to advocate for themselves in the process of seeking services and supports. Each campaign tries to incorporate each of the five operational tactics.

## Advocacy

As a general policy, representatives of the Elder Initiative attempt to secure "seats at the table" of community organizations, service providers, government advisory committees and commissions, and other relevant groups. Speakers, knowledgeable about the available data and the unique issues facing LGBT older adults, are provided whenever and wherever possible to these groups. Membership on boards, committees and commissions are actively sought out in order to assure that the communities' voices are heard.

As part of each sub-topic campaign, advocacy efforts specific to that issue are initiated. In a campaign addressing the issue of cognitive impairment in LGBT older adults, representatives from the EI and collaborating partner organizations provided testimony to state planning committees. The goal in this case was to secure the inclusion of LGBT older adults in the Pennsylvania State Plan on Alzheimer's. Inclusion in that Plan would start the process of data collection, outreach efforts and funding specific to the needs of LGBT older adults with memory loss, dementia and Alzheimer's disease. This advocacy effort is ongoing.

## Education

Workshops, seminars, panel discussions, and community forums are developed and presented throughout the year. These programs may be offered either as a stand-alone event or as part of a larger conference. Each program features experts in the field who discuss the designated topic. Community assets are recruited to provide expert information and to promote and discuss the issue within their own constituencies. In the campaign focusing on cognitive impairment, the Alzheimer's Association, the Mazzoni LGBT Health Center (Philadelphia), and the Penn Memory Center, part of Penn Medicine, the University of Pennsylvania Health System, collaborated on the program.

Education programs are also designed to address the key issue of social networking. They provide a safe and welcoming setting for LGBT older adults to meet new people, share experiences and build community. Many of these programs feature congregate meals, an especially important opportunity for social engagement.

## Information Dissemination

The LGBTEI website is a key asset for the organization. This website provides information on

LGBT issues as well as the ongoing education and advocacy work of the organization. A multi-tiered communications strategy has evolved to disseminate information on each of the LGBTEI's educational and advocacy projects. In addition, the website provides links to social media platforms, an e-newsletter, and information-driven articles that appear in both print and electronic media.

For each campaign topic, information is blogged on the website, articles are placed in branded columns, and press releases are issued. Each education program is advertised in print and e-media, on social media platforms through links to the website, in e-blasts, notices in the e-newsletter, and distributed via printed flyers. Collaborating organizations and community partners promote each education program through their own communications platforms.

Following education events, press releases and/or articles are issued and summaries of the event are posted on the website and highlighted in social media. In cases where the event is videotaped, such as the cognitive issues program, video segments of the presentations are posted to the website and YouTube.

## Referral

Lists of LGBT senior-friendly advocacy, community and service organizations are housed on the website. Resources in categories including housing options and legal and medical services are also listed. In conjunction with each topic addressed in a campaign, lists of relevant resources are compiled and distributed at the education event, included in articles published, and posted to the website.

## Training

The resources, services and systems of care and support for LGBT older adults must be culturally competent as aging LGBT baby boomers begin to access them. The process of training and informing the networks of care providers is an enormous undertaking and requires a paradigm shift in the thinking within those systems. Many organizations, including the LGBTEI with its "Silver Rainbow Project," provide cultural competency training programs for aging service providers.

Current training models include on-site programs, conference sessions and webinars. Other models are being tested to help speed the process of training the network. Limited government and private funding impedes that effort despite advocacy efforts on the national and local levels to create and maintain a funding stream for this training.

Care and service providers are also invited to attend the education programs described above and research and resource information targeted at providers is posted to the website. Webinars and other training programs are listed on the site and featured in the e-newsletter.

## Future Directions: The Intersection of Communities of Interest and Communities of Practice

Integrated provider/community collaborations present great potential for narrowing the health disparities faced by the LGBT older adult population. Currently, the University of Pennsylvania Health System is seeking to develop a "Center of Excellence" that will serve LGBT individuals (see resource list). This "Penn Medicine Program for LGBT Health" seeks to improve the care of LGBT populations by becoming a local and national leader in LGBT patient care, education, research, and advocacy. This program builds upon work initiated by other academic institutions such as Vanderbilt University, the University of California, San Francisco and the University of California, Davis. The University of Pennsylvania recognizes the need to develop a local community of interest to guide the planning and development of this center.

The mission and goals of the University of Pennsylvania program include several dimensions. The LGBT Elder Initiative serves on the advisory board this program. These include cultural competency education for healthcare providers and collaboration with existing local organizations that provide health and social services for LGBT individuals. These organizations include the Mazzoni LGBT Health Center, the William Way Community Center, the Attic Youth Center and the LGBT Elder Initiative.

## Models That Support "Aging in Place"

The LGBTEI tracks the activities of several organizations that promote healthy "aging in place". It also partners with local organizations such as Penn's Village (a local organization that is part of the Village to Village movement) as well as the low income senior housing unit (John C. Anderson Apartments). The following list, "Organizations that support communities of interest," summarizes the mission and activities of these important organizations.

## Organizations That Support Communities of Interest

### Naturally Occurring Retirement Communities

A NORC is a community that was not originally designed for seniors, but that has a large proportion of residents who are older adults (at least 60 years old). These communities are not created to meet the needs of seniors living independently in their homes, but rather evolve naturally, as adult residents age in place. http://www.norcs.org/index.aspx

SAGE Harlem Program is one NORC model serving LGBT older people of color living in Harlem. SAGE Harlem provides culturally and linguistically competent services. In the case of SAGE Harlem, a large number of people moved into an apartment building 30 or 40 years ago, and then stayed. Now elderly, these people make up a large percentage of the population of the building and need services. The program provides services inside the building so people don't need to go out to get them. This model includes three service components: a housing partner, a social worker or case manager, and one or two medical providers, usually a visiting nurse and the nearest hospital.

The goal of these services is to keep people in their own homes as long as possible as opposed to having them go to an institution (SAGE http://www.lgbtagingcenter.org/resources/resource.cfm?r=405#sthash.4RIB1JC4.dpuf).

## LGBT Senior-Friendly Housing Communities

Another model receiving attention is a planned integrated housing-health care-social service model. Several LGBT "senior-friendly" housing developments have been built or are under development. There is a mix of public versus private funding among these developments. The goal is to provide safe, welcoming and affordable housing for LGBT older adults. Many of these developments incorporate access to medical care and social services for residents. Opportunities for social engagement are often provided through collaborations with local LGBT community centers. This model may only be suited to urban areas with significant LGBT populations.

## Neighborhood Support Systems

The Village-to-Village Movement (VtVM) may serve as another model for providing support services for older adults. The model, not specifically LGBT-oriented, centers on neighbors helping each other age in place. The VtVM is a network of community-based organizations that provide services that are not typically supplied by area agencies on aging, senior centers, advocacy groups, and others in the aging services network.

Nationally, there are 120 villages in operation with 100 in development. Over 20,000 people belong to villages. Most villages are supported by volunteers who deliver a variety of services and programs. Each village has a unique personality in that each sets its own goals and services based on their community's needs and preferences. All of the villages are established to help people remain independent and age successfully in their own homes. http://www.vtvnetwork.org.

## Academic Community Partnerships

Integrated provider/community collaborations present great potential for narrowing the health disparities faced by the LGBT older adult population. The University of California Davis Health System and Vanderbilt University School of Medicine are two pioneer models. The University of Pennsylvania's "Penn Medicine Program for LGBT Health" is a more recent effort based on a fully integrated approach throughout the institution and between the institution and the community. Its mission is to improve the care of LGBT populations by becoming a local and national leader in LGBT patient care, education, research, and advocacy. http://www.pennmedicine.org/lgbt/.

The rationale for the Program is that LGBT individuals, and in particular transgender people, face provider and health system barriers to care. Provider level barriers include negative beliefs and actions toward LGBT patients and gaps in knowledge about the health concerns facing the LGBT population. Health system barriers include inequitable health insurance plans and hospital/clinic policies and practices.

## Conclusion

LGBT older adults, due to lifetimes of stigmatization, marginalization, discrimination, and criminalization, face significant health disparities and obstacles to access to the care and services that they need in order to age successfully. Clinicians who seek to improve health outcomes for this population need to develop a full spectrum of professional knowledge and skills. Efforts to improve care require that we improve the quality of data on demographics, health disparities, and the effectiveness of interventions to improve health outcomes. Care also needs to be improved at the systems level by ensuring that all health and social services provided to LGBT older adults are culturally competent. LGBT older adults and the communities in which they live must be active partners in building capacity for needed services. Clinicians must engage in dialogue within their communities of practice as well as key communities of interest in order to achieve these ends.

# References

1. Lave J, Wenger E. Situated learning: legitimate peripheral participation. Cambridge: Cambridge University Press; 1991.
2. IOM (Institute of Medicine).2011. The health of lesbian, gay, bisexual and transgender people: Building a foundation for better understanding. Washington, DC: The National Academies Press.
3. Gates GJ. How many people are lesbian, gay, bisexual and transgender? 2011. [8 November 2015]. Available from: http://www.escholarship.org/uc/item/09h684x2.
4. Gates GJ, Cooke AM. United States Census Snapshot: 2010. 2011. UCLA: The Williams Institute. Available from: https://escholarship.org/uc/item/4j23r1rx
5. Administration on Aging. Aging statistics: Department of Health and Human Services [23 Feb 2014]. Available from: http://www.aoa.gov/AoARoot/Aging_Statistics/.
6. Gates GJ, Newport F. Special report: 3.4% of U.S. adults identify as LGBT: inaugural Gallup findings based on more than 120,00 interviews. Princeton, NJ: Gallup; 2012. [5 May 2015]. Available from: http://www.gallup.com/poll/158066/special-report-adults-identify-lgbt.aspx.
7. Gates GJ. Sexual minorities in the 2008 general social survey: coming out and demographic characteristics. 2010. UCLA. The Williams Institute. [8 November 2015]. Available from: https://escholarship.org/us/item/9k77z7d4.
8. Fredriksen-Goldsen KI, Kim HJ, Emlet CA, Muraco A, Erosheva EA, Hoy-Ellis CP, et al. The aging and health report: disparities and resilience among lesbian, gay, bisexual, and transgender older adults. Seattle, WA: Institute for Multigenerational Health; 2011.
9. IOM (Institute of Medicine).2011. The health of lesbian, gay, bisexual and transgender people: Building a foundation for better understanding. Washington, DC: The National Academies Press.
10. Snyder JE. Trend analysis of medical publications about LGBT persons: 1950-2007. J Homosex. 2011;58(2):164–88.
11. Kelly UA. Integrating intersectionality and biomedicine in health disparities research. Adv Nurs Sci. 2009;32(2):E42–56.
12. Fredriksen-Goldsen KI, Kim HJ, Barkan SE, Muraco A, Hoy-Ellis CP. Health disparities among lesbian, gay, and bisexual older adults: results from a population-based study. Am J Public Health. 2013;103(10):1802–9.
13. MetLife Mature Market Institute. Still out, still aging: the MetLife study of lesbian, gay, bisexual, and transgender baby boomers. Westport, CT: MetLife Mature Market Institute; 2006.
14. Women's Health Initiative [1 May 2014]. Available from: lgbtdata.com.
15. Valanis BG, Bowen DJ, Bassford T, Whitlock E, Charney P, Carter RA. Sexual orientation and health: comparisons in the women's health initiative sample. Arch Fam Med. 2000;9(9):843–53.
16. Wallace SP, Cochran SD, Durazo EM, Ford CL. The health of aging lesbian, gay and bisexual adults in California. Policy Brief UCLA Cent Health Policy Res. 2011;(Pb2011-2):1–8.
17. McNair RP, Hegarty K. Guidelines for the primary care of lesbian, gay, and bisexual people: a systematic review. Ann Fam Med. 2010;8(6):533–41.
18. Bardach SH, Rowles GD. Geriatric education in the health professions: are we making progress? Gerontologist. 2012;52(5):607–18.
19. Saunders MJ, Yeh CK, Hou LT, Katz MS. Geriatric medical education and training in the United States. J Chin Med Assoc. 2005;68(12):547–56.
20. Abellan van Kan G, Rolland Y, Houles M, Gillette-Guyonnet S, Soto M, Vellas B. The assessment of frailty in older adults. Clin Geriatr Med. 2010;26(2):275–86.
21. Emlet CA, Fredriksen-Goldsen KI, Kim HJ. Risk and protective factors associated with health-related quality of life among older gay and bisexual men living with HIV disease. Gerontologist. 2013;53(6):963–72.
22. Bockting WO, Miner MH, Swinburne Romine RE, Hamilton A, Coleman E. Stigma, mental health, and resilience in an online sample of the US transgender population. Am J Public Health. 2013;103(5):943–51.
23. Van Sluytman LG, Torres D. Hidden or uninvited? A content analysis of elder LGBT of color literature in gerontology. J Gerontol Soc Work. 2014;57(2–4):130–60.
24. Woody I. Aging out: a qualitative exploration of ageism and heterosexism among aging African American lesbians and gay men. J Homosex. 2014;61(1):145–65.
25. Conron KJ, Scott G, Stowell GS, Landers SJ. Transgender health in Massachusetts: results from a household probability sample of adults. Am J Public Health. 2012;102(1):118–22.
26. The Henry J. Kaiser Foundation: the burden of out-of-pocket health spending among older versus younger adults: analysis from the consumer expenditure survey, 1998-2003; 2007 [1 July 2014]. Available from: http://kff.org/health-costs/issue-brief/the-burden-of-out-of-pocket-health/.
27. The Henry J. Kaiser Family Foundation: summary of the Affordable Care Act 2013 [1 July 2014]. Available from: http://kff.org/health-reform/factsheet/summary-of-the-affordable-care-act/.
28. MetLife Mature Market Institute. Still out, still aging: the MetLife study of lesbian, gay, bisexual, and transgender baby boomers. [4 May 2014]. Available from: https://www.metlife.com/mmi/research/still-out-still-aging.html#findings.
29. Finkenauer S, Sherratt J, Marlow J, Brodey A. When injustice gets old: a systematic review of trans aging. J Gay and Lesbian Soc Serv. 2012;24(4):311–30.

30. Steinman MA, Lee SJ, John Boscardin W, Miao Y, Fung KZ, Moore KL, et al. Patterns of multiple morbidity in elderly veterans. J Am Geriatr Soc. 2012;60(10):1872–80.

31. The National Resource Center on LGBT Aging. Inclusive questions for older adults: a practical guide to collecting data on sexual orientation and gender identity [5 May 2014]. http://www.lgbtagingcenter.org/resources/resources.cfm?s=4

32. Fredriksen-Goldsen KI, Hoy-Ellis CP, Goldsen J, Emlet CA, Hooyman NR. Creating a vision for the future: key competencies and strategies for culturally competent practice with lesbian, gay, bisexual, and transgender (LGBT) older adults in the health and human services. J Gerontol Soc Work. 2014;57(2–4):80–107.

33. King M, Semlyen J, Tai SS, Killaspy H, Osborn D, Popelyuk D, et al. A systematic review of mental disorder, suicide, and deliberate self harm in lesbian, gay and bisexual people. BMC Psychiatry. 2008;8:70.

34. Fredriksen-Goldsen KI, Cook-Daniels L, Kim HJ, Erosheva EA, Emlet CA, Hoy-Ellis CP, et al. Physical and mental health of transgender older adults: an at-risk and underserved population. Gerontologist. 2014;54(3):488–500.

35. Savasta AM. HIV: associated transmission risks in older adults--an integrative review of the literature. J Assoc Nurses AIDS Care. 2004;15(1):50–9.

36. Lindau ST, Schumm LP, Laumann EO, Levinson W, O'Muircheartaigh CA, Waite LJ. A study of sexuality and health among older adults in the United States. N Engl J Med. 2007;357(8):762–74.

37. Dolcini MM, Catania JA, Stall RD, Pollack L. The HIV epidemic among older men who have sex with men. J Acquir Immune Defic Syndr. 2003;33 Suppl 2:S115–21.

38. Adekeye OA, Heiman HJ, Onyeabor OS, Hyacinth HI. The new invincibles: HIV screening among older adults in the U.S. PLoS One. 2012;7(8), e43618.

39. Schick V, Herbenick D, Reece M, Sanders SA, Dodge B, Middlestadt SE, et al. Sexual behaviors, condom use, and sexual health of Americans over 50: implications for sexual health promotion for older adults. J Sex Med. 2010;7 Suppl 5:315–29.

40. Cotten SR, Anderson WA, McCullough BM. Impact of internet use on loneliness and contact with others among older adults: cross-sectional analysis. J Med Internet Res. 2013;15(2), e39.

41. CDC-HIV/AIDS-Statistics and surveillance. HIV/AIDS Surveillance Report. 2011. [4 November 2014]. Available from: http://www.cdc.gov/hiv/library/reports/surveillance/2011/surveillance_Report_vol_23.html

42. Rowen TS, Breyer BN, Lin TC, Li CS, Robertson PA, Shindel AW. Use of barrier protection for sexual activity among women who have sex with women. Int J Gynaecol Obstet. 2013;120(1):42–5.

43. Abrass CK, et al. Summary report from the human immunodeficiency virus and aging consensus project: Treatment strategies for clinicians managing older individuals with the immunodeficiency virus. J Am Geriatr Soc, 2012; 60(5):974–9.

44. Centers for Disease Control and Prevention. Diagnosis of HIV infection among adults age 50 years and older in the United States and dependent areas. 2007–2010. HIV surveillance supplemental report 2013. [8 November 2014]. Available from: http://www.cdc.gov/hiv/topics/survelliance/resources/reports/#supplemental.

45. Linley L, Prejean J, An Q, Chen M, Hall HI. Racial/ethnic disparities in HIV diagnosis among persons 50 years and older in 37 US States, 2005–2008. Am J Public Health. 2012;102(8):1527–34.

46. Levy BR, Ory MG, Crystal S. HIV/AIDS interventions for middle and older adult: current status and challenges. J Acquir Immune Defic Syndr. 2003;33 Suppl 2:S59–67.

47. Greene M, Justice AC, Lampiris HW, Valcour V. Management of human immunodeficiency virus infection in advanced age. JAMA. 2013;309(13): 1397–405.

48. Perez JL, Moore RD. Greater effect of highly active antiretroviral therapy on survival in people aged > or + 50 years compared with younger people in an urban observation cohort. Clin Infect Dis. 2003; 36(2):212.

49. Blanco JR, Caro-Murillo AM, Castano MA, Olalla J, Domingo P, Arazo P, et al. Safety, efficacy, and persistence of emtricitabine/tenofovir versus other nucleoside analogues in naive subjects aged 50 years or older in Spain: the TRIP study. HIV Clin Trials. 2013;14(5):204–15.

50. Ghidei L, Simone M, Salow M, Zimmerman K, Paquin A, Skarf L, et al. Aging, antiretrovirals, and adherence: a meta analysis of adherence among older HIV-infected individuals. Drugs Aging. 2013;30(10):809–19.

51. Silverberg MJ, Leyden W, Horberg MA, DeLorenze GN, Klein D, Quesenberry CPJ. Older age and the response to and tolerability of antiretroviral therapy. Arch Intern Med. 2007;167(7):684–91.

52. Greene M, Steinman MA, McNicholl IR, Valcour V. Polypharmacy, drug-drug interactions, and potentially inappropriate medications in older adults with human immunodeficiency virus infection. J Am Geriatr Soc. 2014;62(3):447–53.

53. McGinnis KA, Justice AC, Kraemer KL, Saitz R, Bryant KJ, Fiellin DA. Comparing alcohol screening measures among HIV-infected and -uninfected men. Alcohol Clin Exp Res. 2013;37(3):435–42.

54. Baker JV, Peng G, Rapkin J, Abrams DI, Silverberg MJ, MacArthur RD, et al. CD4+ count and risk of non-AIDS diseases following initial treatment for HIV infection. AIDS. 2008;22(7):841–8.

55. Neuhaus J, Angus B, Kowalska JD, La Rosa A, Sampson J, Wentworth D, et al. Risk of all-cause mortality associated with nonfatal AIDS and serious non-AIDS events among adults infected with HIV. AIDS. 2010;24(5):697–706.

56. Rosenthal E, Pialoux G, Bernard N, Pradier C, Rey D, Bentata M, et al. Liver-related mortality in human-immunodeficiency-virus-infected patients between 1995 and 2003 in the French GERMIVIC Joint Study Group Network (MORTAVIC 2003 Study). J Viral Hepat. 2007;14(3):183–8.

57. Moyer VA. Screening for hepatitis C infection in adults: U.S. Preventive Services Task Force recommendation statement. Ann Intern Med. 2013;159(5):349–57.

58. Smith BD, Patel N, Beckett GA. Hepatitis C virus antibody prevalence, correlates and predictors among persons born from 1945 through 1965, United States, 1999-2008. San Francisco, CA: American Association for the Study of Liver Diseases; 2011.

59. Tyerman Z, Aboulafia DM. Review of screening guidelines for non-AIDS-defining malignancies: evolving issues in the era of highly active antiretroviral therapy. AIDS Rev. 2012;14(1):3–16.

60. Oster AM, Sullivan PS, Blari JM. Prevalence of cervical cancer screening in HIV-infected women in the United States. J Acquir Immune Defic Syndr. 2009;51(4):430–6.

61. Grant JM, Mottet LA, Tanis J, Harrison J, Herman JL, Keisling M. Injustice at every turn: a report of the National Transgender Discrimination Survey. Washington, DC: National Center for Transgender Equality, National Gay and Lesbian Task Force; 2011.

62. Rotondi NK, Bauer GR, Scanlon K, Kaay M, Travers R, Travers A. Nonprescribed hormone use and self-performed surgeries: "do-it-yourself" transitions in transgender communities in Ontario, Canada. Am J Public Health. 2013;103(10):1830–6.

63. Cruz TM. Assessing access to care for transgender and gender nonconforming people: a consideration of diversity in combating discrimination. Soc Sci Med (1982). 2014;110:65–73.

64. Stroumsa D. The state of transgender health care: policy, law, and medical frameworks. Am J Public Health. 2014;104(3):e31–8.

65. Department of Health and Human Services. Office for Civil Rights [cited 1 Apr 2014]. Available from: http://www.hhs.gov/ocr/office/index.html.

66. Gooren LJ. Clinical practice. Care of transsexual persons. N Engl J Med. 2011;364(13):1251–7.

67. Van Caenegem E, Wierckx K, Taes Y, Dedecker D, Van de Peer F, Toye K, et al. Bone mass, bone geometry, and body composition in female-to-male transsexual persons after long-term cross-sex hormonal therapy. J Clin Endocrinol Metab. 2012;97(7):2503–11.

68. Maycock LB, Kennedy HP. Breast care in the transgender individual. J Midwifery Womens Health. 2014;59(1):74–81.

69. Gooren LJ. Management of female-to-male transgender persons: medical and surgical management, life expectancy. Curr Opin Endocrinol Diabetes Obes. 2014;21(3):233–8.

70. Hoffman BR. The interaction of drug use, sex work, and HIV among transgender women. Subst Use Misuse. 2014;49(8):1049–53.

71. Hoffman B. An overview of depression among transgender women. Depress Res Treat. 2014;2014:394283.

72. U.S. Department of Health and Human Services: Community Living Initiative [4 May 2014]. Available from: http://www.hhs.gov/od/community/index.html.

73. U.S. Department of Health and Human Services-Agency for Community Living: 2013 to 2018 Strategic Plan.

74. Cantor MH, Brennan M. Social care of the elderly: The effects of ethnicity, class and culture. New York: Springer; 2000.

75. NORCs: an aging in place initiative [5 May 2014]. Available from: http://www.norcs.org/index.aspx.

76. Village to Village Network [5 May 2014]. Available from: http://vtvnetwork.org/.

77. LGBT housing for seniors opens in the heart of the Philadelphia Gayborhood [press release]. 24 Feb 2014.

78. Vitaliano PP, Zhang J, Scanlan JM. Is caregiving hazardous to one's physical health? A meta-analysis. Psychol Bull. 2003;129(6):946–72.

79. Richardson TJ, Lee SJ, Berg-Weger M, Grossberg GT. Caregiver health: health of caregivers of Alzheimer's and other dementia patients. Curr Psychiatry Rep. 2013;15(7):367.

80. Older Americans 2012: key indicators of well-being. 2012: Federal Interagency Forum on Aging Related Statistics.

81. Cantor MH, Brennan M, Shippy RA. Caregiving among older lesbian, gay, bisexual, and transgender New Yorkers. Final report. Washington, DC: National Gay and Lesbian Task Force Policy Institute; 2004.

82. De Vries B, Hoctel P. The family and friends of older gay men and lesbians. In: Teunis N, Herdt G, editors. Sexual inequalities and social justice. Berkeley, CA: University of California Press; 2007. p. 213–32.

83. Lambda legal: after DOMA: family & medical leave act for non-federal employees [1 May 2014]. Available from: http://www.lambdalegal.org/publications/after-doma-fmla.

84. Cheese, Big. imProving the Lives of LgBt oLder AduLts. 2010.

85. SAGE: It's about time: LGBT aging in a changing world: Fourth national conference on LGBT aging conference report: policy recommendations. SAGE fourth annual conference on LGBT aging; 2009. [4 November 2014]. Available at: http://www.sageusa.org/files/SAGE%20Fourth%20National%20Conference%20Findings%20-%202009.pdf

86. United States vs. Windsor [cited 1 May 2014]. Available from: www.en.wikipedia.org/wiki/United_States_v._Windsor.

87. Cray A. Same-sex spouses now recognized for Medicare eligibility and enrollment 2014 [1 May

2014]. Available from: www.thinkprogress.org/lgbt/2014/04/03/3422602/medicare-same-sex-couples/.

88. Quick take: who benefits from the ACA Medicaid expansion? 2012 [1 May 2014]. Available from: www.kff.org/health-reform/fact-sheet/who-benefits-from-the-aca-medicaid-expansion/.

89. Ellis B. CNN Money: nursing home costs top $ 80,000 per year [1 July 2014]. Available from: http://money.cnn.com/2013/04/09/retirement/nursing-home-costs/index.html.

90. Silveira MJ, Wiitala W, Piette J. Advance directive completion by elderly Americans: a decade of change. J Am Geriatr Soc. 2014;62(4):706–10.

91. Buckey JW, Browning CN. Factors affecting the LGBT population when choosing a surrogate decision maker. J Soc Serv Res. 2013;39(2):233–52.

92. Stiff M. Breaking down barriers: an administrator's guide to state law and best policy practice for LGBT healthcare access. In: Foundation HRC, editor. 2009.

93. Orel N. Community needs assessment: documenting the need for affirmative services for LGB older adults. In: Kimmel D, Rose T, David S, editors. Lesbian, gay, bisexual and transgender aging:

Research and clinical perspectives. New York: Columbia University Press; 2006. p. 227–46.

94. Johnson MJ, Jackson NC, Arnette JK, Koffman SD. Gay and lesbian perceptions of discrimination in retirement care facilities. J Homosex. 2005;49(2):83–102.

95. Frazer S. LGBT health and human services needs in New York State. 2009.

96. Jihanian LJ. Specifying long-term care provider responsiveness to LGBT older adults. J Gay Lesbian Soc Serv. 2013;25(2):210–31.

97. The NSCLC advocates for improved nursing home standards, including protections for LGBT residents [press release]. 2012.

98. Sullivan KM. Acceptance in the domestic environment: the experience of senior housing for lesbian, gay, bisexual, and transgender seniors. J Gerontol Soc Work. 2014;57(2–4):235–50.

99. Administration on aging: diversity [4 May 2014]. Available from: http://www.aoa.gov/AoA_programs/Tools_Resources/diversity.aspx.

100. Kaye HS. Toward a model long-term services and supports system: state policy elements. Gerontologist. 2014;54(5):754–61.

# Adult Mental Health

# 13

## Christopher M. Palmer and Michael B. Leslie

## Purpose

The purpose of this chapter is to review mental health issues that occur more commonly in the LGBT community, discuss the interface of the mental health field with the LGBT community, especially in terms of etiology of sexual orientation and gender identity, and discuss unique aspects of relationships in the LGBT community and how they can affect both mental and physical health.

## Learning Objectives

This chapter will prepare learners to:

- Describe mental health concerns that occur more commonly in the LGBT population *(KP4, PC5)*.
- Describe theories of the etiology of sexual orientation and gender identity *(KP3)*.
- Discuss unique aspects of relationships in the LGBT community and how these can affect both physical and mental health *(PC5)*.

C.M. Palmer, M.D. (✉) • M.B. Leslie, M.D.
Department of Psychiatry, McLean Hospital/Harvard Medical School, 115 Mill Street, Belmont, MA 02478, USA
e-mail: cpalmer@partners.org; mleslie@partners.org

- Discuss mental health treatment issues that are specific to the LGBT community *(PC5, PC6)*.

## Gender and Sexuality from the Perspectives of Culture, History, and Mental Health

The perspective of psychiatrists on people with minority sexual orientations and gender identities has evolved over time. Since the 1970s, there has been an emerging consensus within the psychiatric community that homosexuality is not a disease—rather, it is a normal variation of human sexual experience. At this point, every major mental health, public health, and medical professional organization has issued a position paper affirming that homosexuality is a normal variation of sexuality and opposing discrimination based upon it.

The perspective of the American Psychiatric Association (APA) on gender is somewhat more complex. The current, fifth, edition of Diagnostic and Statistical Manual of the American Psychiatric Association includes the diagnosis of "gender dysphoria," which focuses on the distress and impaired functioning that some transgender and gender non-conforming people may experience due to their gender identity [1]. In a statement regarding the diagnosis of "gender dysphoria," the APA clarifies that "gender

© Springer International Publishing Switzerland 2016
K.L. Eckstrand, J.M. Ehrenfeld (eds.), *Lesbian, Gay, Bisexual, and Transgender Healthcare*,
DOI 10.1007/978-3-319-19752-4_13

nonconformity is not, in itself, a mental disorder." In response to concerns that this diagnosis is reminiscent of "ego-dystonic homosexuality" (which was removed from the DSM in 1987) in that it pathologizes the effects of social prejudice, the APA contends that there is a need for a diagnosis related to gender variance so that insurers will cover medically necessary treatment [2].

It is useful to contextualize our discussion of gender, sexuality, and mental health within a larger framework of cultural perspectives on sexuality and gender. Same-sex attraction, behavior, and love have existed from the beginning of history, as have infinitely varied gender identities. Different cultures, however, have viewed sexuality and gender in radically different ways. This is not simply a matter of a culture being "accepting" or "rejecting" of "LGBT" people; the very language and cognitive framework used to think about sexuality and gender is culturally specific. Some cultures embrace more than two genders (such as "two-spirit" people within many Native American societies); others normalize (for example, pederasty in Ancient Greece) or even mandate (for example, the male initiation rituals of the Sambia in Papua New Guinea) homosexual activity. The very framework that we use to think about sexuality and gender—indeed, the concepts of "sexuality" and "gender" themselves—are culturally specific and far from universal.

Many sociologists contend that the modern idea of "homosexuality" as a stable, discrete, sexual orientation emerged in Western cultures in the nineteenth century—around the same time that psychiatry emerged as a separate field of medicine [3]. Prior to this time, homosexual acts were primarily viewed through the lens of Christian moral teachings as aberrant and immoral behaviors. During the nineteenth century, physicians became interested in same sex attraction as a clinical problem, and both the modern concept of "homosexuality" and its medical pathologization began.

Psychiatrists were among the first clinicians to study sexual orientation and gender identity. It is sometimes overlooked that these early investigators were not universally pathologizing. In his *Three Essays on Sexuality*, Sigmund Freud, a founder of psychoanalysis, contended that humans are born with pluripotent libido that can develop in many different ways based on societal taboos and relational events [4]. Writing to an American mother in 1932, Freud reassured her that homosexuality was "nothing to be ashamed of, no vice, no degradation, it cannot be classified as an illness, but a variation of sexual function." Freud opposed attempts to change a patient's sexual orientation on the grounds that it was unlikely to succeed and felt the role of therapy was to help the patient "gain harmony, peace of mind, full efficiency, whether he remains a homosexual or gets changed" [5]. Unfortunately, subsequent psychoanalysts took a far more negative perspective, viewing homosexuality as a pathological condition caused by family problems and developmental failures. This perspective informed the inclusion of homosexuality as a mental disorder in the first and second versions of the American Psychiatric Association's Diagnostic and Statistical Manual.

Subsequent authors, such as Havelock Ellis, and researchers, including Alfred Kinsey and Evelyn Hooker, expanded psychiatry's perspective on variations in human sexual behavior. These and other pioneers, along with the emergence of the gay rights movements in the years after the 1969 Stonewall uprising, led both psychiatrists and society at large to re-evaluate their understanding of homosexuality as a pathological condition. The American Psychiatric Association declassified homosexuality itself as a mental disorder in 1973, and finally removed the last vestiges of this diagnosis ("ego-dystonic homosexuality," or a patient's distress with their own sexual orientation) in 1987.

## The Etiologies of Sexual Orientation and Gender Identity

### Context and Controversies

The causes of varying sexual orientations and gender identities have been widely studied over the past 150 years. While numerous etiological theories—some rigorously evidence based, and others dubiously speculative in nature—have been proposed, none have proven conclusively a primary determining factor for sexuality and/or gender. At this point, a variety of causative factors have been identified; it appears likely that both sexuality and gender are determined by a combination of genetic, hormonal, psychological, and social factors.

Exploration of the etiology of sexual orientation and gender identity is inherently controversial and often politically fraught. Careful attention must be paid to the possibility of bias. Identical theories can be used to support radically different agendas; conviction in the primacy of biological causes fueled the horrific genocide of gender and sexuality minorities in Nazi Germany but also underpins (either implicitly or explicitly) many contemporary arguments for LGBT equality. Cross-national research suggests that those who espouse a biological explanation for homosexuality tend to hold significantly more positive attitudes towards it [6]. Historically, investigators have often (again, either implicitly or explicitly) assumed that homosexuality and transgender identity are theoretical, evolutionary, or social conundrums in need of explanation while assuming that heterosexuality and cis-gender identity represent a normative, even "default," developmental state. It is our opinion (and the current scientific consensus) that any coherent etiological theory must start from a neutral position regarding outcome and explain the full diversity of sexual orientations or gender identities.

## Biological Theories

With that important context noted, there have been a variety of empirical studies exploring the role of biological factors in determining sexual orientation and gender identity. Twin studies have generally demonstrated a greater concordance in sexual orientation in monozygotic than dizygotic twins [7]. A 2010 study of 7600 adult twin pairs in Sweden found that same-sex behavior in both men and women was explained strongly by individually specific environmental sources (such as peer groups, sexual experiences,

illnesses, and traumas) and somewhat less strongly by heritable factors. Sexuality in men demonstrated a statistically non-significant trend towards a stronger effect of heredity effects than women. Environmental variables shared by each twin (such as familial environment and societal attitudes) had a weak effect in female twins and none at all in men. Although wide confidence intervals necessitate cautious interpretation, the results are consistent with moderate familial (primarily genetic) effects, and moderate to large effects of the non-shared environment on same-sex sexual behavior [8].

Chromosome linkage studies of sexual orientation have indicated the presence of multiple contributing genetic factors throughout the genome. Beginning with Dean Hamer and colleague's widely reported study in 1993, multiple investigators have suggested that particular allelic variations in a distal region of the X-chromosome (known as Xq28) may be associated with male homosexuality that follows a maternal inheritance pattern [9]. Subsequent studies have revealed additional alleles that may be associated with male homosexuality, and animal studies confirm clear genetic control of courtship behaviors in the common fruit fly [10]. The genetic explanation for variance in sexual orientation and gender identity is further supported by a number of subtle physical differences, including differences in the relative lengths of certain fingers, direction of hair whirl pattern, and a greater tendency towards left-handedness for both gay men and lesbian women.

A variety of other biological factors appear to contribute to sexual orientation, especially in men. Birth order appears to play a significant role; each additional older brother increases the odds of a man being gay by 33 %. It has been controversially hypothesized that male fetuses provoke a maternal immune reaction that becomes stronger with each successive male fetus and that interferes with masculinization of the fetal brain [11]. It has been reported that women related to homosexual men tend to have more children than women related to heterosexual men, and that women related to homosexual men through their own mothers tend to have more offspring than those related to homosexual men through their fathers. Based on this observation, researchers have hypothesized the existence of X-linked genes that promote both maternal fertility and homosexuality in male offspring. A number of neuroanatomical differences have been correlated with variance in sexual orientation and gender identity, including (most famously, but also quite controversially) several nuclei in the anterior hypothalamus [12]. Finally, there are multiple theories that link variations in prenatal hormonal milieu with adult sexual orientation and gender identity.

## Evolutionary Theories

A variety of hypotheses have been proposed to explain the evolution and maintenance of homosexuality among humans, given its apparent reproductive (and thus evolutionary) disadvantage. Some scholars have suggested that while the genes predisposing to homosexuality reduce homosexuals' reproductive success, they may confer some advantage in heterosexuals who carry them (such as the increased female fecundity described above). Alternatively, the theory of kin selection (colloquially referred to as the "gay uncle" hypothesis) posits that childless people may nonetheless increase the prevalence of their family's genes in future generations by providing resources (food, supervision, defense, shelter, etc.) to the offspring of their closest relatives.

## Psychoanalytic Theories

In addition to biological, genetic, evolutionary, and social approaches, psychoanalytic theory has richly and usefully addressed questions of sexuality and gender. In his *Three Essays on the Theory of Sexuality*, Sigmund Freud presented a theory of psychosexual development that attempted to explain the process by which people eventually develop adult sexual attractions. In contrast to essentialist perspectives of modern geneticists, Freud argued that infants are born "polymorphously perverse"—meaning that a wide variety of experiences could potentially produce libidinal gratification. Largely unconscious and often relational crises (including the Oedipal crisis and castration anxiety) pushed the omni-sexual infant through a series of developmental stages (famously termed oral, anal, phallic, latency, and genital) towards mature adult sexuality. Freud felt that this was a universal model of psychosexual development that could explain all manifestations of adult human sexuality [4]. Subsequent psychoanalytic theorists have continued to offer nuanced and complex ways to understand the diversity of sexualities and gender identities, albeit with varying degrees of pathologization and prejudice. Several "pop psychology" theories—such as the role of the over-bearing mother and the passive, absent father in "turning" sons gay—have been debunked.

Contemporary psychoanalytic perspectives on sexuality and gender are informed by deconstructionist philosophy, third wave feminism, and the LGBTQ civil rights movement. In 1990, Judith Butler argued in her ground-breaking work *Gender Trouble* that the apparent "normal" coherence of sex, gender, and sexuality is, in fact, a construction of culture [13]. For a somewhat clichéd example, consider a butch-acting, heterosexual, biologically male, cowboy. The coherence of his identity is constructed by the repetition of "stylized actions" over time—walking with a swagger, drinking beer, riding horses, and sleeping with women. From our perspective within American culture, we take for granted that these behaviors and traits comprise a distinct and coherent identity; in fact, they are produced by our culture itself. Our cowboy creates his identity as a butch, straight man by engaging in the consistent and predictable repetition of stylized actions; in this sense, gender is "performative." It is important to note that this is not a voluntary, flexible, or even fully conscious performance. Butler contends that social "regulative discourses" ranging from the benign (e.g. dressing male infants in blue onesies) to the horrifying (e.g. the murders of Matthew Shepherd or Brandon Teena) coerce people to perform normative behaviors and thereby manifest a congruent gender, sex and sexuality. Thus, Butler contends that gender itself is a product of a social regulative discourse—and that gender does not exist as an essential, innate entity [13].

Other psychoanalysts take a less radical position. Jessica Benjamin, for example, argues that the existence of gender is paradoxical; in some contexts it is "thick and reified," while in others, it is "porous and insubstantial." Benjamin suggests that, beyond describing actual individual identity, gender is an abstract, fundamental concept that determines the very framework of our thinking, thereby defining the categories that might be used to deconstruct it. Thus, the binary opposition of conceptual "maleness" and "femaleness" is superordinate to any concrete relationships or actual identities. Ultimately, Benjamin contends that gender exists in infinitely complex and ambiguous formations, and that our ability to understand this complexity and play with it actually contributes to our creativity [14].

## Essentialism and Mutability of Sexuality and Gender

Finally, all theories of sexuality and gender offer an implicit (or sometimes explicit) position on the essentialism and mutability of these entities. Genetic theories imply an immutability that is useful in civil rights litigation but contradicts the lived experience of some individuals, especially (but certainly not exclusively) lesbian women. In sharp contrast; Freud began from a position of nearly complete mutability; the infant has a libido, but its object changes through the course of development. Butler and Benjamin offer sophisticated and useful critiques of the very ideas of "gender" and "sexuality" rooted in philosophical and feminist perspectives. Behavioral psychologists in the 1960s (famously led by John Money) contended that gender identity in children is fluid and largely determined by rearing; this now discredited theory led to the castration of male children with penile malformations and their subsequent assignment to female gender and rearing, often with tragic results. Experts on the treatment of children born with differences of

sex development now recommend an approach that is less interventionist and more flexible, individualized, and evidence-based [15]. There is also nearly universal clinical consensus that sexual orientation and gender identity cannot be changed by direct psychotherapeutic interventions. So-called "conversion" (or "reparative") therapies are not evidence-based treatments; they cause more psychological stress than they alleviate and they fail to produce meaningful changes in orientation or identity. "Conversion" treatments are opposed on scientific, clinical, and ethical grounds by all relevant American professional organizations, including the American Medical Association, the American Psychiatric Association, the American Academy of Pediatrics, the American Psychological Association, the National Association of Social Workers, the American Association for Marriage and Family Therapy, and the American Psychoanalytic Association.

## Mental Health Issues in the LGBT Population

### Reasons for Mental Health Disparities

Adults with minority gender identities and sexual orientations clearly experience an increased risk for many mental health conditions, including mood and anxiety disorders, PTSD, substance use disorders, body dysmorphic and eating disorders, and personality disorders. Of note, there is no clear difference in the prevalence of schizophrenia or bipolar disorder. The exact magnitude of the relative risk varies by population and will be discussed below in further detail. Several factors contribute to the increased prevalence of mental illness in the LGBT population.

### Minority Stress

The theory of minority stress was developed to explain why minority individuals (including sexuality and gender minorities) often suffer physical and mental health experience disparities compared to their peers in majority groups. A large body of evidence now supports the assertion that LGBT people face difficult social situations that lead to poor health, including prejudice and discrimination, unequal socioeconomic status, and limited access to healthcare. In general, evidence does not support the hypothesis that LGBT individuals are inherently susceptible to health problems; environmental factors explain minority health disparities better than do genetic factors [16–18].

Minority stress theory suggests that, for LGBT people, repeated difficult social situations constitute stressors that contribute to health disparities. These stressors can be separated into two major types, external and internal. External stressors (sometimes termed "distal") include experiences with prejudice, rejection, and discrimination. In time, these external stressors can lead to internal (or "proximal") stressors, including internalized homophobia, remaining in the closet, and vigilance and anxiety about prejudice. Together, internal and external stressors accumulate over time, leading to chronically high levels of stress that cause poor health outcomes [18]. Minority stress theory is supported by numerous empirical studies [19].

Several studies have demonstrated a link between external stressors and health disparities. Compared with heterosexual peers, LGBT adults more frequently report both lifetime and day-to-day experiences with discrimination; much of this difference can be attributed to their sexual orientation. Perceived discrimination is associated with worse quality of life and indicators of psychiatric morbidity. Controlling for differences in discrimination experiences reduces significantly the association between psychiatric morbidity and sexual orientation for LGBT adults [20].

## Internalized Sexual Prejudice

Minority stress theory suggests that internal stressors underlie many of the health disparities facing the LGBT community. One such internal stressor is internalized sexual prejudice, commonly known as "internalized homophobia." Internalized sexual prejudice refers to the negative beliefs, stereotypes, stigmas, and prejudices about homosexuality and LGBT identity held by

LGBT people about themselves, whether or not they identify as LGBT. Internalized sexual prejudice creates a conflict between a person's idealized self-image and his or her actual sexual orientation. The person may not be fully consciously aware of this conflict. People with high levels of internalized sexual prejudice tend to hold negative views of their own sexual orientation, ranging from mild discomfort to outright disapproval. This chronic internal conflict and negative self-judgment leads to chronic anxiety, depression, repression of sexual desire, forced attempts at heteronormative behavior, and desperate attempts to change one's sexual orientation. It is also likely related to the high rate of self-harm behaviors, substance use, risk-taking behaviors, and suicide among LGBT youth and adults [21]. Historically, internalized sexual prejudice was diagnosed as "ego-dystonic homosexuality" until its removal from the DSM in 1987. As previously discussed, this diagnosis was used to justify psychotherapy designed to change a patient's sexual orientation. This kind of "reparative" therapy has now been refused by all of the major professional mental health associations. Both clinical experience and the evidence base instead support helping an LGBT person to resolve their internalized sexual prejudice rather than try (in vain) to change their sexual orientation. Internalized sexual prejudice can be mitigated with education, social relationships, life experiences, and psychotherapy.

## Co-occurring Risk Factors

Minority stress theory and internalized sexual prejudice contribute to the significant mental health disparities facing people with minority gender identities and sexual orientations. A slightly different perspective can be gained through examining discrete risk factors for poor mental health outcomes. Many of these risk factors affect both heterosexual and LGBT people: poor family or social support, lack of education, homelessness, substance use, chronic physical illness, psychiatric disorders, discrimination, and hate crimes. While heterosexuals experience these stressors, they are far more prevalent among LGBT persons [22].

## Suicide

Adults with minority gender identities and sexual orientations are clearly at increased risk of deliberate self-harm, attempted suicide, and completed suicide, although exact rates vary among studies and sub-population. Numerous studies have demonstrated rates of suicide attempts among gender and sexuality minorities ranging from 1.5 to 7 times the rate of heterosexual, cis-gendered peers [23]. A very large meta-analysis (including 214,344 heterosexual and 11,971 non heterosexual subjects) found a twofold excess in suicide attempts in adult lesbian, gay and bisexual people [24].

Sub-populations within the LGBT community suffer varied risks of suicide. Gender appears to play a significant factor in determining this risk. Same sex orientation clearly increases the risk of both attempted and completed suicide more for men than for women [23, 24]. Several studies have reported that the gender pattern for suicidal ideation is opposite that for suicide attempts, with risk of suicidal ideation higher among lesbian/bisexual women and risk of suicide attempts higher among gay/bisexual men [23].

While research specifically addressing suicide amongst lesbian and bisexual women is limited, there is solid evidence that, compared with heterosexual women, lesbian and bisexual women are about twice as likely to have attempted suicide; having a "closeted" sexual orientation further increases risk [25].

LGBT people of color in general, and Native Americans and Latinos in particular, may be at increased risk of suicide compared with white LGBT people [25, 26].

Data regarding suicide among bisexual people is limited, although data suggests that bisexual people attempt suicide at nearly three times the rate of heterosexual peers, a rate which is even higher than that suffered by either gay men or lesbian women [27].

Transgender and gender non-conforming adults clearly suffer the greatest risk of suicide among LGBT populations. Unfortunately, relatively sparse data is available regarding the magnitude of this risk, and much of it comes from studies of people who have sought medical or surgical gender affirmation treatments (and thereby represent only one subgroup of a larger population). Various studies estimate that between 10 and 45 % of transgender and gender variant individuals attempt suicide. Particular risk factors include younger age, more severe discrimination, and lack of family support [23].

## Mood Disorders

Numerous studies have demonstrated that people with minority gender identities and sexual orientations suffer a disproportionately high rate of mood disorders, especially major depression. The risk of a gay man developing depression is approximately two to three times that of a heterosexual man. Lesbian women face approximately 1.5 times the risk of straight women. For both men and women, rates are even higher among those who identify as bisexual. The impact of aging on the prevalence of depression is not entirely clear [27, 28].

Studies have not demonstrated that LGBT adults face a significant increase in the risk of experiencing a manic episode or receiving the diagnosis of bipolar affective disorder [29].

The relationship between race/ethnicity and depression within the LGBT population is not entirely clear. One study found that African-American LGB people have significantly lower rates of depression than either Latino or white LGB people. This stands in contrast to the fact that LGBTQ people of color appear to have a higher rate of suicide attempts [26].

More research is needed regarding the prevalence of mood disorders within the transgender and gender non-conforming population. Preliminary findings indicated a markedly elevated risk of depression among transgender individuals [30], perhaps as high as 44.1 %, although likely higher among female-identified individuals [31]. Of note, social stigma was positively associated with psychological distress, but is moderated by peer support from other transgender people [31]. There is ample evidence that depression symptoms improve dramatically with the initiation of gender affirmation treatments, including hormones [32].

## Anxiety Disorders

Research has demonstrated that gender and sexuality minorities are at increased risk of developing an anxiety disorder. Gay men, lesbian women, and bisexual women suffer anxiety disorders at two to three times the rate of same-gendered heterosexuals; lesbian women suffer anxiety disorders at approximately 1.5 times the rate of straight women [27, 28]. This pattern of significantly elevated risk holds roughly for each specific anxiety disorder, including panic disorder, specific phobia, social phobia, and generalized anxiety disorder [28, 29]. Of note, generalized anxiety disorder is clearly related to general societal attitudes. A very large (34,000 subject) study examined the mental health of LGB people in the 14 states that banned same sex marriage in 2004. LGB subjects in states that banned same sex marriage displayed a 248 % increase in generalized anxiety disorder, compared to no significant increase in the comparable control group (from states which did not pass marriage bans) [33].

There is a suggestion that the prevalence of anxiety disorders may decrease with age [26]. The relationship between race/ethnicity and anxiety among LGBT people is not clear. More research is needed regarding the prevalence of depression within the transgender and gender non-conforming population.

## Post-traumatic Stress Disorder

All minority gender identity and sexual orientation groups experience high rates of discrimination and bias crimes, as well as corresponding high rates of post-traumatic stress disorder.

LGBT people are more likely than almost any other minority group in the United States to be victimized in a hate crime. According to a 2010 analysis of FBI hate crime data and US Census population statistics by the Southern Poverty Law Center, LGBT people account for more than 17 % of all hate crimes victims. LGBT people are victimized at 2.4 times the rate of Jewish Americans, 2.6 times the rate of African Americans, 4.4 times

the rate of Muslim Americans, 13.8 times the rate of Latinos, and 41.5 times the rate of non-gay whites [34]. One study suggests that double minority status does not necessarily increase the risk; African-American and Latino LGB people were no more likely than Caucasian LGB people to experience a prejudice event [35]. The incidence of hate crimes against transgender communities is even higher than that facing sexual orientation minorities; these crimes tend to be particularly brutal, sexual, and lethal.

Given that lesbian, gay, and bisexual people suffer more traumatic events than their heterosexual peers, it is not surprising that they develop PTSD much more frequently, as well. Using data obtained from a very large, representative, national survey, Roberts and colleagues determined that lesbian women, gay men, bisexual women, and heterosexuals who reported any same-sex sexual partners over their lifetime had approximately twice the risk of developing PTSD than that of exclusively heterosexual people. This higher risk was largely accounted for by sexual orientation minorities' greater exposure to violence, exposure to more potentially traumatic events, and earlier age of trauma exposure. Roberts and colleagues conclude there is an urgent need for both violence prevention and trauma treatment programs for sexual orientation minorities [36].

Anti-gay prejudice is often intertwined with prejudice against gender non-conformity. Gordon and Meyer contend that careful consideration of anti-LGBT bias must include a thoughtful analysis of both transphobia and homophobia [37]. Transphobia is widespread and severe, even in progressive states and within the LGB community. The Massachusetts findings from a 2009 survey by the National Center for Transgender Equality and the National Gay and Lesbian Task Force indicated that 58 % of transgender adults were verbally harassed in a place of public accommodation, 22 % of transgender adults were denied equal treatment by a government agency or official, and 24 % of transgender adults suffered police harassment [38]. While data on prejudice against transgender and gender non-conforming people is sparse, multiple studies suggest rates of discrimination events approaching 60 % and bias crimes approaching 25 % [39]. There is no conclusive data regarding risk of PTSD among gender identity minorities, although one would expect rates exceeding that of the larger LGBT community.

## Disorders of Body Image and Eating

Multiple studies have demonstrated that sexual orientation is a robust risk factor for eating disorders in men, increasing the risk that sexual orientation minority men will develop anorexia or bulimia [40, 41]. This holds true across different racial and cultural groups [40]. Multiple studies suggest that sexual minority men represent a disproportionate percentage—perhaps as high as 42 %—of men seeking treatment for eating disorders. The reasons for this disparity are not entirely clear, although a sociocultural explanation has been proposed which suggests that men may feel pressure to obtain a lean physique in order to attract a male partner, as men tend to emphasize physical appearance when selecting mates [42]. This theory receives support from the fact that being in a stable relationship seems to be a protective factor for restrictive disordered eating in sexual minority men [43], while attending a gay recreational group increases risk [40].

In most studies, same-sex orientation is associated with increased male body dissatisfaction, body image distortions, fear of being fat, and drive for thinness. Gay men are also more likely than heterosexual men to hold distorted cognitions about the importance of having an ideal physique [44]. Ironically, at the same time that gay men are striving to be lean, they are also beset with fears of being too skinny, a condition termed "muscle dysmorphia." Evidence suggests that gay men aspire to a more muscular body ideal than do heterosexual men [45]. This muscular ideal may have developed in response to wasting observed in gay men suffering during the early days of the AIDS epidemic, although the idealization of a hyper-masculine body type certainly predates this period. Compared to other forms of body dysmorphic disorder, muscle dys-

morphia is associated with higher rates of substance use, especially anabolic steroid use, and suicide attempts [46]. Distortions of male body image and related disordered eating and exercise behaviors are often called the "Adonis complex," the title of a book on this subject by Pope and Phillips [47].

There is greater controversy regarding the relationship between sexual orientation and risk for eating disordered behaviors in women. Applying the sociocultural perspective to sexual minority women, some researchers have proposed that they may be less prone to eating disorders because they do not share with heterosexual women the pressure to attract a male partner [42]. Studies, however, have yielded conflicting results. While some have found that lesbian women suffer from lower levels of body dissatisfaction and eating disorders, others have found no difference in eating disorder prevalence [40]. In their study on women's mental health, Koh and Ross found that lesbian women were significantly less likely than either straight or bisexual women to want to lose weight [25]. Nevertheless, lesbian women were slightly more likely than straight women to have an eating disorder. In contrast, bisexual women were twice as likely to have or have had an eating disorder compared with lesbian women.

There are no solid data regarding the prevalence of eating disorders among transgender and gender non-conforming adults.

## Substance Use Disorders

Sexual orientation and gender identity minorities experience elevated rates of substance use disorders, although the risk is fairly specific to each substance and each sub-population. Intersectionality of identity plays a significant but nuanced role; for example, sexual minority women of color may have greater risks than either heterosexual women of color and or white lesbian women and bisexual women. Sexual minority men of color, on the other hand, appear to face lower risk than white gay and bisexual men [48].

Tobacco use in general, and smoking in particular, represents a major health hazard within the LGBT community. A systematic review paper found that gay men appear to have between 1.1 and 2.4 times the odds of smoking compared to straight men. Lesbian women have between 1.2 and 2.0 times the odds of smoking compared to straight women. Younger women smoke more than older women; researchers speculate that the younger women are more likely to socialize in bars, which might explain the difference. Bisexual women have the very highest rate of tobacco use—approaching 40 %—of any sexuality minority group. Almost no data exists regarding the rate of nicotine use among transgender and gender non-conforming people [49, 50].

With regards to alcohol, multiple studies suggest that lesbian women face a markedly increased risk of developing alcohol use disorder, with a lifetime prevalence that ranges from about three to six times that of heterosexual women. Minority sexual orientation conveys a smaller risk for men; the odds ratio of alcohol dependence for gay men (vs. heterosexual men) ranges from about 1.25 to 2 [25, 24, 51]. Further research is needed regarding the prevalence of alcohol use among transgender and gender non-conforming individuals.

Studies suggest that gay men and lesbian women both experience elevated risks of illicit substance use [51]. While different studies demonstrate varying findings, a meta-analytic review suggests a relative risk of 2.41 for gay or bisexual men and 3.50 for lesbian or bisexual women compared with heterosexual peers [24]. In general, bisexuality is associated with a higher risk than same-sex orientation [26]. In general, LGBT individuals are much more likely than heterosexual, cis-gendered people to abuse methamphetamine and cocaine or crack [52].

Relatively little is known about the substance use behaviors of transgender and gender non-conforming individuals, as national substance use surveillance systems and epidemiological surveys predominantly assume that all participants are cis-gender. Transgender women do appear more likely than trans-men or cis-gendered individuals to endorse primary methamphetamine use [53]. It is also known that desperation drives some transgender individuals to seek black market gender affirmation treatments, including hormones of dubious provenance and quality [54].

There is evidence that LGBT-specific substance abuse treatment programs may demonstrate greater effectiveness than treatment as usual [55].

## Personality Disorders

Personality disorders describe a relatively inflexible and maladaptive pattern of thinking and feeling about oneself and others that significantly and adversely affects how an individual functions in many aspects of life. Volumes have been written discussing the etiology of personality disorders. At this point, most experts would concur that personality disorders result from a mixture of genetic and environmental factors, including subtle differences in underlying neuroanatomy and brain function, inborn temperament, early attachment patterns, and life experiences.

There exists only a modicum of data describing the frequency and nature of personality disorders among people with minority sexual orientations and gender identities. Historically, people with personality disorders were viewed with clinical hopelessness and treated with disdain. While strong evidence now suggests that personality disorders respond to treatment and can improve over time, clinical bias persists. Given the health disparities and clinical bias suffered by LGBT people, any research on the intersection of personality disorders and sexual orientation/gender identity must be evaluated thoughtfully from the perspective of potential bias. LGBT people with personality disorders are a doubly marginalized population.

A number of studies in the late 1980s and early 1990s examined the sexual orientations of men and women with diagnosed borderline personality disorder (BPD). In general, these studies found elevated rates of homosexual or bisexual orientation, with a markedly larger effect observed in men than in women. Using a variety of study designs (including chart review and interview-based methodologies) in a variety of settings (inpatient and outpatient), authors have found rates of homosexual orientation among borderline men ranging from approximately 16 % [56, 57] to approximately 50 % [58, 59]. Rates of same-sex attraction among borderline women ranged from 1 % [56] to approximately 15 % [59, 58].

A more thorough assessment of the relationship between sexual orientation and borderline personality disorder was published in 2008 from the data set of the McLean Study of Adult Development. Subjects with BPD were about twice as likely as comparison subjects to report either homosexual/bisexual orientation or intimate same-sex relationships. Somewhat surprisingly, gender did not significantly affect sexual orientation; 29.8 % of men and 26.6 % of women with BPD reported homosexuality/bisexuality, a non-significant difference. People with BPD were three times more likely than comparison subjects to report changing the gender of intimate partners, but not their own sexual orientation, during the follow-up period. The authors concluded that same-gender attraction and intimate relationship choice is an important interpersonal issue for a significant minority of borderline men and women [60]. Subsequent authors have found a similar frequency of minority sexual orientations among women with confirmed diagnoses of BPD [61].

Cluster C personality disorders do not appear to occur with significantly different frequencies among sexual orientation or gender identity minorities [27].

While the co-occurrence of personality and substance use disorders is common regardless of sexual orientation, borderline personality disorder, obsessive-compulsive personality disorder, and avoidant personality disorder appear to be two to three times more common among people with minority sexual orientations receiving addiction treatment than their heterosexual peers [62].

A few recent studies have explored the matrix of core identity instability (often postulated as a core aspect of BPD), sexuality and gender iden-tity issues (commonly faced by LGBT people), and clinician bias. Individuals struggling through the process of coming out experience a transformation in their core identity, but this is by no means synonymous with borderline identity instability. Some have argued that possessing a homosexual orientation in a heteronormative society could increase identity conflict and support the increased prevalence of BPD among LGBT people. It is also possible that LGBT people, particularly gay and bisexual men, might be exposed to traumatic stressors that have been linked to BPD in women [63]. Still others question whether the apparent increased prevalence of BPD in gay and bisexual men primarily reflects diagnostic bias among clinicians. Evidence suggests that clinicians are more likely to diagnosis identical symptoms as BPD in women than in men; perhaps this bias is extended to gay or bisexual men if they are perceived as being feminine or violating heteronormative masculine ideals. A recent study explored the impact of clinician perspective on the complex diagnostic matrix of personality and sexuality/gender identity using a hypothetical case with a patient whose problems resembled BPD symptoms but were also consistent with a sexual identity crisis. The authors found an effect of sexual orientation for male clients, but not female clients. Male clients whom therapists perceived likely to be gay or bisexual were more likely to be diagnosed with BPD. Therapists were more confident and willing to work with female clients and gave them a better prognosis [64].

The relationship between minority gender identity and personality disorders has received little rigorous evaluation. The challenges of growing up in a transphobic society and experiences of trauma might contribute to an increased prevalence of borderline symptomatology among gender non-conforming and transgender communities, although this has not yet been demonstrated beyond the level of conjecture. One study exploring the frequency of gender dysphoria among women with confirmed BPD found no significant difference from women in a diagnostically heterogeneous clinical control group. The authors conclude that frank gender dysphoria is not a particular salient aspect of the identity issues with which female patients with BPD struggle [61].

## Relationships

Why discuss relationships in the mental health section? As has been written in so many other books and publications over the past 100 years, it's not due to the assumption that all same-sex couple relationships are pathological, or that our relationships with our mothers "caused" us to be this way. It's also not due to the assumption that LGBT people don't have normal, healthy relationships. Obviously, these assumptions are incorrect as will be discussed. However, there can be challenges in same-sex couple relationships and also in the way that families and friends relate to LGBT people, and vice versa. People who are struggling with their sexual identity may have profound problems with relationships, sometimes living secret lives and feeling completely alone because no one knows. The gay and lesbian communities have their own unique identities, which in many ways affect friendships, romantic relationships, and sexual relationships. But again, why is this important? It's important because relationships, both sexual and non-sexual, can have a profound impact on mental health, and also physical health. Additionally, mental health problems, in turn, can have a profound impact on relationships and their stability. As discussed, the LGBT communities have higher rates of many psychiatric and psychological problems, which in turn may adversely affect relationships. Finally, some sexual behaviors, such as having multiple sexual partners (often labeled "promiscuity"), can be seen as a sign of mental illness, such as Bipolar Disorder or a "sex addiction." It's important to discuss some cultural differences between the LGBT community from the heterosexual community in order to inform thinking about these behaviors as either a "symptom" or simply a cultural difference.

Entire books have been written on all of the nuances of relationships in the LGBT community. Therefore, this section will undoubtedly fall short in many ways, as it is not intended to be a compendium on all of the different types of relationships and the ways in which they might be unique for our community. Some of the information included may seem pretty basic for anyone involved with the LGBT community. It is included here for those medical professionals who may not be familiar with some aspects of the community, in the hopes that this will make them aware of common themes and issues in the LGBT community. Hopefully, this will enhance their cultural competence so that they can be more effective as healthcare practitioners. Although there is a significant amount of research on the correlation of relationships and health, much of it has been done with the heterosexual population. This section will review some of this literature, making the assumption that the effects seen in the heterosexual community are likely to be seen in the LGBT community. When possible, however, research that is specific to our community will be included and reviewed. Finally, some of the unique aspects of relationships for the LGBT community will be discussed as a basis for understanding some of the challenges and opportunities facing our community, and to provide a framework of topics for possible discussion between patients and healthcare workers.

## Relationships and Health

Throughout history, finding or experiencing romantic love has often been associated with happiness, and unrequited love and isolation have often been associated with depression and despair. So for most people, it seems simply intuitive that relationships, especially sexual and romantic ones, are correlated with happiness or depression. Most people assume that it is a simple cause and effect relationship, meaning that good relationships lead to happiness, and bad relationships or the absence of a relationship leads to depression.

Over the past 100 years, there has been much research on the correlation between relationships, especially marriage, and both physical and mental health. It is thought that close relationships and/or enhanced social networks have beneficial effects on stress response, immune system functioning, cardiovascular reactivity, blood pressure, inflammation, and other factors [65]. Some of the earliest research in this area began in 1890, when the National Center for Health Statistics began publishing reports on mortality based on marital status, and numerous subsequent studies based on this data found that married people, independent of race or gender, lived longer on average than those who were single, widowed, or divorced [66]. Abel-Smith and Titmuss [67] looked at data from England and found that those that were married utilized health services less frequently than those who were not. Pollack [68] reviewed the literature on marriage status and mental health service utilization and concluded the following: "The relationship between marital status and mental disorders has been extensively studied over the years. In the large number of studies that have measured the rate at which persons in specific marital status categories have come under psychiatric care, the patterns have been remarkably similar. The rate for married persons has been consistently the lowest, while the rates for separated and divorced persons have been the highest, with rates for single and widowed persons somewhere between these extremes." The French sociologist, Emile Durkheim, was one of the first people to study and report on the correlation of social relationships and mortality from a specific cause: suicide. In his book, Suicide: A Study in Sociology [69], he reported that those who were not married or didn't have children were more likely to commit suicide than those who were married or had children. In recent years, the research has continued to look at marital status, but has also focused on more inclusive forms of social connections. It has been shown that the more close relationships a person has, the less likely they are to get a common cold or have symptoms of infection [70]. Being married and/or having a close confidant has been shown to decrease cardiac mortality compared to individuals who have neither of these [71, 72]. In a large study looking at over 1.2 million cancer patients, being married was found to increase the chances of survival from cancer,

with an effect size similar to that of adjuvant chemotherapy [73]. DeKlyen et al. [74] looked at new, heterosexual parents in the Fragile Families and Child Wellbeing Study and compared those that were married, cohabiting, not cohabiting but romantically involved, and not romantically involved to see if there were differences in mental health and behavioral problems among the groups. They found that married people had the lowest rate of mental health problems and that the prevalence increased in the groups in the following order: those who were cohabiting; those who were romantically involved, but not cohabiting; and those who were not romantically involved. This study suggests that the level of commitment, or at least the frequency of contact in a romantic relationship, effects mental health status. Hughes and Waite [75] looked at marital biography and health in mid-life. They found that marriage protected against a variety of health conditions, and that marriage disruption (divorce or death) damages health, with the effects still evident years later.

Most people assume from the above referenced studies that close relationships lead to improved physical and mental health. However, the above studies simply show a correlation, and as commonly known, correlation does not necessarily confirm causation. Two studies call into question this cause and effect relationship. The first study [76] looked at 5877 individuals who completed questionnaires about the age of onset of 14 DSM-III-R lifetime diagnoses and the ages of first marriage and divorce, and then created survival models for the marriages based on preexisting psychiatric diagnoses. This study found that people with psychiatric disorders are more likely to get a divorce and that they remain married for a shorter period of time than those who don't have a psychiatric diagnosis. The second study looked at over 46,000 people from 19 countries and analyzed the effect of 18 different psychiatric disorders on probability of getting married or staying married [77]. They found that 14 of the 18 mental disorders studied were associated with a lower likelihood of ever getting married, and that all 18 disorders were associated with a greater risk of divorce. Therefore, in the prior correlational studies, it's not surprising that people who were divorced had higher rates of psychiatric diagnoses. It may be that psychiatric disorders lead to divorce as opposed to the other way around.

In the end, although the distinction of cause and effect is unclear, what is clear is that intimate relationships and strong friendships are important to both physical and mental health, whether they directly cause the improvement in health, or whether they are simply an indication or "symptom" of health. It may be that this is simply a positive feedback cycle, whereby they are both continuously influencing each other.

Much of the research cited above refers to marriage, which until only recently was not an option for many in the LGBT community. Within the LGBT communities, some feel passionately that marriage is a "heterosexist" institution, and would prefer to have nothing to do with it. Others feel that it has been used to oppress women, or oppress people's normal sex drives and behaviors. In the end, it's very likely that marriage, as commonly defined in Western societies, is not what is healing, but that close relationships, whether in the context of a marriage or not, are what heal, or at least are correlated with health.

The discussion so far has illustrated why relationships, both sexual and non-sexual, are important to mental and physical health. This section will now delve into some of the ways that relationships for LGBT people can be affected by issues that are specific to our community.

## Relationships with Families of Origin

There can be many issues for LGBT people in how they relate to their families of origin, given that their "difference" is often initially hidden, and many families, religions, and cultures have at least some degree of homophobia and transphobia. Most LGBT youth feel forced to keep their difference private or secret, at least for a period of time. The "difference" is almost always much more than just sexual attraction. It can feel all-encompassing to a person's existence, and in many ways, it is. It includes not only sexual

thoughts when one is aroused, but also feelings of love, intimacy, and connection. It includes innumerable aspects of how a person relates to the world and his/her own body. Gender non-conformity not only applies to transgender youth, but oftentimes to LGB youth as well. Gay boys may want to cross their legs "like a girl." Lesbian girls may feel uncomfortable wearing a dress. For transgender youth, the differences are much greater and pervade seemingly every aspect of life. Yet, most of these youth will try desperately to hide their differences. They become hyper-aware of what others might perceive, fearing that if they don't keep up their guard, they will be exposed. It includes innumerable day-to-day experiences: the way they talk, the way the walk, glances at other people, pausing to look at a picture in a magazine, fear that the way they throw a ball may give them away, fear that wearing a certain colored shirt may be "too feminine," etc. When they feel that someone may have seen something that might expose them, they can go into a panic: fearing shame, humiliation, disgust, or rejection. This experience often leads an individual to feel completely isolated, terrified, and ashamed. These youth often distance themselves from others, including their families of origin, for fear of exposure. Despite their desperate loneliness and longing for connection, they feel compelled to push people away, or at least keep some distance, usually because they feel certain that they will be rejected if they allow people to get close to them. This process just adds to the feelings of guilt and shame, as they can't explain to their friends and loved ones why they are distancing themselves. For many, the perceived rejection extends to God as well. So oftentimes, LGBT youth may feel there is truly nowhere to turn for help. Some will go to great lengths to "make up" for these perceived deficiencies. They will try to be "perfect" in other ways. They may work hard in school, and sometimes put unreasonable expectations on themselves. They may immerse themselves into sports, and be devastated with losses. They may try to look perfect by dieting, working out, or dressing impeccably. They may try anything to make themselves "lovable." Even though these youth may be loved, they oftentimes don't believe it. The mental health consequences of years of this experience are undeniable—higher rates of depression, suicide, substance abuse, etc. Sadly, these core beliefs can be ingrained in a person for life. Even after coming out, some people continue to have a deep-seated fear that they are unlovable, and this can affect their relationships for decades. Even when they rationally know that their difference doesn't make them any less worthy or lovable than others, these beliefs may crop up again years later, especially during times of stress or difficulty.

Even after coming out, problems can persist with families of origin. In many ways, coming out involves a whole process of learning about and acclimating to a new culture: the specific LGBT culture in which one comes out. Although there are innumerable variations, there are almost always differences from the culture in which one was raised. In many ways, this is exciting and freeing, allowing the individual to finally be himself or herself, oftentimes for the first time. In other ways, it can be confusing, disorienting, and disheartening, as some people may feel they don't belong, or may miss some of the aspects of their prior life and relationships. They may fear that the people in their life up to that point will judge them, or simply not understand. Many LGBT people fear discussing sexual issues openly with friends or family. Even when they do, the support they receive is sometimes not seen as helpful as it is by heterosexuals. Friedman and Morgan [78] interviewed 229 college women about times when they went to friends or parents for issues related to their sexuality. Interestingly, they did not find a difference in how often sexual-minority women and heterosexual women sought support from friends or parents, but they did find that sexual-minority women perceived both parents and friends' responses as less helpful than did heterosexual participants.

A significant challenge for many LGBT people, therefore, is the ability to integrate their life with their family of origin and the values of their upbringing. After many people come out, there is a period of questioning some of the values they were taught as children, particularly religious beliefs. In many ways, this can be a wonderful opportunity for individuals to grow. They can consider their beliefs and values as adolescents or adults, with more knowledge and life experience than they had as children. However, problems can occur when individuals end up feeling completely disconnected from their past life and the people who were part of it. In extreme cases, they may be "disowned" by their family of origin, or they may "disown" or "disconnect" from them. This can sometimes leave a person feeling uprooted, lost, and alone.

In addition to the innumerable problems encountered by LGBT individuals, the family members themselves often have difficulty adjusting to the individual who comes out. Just as the individuals may have needed time to accept themselves and integrate this information with everything else they have been taught and believed to be true, the family members may also need time. Many can experience depression, anger, disbelief, and other complicated feelings in response to learning of their family member's sexual orientation or gender identity. Many parents describe a period of mourning, feeling that they have "lost" the child they thought they had known. An important consideration is referral of family members to support groups, such as Parents, Families, and Friends of Lesbian women and Gays (PFLAG) or mental health services, given that acceptance by family members has a significant, beneficial effect on reducing depression and suicide in LGBT individuals [79].

## Friends

For some in the LGBT community, there are no differences in friendships compared to their heterosexual counterparts. Friends may come from a variety of sources, such as school, work, neighborhood, or other acquaintances, without regard to sexual orientation, gender identity, or other factors. However, for most in the LGBT community, there is often a need or comfort in being with people who are similar. Many people fear judgment or discomfort from the heterosexual community regarding their differences, or they just prefer to be with people who have similar experiences. It can be comforting to share common experiences. It can be helpful to get advice or feedback from people who are in a similar position, whether it's advice about dating, sex, coming out to people at work, or other issues. It can be helpful to talk about stigma and experiences of discrimination with people who understand, and may have had similar experiences. So for many in the LGBT community, they seek out a group of friends who are similar to themselves: gay men tend to seek a group of gay male friends, lesbian women tend to seek a group of lesbian friends, M-F trans may seek a similar group, etc. While none of these tendencies is absolute, and almost all people in all groups have friends that are exceptions to these trends, the trends do appear to be real. Galupo [80] interviewed heterosexual, gay, lesbian, and bisexual people about their friendships and found that "heterosexual women and men primarily developed friendships of similarity, with relatively few friendships experienced in a cross-orientation (5.50 %), cross-sex (28.06 %), or cross-race (17.11 %) contexts. In contrast, bisexual women and men reported more cross-orientation (79.55 %), cross-sex (32.99 %), and cross-race (23.13 %) friendships. Likewise, lesbian women and gay men reported cross-orientation (53.03 %) cross-sex (23.73 %), and cross-race (25.77 %) friendships." Although the LGB people had more diversity in their friendships, it's actually somewhat surprising that in this sample of gay men and lesbian women, 47 % reported that they did not have any heterosexual friends and, overall, they had fewer cross-sex friends than the heterosexuals did. Nardi [81] found that 82 % of gay men reported that their "best friend" was another gay or bisexual man. This is consistent with research that suggests that many people, not just in the LGBT community, choose friends who share similar attitudes, beliefs, and health behaviors. Bahns et al. [82] looked at college students at large and small campuses and, interestingly, found this to be the case especially when people have a larger and more diverse pool of people from which to choose friends. In other words, when people have more choices of potential friends, they tend to choose people who are similar to themselves. Consistent with this theme, in the heterosexual community, heterosexual women tend to choose friends who are also heterosexual women, and heterosexual men tend to choose friends who are heterosexual men [83].

One of the things that differentiates patterns of friendships in the heterosexual community from those in the LGB community is that same-sex friends are also potential sexual partners in the LGB community. One question that sometimes arises in these friendships is whether there is sexual tension in the friendship, and whether the two people can remain "just friends." This same issue comes up in the heterosexual community when a man and a woman develop a friendship, and can often be a source of concern for a partner or significant other. Surprisingly, little, if any, research has been done in this area for gay men and lesbian women, but research has been done in the heterosexual community. Kaplan and Keys [84] looked at heterosexuals in cross-sex friendships and found that 58 % of them reported some degree of sexual attraction to each other. Afifi and Faulkner [85] looked at heterosexual, cross-sex friendships in college students and found that approximately half of them had included sexual contact at some point in an otherwise platonic friendship.

When there is sexual attraction or tension in a platonic friendship, there are some debates about whether this is a benefit or burden. Some argue that it adds spice to the relationship and makes it more stimulating and enjoyable, even if sexual activity is never included. Others argue that it may result in feelings of longing, jealousy, or depression. Belske-Rechek et al. [86] tried to answer this question by interviewing heterosexual adults aged 18–55 who had at least one cross-sex friendship. Although most respondents reported more benefits than costs to the relationships overall, they more commonly reported that sexual attraction was a cost more than a benefit, often causing problems with their current romantic partner, such as jealousy. Those who reported attraction to a current cross-sex friend reported less satisfaction with their current romantic relationships. Although no research has been published in this area that is specific to the LGBT community, it is not difficult to imagine that some of these issues may also be relevant.

Although there is no published data on friendships in the LGBT communities and how often there is sexual attraction or sexual activity between friends, anecdotal experience suggests that these things are certainly not uncommon. Many gay and lesbian friendships begin because at least one person is sexually attracted to the other. It may be the reason they initially approach the person at a club or party. Oftentimes, the other person isn't interested in a sexual relationship, so they pursue a friendship instead. Sometimes, they date first, come to realize that they aren't a match for a romantic relationship, but make great friends. Other times, one person is already involved with someone else, so they pursue a friendship instead. Many times, these lead to fantastic friendships without complications that can last a lifetime. However, the attraction can sometimes lead to complications or strains in the relationship. The person who is attracted to the other may experience the dysphoria and frustration of unrequited love. They may spend years in the friendship hoping the other person's feelings will change. The recipient of the attraction may feel guilty or sad about the other person's hurt, oftentimes knowing about the unspoken attraction. If either one is dating or has a partner, the partner may become jealous and question the motivations of the friendship. Additionally, when trouble arises with a romantic partner or new dating relationship, the person may naturally want to discuss this with others, including a friend who happens to be sexually attracted. This is where it can sometimes get complicated, as the friend may give advice that is at least somewhat biased by his or her own feelings. For example, the friend may feel that the other friend deserves better and should move on to another relationship, instead of supporting the friend to work through relationship issues with the partner. The friend may also see it as the opportunity he/she has been waiting for to finally be together romantically. The friend may undermine new romantic relationships by not being as supportive as possible, or insinuating again that the person could do better. This can occur due to jealousy on many

fronts: jealous that he/she can't have you, jealous that he/she doesn't have a significant other and now you do, jealous of the new significant other and wanting him or her for self, or jealous, afraid, or resentful that now you will be less available as a friend because you will be spending more time with the new love and less time with him/her. Again, these are not universal rules that apply to all LGBT friendships, and are much less relevant to LGBT people who are in stable, long-term relationships. But they can occur, and they can have effects on the stability of new relationships and on the support that LGBT people feel from their social network for their romantic relationships. Given that stability of relationships and social networks are important to health, these issues are at least worth keeping in mind and exploring with patients when appropriate.

One unique type of friendship in the gay community is the friendship between a gay man and a heterosexual woman. Popular media has highlighted examples of such friendships in television shows such as "Will and Grace" and "Sex and the City." A unique aspect of these friendships is that both friends know that sex is unlikely to occur in the relationship, and they are not competing for the same sexual partners. This sets this type of relationship apart from many others. Some small studies have been done with these heterosexual women (sometimes referred to as "fag hags" or "fruit flies") and the gay men with whom they are friends to discern what is unique and advantageous about these friendships. Many of these women feel that gay men provide attention to them that heterosexual men don't provide [87–89]. They report feeling valued for their personality, as opposed to their sexuality or their body, when they are with their gay friends. Grigoriou [88] in her 2004 paper, "Friendship between gay men and heterosexual women: An interpretive phenomenological analysis," described how many women feel a sense of honesty and safety when interacting with their gay male friends, as opposed to their women friends or heterosexual males. She also interviewed gay men about their perspectives on these friendships, and found that many of them found these friends to be particularly trustworthy sources of information and support, especially regarding dating and relationship advice. Some of these gay men clearly favored the friendships they had with heterosexual women over friendships with other gay men. "Some participants talked about pretence, sarcasm and 'bitchiness' in the gay world and they described their friendships with other gay men as affected by these characteristics." Russell et al. [90] interviewed gay men and straight women about these friendships. They also found that straight women perceived dating advice from a gay man to be more trustworthy than similar advice offered by a straight man or woman, and found that gay men perceived dating advice offered by a straight woman to be more trustworthy than advice offered by a lesbian woman or another gay man.

Friendships in the LGBT community can sometimes include sex and other forms of physical intimacy. "Friends with benefits" and "fuck buddies" are two common terms used to describe friendships that include sex on a regular basis, with the former term implying more emphasis on the friendship and less on the sex, and the latter term implying more emphasis on the sex, and less on the friendship, or sometimes not including friendship at all, but just a regular sexual partner without commitment. These are usually distinguished from "dating," which usually implies the pursuit of a more serious relationship. Certainly, these sexual friendships can be seen in the heterosexual community as well, but they appear to be much more common in the LGBT communities. As a healthcare practitioner, it's important not to make automatic judgments, moral or otherwise, about these relationships. For some, it's a way to express love or affection for a friend, while acknowledging that the relationship is unlikely to progress into a long-term relationship. Others may seek out such relationships while they are still looking for a longer-term relationship, feeling that it's safer and more comfortable to have a regular, sexual partner who is also a friend, as opposed to random strangers. It may also be a way to feel connected to someone in a more meaningful way and deal with loneliness. Some may have given up on the idea of a long-term, committed relationship and may have several friends with benefits as way of life. And some may be in long-term, committed relationships that are not monogamous, and may feel these friendships are a safer and more comfortable way to "play" outside of their primary relationship. These are just some of the innumerable reasons that people may choose to pursue sexual friendships. While some people can have several of these friendships without complications, it is probably more common to find that these relationships often include some degree of complication. Sometimes someone wants more at the outset, but feels this is all that is being offered. Or feelings may change and grow stronger as the friendship and intimacy progress. Sometimes, someone moves on to another friend or relationship, leaving the other person hurt. Sometimes, people's interest in the sexual component of the friendship simply wanes, and they want less sex or less contact. Sometimes, there isn't open communication about the other people that are involved, and people may feel betrayed or get hurt. In the end, it's important that the two friends communicate openly about their desires and expectations, and the way these are changing and evolving over time. Needless to say, this is easier said than done. Given the high degree of judgment from friends and families about such relationships, many people often find that they don't have as many sources of support for discussing these relationships. Therefore, it's important for medical practitioners to be aware of these types of relationships and ask about them overtly in order to let the patient know that you are open to discussing them without judgment.

In addition to friendships that include sex, it is increasingly common for LGBT friends to express physical affection without the expectation of sex or the feeling of any boundary violation with their romantic partners. This is commonly seen in dance clubs, where friends might kiss or "make out" with each other, or "dirty dance" with each other, but without any expectation of sex or anything other than friendship outside of the club. This can be seen among and between lesbian women and gay men, and also between gay men and their heterosexual, female friends. While, in theory, it could also include heterosexual men, this appears to be much less common. For many, it's a fun way to celebrate the night and let loose. Many people can do this without complication, but again, for some, there can be unspoken desires or feelings. The other friends present may suspect that more might be occurring outside of the club. Or they may get jealous that one of the friends isn't doing the same thing with them. Some romantic partners may become jealous if they witness it or hear about it, or question the stability of the relationship, but other partners may simply accept it as part of the culture.

## Monogamy, or Not

Before discussing the topics of dating and long-term, committed relationships, it's important to address the issue of monogamy, as this can be a contentious and controversial topic. It is often used to stigmatize gay male sexual behavior. There are people who hold passionate positions on both sides of the issue. Many gay men have argued for decades that monogamy is a hetero-sexist, Christian-based ideal that is not relevant to the gay community. Given that the Christian-right has a long history of attacking the LGBT community, while also pursuing an agenda of promoting monogamy, it's not difficult to see how these messages could be paired with each other, and both could be seen as undesirable. Society also has a long history of instilling guilt and shame on the gay community for any sexual behavior, so most of us have had to work hard to detach ourselves from these value systems, and create something on our own. For some, the way out of the model of 'guilt and shame for any sexual behavior' is 'anything goes.' While this can work for some people, it doesn't work for everyone. Some in the community feel a strong need for a long-term, committed, monogamous relationship. They may be searching for "the one," or may feel that they've found him or her. The movement for equal marriage rights for the gay community is certainly a testament to the desire of many in our community to engage in long-term, committed, monogamous relationships.

There are evolutionary theories that support the role of monogamy in order to maximize survival of offspring. There are many obvious advantages to having two parents over one—while one is protecting and nurturing the children, the other can hunt or gather food, for instance. This is not restricted to humans, either. There are at least 11 other animal species that engage in monogamous pairing: swans, penguins, black vultures, French angelfish, wolves, albatrosses, termites, prairie voles, turtle doves, schistosoma mansoni worms, and bald eagles. Some of these species are monogamous with their mate for life, while others are serially monogamous. Gibbons, once thought to be monogamous, remain together for life to raise offspring, but will have sex outside of the relationship. Looking at this list of species, one can see that it includes not only primates, but also some relatively simple organisms, such as worms. Therefore, it suggests that there are primitive brain regions or other regulatory mechanisms that control sexual mating and lead some organisms to be monogamous. Many scientists are studying these animals to learn more about mating behaviors. Even though most people aren't thinking about raising children at the same time that they are having sex, these biological drives are almost certainly influencing sexual behavior and feelings. Given the strong urge in many humans for monogamy, it's not difficult to imagine that, at least for these particular individuals, that it might be a biological drive, as opposed to religious or cultural upbringing, that is guiding their desire for monogamy.

However, most animals do not have monogamous mating patterns [91], so it's plausible that humans also may not be inherently monogamous. History is replete with examples of humans practicing polygamy, polyandry, and/or being unfaithful to their spouses. Throughout literature as far back as Greek Mythology, a frequently described human dilemma is that of infidelity. Zeus was often cheating on his wife, Hera, but she was also incredibly jealous and rageful for each occurrence.

So it's possible that some humans are biologically wired toward monogamy, and others simply are not. It's conceivable that monogamy, like so many other human, biologically-driven traits, such as introversion versus extroversion, is something that is expressed on a continuum, with some people being born with a drive to be very monogamous and others with a drive to have multiple sexual partners. As much as many people want to frame this as a moral issue, it may be that it is neither good nor bad, it's just the way people are born. This shouldn't be confused with lying or cheating in order to achieve having multiple sexual partners, which can certainly be hurtful and unnecessary. Regardless of whether people are inclined to practice monogamy or not, it's important that they find partners with whom they can share this information, and vice versa. Ideally, we as a community and as healthcare practitioners can refrain from judging either position, realizing that monogamy is a couple's or individual's choice, or possibly biological drive.

## Dating and Hook Ups

Dating? A one-night stand? A hook-up? There is a spectrum of sexual behavior and relationship-seeking in the LGBT communities that can sometimes be difficult to define. At one end of the spectrum is "dating," in which people are seeking a more serious relationship. This is sometimes in pursuit of a long-term, committed, monogamous relationship (i.e. looking for "the one"), but at other times it's done in pursuit of a boyfriend or girlfriend, with no expectation of something monogamous or long-term. At the other end of the spectrum is finding someone for quick sex, sometimes without any conversation at all. And there can be everything in between—friends with benefits, fuck buddies, sex with people you meet while on vacation, sex with an "ex," etc. The reason to discuss all of these types of sex and romance together is because oftentimes, the two people may be looking for different things. For example, one person may think he is going on a "date" and the other person thinks it's just a "hook up," a term commonly used to describe one-time sex or sexual activity.

As differences in sexual orientation are increasingly accepted, it's becoming more common and easier than ever to date openly. More and more LGBT people are coming out in middle school and high school and begin dating at the same time as their heterosexual peers. For many of these individuals, their dating stories are similar to heterosexuals and, quite frankly, there's not much more to say about their stories, because they are so "normal." They involve the usual stories of courtship, dating, working out relationships, etc. Straight friends and family may get involved with advice, or helping to set them up with other LGBT people they know. The dates themselves can also be quite "normal," especially in larger cities, where public displays of affection between same-sex couples, such as kissing or holding hands while walking down the street, is increasingly commonplace. So for some in the LGBT community, there are no significant differences from heterosexuals regarding dating, finding sex, or finding love.

For better or worse, this isn't the case for the majority of LGBT people. For many, finding dates or sexual partners is accomplished by networking within their LGBT social network, seeking out places where other LGBT people go, such as dance clubs or bars, or using online sites or mobile phone applications ("apps"). Again, all of this can be similar to the heterosexual community, but there are some differences that are important to mention.

One of the biggest differences is the number of sexual partners, and the types of sexual partners, that gay men have, on average, relative to other groups. This applies to other groups of people who have sex or romantic relationships with gay men, including some bisexual, transgender, and queer individuals. Many people refer to having multiple sexual partners as "promiscuity," which has negative connotations and often comes with moral judgments. Some gay men experience this as one of the negative aspects of gay life, although others clearly celebrate this part of gay culture. Why mention this? It's not meant to imply that this difference is bad or wrong. It's also not meant to imply that this applies to all gay men, as it clearly does not [92]. But this "difference" has many health implications. It is often associated with or inter-related with the following issues that can be problematic:

1. It is often assumed to be pathological by many mental health professionals.
2. It sometimes puts individuals at higher risk for HIV and other sexually transmitted diseases.
3. It is sometimes inter-related with drug and alcohol use.

Without any guidelines or studies addressing how to think about this issue, clinicians are left to make their own assessments and recommendations. Unfortunately, many clinicians have some degree of homophobia [93]. This can influence how gay sex is viewed and how "promiscuity" might be addressed. Additionally, many in the gay community keep this information private or secret from their healthcare professionals [94, 95], or even from friends in the LGBT community, likely because of fear of judgment. Dating and sex can have a significant impact on a person's mental or physical health, so should be topics of discussion, at least in some situations. Healthcare professionals, therefore, need to be aware of these differences so that they can initiate conversations with their patients about these issues when appropriate.

Although the issue of gay "promiscuity" has not been evaluated by rigorous, epidemiologic studies, there are at least three significant sources of research that have looked at this issue. In 1967, the National Institute of Mental Health established a Task Force on Homosexuality, which concluded that more research on homosexuality was needed, and subsequently reached out to the Institute for Sex Research (formerly headed by Alfred Kinsey) to do a comprehensive study. Alan Bell and Martin Weinberg led a survey study of 686 gay men, 293 lesbian women, 337 heterosexual men and 140 heterosexual women living in San Francisco. In 1978, they published the book, "Homosexualities: A Study of Diversity Among Men and Women," in which they reported some of the findings of these studies [96]. They reported that 28 % of gay men had over 1000 sexual partners in their lifetime, almost half had over 500, another third had between 100 and 500, and over 90 % had at least 25. Most of the sexual encounters were with strangers. They reported that women were more likely to be monogamous than men, and that most lesbian women had fewer than 10 same-sex, sexual partners in their lifetime, with little sex between strangers. The biggest criticism of this study is that it was not a representative sample of the population; it was conducted only in San Francisco during the pre-HIV era, where gay clubs and bath houses were innumerable.

In 1989, Fay et al. [97] re-analyzed survey data from 1970 of 1450 American men over the age of 21 (originally done by The Kinsey Institute for Sex Research) to try to determine what percentage of the American population were men who had sex with men and the number of sexual partners that these men reported (primarily to estimate the impact of the AIDS epidemic). It should be noted that 21 % of the surveys from this study had incomplete or absent responses regarding same-gender sexual contact, so the researchers imputed responses and included these in their analyses. Looking at men who reported having sex with other men either "occasionally" or "fairly often," and having at least one sexual contact with a man after age 20 (which would likely be an estimate of the "gay" or "bisexual" male population), they found that 1.9 % ($N=28$) of the sample met this criteria by direct report, and after adjusting for incomplete surveys, they imputed an estimate of 3.3 % ($N=48$) of the sample. The small sample sizes should be noted. When looking at the number of sexual partners, they estimated that 2.1 % of the entire sample, or 64 % of the "gay or bisexual" men, reported five or more male partners during their lifetime, and 1.2, or 36 % of the "gay or bisexual" men, reported having ten or more male sexual partners during their lifetime. Of this latter group, 4 reported 20 lifetime partners, 1 reported 50, and 2 reported greater than 100 partners (8 %, 2 %, and 4 % of the "gay or bisexual" population, respectively). The biggest limitations of this study are that a significant portion of the data

**Table 13.1** Mean number of sexual partners

|  | Past year | Past 5 years | Since age 18 |
|---|---|---|---|
| Men who reported same-gender partners since age 18 | 2.3 | 12.2 | 44.3 |
| Men who denied any same-gender partners since age 18 | 1.8 | 4.9 | 15.7 |
| Women who reported same-gender partners since age 18 | 3.8 | 7.6 | 19.7 |
| Women who denied same-gender partners since age 18 | 1.3 | 2.2 | 4.9 |

Adapted from Laumann et al. [98], p. 315

(almost half of the "gay or bisexual" men) was missing and "imputed" by the researchers, and the sample size of "gay or bisexual" men was quite small. Nonetheless, this study is often cited as evidence that Bell and Weinberg's study was clearly flawed and overestimated how commonly gay men have multiple sexual partners.

A more recent survey also looked at the number of sexual partners over a lifetime, and its findings were reported in the book, "The Social Organization of Sexuality: Sexual Practices in the United States" [98]. Over 3000 people were interviewed, of which 8.9 % of the women and 10 % of the men reported at least some "same-gender sexuality." They calculated the mean number of sexual partners in the past year, the past 5 years, and since age 18 and reported their results as follows (Table 13.1).

In this sample, heterosexual women had the fewest number of sexual partners, followed by heterosexual men, followed by lesbian or bisexual women, followed by gay or bisexual men.

Where do all of these men meet each other? In the past, gay men typically met other men, for sex or dates, in a variety of places, some common and ordinary places such as their place of work, school, support groups, gay bars, or clubs, but also in "seedier" places such as bath houses, rest stops along highways, public bathrooms, etc. For some, these latter places just added to the sense of shame and secrecy of being gay. One gay man summarized coming out as, "making a commit-

ment to going to sleazy places in order to have sex with other men." Certainly, not all of these places were "sleazy," and not all gay men had this impression of these places, but this was not an uncommon perception. This mindset likely contributed to the perception of what it meant to be gay. With the advent of the Internet and mobile phones came new, easier ways to meet other gay men. Liau et al. [99] did a meta-analysis of studies looking at men who had sex with men (MSM) who were recruited "offline" and found that 40 % of them had used the Internet as a venue for seeking sex partners. Garofalo et al. [100] looked at young MSM (ages 18–24) and found that 68 % of the sample had gone online to meet a sexual partner and 48 % of them had actually found a sexual partner online. Most of the young MSM report using the Internet to look for longer-term relationships, but are often frustrated by men who are interested in just sex [101]. Internet sites, such as Match.com, are often used for dating. Other sites, such as ManHunt or the Craigslist personals, are more often used for finding one-time, sexual partners. Increasingly, mobile phone apps are the primary way that gay men meet each other. Grindr, Scruff, and other phone apps allow gay men to connect with other gay men. Grindr, first launched in 2009, claims they are "the world's largest all-male, location-based, social network" and boast "over four million users in 192 countries" [102]. The Grindr app locates 100–300 other gay men who are in close proximity to the user and are currently online. This allows gay men to connect with others who are also looking for some type of immediate interaction, whether it's chatting on the app, looking for dates, looking to get together for sex, or sometimes looking to buy or sell drugs. So if a gay man is traveling to another city, he can easily connect with other gay men who are nearby, even staying in the same hotel. To many people, this is an entirely new world. It is commonly a world that is kept secret from the heterosexual community, and from healthcare practitioners, for fear of judgment.

According to the Centers for Disease Control [103], new HIV infections are highest among 25–34 year old MSM, followed by 13–24 year old MSM. Between 2008 and 2010, there was a

12 % increase in new infections in the United States. Research has been done looking at online communications and risky sexual behavior, primarily in an effort to better understand the risk of HIV transmission. Some research suggests that when men meet each other online as opposed to a bar or club, they are more likely to report higher levels of sexual risk behaviors, such as multiple sexual partners and inconsistent condom use [104–106]. Research suggests that when MSM meet other men online, they are more willing to express inhibited sexual desires and have a heightened sense of trust and intimacy [107, 108]. Garafalo [100] found that only 53 % of young men (ages 16–24) who found sexual partners online used condoms consistently.

So what does all of this mean? Unfortunately, this phenomenon has not been adequately studied or addressed by the medical community in order to create any guidelines for clinicians to think about this issue regarding mental health. It has been studied in efforts to reduce HIV transmission, but these studies don't address how to think about the mental health aspects of having multiple sexual partners. Therefore, it's up to individual clinicians to decide how to interpret having multiple sexual partners, and unfortunately, there is wide variability in how this is interpreted. These statistics make many people uncomfortable. They are most commonly cited by the Christian Right to vilify homosexuality. Therefore, some in the LGBT community would rather ignore these statistics, or discredit them. However, this fails to acknowledge a phenomenon in our culture, one that has implications for relationships and both physical and mental health. Although there are no data on how mental health practitioners view this aspect of gay culture, anecdotal experience suggests that many mental health practitioners interpret having multiple sexual partners as pathological. It can sometimes be seen as a symptom of Bipolar Disorder or Borderline Personality Disorder, in which hyper-sexuality and promiscuity can be symptoms. Other clinicians may see this behavior as representing a psychological disturbance, searching for something missing in their lives, or "acting out" in some way. Still others will call it "sex addiction." Although this is not a diagnosis recognized in DSM-5, there are treatment groups for "sex addicts" around the country for this perceived "illness." Some view this as a consequence of decades of oppression and being denied the right to marry. Some see gay men as feeling angry toward other gay men after having been treated poorly or as a sexual object, so they simply reenact what was done to them and use other men as sex objects and nothing more. Others see it as desperate loneliness and longing for connection—"looking for love in all the wrong places," so to speak. There are innumerable other interpretations for this behavior. For better or worse, if a gay man seeks mental health treatment for any reason and reveals this behavior to the mental health practitioner, this sexual behavior may very well become a focus of treatment. It would not be uncommon for a clinician to view this as a symptom of an illness that he may not have (such as Bipolar Disorder), and inappropriately treat him with medication for such a disorder. The clinician may view it as a maladaptive way of coping with depression, anxiety, or low self-esteem, and a goal of treatment would be to reduce or eliminate this behavior. Some clinicians have been known to target the "hypersexuality" itself and prescribe high doses of antidepressants or hormonal therapy, primarily to decrease libido and decrease sexual behavior [109].

So there are numerous psychological and psychiatric explanations for having multiple sexual partners, most of which are pathological. But if the prevalence of this phenomenon is not uncommon in gay men, another possible explanation is that it is a normal, healthy part of being a gay man, at least for some. It may be that men, on average, are much less inclined to monogamy and have higher libidos than women, so gay men are having sex more often and with more partners than other groups. It may be that whatever causes a man to be gay, whether it's genetic, environmental, or something else, also increases the probability that he will desire multiple sexual partners. It may be that this is a learned behavior in the gay community that just perpetuates itself, and is simply a cultural, not pathological, trait. Given the impact this behavior can have on mental and physical health, further research is certainly needed to inform clinical care.

Not all gay men are having sex with multiple partners, or even having sex at all. Kanouse et al. [92] found that 13 % of homosexual and bisexual men reported no sexual partners in the previous year. Some gay men have monogamous boyfriends. And some gay men, as will be discussed in the next section, are in long-term relationships.

What about lesbian women? Much less research has been done on lesbian dating and hooking up, given the dramatically lower prevalence of HIV and other STD's, which is the basis for much of the research on gay men's sexual behavior. Loulan [110] surveyed 1566 lesbian women and found that 43 % of lesbian women had been abstinent for a year or longer. The data regarding numbers of sexual partners, as cited earlier, suggest that lesbian women typically have similar numbers of partners to that of heterosexuals, and that one-time sex is much less common than is seen among gay men. The dating world of lesbian women seems to be much more focused on relationships than on sex, and in this way, may be more similar to that of heterosexuals and pose fewer health risks than seen in the gay male population [111].

## Long-Term Relationships and Families

As already reviewed in the section "Relationships and Health", numerous health benefits have been correlated with marriage, and to a lesser extent, co-habitation with a romantic partner. In 2001, the Netherlands was the first county in the world to legally recognize same-sex marriage. In 2003, the Massachusetts' Supreme Judicial Court ruled that denying same-sex couples the right to marry was unconstitutional. After the court ruling, same-sex couples, at least in Massachusetts, could legally marry for the first time in US history beginning in 2004. Shortly thereafter, numerous states passed constitutional amendments banning same-sex marriage. Over the ensuing decade, however, a number of states have followed the lead of Massachusetts and allowed same-sex marriage. In 2015, the United States Supreme Court overturned all state constitutional amendments banning same-sex marriage, and upheld the right of same-sex couples to legally marry throughout the country.

This revolution in equal marriage rights has galvanized the gay rights movement in many ways. Many in the LGBT community are excited to finally see full and complete acceptance of our relationships by an increasing number of people in our society, and to finally receive the same legal and financial benefits of marriage that heterosexuals receive. This may have long-term effects on our community, our ability to integrate our lives within society and families, and ultimately the mental and physical health of our community. Riggle, Rostosky, and Horne [112] looked at the effects of legally recognized relationships on the well-being of gay and lesbian people. They found that people in committed or legally recognized relationships reported less psychological distress (i.e., internalized homophobia, depressive symptoms, and stress) and more well-being (i.e., the presence of meaning in life) than single participants. Wight et al. [113] looked at the effects of same-sex legal marriage in California on psychological well-being in people who participated in the California Health Interview Survey. They found that same-sex married lesbian, gay, and bisexual people were significantly less distressed than lesbian, gay, and bisexual people not in a legally recognized relationship and that married heterosexuals were significantly less distressed than non-married heterosexuals. Furthermore, they found that psychological distress was not significantly distinguishable among same-sex married lesbian, gay, and bisexual persons; lesbian, gay, and bisexual persons in registered domestic partnerships; and heterosexuals.

Sadly, the marriage rights movement has also had adverse effects on our community, given that some states went to great efforts to pass constitutional amendments banning same-sex marriage, resulting in increased overt expression of homophobia in some of these states. Hatzenbuehler et al. [33] compared LGB people living in states that passed amendments to LGB people living in other states, and also to heterosexuals in the same states. They reported that psychiatric disorders, as defined by the Diagnostic and Statistical Manual of Mental Disorders, Fourth Edition (DSM-IV), increased significantly in LGB people living in states that banned gay marriage. They reported that mood disorders increased by 36 %, generalized anxiety disorder increased by 248 %, alcohol use disorder increased by 42 %, and psychiatric comorbidity increased by 36 %. These psychiatric disorders did not increase significantly among LGB people living in states without constitutional amendments and they found no evidence for increases of the same magnitude among heterosexuals living in the states with the constitutional amendments.

The 2010 US Census reported that there were 131,729 same-sex married couple households and 514,735 same-sex unmarried partner households residing in the United States, an 80 % increase in the number of same-sex partner households since the US Census in 2000 [114]. Given that some same-sex couples are not comfortable revealing their sexual orientation to the government, it is likely that these figures underreport the actual number of same-sex couple households. Nearly 2/3 of the same-sex marriages or registered partnerships are lesbian couples and 1/3 are gay male couples [115]. For many of these couples, their lives and relationships are identical to those of heterosexuals, so it's the usual issues of working out problems with each other, doing household chores, paying bills, socializing with friends and families, etc. Are there any significant differences? Roisman et al. [116] tried to answer this question by conducting a study with committed gay male and lesbian couples and comparing them to committed and non-committed heterosexual couples. They did multiple levels of analysis of self-reports, partner reports, laboratory observations, attachment, and measures of physiological reactivity during couple interactions. In the end, they found no differences between the committed same-sex couples and the committed heterosexual couples, with one exception—lesbian women were especially effective at working together harmoniously in laboratory observations. Kurdeck [117] followed couples over the first 10 years of co-habitation to evaluate the stability of the relationship and any

changes. Participants were both partners from couples that were lesbian, gay, heterosexual without children, and heterosexual with children. He found that relative to the other couples, lesbian couples had the highest levels of relationship quality over all assessments. The pattern of change in relationship quality varied by type of couple: lesbian and gay couples showed no change, those of heterosexual couples without children showed an early phase of accelerated decline followed by a leveling off, and those from heterosexual couples with children showed an early phase of accelerated decline followed by a second phase of accelerated decline. Both of these studies suggest that lesbian relationships appear to be the most harmonious.

The question of monogamy often comes up in regards to same-sex couples. Gay men are often thought to be in non-monogamous relationships. Hoff et al. [118] looked at 566 gay couples in San Francisco and asked about their relationship status—monogamous, open, or discrepant. They found that about half of the couples were monogamous and the other half had agreed to have an open relationship. Only 8 % were discrepant, meaning they didn't agree. It should be noted that the couples that reported being non-monogamous were open with each other about this; they presumably weren't lying to or cheating on each other. The question of monogamy in lesbian relationships is asked much less frequently, and unfortunately, there are no studies looking at this issue for lesbian relationships. One issue that does sometimes come up for lesbian relationships is the issue of reduced sexual frequency, or "lesbian bed death," a term coined by Drs. Pepper Schwartz and Phillip Blumstein in the book, American Couples: Money-Work-Sex [119]. When they asked couples how often they "had sex," they found that only about 1/3 of lesbian women in relationships of 2 years or longer had sex once a week or more, 47 % of lesbian women in long-term relationships had sex once a month or less, but only 15 % of heterosexual couples reported having sex once a week or less. Subsequent studies have also found that the frequency of sex is lowest among lesbian couples compared to other types of couples. However, Blair and Pukall [120] looked at same-sex couples (both male and female) and heterosexual couples and found that when the couples did have sex, lesbian women spent the most time on each sexual encounter compared to the other groups. They argue that it's the quality of sex that counts, not the frequency.

Despite the increases in same-sex coupling and marriage rights, the proportion of LGB people with children is decreasing [121]. This is thought to be due to LGB people coming out earlier in life and, therefore, fewer of them are engaging in heterosexual relationships prior to coming out and having children from those relationships. According to responses from the 2008 General Social Survey, 19 % of gay and bisexual men and 49 % of lesbian women and bisexual women report having a child [122]. Childbearing is substantially higher among racial and ethnic minorities. While the childbearing rates are decreasing, the proportion of same-sex couples who have adopted children has nearly doubled from 10 to 19 % between 2000 and 2009 [121]. Overall, according to Census data, in 2000, about 63,000 same-sex couples were raising children, and in 2010, it's up to 110,000.

These trends are exciting for the LGBT communities. If, in fact, social acceptance of our differences and our ability to engage in meaningful relationships and connections with other people can be protective against mental health problems, these recent trends will likely help our community and hopefully normalize our rates of mental health issues with the rest of the population.

## Assessment and Treatment of the LGBT Population

### General Principles

People with minority sexual orientations and gender identities suffer from the same types of psychiatric illness as do the general population, although often at higher rates. The principles of psychiatric care are therefore the same, regardless of a particular patient's identity. An attitude of gentle curiosity balanced with compassion for a person's suffering and respect for their experience and strength underlies all effective psychiatric interventions. Providers should not feel daunted by the specialized mental health needs of LGBT patients!

As with all health care encounters, our patients are our best teachers. We've all had the uncomfortable experience of feeling "caught" in our own ignorance about a particular patient's situation—whether our lack of knowledge involves the medical nuances of an HIV regimen or which pronouns to use when referring to a gender nonconforming spouse. It's more comfortable to feel like an "expert," but given our diverse communities and the explosion of specialized medical knowledge, achieving a state of generalized "expertise" represents more of an ideal than a reality. When feeling "caught" in our own ignorance, it generally works best to acknowledge the gap in our knowledge base and enlist the patient's experience and available medical resources in a transparent and timely manner. Patients don't expect us to be perfect.

## The Treatment Relationship and the Provider's Identity

Any treatment interaction involves two people, each of whom has two identities: a private, perhaps unrealized, core identity and the persona which they choose to present within the relationship. This extends to matters of sexual orientation and gender identity. Consider the example of a male patient who has unprotected sex "on the down low" with other men but chooses to keep this behavior a secret from his wife and family. Imagine that his PCP, on the other hand, proudly identifies as a married lesbian woman in her private life. Perhaps both are parents, though by very different routes. Does she, either directly or indirectly, convey her minority sexual orientation? Does he assume (based on her wedding band and the family photos in her office) that she is straight? Will this man disclose his high risk sexual behavior and receive the medical care that he needs?

While this example is extreme, it highlights the complicated matrix of identity and disclosure that takes place within any treatment relationship.

LGBT patients are constantly "scanning for safety," attempting to discern whether a person is a role model, a supportive ally, a neutral figure, a moralizing critic, or a homophobic threat [123]. This extends to interactions with health care providers, about whom LGBT patients often feel an apprehensive curiosity. Patients may try to alleviate these emotions through direct inquiry, indirect inquiry (such as leading questions), or through direct investigation (made easier with the advent of the internet) [124].

Conversely, providers may choose to keep their identity private or disclose it in either a direct or an indirect manner. Disclosure may occur by accident (such as a patient reading a wedding announcement in the newspaper). Unfortunately, there are no hard and fast rules to guide the provider in making this decision. Self-disclosure of a provider's identity can sometimes help patients who are struggling with coming out and would like to normalize their experience, but it comes with the risks of over-identification and subtle boundary challenges (in either direction). Ultimately, providers must consider (1) the best interests of their patient, (2) their comfort with their own sexual or gender identity, (3) their training and theoretical position, and (4) their need for privacy vs. their wish to integrate various aspects of their identity (sexual, gender, personal, professional) [124].

The real—and perceived—identity of both patient and therapist can significantly affect a treatment relationship. Levounis and Anson have proposed the following matrix to highlight common themes involving identity that can arise in the patient-provider dyad (Table 13.2).

LGBT patients who work with self-identified LGBT providers may find useful rapport, familiarity, and understanding, but the provider should be wary of making assumptions about the patient or over-identifying with their problems. Similarly, a concordant straight dyad may experience an easy rapport but also collude in avoiding active issues of sexuality and gender. A straight provider caring for an LGBT patient may have to work to gain the patient's trust and become more culturally competent. Finally, LGBT providers need to consider that straight patients may experience complicated feelings (potentially including embarrassment, guilt, discomfort, or homophobia) during their interactions.

## Coming Out

"Coming out" or "coming out of the closet" refers to the process of disclosing one's sexual orientation and/or gender identity. Coming out is a highly individual and uniquely personal experience influenced by one's personality, development, resources, family, social environment, and cultural background. There is no single "correct" or "best" way to come out.

The process of coming out as LGBT to oneself and others can be understood as a developmental process that proceeds through a series of milestones. There are a variety of different models explaining the emergence of positive self-identity among people with a minority sexual orientation or gender identity. Models of lesbian, gay, and bisexual identity development generally

**Table 13.2** Patient-provider dryad

|  | LGBT patient | Straight patient |
|---|---|---|
| LGBT provider | Rapport vs. over-identification | Understanding vs. shame |
| Straight provider | Trust vs. mistrust | Openness vs. closure |

Adapted from Levounis and Anson [124]

include variations of the following milestone events:

- Feeling different from peers
- Same-sex attractions
- Questioning assumed heterosexuality
- Experimenting with sexual behaviors
- Self-identification
- Disclosure
- Romantic relationships
- Self-acceptance and synthesis [125]

A somewhat similar model describing the "states of transgender emergence" has been proposed by Arlene Ishtar Lev:

- Awareness
- Seeking information/reaching out
- Disclosure to significant others
- Exploration: Identity and self-labeling
- Exploration: Transition issues/possible body modification
- Integration: Acceptance and post-transition issues [126]

Lev is careful to avoid a proscriptive model of identity formation, noting that the narrative of "woman trapped in a man's body" (or vice-versa), while expected by many clinicians, simply reinforces the gender binary and does not describe the actual lived experience of many transgender and gender non-conforming individuals [126].

The importance of coming out may be changing over time; as homophobia and transphobia abates, LGBT people may be feeling less pressure to define their identity or announce it publicly. This trend towards more flexible and nuanced patterns of identity is particularly evident among young adults, who are embracing a range of sexualities and genders (including pan-sexuality and gender non-conformance in addition to LGBT identities) with ease and frequency that often surprises older LGBT people. For a fortunate minority of young people, the focus has shifted from defining oneself in a hostile environment to simply being oneself in a more tolerant one.

## Assessment and Treatment of LGBT Patients

The mental health assessment of LGBT patients is not fundamentally different from that of non-LGBT patients. However, given the specific mental health risks faced by LGBT people, it is useful to keep in mind some general principles and questions:

1. Create a welcoming practice: Consider the overall experience of LGBT patients seeking care in your practice. Creating a safe space will help patients feel comfortable and share critical information. Do you have pride symbols, "safe space" stickers, or LGBT-themed magazines in the waiting area? Are front office staff trained on how to maintain a safe and welcoming environment? Do you have a gender neutral bathroom for trans patients?
2. Practice forms: The paperwork that patients complete can set the tone for an encounter. Inclusive intake forms generally ask the following questions:
   (a) What is your gender? (options include male, female, transgender [male to female], transgender [female to male], gender non-conforming, other, and declines to answer)
   (b) What sex were you assigned at birth? (options include male, female, or something else)
   (c) What is your sexual orientation? (options include heterosexual, gay, lesbian, bisexual, queer, other, and declines to answer)
   (d) What sex/gender are your sexual partners? (Check all that apply—options include none, male, female, or transgender)
3. Language: follow the patient's example in using words to describe sexual orientation and gender identity. If you are uncertain, ask directly—for example, "What name would you like me to use when addressing you? What pronouns would you like me to use when speaking about you with other providers?"

4. Screening: LGBT people face elevated risks of most mental health conditions. This is largely due to internalized sexual prejudice and minority stress. Be sure to screen thoroughly for conditions that pose an increased risk for members of this population.
5. Trans-specific issues: familiarize yourself with the World Professional Association for Transgender Health's Standards of Care document (available online at www.wpath.org)

# References

1. American Psychiatric Association. Diagnostic and statistical manual of mental disorders. 5th ed. Arlington, VA: American Psychiatric Association; 2013.
2. Association AP. DSM5.org. [Online]. 2013 [cited 21 Apr 2014]. Available from: http://www.dsm5.org/Documents/Gender%20Dysphoria%20Fact%20Sheet.pdf.
3. Foucault M. The history of sexuality, volume 1: An introduction. London: Allen Lane; 1976.
4. Freud S. Three essays on the theory of sexuality. 1962nd ed. New York: Basic; 1905.
5. Freud S. Letter to an American mother (1935). Am J Psychiatry. 1951;107(10):786–7.
6. Ernulf K, Innala S, Whitam F. Biological explanation, psychological explanation, and tolerance of homosexuals: a cross-national analysis of beliefs and attitudes. Psychol Rep. 1989;65(3):1003–10.
7. Bailey J, Pillard R. A genetic study of male sexual orientation. J Theor Biol. 1997;185(3):373–8.
8. Langstrom N, Rahman Q, Carlstrom E, Lichtenstein P. Genetic and environmental effects on same-sex sexual behavior: a population study of twins in Sweden. Arch Sex Behav. 2010;39(1):75–80.
9. Hamer D, Hu S, Magnuson V, Hu N, Pattanucci A. A linkage between DNA markers on the X chromosome and male sexual orientation. Science. 1993;261(5119):321–7.
10. Park D, Choi D, Lee J, Lim D, Park C. Male-like sexual behavior of female mouse lacking fucose mutarotase. BMC Genet. 2010;11:62.
11. Blanchard R, Klassen P. H-Y antigen and homosexuality in men. J Theor Biol. 1997;185(3):373–8.
12. LeVay S. A difference in hypothalamic structure between heterosexual and homosexual men. Science. 1991;253(5023):1034–7.
13. Butler J. Gender trouble: feminism and the subversion of identity. New York: Routledge; 1990.
14. Benjamin J. In defense of gender ambiguity. Gend Psychoanal. 1996;1(1):27–43.
15. Lee P, Houk C, Ahmed S, Hughs I. Consensus statement on management of intersex disorders. Pediatrics. 2006;118(2):e488–500.
16. Dohrenwend B. Social status and psychological disorder: an issue of substance and an issue of method. Am Sociol Rev. 1966;31(1):14–34.
17. Dohrenwend B. The role of adversity and stress in psychopathology: some evidence and its implications for theory and research. J Health Soc Behav. 2000;41(1):1–19.
18. Meyer I. Prejudice and discrimination as social stressors. In: Meyer I, Northridge M, editors. The health of sexual minorities. Washington, DC: APA; 2007. p. 242–67.
19. Pascoe E, Richman L. Perceived discrimination and health: a meta-analytic review. Psychol Bull. 2009;153(4):531–54.
20. Mays V, Cochran S. Mental health correlates of perceived discrimination among LGBT adults in the United States. Am J Public Health. 2001;91(11):1869–76.
21. Newcomb M, Mustanski B. Internalized homophobia and internalizing mental health problems: a meta-analytic review. Clin Psychol Rev. 2010;30:1019–29.
22. Suicide Prevention Resource Center [Online]. Newton, MA: Education Development Center; 2008 [cited 21 Apr 2014]. Available from: http://www.sprc.org.
23. Haas A, Eliason M, Mays V, et al. Suicide and suicide risk in lesbian, gay, bisexual, and transgender populations: review and recommendations. J Homosex. 2011;58:10–51.
24. King M, Semlyan J, Tai S, Killaspy H, Osborn D, Popelyuk D, et al. A systematic review of mental disorder, suicide, and deliberate self harm in lesbian, gay and bisexual people. BMC Psychiatry. 2008;8(70):e1–17.
25. Koh A, Ross L. Mental health issues: a comparison of lesbian, bisexual and heterosexual women. J Homosex. 2006;51(1):33–57.
26. Meyer I, Dietrich J, Schwartz S. Lifetime prevalence of mental disorders and suicide attempts in diverse lesbian, gay, and bisexual populations. Am J Public Health. 2008;98(6):1004–6.
27. Bolton SL, Sareen J. Sexual orientation and Its relation to mental disorders and suicide attempts: findings from a nationally representative sample. Can J Psychiatry. 2011;56(1):35–43.
28. Bostwick W, Boyd C, Hughes T, McCabe S. Dimensions of sexual orientation and the prevalence of mood and anxiety disorders in the United States. Am J Public Health. 2010;100(3):468–75.
29. Cochran S, Mays V. Lifetime prevalence of suicide symptoms and affective disorders among men reporting same-sex sexual partners: results from NHANES III. Am J Public Health. 2000;90(4):573–8.
30. Hoffmann B. An overview of depression among transgender women. Depress Res Treat. 2014;2014:1–9.

31. Bockting W, Miner M, Swinburne Romine R, Hamilton A, Coleman E. Stigma, mental health, and resilience in an online sample of the US transgender population. Am J Public Health. 2013;103(5): 943–51.

32. Gorin-Lazard A, et al. Hormonal therapy is associated with better self-esteem, mood, and quality of life in transsexuals. J Nerv Ment Disord. 2013;201:996–1000.

33. Hatzenbuehler ML, McLaughlin KA, Keyes KM, Hasin DS. The impact of institutional discrimination on psychiatric disorders in lesbian, gay, and bisexual populations: a prospective study. Am J Public Health. 2010;100:452–9.

34. Potok M. Southern Poverty Law Center. [Online]. 2010 [cited 21 Apr 2014]. Available from: http://www.splcenter.org/get-informed/intelligence-report/browse-all-issues/2010/winter/anti-gay-hate-crimes-doing-the-math.

35. Alessi E, Martin J, Gyamerah A, Meyer I. Prejudice-related events and traumatic stress among heterosexuals and lesbian women, gay men and bisexual women. J Aggression Maltreat Trauma. 2013;22(5):510–26.

36. Roberts A, Austin S, Corliss H, Vandermorris A, Koenen K. Pervasive trauma exposure among US sexual orientation minority adults and risk of post-traumatic stress disorder. Am J Public Health. 2010;100(12):2433–41.

37. Gordon A, Meyer I. Gender nonconformity as a target of prejudice, discrimination, and violence against LGB individuals. J LGBT Health Res. 2007;3(3):55–71.

38. National Center for Transgender Equality and the National Gay and Lesbian Task Force. Findings of the National Transgender Discrimination Survey. [Online]. 2009 [cited 21 Apr 2014]. Available from: http://www.endtransdiscrimination.org/PDFs/ntds_state_ma.pdf.

39. Lombardi E, Wilchins R, Priesing D, Malouf D. Gender violence: transgender experiences with violence and discrimination. J Homosex. 2001;42(1):89–101.

40. Feldman M, Meyer I. Eating disorders in diverse lesbian, gay, and bisexual populations. Int J Eat Disord. 2007;40(3):218–26.

41. Russell C, Keel P. Homosexuality as a specific risk factor for eating disorders in men. Int J Eat Disord. 2002;31:300–6.

42. Seiver M. Sexual orientation and gender as factors in socioculturally acquired vulnerability to body dissatisfaction and eating disorders. J Consult Clin Psychol. 1994;62:252–60.

43. Brown T, Keel P. The impact of relationships on the association between sexual orientation and disordered eating in men. Int J Eat Disord. 2012;45(6):792–9.

44. Kaminski P, Chapman B, Haynes S, Own L. Body image, eating behaviors, and attitudes toward exercise among gay and straight men. Eat Behav. 2005;6:179–87.

45. Yelland C, Tiggemann M. Muscularity and the gay ideal: body dissatisfaction and disordered eating in homosexual men. Eat Behav. 2003;4:107–16.

46. Pope C, Pope H, Menard W, Fay C, Olivardia O, Phillips K. Clinical features of muscle dysmorphia among males with body dysmorphic disorder. Body Image. 2005;2(4):395–400.

47. Pope H, Phillips K. The Adonis complex: the secret crisis of male body obsession. New York: Free; 2000.

48. Mereish E, Bradford J. Intersecting identities and substance use problems: sexual orientation, gender, race, and lifetime substance use problems. J Stud Alcohol Drugs. 2014;75:179–88.

49. Lee JG, Griffin G, Melvin C. Tobacco use among sexual minorities in the USA, 1987 to May 2007. Tob Control. 2009;18:275–82.

50. American Lung Association. Disparities in lung health series. [Online]. 2010 [cited 26 Apr 2014]. Available from: http://www.lung.org/assets/documents/publications/lung-disease-data/lgbt-report.pdf.

51. Cochran S, Sullivan J, Mays V. Prevalence of mental disorders, psychological distress, and mental health services use among lesbian, gay, and bisexual adults in the United States. J Consult Clin Psychol. 2003;71(1):53–61.

52. Cochran B, Cauce A. Characteristics of lesbian, gay, bisexual, and transgender individuals entering substance abuse treatment. J Subst Abuse Treat. 2006;30:135–46.

53. Flentje A, Heck N, Sorensen J. Characteristics of transgender individuals entering substance abuse treatment. Addict Behav. 2014;39:969–75.

54. Benotsch E, Zimmerman R, Cathers L, McNulty S, Pierce J, Heck T, et al. Non-medical use of prescription drugs, polysubstance use, and mental health in transgender adults. Drug Alcohol Depend. 2013;132:391–4.

55. Senreich E. LGBT specialized treatment: are specialized LGBT program components helpful for gay and bisexual men in substance abuse treatment? Subst Use Misuse. 2010;45:1077–96.

56. Stone M. The fate of borderline patients. New York: Guilford; 1990.

57. Paris J, Zweig-Frank H, Guzder J. Psychological factors associated with homosexuality in males with borderline personality disorder. J Pers Disord. 1995;9:56–61.

58. Zubenko G, George A, Soloff P, Schultz P. Sexual practices among patients with borderline personality disorder. Am J Psychiatry. 1987;144(6):748–52.

59. Dulit R, Fyer M, Miller F, Sacks M, Frances A. Gender differences in sexual preference and substance abuse of inpatients with borderline personality disorder. J Pers Disord. 1993;7:182–5.

60. Reich D, Zanarini M. Sexual orientation and relationship choice in borderline personality disorder over ten years of prospective follow-up. J Pers Disord. 2008;22(6):564–72.

61. Singh D, McMain S, Zucker K. Gender identity and sexual orientation in women with borderline personality disorder. J Sex Med. 2011;8:447–54.

62. Grant J, Flynn M, Odlaug B, Schreiber L. Personality disorders in gay, lesbian, bisexual, and transgender chemically dependent patients. Am J Addict. 2011;20(5):405–11.

63. Kalichman S, Benotsch E, Rompa D, Gore-Felton C, Austin J, Luke W. Unwanted sexual experiences and sexual risks in gay and bisexual men: associations among revictimization, substance use, and psychiatric symptoms. J Sex Res. 2001;38:1–9.

64. Eubanks-Carter C, Goldfriend M. The impact of client sexual orientation and gender on clinical judgements and diagnosis of borderline personality disorder. J Clin Psychol. 2006;62:751–70.

65. Berkman L. Social networks and health. In: World Health Organization conference, Geneva. 2010.

66. Somers A. Marital status, health, and use of health services: an old relationship revisited. JAMA. 1979;241:1818–22.

67. Abel-Smith B, Titmuss R. The cost of the National Health Service in England and Wales Cambridge. Cambridge: Cambridge University Press; 1956.

68. Pollack E. Mental health indices of family health. World Health Statistics Report. 1975.

69. Durkheim E. Suicide: a study in sociology. London: Free; 1951.

70. Cohen S, Doyle WJ, Skoner DP, Rabin BS, Gwaltney Jr JM. Social ties and susceptibility to the common cold. JAMA. 1997;25(277):1940–4.

71. Williams RB, Barefoot JC, Califf RM, Haney TL, Saunders WB, Pryor DB, Hlatky MA, Siegler IC, Mark DB. Prognostic importance of social and economic resources among medically treated patients with angiographically documented coronary artery disease. JAMA. 1992;267(4):520–4.

72. Berkman LF, Leo-Summer L, Horwitz RI. Emotional support and survival following myocardial infarction. Ann Intern Med. 1992;117(12):1003–9.

73. Aizer AA, Chen MH, McCarthy EP, Mendu ML, Koo S, White TJ, et al. Marital status and survival in patients with cancer. J Clin Oncol. 2013;31(31):3869–76.

74. DeKlyen M, Brooks-Gunn J, McLanahan S, Knab J. The mental health of married, cohabiting, and non-coresident parents with infants. J Public Health. 2006;96(10):1836–41.

75. Hughes ME, Waite LJ. Marital biography and health at mid-life. J Health Soc Behav. 2009;50(3):344–58.

76. Kessler R, Walters E, Forthofer M. The social consequences of psychiatric disorders, III: Probability of marital stability. Am J Psychiatry. 1998;155:1092–6.

77. Breslau J, Miller E, Jin R, Sampson NA, Alonso J, Andrade LH, et al. A multinational study of mental disorders, marriage, and divorce. Acta Psychiatr Scand. 2011;124(6):474–86.

78. Friedman CK, Morgan EM. Comparing sexual-minority and heterosexual young women's. J Youth Adolesc. 2009;38(7):920–36.

79. Ryan C, Huebner D, Diaz RM, Sanchez J. Family rejection as a predictor of negative health outcomes in white and Latino lesbian, gay, and bisexual young adults. Pediatrics. 2009;123(1):346–52.

80. Galupo M. Cross-category friendship patterns: comparison of heterosexual and sexual minority adults. J Soc Pers Relat. 2009;26(6-7):811–31.

81. Nardi P. Gay men's friendships. Chicago, IL: University of Chicago Press; 1999.

82. Bahns AJ, Pickett KM, Crandall CS. Social ecology of similarity: big schools, small school and social relationships. Group Process Intergroup Relat. 2011;15(1):119–31.

83. Monsour M. Women and men as friends: relationships across the life span in the 21st century. Mahwah, NJ: Lawrence Erlbaum; 2002.

84. Kaplan C, Keys D. Sex and relationship variables as predictors of sexual attraction in cross-sex platonic friendships between young heterosexual adults. J Soc Pers Relat. 1997;14(2):191–206.

85. Afifi SL, Faulkner W. On being 'just friends': the frequency and impact of sexual activity in cross-sex friendships. J Soc Pers Relat. 2000;17(2):205–22.

86. Bleske-Rechek A, Somers E, Micke C, Erickson L, Matteson L, Stocco C, Schumacher B, Ritchie L. Benefit or burden? Attraction in cross-sex friendship. J Soc Pers Relat. 2012;29:569–96.

87. Castro-Convers K, Gray LA, Ladany N, Metzler AE. Interpersonal contact experiences with gay men: a qualitative investigation of "fag hags" and gay-supportive heterosexual men. J Homosex. 2005;49:47–76.

88. Grigoriou T. Friendship between gay men and heterosexual women: an interpretive phenomenological analysis. London: London South Bank University, Families and Social Capital ESRC Research Group; 2004.

89. Moon D. Insult and inclusion: the term fag hag and gay male community. Soc Forces. 1995;74:487–510.

90. Russell EM, DelPriore DJ, Butterfield ME, Hill SE. Friends with benefits, but without sex: straight women and gay men exchange trustworthy mating advice. Evol Psychol. 2013;11(1):132–47.

91. Barash JE, Lipton DE. The myth of monogamy. New York: WH Freeman; 2001.

92. Kanouse DE, Berry SH, Gorman EM, Yano EM, Carson S. Response to the AIDS epidemic: a survey of homosexual and bisexual men in Los Angeles County. Santa Monica, CA: RAND; 1991.

93. Fitzpatrick R, Dawson J, Boulton M, McLean J, Hart G, Brookes M. Perceptions of general practice among homosexual men. Br J Gen Pract. 1994;44(379):80–2.

94. Gerbert B, Bleecker T, Bernzweig J. Anybody talking to physicians about acquired immunodeficiency syndrome and sex? A national survey of patients. Arch Fam Med. 1993;2(1):45–51.

95. Nusbaum CD, Hamilton MR. The proactive sexual health history. Am Fam Physician. 2002;66(9):1705–12.

96. Bell MS, Weinberg AP. Homosexualities: a study of diversity among men and women. South Melbourne: Macmillan; 1978.

97. Fay RE, Turner CF, Klassen AD, Gagnon JH. Prevalence and patterns of same-gender sexual contact among men. Science. 1989;243:338–48.

98. Laumann EO, Gagnon JH, Michael RT, Michaels S. The social organization of sexuality: sexual practices in the United States. Chicago, IL: University of Chicago Press; 1994.

99. Liau A, Millett G, Marks G. Meta-analytic examination of online sex-seeking and sexual risk behaviour among men who have sex with men. Sex Transm Dis. 2006;33:576–84.

100. Garofalo R, Herrick A, Mustanski BS, Donenberg GR. Tip of the iceberg: young men who have sex with men, the Internet, and HIV risk. Am J Public Health. 2007;97:1–6.

101. Kubicek K, Carpineto J, McDavitt B, Weiss G, Kipke MD. Use and perceptions of the internet for sexual information and partners: a study of young men who have sex with men. Arch Sex Behav. 2011;40:803–16.

102. Grindr. [Online]. 2014 [cited 11 Apr 2014]. Available from: http://grindr.com/learn-more.

103. Centers for Disease Control—HIV Incidence. [Online]. 2010 [cited 11 Apr 2014]. Available from: http://www.cdc.gov/hiv/statistics/surveillance/incidence/.

104. Benotsch EG, Kalichman S, Cage M. Men who have met sex partners via the Internet: prevalence, predictors, and implications for HIV prevention. Arch Sex Behav. 2002;31(2):177–83.

105. Ogilvie GS, Taylor D, Trussler T, Marchand R, Gilbert M, Moniruzzaman A, et al. Seeking sexual partners on the internet: a marker for risky sexual behaviour in men who have sex with men. Can J Public Health. 2008;99(3):185–8.

106. Bull SS, McFarlane M, Rietmeijer C. HIV and sexually transmitted infection risk behaviors among men seeking sex with men online. Am J Public Health. 2001;91(6):988–9.

107. Ross MW. Typing, doing, and being: sexuality and the internet. J Sex Res. 2005;42(4):342–52.

108. Bauermeister J, Giguere R, Carballo-Dieguez A, Ventuneac A, Eisenberg A. Perceived risks and strategies employed by young men who have sex with men when seeking online sexual partners. J Health Commun. 2010;15(6):679–90.

109. Kafka M. Hypersexual disorder: a proposed diagnosis for DSM-V. Arch Sex Behav. 2010;39:377–400.

110. Loulan J. Research on the sex practices of 1,566 lesbian women and the clinical implications. Women Ther. 1988;7:221–34.

111. Nichols M. Lesbian relationships: implications for the study of sexuality and gender. In: McWhirter DP, Sanders SA, Reinisch JM, editors. Homosexuality/heterosexuality: concepts of sexual orientation. New York: Oxford University Press; 1990. p. 350–64.

112. Riggel EDB, Rostosky SS, Horne SG. Psychological distress, well-being, and legal recognition in same-sex couple relationships. J Fam Psychol. 2010;24(1):82–6.

113. Wight RG, LeBlanc AJ, Badgett MVL. Same-sex legal marriage and psychological well-being: findings from the California Health Interview Survey. Am J Public Health. 2013;103(2):339–46.

114. US Census Bureau. [Online]. 2011 [cited 4 Apr 2014]. Available from: http://www.census.gov/newsroom/releases/archives/2010_census/cb11-cn181.html.

115. Badgett MV, Herman JL. Patterns of relationship recognition by same-sex couples in the United States. Los Angeles, CA: Williams Institute; 2011.

116. Roisman GI, Clausell E, Holland A, Fortuna K, Elieff C. Adult romantic relationships as contexts of human development: a multimethod comparison of same-sex couples with opposite-sex dating, engaged, and married dyads. Dev Psychol. 2008;44(1):91–101.

117. Kurdek L. Change in relationship quality for partners from lesbian, gay male, and heterosexual couples. J Fam Psychol. 2008;22(5):701–11.

118. Hoff C, Beougher S, Chakravarty D, Darbel L, Neilands T. Relationship characteristics and motivations behind agreements among gay male couples: differences by agreement type and couple serostatus. AIDS Care. 2010;22(7):827–35.

119. Schwartz P, Blumstein P. American couples: money, work, sex. New York: William Morrow; 1983.

120. Blair K, Pukall C. Sexual orientation & gender differences in the duration of sexual activity within same-sex and mixed-sex relationships. In: International Association of Relationships Research, July, Chicago; 2012.

121. Gates G. Family formation and raising children among same-sex couples. Los Angeles, CA: Williams Institute, National Council on Family Relations; 2011.

122. General Social Survey. [Online]. 2008 [cited 11 Apr 2014]. Available from: http://www3.norc.org/gss+website/.

123. Garramone P. PFLAG speaks about experiences with LGBTQ youth. Greater Boston PFLAG Connections. 2014.

124. Levounis P, Anson A. Sexual identity in patient-therapist relationships. In: Levounis P, Drescher J, Barber M, editors. The LGBT casebook. Washington, DC: American Psychiatric Association; 2012.

125. Cohen K, Savin-Williams R. Coming out to self and others. In: Levounis P, Drescher J, Barber M, editors. The LGBT casebook. Washington, DC: American Psychiatric Association; 2012.

126. Lev A. Transgender emergence: therapeutic guidelines for working with gender-variant people and their families. New York: Routledge; 2004.

# Sexually Transmitted Infections in LGBT Populations

# 14

Andrew J. Para, Stephen E. Gee, and John A. Davis

## Learning Objectives

- Describe the epidemiology of STIs in the LGBT community *(PC5)*
- Discuss how risk for different STIs varies by sexual behavior *(KP4, PC5)*
- List the different treatment and management strategies for various STIs *(PC5, PC6)*

A.J. Para, M.D. (✉)
Department of Medicine, Northwestern University Feinberg School of Medicine, Chicago, IL 60611, USA
e-mail: Andrew.para@osumc.edu

S.E. Gee, M.D.
Department of Obstetrics and Gynecology, Ohio State University College of Medicine, Columbus, OH 43201, USA
e-mail: stephen.gee@osumc.edu

J.A. Davis, M.D., Ph.D.
Department of Infectious Diseases, Ohio State University College of Medicine, 370 West Ninth Avenue, 155A Meiling Hall, Columbus, OH 43201, USA
e-mail: john.davis@osumc.edu

## Introduction

### LGBT Populations and Sexually Transmitted Infections

As mentioned elsewhere in this text, LGBT persons are estimated to make up some 5–10 % of the US population, yet are at disproportionately increased risk of many health conditions. One of the areas in which this was initially appreciated was with sexually transmitted infections (STI), particularly in men who have sex with men (MSM). For example, MSM accounted for about 50 % of all new HIV infections in 2011 [1]. In the same year at CDC STD Surveillance Network sites, 72 % of newly diagnosed primary and secondary syphilis was in MSM [2]. We begin this chapter with a discussion of sexual behavior and how to elicit appropriate information in a sexual history. We then discuss, briefly, the limitations presented by the literature that focuses more on behavior than on identity, and how identity plays a role in STI transmission via networks. The next major section of this chapter is a discussion of the epidemiology, clinical presentation, treatment, and prevention of the key STI pathogens. The final section deals with the common clinical syndromes encountered in STI, including the diagnostic approach to each.

One other caveat: as is evident by the references and discussion that follow, the literature has

© Springer International Publishing Switzerland 2016
K.L. Eckstrand, J.M. Ehrenfeld (eds.), *Lesbian, Gay, Bisexual, and Transgender Healthcare*,
DOI 10.1007/978-3-319-19752-4_14

been dominated by STI in MSM, to the relative exclusion of any other LBT populations. Where possible, we have included discussion of the extant literature on women who have sex with women (WSW), lesbian, bisexual, and trans populations.

## Sexual Behavior and STI Risk

The distinctions amongst sex, gender, and sexuality are particularly important in the discussion about STI and STI risk. It is imperative to note that an individual's sexual behavior—not identity—is the primary determinant of his or her risk of STI exposure and acquisition. Some providers will make decisions about screening based either on how a patient identifies (e.g., "Only gay patients need to be screened for HIV"), or worse, based on how the provider *perceives* their identification/sexual orientation (e.g., "Well, I wouldn't screen him for HIV because he doesn't seem gay"). Whether a man identifies as "gay" or "straight", it is clear that if that man participates in unprotected receptive anal intercourse with another man (amongst other behaviors), there is a higher risk of acquisition of HIV, and that man should be screened for HIV. The sexual history, then, should focus on behavior first. If a clinician can clarify patients' specific sexual acts, he/she can appropriately assess their potential sites of infection and pathogen exposures.

Consider a self-identified straight male who regularly has insertive oral and anal sex with other men. These *behaviors* put him at risk for urogenital STI acquisition from his male sexual partner(s) regardless of his discordant sexual identity. A different self-identified straight male may have insertive *and* receptive oral and anal sex with other men. This man is thus at risk for STI exposure at his pharynx and anorectum in addition to his urogenital tract. Even though both of these men identify as straight and have sex with other men, their individual STI risks are different. Now consider a self-identified straight male who only participates in receptive oral and anal sex with other men but also has penetrative oral and vaginal sex with women. This man is at risk for urogenital, pharyngeal, and anorectal STI acquisition. However, he is likely exposed to different types of pathogens at his urogenital tract in comparison to his pharynx and anorectum based on the variability of pathogens that affect WSM versus MSM. It may seem challenging and cumbersome to delve into the details of patients' sexual activities but these specific behaviors differentiate patients' risks on an individual basis and permit appropriate risk reduction counseling and screening. It is thus important that culturally competent providers become comfortable with discussing sex and sexual behaviors with *all* of their patients.

## Behavior Versus Sexual Orientation

The terms "MSM" and "WSW" have been widely incorporated into sexual health literature because of their inherent objectivity in differentiating populations of sexual minorities from their heterosexual counterparts. This methodology was intended to give researchers the advantage of generalizing a non-heterosexual population based solely on its members' sexual behaviors without implicating their social variability. As stated previously, sexual behavior is what primarily determines STI risk. However, opponents of this research model argue that this cultural stripping inhibits effective interpretation of data associated with specific sexual behaviors as an individual's sexual identity and behavior are intrinsically interconnected [3, 4]. From a health care provider's perspective, it is important to note that subpopulations of MSM (e.g. openly gay men versus men "on the DL") may have different social networks, may engage in different specific sexual behaviors, and, thus, may have different STI risks. This point highlights the need for clinicians to assess patients' sexual identities *and* behaviors when taking sexual histories. Further, research strategies that assess the variance within "MSM" and "WSW" from population perspective are needed so health care providers can recognize the risks associated with specific sexual identities within the generalized MSM and WSW groups.

# A Discussion of Key Pathogens

## Human Immunodeficiency Virus

### Epidemiology

Human immunodeficiency virus (HIV), the etiologic agent of the Acquired Immunodeficiency Syndrome (AIDS), infects approximately 2.3 million people globally and 50,000 people in the United States annually [5, 6]. While treatment standards and implementation differ markedly for developed versus developing nations, overall our ability to treat HIV (with highly active antiretroviral therapy, or HAART) has improved the overall survival of those infected with HIV. With mortality rates lower than incidence rates, the prevalence of HIV has increased overall, and there are an estimated 35.3 million people globally, and 1.1 million people in the US, living with HIV [5, 6].

HIV is an infection that is disproportionately represented in those with barriers to access of health care. The largest proportion of those newly diagnosed with HIV and living with HIV overall are MSM. In addition, racial/ethnic minority populations are overrepresented in HIV infections. According to Centers for Disease Control and Prevention (CDC) data, MSM, while only 2–5 % of the US population, accounted for 63 % of all new HIV infections in 2010 [7]. Likewise, African-American males are infected with HIV at an eightfold higher rate than white males [8]. The highest rate of HIV infection is currently in young (ages 13–24) MSM of color [8].

It is also important to note that accurate statistics for HIV infection are somewhat compromised by barriers to testing (see Clinical Presentation and Diagnosis, below). The CDC estimates that 16 % of those currently living with HIV in the US are unaware of their diagnosis [6]. There are also data to show that this fact has implications for the propagation of HIV in communities (see Prevention, below).

### Clinical Presentation

HIV is a retrovirus that replicates in host immune cells (primarily CD4+ T cells) and, as a part of viral replication, causes destruction of many of those cells. HIV infection and the host response

are dynamic, with most infected individuals mounting a robust, but ultimately ineffective immune response. After infection, an initial high viral load is usually brought under some level of control, while destruction and regeneration of immune cells reaches a steady state. When this process shifts in favor of viral replication, the immune system deteriorates and opportunistic infections (OIs) may ensue. In the absence of effective immune reconstitution, infections may progress unchecked, leading to morbidity and, ultimately, mortality. This process is summarized graphically in Fig. 14.1.

Clinical manifestations depend primarily on when in the course of infection a patient is encountered. In the initial viremic phase (acute HIV), symptomatic patients often present with a mononucleosis-like syndrome (fevers, generalized lymphadenopathy, occasionally with sore throat). However, approximately half of all individuals infected with HIV may be asymptomatic, even in the acute phase of the illness [9]. In advanced HIV disease (AIDS), symptoms such as fever, night sweats, weight loss, and inappetance are common. Likewise, as patients with advanced HIV disease are at risk for opportunistic infections, symptoms of OI may predominate, based on pathogen and/or site of infection. Common clinical syndromes encountered with OI in AIDS include meningitis/encephalitis, pneumonia, gastroenteritis/colitis, and undifferentiated fever.

### Diagnosis

The United States Preventive Services Task Force (USPSTF) has issued recommendations for screening patients for HIV (see Table 14.1) [10]. The standard testing protocol includes use of an HIV enzyme-linked immunosorbent assay (ELISA) for initial screening, and then Western blot for confirmatory testing. As both of these rely on an immune response (antibody formation), neither is sensitive for screening for acute HIV. For acute HIV, nucleic acid testing or antigen testing would be more appropriate. Screening may sometimes lead to an "indeterminate" result. In such cases, though there are many causes of a false positive ELISA (and occasionally even a

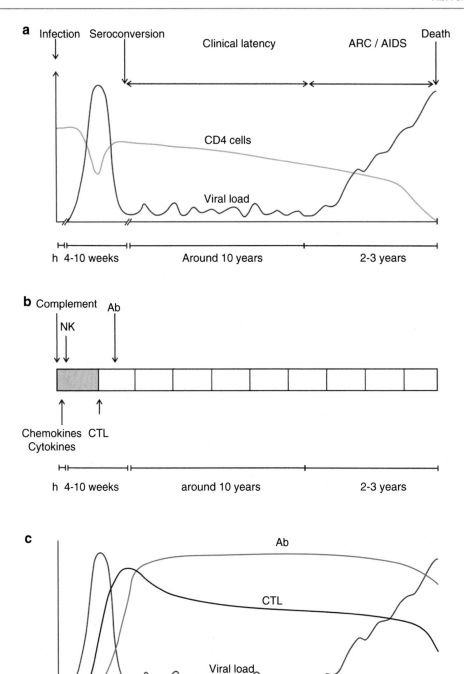

**Fig. 14.1** This graph depicts the natural history of HIV infection without antiretroviral therapy. Note initial surge in viral load at disease onset. Over time, the CD count declines and there is an associated, steep rise in the viral load when CD4 numbers are depleted. As the CD4 count is depleted, patients are at increased risk for opportunistic infections and certain malignancies

**Table 14.1** United States Preventive Services Task Force (USPSTF) Guidelines for screening patients for HIV

| Recommended Populations for Screening |
| --- |
| Adolescents and adults aged 15–65 |
| Younger adolescents and older adults at increased risk for infection |
| Pregnant women |
| Populations at Higher Risk |
| Men who have sex with men (MSM) |
| Active injection drug users |
| Those who are being tested for other sexually transmitted infections (STI) |

false positive Western blot), it is usually best to repeat the testing process in a few weeks to see if there has been evolution of an immune response.

## Treatment

Treatment of HIV is complex and rapidly evolving; thus, a thorough discussion of management of HIV is beyond the scope of this chapter, and only key points are mentioned here. The Department of Health and Human Services (DHHS) produces and maintains guidelines for the treatment of both HIV and opportunistic infections associated with HIV [11, 12]. Guidelines for treatment as of the writing of this chapter are summarized in Table 14.2. In general, treatment should consist of three antiretroviral agents, from at least two different classes of medication (Table 14.2B). Treatment should be initiated as close to the time of diagnosis as possible, with the possible exception of those who are concomitantly diagnosed with an opportunistic infection. In the case of a diagnosis in the setting of OI, data are clear about the need for early HAART in some infections (e.g., tuberculosis), but equivocal in others. It is clear, however, that early therapy confers a morbidity and mortality benefit, especially when treatment forestalls the onset of immune compromise. It is also clear that treatment, once started, should not be interrupted. Even transient interruption of therapy and other episodes of non-adherence to an established regimen increase the risk of virologic resistance, virologic failure, and immunologic failure.

Guidelines are also available for the primary care physician to help guide the care of the patient with HIV who is establishing care and who presents for maintenance of care. These are generated and reviewed regularly by the HIV Medical Association of the Infectious Diseases Society of America [13].

## Prevention

HIV prevention has been studied extensively using many approaches, including many behavioral and biomedical methods. Behavioral methods (such as encouraging testing, and safer sex practices) have been part of prevention efforts from the time the HIV transmission cycle was elucidated, though results of such efforts have been disappointing overall. More recently, biomedical methods, especially pre-exposure prophylaxis (PrEP), have shown promising results in both rates of HIV prevention and rates of in-study adherence. One study in particular merits mention here. The iPrEx study looked at the effect of daily tenofovir/emtricitabine (Truvada) in the prevention of HIV acquisition in MSM and transgender women (MTF) who have sex with men. The study showed that PrEP reduced the acquisition of HIV 47 % in all those who were assigned to receive it, and was even more effective (93 %) in those who demonstrated adherence to the PrEP regimen (detectable levels of medication in the blood) [14]. Other studies of the PrEP approach have yielded similar results. Studies are currently underway to see if other dosing strategies provide equal (or better) rates of prevention.

When providing prevention counseling to an individual patient, it is helpful to target risk mitigation, leading to an open and frank conversation about what the patient feels are realistic expectations. It is important to note that patients may engage in many such behaviors to limit their risk of HIV acquisition, including serosorting, seroadaptation, and PrEP. Ultimately, the strategies that are employed are individual, and these should be discussed regularly with each sexually active patient.

Lastly, the role of prevention with the patient living with HIV should also be discussed. From data in the last decade from the CDC, it has been shown that knowing one's status can have an impact on transmission of HIV. As many states have laws pertaining to sexual acts and the need to disclose HIV status, it is also important for providers to be aware of pertinent laws/statutes and to discuss them with their patients who have

**Table 14.2** Department of Health and Human Services (DHHS) guidelines for when to initiate treatment (A) and what to initiate (B) in the treatment of persons living with HIV

| A. When to Treat | | |
|---|---|---|
| Clinical condition | Recommendation | Strength of recommendation |
| *For patients who are HIV+, to prevent progression and complications of disease* | | |
| CD4 > 500 cells/mm³ | Treat | BIII |
| CD4 350–500 cells/mm³ | Treat | AII |
| CD4 < 350 cells/mm³ | Treat | AI |
| *For patients who are HIV+, to prevent transmission of HIV* | | |
| Risk group | Strength of recommendation | |
| Heterosexuals | AI | |
| Perinatal/Pregnancy | AI | |
| Other | AIII | |

| B. What to Start | | | |
|---|---|---|---|
| Recommended (AI) | Backbone | Plus other agent | |
| | TDF/FTC | DRV/r | PI-based regimen |
| | TDF/FTC | ATV/r | |
| | TDF/FTC | EFV | NNRTI-based regimen |
| | TDF/FTC | RAL | INSTI-based regimen |
| | TDF/FTC | EVG/COBI | |
| | TDF/FTC | DTG | |
| | ABC/3TC | DTG | |
| Recommended only for patients with a pre-ART plasma HIV RNA <100,000 copies/mL | | | |
| | ABC/3TC | EFV | |
| | TDF/FTC | RPV | |
| | ABC/3TC | ATV/r | |

| Notes | |
|---|---|
| 1. ABC-containing regimens should only be used for patients who test negative for HLA-B*5701 | |
| 2. The combination TDF/FTC/RPV should only be used in patients with a pre-treatment CD4 of >200 cells/mm³ | |
| 3. The agents FTC and 3TC may be used interchangeably | |
| (1) DHHS guidelines, available at http://aidsinfo.nih.gov | |
| Strength of recommendation | A = strong, B = moderate, C = optional |
| | I = data from randomized controlled trials; II = data from well-designed, non-randomized trials or observational cohort studies with long-term follow up; III = expert opinion |

HIV. It is also important to discuss with patients with HIV that they are still at risk for other STI (as noted elsewhere in this chapter) and should thus be screened appropriately for STI.

## Chlamydia trachomatis

### Epidemiology

*Chlamydia trachomatis* (CT) is a small obligate intracellular Gram-negative bacterium that causes a wide spectrum of disease. From a sexual health perspective, the most important CT serotypes are D-K, which are known to cause the common chlamydial genitourinary syndromes. CT has been the most commonly reported STD to the US Center for Disease Control (CDC) since 1994, and more than 1.4 million cases of CT infections were reported in the US in 2012 [15]. Yearly incidence of CT infections has been increasing for the past 20 years, which may partially be due to improved population screening strategies. Within the context of the LGBT population, there is significant data available on CT infections affecting

MSM. Approximately 6–22 % (variation based on site) of MSM who received care at the CDC STD Surveillance Network clinics in 2012 were infected with CT [15]. Unfortunately, little data is available on the association between female-to-female sexual contact and CT transmission. Some self-identified lesbians and other WS(M)W also have oral, insertive vaginal, and/or insertive anal sex with men, however, and these sexual behaviors put these populations of women at risk for CT exposure and infection.

## Clinical Presentation

The most common sites of CT inoculation are the cervix, urethra, anorectum, pharynx, and conjunctivae. Depending on the site and host, a majority of those infected with CT are asymptomatic. Current literature shows that CT urethritis in men can be asymptomatic in over 80 % of those infected [16, 17]. Two studies done in San Francisco, California and Columbus, Ohio independently found that 85 % of rectal CT infections in MSM were asymptomatic [18, 19]. Similarly, as much as 80 % of female urogenital CT infections are asymptomatic [20]. Asymptomatic CT infections in the female urogenital tract put patients at risk for complications as severe as infertility, pregnancy complications, and chronic pain secondary to pelvic inflammatory disease (PID) if left untreated. Further, asymptomatic carriers of CT at any anatomical site serve as an unknowing reservoir of CT transmission and spread.

Symptomatic urogenital CT infection in men most commonly manifests as urethritis (see Urethritis below). A small minority of these men develops prostatitis or epididymitis from urethral spread. MSM who participate in receptive anal intercourse can develop CT proctitis (infection of the anorectum). Symptomatic urogenital infection in women most commonly presents as cervicitis (see Cervicitis below). Some female patients with cervicitis develop a concurrent CT urethritis, while others develop urethritis without a corresponding cervicitis. CT proctitis in women can result from either direct receptive anal intercourse with an infected male or from self-inoculation by infected cervicovaginal secretions. Urogenital CT infection in women can progress to PID, a process characterized by inflammation of the uterine lining, fallopian tubes, ovaries, and/or adjacent pelvic organs, in approximately 10 % of untreated cases [20]. CT conjunctivitis can occur in men or women either by direct or indirect (via the hands) inoculation by infected urogenital secretions. Although CT can infect the pharynx, it is not known to be a major cause of symptomatic pharyngitis. A systemic autoimmune process called reactive arthritis (Reiter's syndrome) is characterized by recent urogenital CT infection, ocular inflammation (usually conjunctivitis), and a large joint polyarthritis.

## Diagnosis

Nucleic acid amplification testing (NAAT) has largely replaced culture for all sites, and is the preferred diagnostic method for genitourinary CT infections in both men and women. For women, a vaginal swab for NAAT is currently the most sensitive and specific specimen collection method for CT detection, though first-catch urine, endocervical swabs, and urethral swabs are also viable specimens in women [21]. A first-catch urine sample for NAAT is the preferred collection method for urogenital CT infection in men [22]. A urethral swab is a viable alternative but is typically less comfortable for the patient. For men at risk for rectal CT, many laboratories have been approved for rectal NAAT specimens under the Clinical Laboratory Improvement Amendment (CLIA) regulations despite its lack of FDA approval. There are currently no recommendations for routine NAAT of pharyngeal specimens in men or women; although, the pharynx is likely a contributing reservoir for the spread of CT.

As mentioned above, the majority of CT cases are asymptomatic. Therefore, screening patients based on their sexual behaviors is imperative, as swabbing at one inoculable site does not indicate CT positivity or negativity at a different location. Kent et al. found that 53 % cases of rectal CT in MSM would have been missed if patients were screened only with urogenital samples [18]. This finding highlights the importance of routinely screening patients for CT at susceptible sites based on an individual's sexual behavior.

## Treatment

According to the 2010 CDC treatment guidelines, 1 g of azithromycin in one dose or 100 mg of doxycycline taken twice daily for 7 days are equally effective in treating a non-LGV chlamydial infection [22]. Other macrolides or fluoroquinolones are alternative therapies but may be less effective. The one-time-dose of azithromycin is preferable for patients in whom medication noncompliance may be an issue, but gastrointestinal distress and subsequent medication loss with emesis must be considered. If diagnosed with CT, patients are recommended to abstain from further sexual activity for 7 days and until all symptoms have diminished. When a patient is diagnosed with CT, all sexual partners of the patient within the past 60 days should be contacted and recommended for testing at susceptible sites. Infected patients should follow-up with their provider in approximately 3 months for retesting regardless of whether they believe their sexual partner(s) were screened and treated appropriately. Contrary to *Neisseria gonorrheae* (GC), little concern exists for the development of antibiotic resistance in CT.

## Lymphogranuloma Venereum

Lymphogranuloma venereum (LGV) is a particular form of invasive CT disease, commonly manifest as proctitis and suppurative inguinal adenopathy, and is typically caused by L1–L3 serovars of CT. Clusters of LGV have been reported in MSM, most often in the context of a sexual network, though it should be noted that many cases can be traced back to en endemic exposure (e.g., travel to endemic tropical/subtropical area). Overall, rates of LGV are higher amongst MSM than in the general population. It is unclear whether this represents an increase in the prevalence of the LGV-causing serovars in MSM, or the increased incidence of CT in MSM, as has also been reported when compared with other populations. For LGV, the standard treatment is oral doxycycline, 100 mg, taken twice daily for 21 days.

## *Neisseria gonorrheae* (Gonorrhea)

### Epidemiology

*Neisseria gonorrheae*, or gonococcus (GC), is a diplococcal, Gram-negative bacterium that exhibits a similar spectrum of disease as *Chlamydia trachomatis* (CT). GC is the second most common bacterial sexually transmitted pathogen following CT. Over 330,000 GC infections in the US were reported to the CDC in 2012 [15]. Interestingly, the lowest recorded GC infection rate was in 2009, yet GC prevalence rates over 2010–2012 progressively increased. This trend highlights both the impact of improved screening strategies and the possibility of increasing GC burden in the US population. Similar to CT, data shows that MSM are disproportionately affected by GC. A study looking at the rates of GC in San Francisco from 1999 to 2008 showed that 72 % of GC infections were detected in MSM [23]. Approximately 10–30 % of MSM (variability based on location) screened through the CDC STD Surveillance Network tested positive for GC in 2012 [15]. Again, similar to CT, female-to-female transmission of gonococcal infections is not well documented. WS(M)W and self-identified lesbians can have sex with men, however, and put themselves at risk for pharyngeal, urogenital, and anorectal GC acquisition.

### Clinical Presentation

Symptomatic GC infection exhibits considerable clinical overlap with symptomatic CT infections. Urogenital infections in men are likely to present as urethritis (see Fig. 14.2), which can spread locally to cause prostatitis or epididymitis. Contrary to CT, GC urethritis is largely symptomatic in men. In a study assessing around 1800 cases of GC urethritis, only 10.2 % were entirely asymptomatic [24]. Female urogenital infections are likely to present as cervicitis (most common), urethritis, or a combination of both. A majority of female urogenital GC infections are asymptomatic [25]. Urogenital GC in women can progress to pelvic inflammatory disease (PID), a process characterized by inflammation of the upper female genital tract (i.e. uterine lining, fallopian tubes, ovaries) and other pelvic organs [26].

**Fig. 14.2** This image shows the polymorphonuclear cells seen histologically in bacterial urethritis. Note the associated Gramnegative diplococci characteristic of an infection with *Neisseria gonorrhoeae*

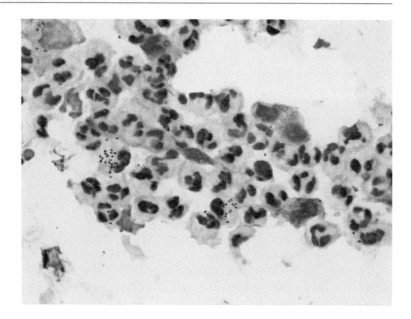

The risk of progression of asymptomatic urogenital GC in women to PID and its associated morbidities is a serious concern for those infected. This highlights the need for sufficient screening and treatment of women at risk for GC acquisition.

Proctitis (infection of the anorectum) can occur in both men and women and is largely asymptomatic in both sexes. As mentioned above, Kent et al. showed that approximately 85 % of rectal gonococcal infections in their San Francisco MSM study population were asymptomatic [18]. Rectal GC in females occurs from either direct inoculation from an insertive male sexual partner or from autoinoculation by infected cervicovaginal fluids [27]. Pharyngeal gonorrhea is mostly asymptomatic and may be a concerning source of pathogen transmission and spread in the sexually active population.

Although rare, disseminated infection can present in men and women as gonococcal bacteremia with migratory polyarthritis, tenosynovitis, and/or cutaneous lesions. GC is the most common cause of polyarthritis in sexually-active, healthy young adults.

## Diagnosis

The diagnostic approach to anogenital GC infections is largely comparable to CT. Nucleic acid amplification testing (NAAT) is recommended and approved by the FDA for the detection of urogenital gonococcal infections in both men and women [22]. In women, vaginal and endocervical swabs and urine can be used for NAAT. In men, viable NAAT collection methods include a urethral swab or urine. Using urine for NAAT may be easier for providers and more comfortable to patients in comparison to direct urogenital swabs. Of note, in symptomatic men, Gram stain of a urethral specimen is a specific and sensitive method of diagnosing urogenital GC; however, its sensitivity diminishes if the patient is asymptomatic [22]. Although not officially approved by the FDA, NAAT can also be used for the detection of rectal or pharyngeal gonococcal infections in men and women when laboratories receive independent authorization to perform these diagnostic tests. The specific NAAT kit used is relevant for the detection of pharyngeal and rectal specimens as commensal Neisseria flora can generate false-positive results in certain kits.

Providers should be aware of the need for antibiotic susceptibility testing when patients experience possible treatment failure (i.e. persistent symptoms after completion of prescribed antibiotic course) as these cases may represent instances of antibiotic-resistance. Antibiotic susceptibility can only be determined from cultured

*Neisseria gonorrhoeae* and not from routine NAAT. Treatment is discussed further in the next section.

## Treatment

Since 2012, the CDC has recommended treating all GC infections with both ceftriaxone 250 mg injected intramuscularly and oral azithromycin 1 g in one dose [22]. GC treatment regimens have varied significantly in the past few decades as it has developed resistance to multiple classes of antibiotics [22]. Rates of resistance to fluoroquinolones rose to levels that led to their removal from recommendation guidelines in 2007. Interestingly, these resistant strains of GC were predominantly found in MSM in the 1990s before spreading more diffusely throughout the population. Cephalosporins (ceftriaxone, cefixime) became the standard of care for GC infection at all anatomical locations following the discontinuation of quinolone utilization. Mirroring the trend seen with fluoroquinolones a few years prior, resistance toward cefixime was seen in sporadic cases of gonococcal infections in MSM in 2011. This finding prompted a national effort by the CDC to maximally reduce the development of cephalosporin resistance. Cefixime was removed from the first-line therapy recommendations for GC. Ceftriaxone is now the only first-line cephalosporin therapy indicated for GC infections. The mandatory addition of azithromycin to ceftriaxone is intended to reduce selection for cephalosporin-resistant strains of GC due to their anti-gonococcal properties. Both of these antibiotics are also effective at eliminating CT in a patient co-infected with GC and CT.

If a patient experiences therapeutic failure with persistent symptoms of GC after antibiotic treatment, a follow-up culture with antibiotic susceptibility testing is indicated as mentioned above. Although many cases of GC infection on follow-up are due to reinfection instead of treatment failure, screening the patient for cephalosporin-resistant strains of GC is important in the context of public sexual health. This is especially important for MSM, who are reported to be at increased risk for resistant infection [29].

## Herpes Simplex Virus

### Epidemiology

Herpes simplex virus type 1 (HSV-1) and herpes simplex virus type 2 (HSV-2) are classically known to cause lifelong, recurrent cutaneous and mucosal ulcerative lesions of the mouth and genitalia. Despite the historical notion that HSV-1 inoculation was limited to the mouth and HSV-2 was limited to the genitals, both HSV-1 and -2 are now known to be present at both sites, and both can cause the clinical syndrome known as genital herpes.

An analysis of data collected from the National Health and Nutrition Examination Survey (NHANES) showed that HSV-1 and HSV-2 affect a significant proportion of the US population [30]. From 2005 to 2010, 53.9 % of those aged 14–49 in the US were seropositive for HSV-1. HSV-2 had a seroprevalence of 15.7 % in the same age range over the same time period. Interestingly, in comparison to data from 1999 to 2004 from the same survey, HSV-1 seroprevalence decreased dramatically in the 14–19 year old age group. This correlates with recent hypotheses that childhood, non-sexual HSV-1 transmission is declining. It is unsurprising that genital HSV-1 infections have become more common as these increasing numbers of HSV-1 seronegative teenagers and young adults practice increasing rates of oral sex [31]. HSV-2 seroprevalence did not change significantly between 1999–2004 and 2005–2010 [30]. Because HSV-1 and -2 are lifelong infections, data on HSV incidence is logistically challenging to obtain, especially in older populations, and is less available than prevalence data.

Within the context of the LGBT population, both HSV-1 and HSV-2 are relevant. A study that looked at NHANES data from 2001 to 2006 showed that 18.4 % of men who had had sex with men in their lifetime were seropositive for HSV-2 [32]. A study done in New York City showed that as many as 32.3 % of their MSM population had serological evidence of HSV-2 infection, highlighting the variability of HSV-2 seroprevalence based on study population and local sexual culture [33]. Data available on HSV-1 in MSM shows a similar trend to that of the general population; rates of anogenital HSV-1 are on the rise [34]. A study assessing the prevalence of HSV in a study population of approximately 400 WSW showed that 46 % were seropositive for HSV-1 and 7.9 % were positive for HSV-2 [35]. The authors of this study emphasized the point that genital HSV-1 may be especially predominant in the WSW population as oral sex is a major component of female-to-female sexual contact. An interesting study assessing HSV-2 seropositivity in self-identified bisexual men showed that HSV-2 infection was significantly associated with the number of lifetime female sexual partners but not with the number of male partners [36]. Thus, heterosexual behaviors were directly implicated in HSV exposure and acquisition in the MSM population.

## Transmission and Acquisition

HSV is transmitted by viral particles shed from the skin or mucosal surface of an infected individual [37]. This viral shedding can occur in the setting of an active HSV outbreak (i.e. ulcerative lesions on the skin or mucosal surface) or asymptomatically. If an individual is suceptible to the virus and is exposed at an inoculable site, he/she can experiene a local, primary "outbreak" as well as develop a latent HSV infection as the virus ascends the nerve roots present in the inoculated tissue and establishes dormancy in the nerve cell bodies. The virus then periodically reactivates, causing intermittent subclinical viral shedding and recurrent cutaneous vesicular/ulcerative lesions at the initial inoculation site.

HSV seropositive patients should be educated on their risk of transmitting HSV to their sexual partner(s). The greatest quantity of viral shedding and thus transmission risk, is associated with sexual activity when active genital (or orolabial) lesions are present [38]. Any type of sexual activity—even body contact involving the affected region—should be avoided by patients with active lesions. However, asymptomatic viral shedding occurs frequently and is likely the cause of the majority of cases of HSV transmission [39]. Data suggests that HSV-2 has a greater tropism than HSV-1 for the anogenital region; this means that it is more likely to establish recurrent

HSV-2 infection in this region [40]. The same holds true for HSV-1 and the orolabial region. Yet, HSV-1 can be acquired genitally from oral secretions. Within the context of the viruses' natural histories, genital HSV-1 sheds asymptomatically less often, causes breakouts less frequently, and exhibits more dramatic decreases in yearly recurrence rates compared to HSV-2 [41].

Patients should be aware that while condoms can be somewhat effective in preventing HSV transmission from asymptomatic viral shedding, any infected mucosal or skin surface can shed viral particles (as a large cutaneous surface area may be innervated by the peripheral nerves infected during the initial inoculation event) [37, 42]. For example, if a patient has a genital HSV infection, he/she may shed the virus from his/her thighs, buttocks, upper abdomen, or perineum in addition to the genitals directly.

Some data suggest that HSV-1 provides some host immunity protection against future acquisition of HSV-2 [39]. However, a patient with a genital HSV-1 infection can become infected with HSV-2 genitally as well [43]. Therefore, it is important for patients to both know their serologic status with respect to HSV-1 and -2 and continue to maintain safe sexual practices regardless of whether or not they have had a genital herpes outbreak as they may only have genital HSV-1.

## Clinical Presentation

The initial, or primary, infection with HSV-1 or -2 and the associated symptoms are typically more severe than the subsequent symptomatic episodes characteristic of recurrent genital herpes [37]. Symptoms of primary infection occur a few days to a week after exposure. Primary HSV infection of the anogenitalia can manifest as local cutaneous lesions (clustered vesicles, unroofed vesicles, or crusted-over lesions), cutaneous pain, pruritus, dysuria, genital discharge, or painful inguinal lymphadenopathy (see Fig. 14.3). Systemic symptoms such as fever, malaise, headache, and muscle aches are also common in both men and women. More serious sequelae of a disseminated primary infection uncontrolled by host immune factors include encephalitis or aseptic meningitis, but these neurological conditions are rare.

**Fig. 14.3** This image depicts a very severe case of genital HSV in a female. Recurrent outbreaks of HSV are typically less extensive than the case shown here

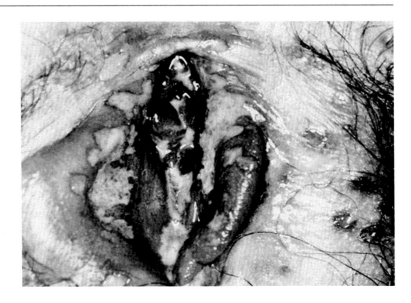

HSV-1 and -2 outbreak recurrences typically occur at the initial site of inoculation with less severe cutaneous symptoms and few to no systemic findings [37]. Some patients may experience a prodrome characterized by tingling or pruritus in the area that later exhibits HSV vesicular lesions. As mentioned above, genital HSV-1 infections are typically milder in course compared to genital HSV-2 [41]. Individuals with HSV-1 or -2 may be entirely asymptomatic and not experience the typical symptoms of a primary infection or recurrent lesions. Others may exhibit signs and symptoms of the primary infection but never experience a recurrent outbreak and vice-versa. Atypical presentations of genital HSV are common and range from fissures to patchy erythema to excoriations. The wide variability in the appearance of genital herpes highlights the need for proper screening and diagnosis of patients with HSV from a public health perspective to decrease transmission and morbidity associated with the disease.

### Diagnosis

Some cases of genital HSV may be diagnosed clinically, though laboratory confirmation is recommended [22]. Serologic testing specifically may play a role in the screening and diagnosis of HSV infection in asymptomatic individuals who may unknowingly transmit the virus to seronegative sexual partners.

The recommended confirmatory testing of an active lesion is HSV PCR performed on a swab of the base of an unroofed vesicular lesion. HSV PCR has proved superior to viral culture in terms of sensitivity, reproducibility, and time until available results [44, 45]. If HSV testing is indicated in a patient without active lesions, serological studies are available to diagnose and differentiate between HSV-1 and -2. Other indications for serologic testing include an atypical or questionable presentation of HSV infection, a negative viral culture or HSV PCR, a history of HSV lesions but no active lesions at the time of presentation, the presence of mostly healed lesions, or a person with an HSV seropositive sexual partner looking to confirm their status after exposure. Serologically differentiating between HSV-1 and -2 at the genital site has implications in quantifying a patient's risk of asymptomatic viral shedding (i.e. risk of transmission to a seronegative partner) and viral acquisition, as mentioned above, depending on the serological statuses of an individual and his/her partner(s).

### Treatment

For recurrent, symptomatic genital herpes by HSV-1 or HSV-2, two treatment strategies are available: episodic and suppressive therapy. Patients with psychosocial issues related to their HSV infection, with serodiscordant sexual partner(s) (even in the absence of outbreaks), or with frequent, painful recurrent episodes of HSV lesions, may benefit from the suppressive approach. Suppressive therapy reduces asymptomatic HSV viral shedding and symptomatic flare-ups, decreasing the risk of HSV transmission to seronegative sexual partners [46]. A typical suppressive regimen would involve acyclovir 400 mg two times per day or valacyclovir 500 mg once per day. Despite its moderately higher cost, valacyclovir may be a preferred regimen when patient noncompliance is an issue as only one dose is administered daily. Current data show that there is little risk of HSV developing antiviral resistance on long-term therapy [47]. If a patient on a suppressive regimen experiences a breakthrough recurrence, following the episodic treatment plan outlined below is appropriate. This treatment regimen conveniently uses the same dosages per pill as the suppressive regimen with a greater number of pills taken each day (see below). Of note, patient's experiencing the more severe primary outbreak may require a longer treatment course [22].

For patients who have less frequent recurrences or who are less concerned with HSV from a psychosocial or sexual transmission standpoint, episodic treatment initiated when lesions appear may be appropriate. A typical treatment regimen would involve acyclovir 500 mg three times per day for 5 days or valacyclovir 500 mg two times per day for 3 days.

As genital HSV-1 infection typically exhibits a milder course compared to genital HSV-2 [41], is serologically more common, has less frequent recurrences, and is asymptomatically shed less often at an anogenital site, suppressive therapy in patients with symptomatic genital HSV-1 may not be indicated, though patient concern may make suppression preferred.

### *Treponema pallidum* (Syphilis)

#### Epidemiology

Syphilis, a disease known since antiquity, is an infection caused by the spirochete *Treponema pallidum*. Given its ability to remain asymptom-

atic and the concern for long-term sequelae, syphilis remains a concern to public health deserving attention. This infection is of particular interest within the LGBT community as it disproportionately affects MSM. Syphilis rates in the US declined throughout the 1990s to a nadir in 1998 of 6993 [48]. Unfortunately the 1999–2000 rates of syphilis increased, predominantly in MSM populations within large metropolitan areas such as New York City [49]. 2000–2003 saw a 19 % increase in the rate of syphilis [50]. These outbreaks often occurred among networks MSM and were aided by newer technologies such as the widespread use of the internet, as was the case with one prominent outbreak in San Francisco from a single internet chat room [51]. Even within MSM, the burden of this disease is disproportionately borne by black, Hispanic, and young MSM [52]. Multiple factors have been proposed as reasons for this increase including rising rates of HIV, less adherence to barrier methods, and lack of education about acquisition and testing for syphilis.

It is important for the provider to educate patients on the ability of syphilis to be spread in manners besides anal and vaginal penetrative sex. In one cohort, 6 % of cases of syphilis were reported in men who denied anal sex and 25 % in those who endorsed consistent condom use. Though syphilis burden is much lower in WSW populations they are also at risk for infection given the transmissibility of *Treponema pallidum* via spread of sexual secretions and cases of syphilis between female partners has been reported in the literature [53].

#### Clinical Presentation

Syphilis is spread via direct contact, typically during sexual intercourse. It is a fairly infectious agent with efficiency of transmission of about 30 %. It is known in medicine as "The Great Imitator" due to its myriad presentations in patients. This section by no means attempts to provide an exhaustive description of possible presentations but instead focuses on the most common presentations of the different stages of infection: primary, secondary, latent, and tertiary.

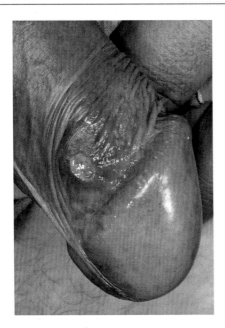

**Fig. 14.4** This image depicts a penile chancre typical of a primary syphilis infection. Note the indurated, erythematous base surrounding the lesion

Primary syphilis is characterized by the classic painless ulcer, or chancre (see Fig. 14.4). The median incubation period between exposure and manifestation of chancre is 21 days. The chancre appears at the site of inoculation and is classically described as 1–2 cm, non-painful, and non-purulent. Many presentations of primary syphilis may stray from this classical presentation and thus a high level of suspicion with low threshold to test should be used with high-risk patients. The chancre may be accompanied by regional lymphadenopathy. There is usually only one chancre; however, among HIV positive patients there have been reports of multiple chancres at presentation. Due to the largely asymptomatic nature of the chancre these can go unnoticed, especially when present in the anus, oropharynx, or vaginal vault as opposed to the labia or penile shaft. The ulcer usually heals within 2–3 weeks. During this period the disease is transmissible and patients should refrain from further sexual contact until treatment is complete.

Secondary syphilis develops in about 25 % of untreated patients and usually manifests within weeks to a few months after the primary infection.

Though it typically appears after resolution of the primary chancre, in immunocompromised patients secondary syphilis may appear sooner. Most patients experience rash as the predominant symptom of secondary syphilis. This rash may take many forms, excepting a vesicular rash, and is classically a maculopapular rash that does not spare the palms and soles (see Figs. 14.5 and 14.6). These are usually reddish brown 0.5–2 cm lesions that may present with or without scale. Some patients develop condyloma lata, or raised, large, white-grey lesions on mucous membranes or perineum, often adjacent to the location of the primary chancre. Condyloma lata can be mistaken for genital warts. These lesions have a very high organism burden and are highly infectious. Other systemic symptoms of secondary syphilis include fever, headache, malaise, sore throat, orogenital mucous patches, and generalized lymphadenopathy. Patients may also experience gastrointestinal symptoms, hepatitis, renal abnormalities, muscle aches, and ocular symptoms such as uveitis.

Without treatment, most cases go on to a latent, non-infectious period. During this period the disease may be spread vertically but not between sexual partners; however, about one-fourth of patients experience a recurrent secondary infection wherein they may transmit the disease. Latent syphilis can be defined as early or late latent infection, with the cutoff point between the two at 1 year. In latent syphilis, often the date of infection is not known, so the cutoff is interpreted with respect to the last known negative test. The dichotomy is important from a public health perspective given that early latent cases may identify sexual partners that should be notified from the last year, while late latent syphilis requires a longer duration of therapy than primary, secondary, and early latent infection.

About one third of untreated patients will go on to develop tertiary syphilitic symptoms. These can develop as soon as a year after infection or more indolently occur even up to 25–50 years later. These are more likely to occur more rapidly or with a more dramatic presentation in HIV-infected patients. Typically syphilis is unable to be transmitted during this stage. Classic manifes-

**Fig. 14.5** This figure shows the palmar rash typical of secondary syphilis

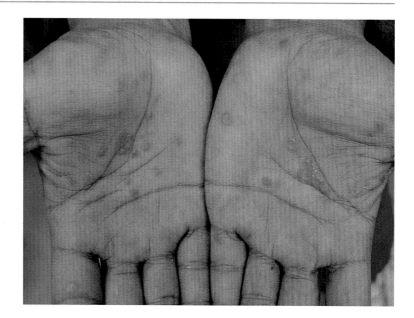

**Fig. 14.6** This figure shows the rash on the soles of the feet typical of secondary syphilis

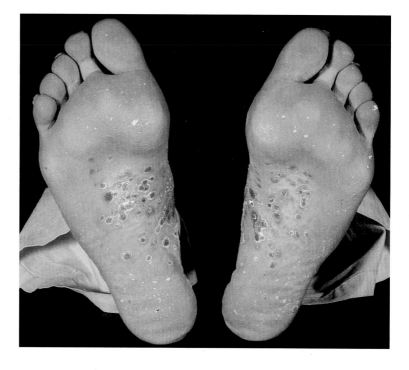

tations of this late stage of infection are gummas, cardiovascular, and neurologic findings. Gummas are the most rare manifestation and present as granulomatous lesions on the skin, bones, or internal organs (see Fig. 14.7). The classic cardiovascular symptom of tertiary syphilis is dilation of the ascending aorta. Neurosyphilis can present with symptoms ranging from meningitis to ocular symptoms (e.g., the Argyll-Robertson pupil), otologic manifestations, and tabes dorsalis. Meningitic symptoms are characteristic of early neurosyphilis and are usually seen in the first 12 months of infection, or after treatment of early syphilis in patients co-infected with HIV.

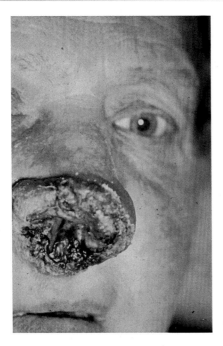

**Fig. 14.7** This image shows a severe gumma on the nose of a man affected by tertiary syphilis

Late neurosyphilis occurs 10–25 years after initial infection and, while it can present with a range of neurologic symptoms, typically includes the classic tabes dorsalis and gummatous parenchymal presentations [54]. Given the varying presentations, late-stage syphilis is an important part of many differential diagnoses and the stage of this presentation has important implications for dosing and duration of treatment.

### Diagnosis

Syphilis is notorious for its difficulty to culture, making live study and direct diagnosis more difficult. The classic method for diagnosis is dark-field microscopy in which the spiral treponemes light up brightly. Unfortunately this technique is not sensitive and it is rarely available in the clinical setting. Indirect serologic assays are the mainstays of syphilis testing and recommended by the CDC for diagnosis of syphilis. There are both non-treponemal and treponemal tests. Non-treponemal tests, such as the rapid plasma reagin (RPR) and the Venereal Disease Research Laboratory test (VDRL), are sensitive but not specific and are used for screening. The more specific treponemal tests, the fluorescent treponemal antibody absorption test (FTA-ABS), the *Treponema pallidum* particle agglutination test (TPPA), and the microhemagglutination-*Treponema pallidum* (MHA-TP), are used as confirmatory testing for those who test positively with screening tests. Newer PCR methods are described but not yet widely available [55]. Both screening and confirmatory tests must be positive for a diagnosis of syphilis. In the case where a patient has already been treated for syphilis, a fourfold or greater increase in non-treponemal titers represents presumptive reinfection.

Neurosyphilis can only be diagnosed via lumbar puncture and direct testing of the CSF. This should be a consideration in any patient who is displaying neurologic or ocular symptoms of syphilis infection, HIV co-infected patients with syphilitic infection of unknown duration, or patients who have failed treatment on a regimen that does not sufficiently cross the blood-brain barrier. Routine testing for neurosyphilis is not advised as early syphilis can have positive CSF findings that do not correlate with later sequelae of neurosyphilis. While CSF VRDL is very specific, its low sensitivity requires other testing including protein, cell count, and CSF-FTA. CSF-FTA is one of the most sensitive tests for neurosyphilis available and is a good test for ruling out neurosyphilis in the general population; however, as with all testing, it should be borne in mind that such a test cannot definitively rule out neurosyphilis, particularly when there is a high pre-test probability of syphilis in the patient under consideration (as may be the case, for example, with MSM populations) [56]. In otherwise healthy patients with symptoms of neurosyphilis, the CDC recommends cut-off of >5 white blood cells per mL of CSF be used to support diagnosis (a cut-off of >20 white blood cells per mL of CSF is recommended for patients with HIV). The results of these tests must be clinically correlated to patient symptoms and overall health. Patients with borderline CSF results often benefit from expert guidance in determining management with treatment versus watchful waiting with serial LPs.

Anytime there is a concern for syphilis, there should also be concern for other STI, especially HIV, and HIV testing is indicated.

## Treatment

Penicillin remains the antibiotic of choice in the treatment of syphilis. There is currently no evidence of penicillin resistance in the organism. The duration and dosage of treatment depends upon the stage and symptoms of disease (see Table 14.3). Alternate regimens do exist for penicillin-allergic patients except in the cases of neurosyphilis or pregnancy, wherein desensitization therapy is the recommended treatment in these groups.

Practitioners should warn patients of the potential for the Jarisch-Herxheimer reaction upon initiation of treatment. Characterized by rash, headache, myalgias, and hypotension, this usually occurs within 1–2 h of treatment and resolves within 24–48 h. It can be managed with antipyretics and analgesics. This reaction is more common in patients who are being treated for early syphilis, those with higher RPR titers, and those who are co-infected with HIV.

Response to treatment and follow-up is somewhat specific to each stage of the disease and can be found in the CDC's Guidelines for STI Treatment [22]. In general, follow-up of non-treponemal testing is done at 6 and 12 months with a desired fourfold drop in titers at 12 months representing cure. More frequent 3-month intervals may be advisable in HIV-infected patients who are more likely to fail treatment. Finally, in patients who are not responding to treatment as expected it may be prudent to test for HIV and to consider to LP for possible CSF involvement.

Sexual partners should be offered testing. Though syphilis transmission is thought to only occur when patients have mucocutaneous lesions, sexual partners of those with latent or tertiary syphilis should still be offered testing. The guidelines for partner testing and treatment can also be found in the CDC Guidelines for STD Treatment.

## Human Papillomavirus

### Epidemiology

The human papillomavirus (HPV) has over 100 serotypes and 75–80 % of sexually active adults acquire some form of genital infection with HPV by age 50 [22]. Named for the visible wart lesions that it causes, it is increasingly appreciated for its role in many forms of cancer (cervical, anal, penile, vaginal, vulvar, oropharyngeal). This section focuses mainly on the manifestation of genital warts. For information on the relationship of HPV to cancer and HPV vaccination please see Chap. 17.

Within the LGBT community there are some special considerations around HPV infection. A common misconception is that WSW are at lower risk for this infection; however, HPV has been seen in WSW with no history of male partners [57]. For WSW who do have male partners, increased number of male partners represents a risk factor for HPV acquisition/infection. There is evidence that insertive toys present a potential risk for HPV transmission [58]. WSW should undergo routine Pap screening. Within the MSM population, 57 % of patients in one study were found to have anal infection with HPV with HPV 16 being the most common agent [59]. Some experts recommend that MSM who engage in receptive anal intercourse should be tested every 3–5 years with anal pap smears [60]. Again both populations may present with anogenital warts.

### Clinical Presentation

Anogenital warts can range in appearance from pink to flesh colored and from flat, smooth lesions to hyperkeratotic raised lesions, to the classic condyloma acuminata (cauliflower-shaped, verrucous lesions, see Fig. 14.8). Though infection is often asymptomatic, patients can present with pruritis, bleeding, pain, or vaginal discharge (see Fig. 14.9). In certain instances, the lesions can become large and interfere with intercourse or defecation.

### Diagnosis

When diagnosing the lesion, careful attention should be given to the size and extent of the lesions. Providers should use anoscopy and/or pelvic examination to search for other lesions outside of the perineal, penile, or vulvar areas. Additionally, the oral cavity should also be examined for lesions. Anogenital warts are usually diagnosed by visual inspection; however, when unclear a biopsy may be performed. Additionally, 5 % acetic acid can be applied to the area to assess for extent of disease, though this is not

**Table 14.3** Pathogen, presentation, and treatment

| Pathogen/Disease | Classic patient complaint(s) | Treatment recommendations |
|---|---|---|
| Genital herpes (HSV-1, HSV-2) | Primary infection: painful anogenital vesicular rash with associated lymphadenopathy and constitutional symptoms (e.g. fever, malaise) Recurrent outbreak: painful anogenital vesicular rash (commonly to lesser extent than primary infection) with surrounding erythema; possible prodrome | Suppressive: acyclovir 400 mg PO BID, valacyclovir 500 mg PO QD Episodic: acyclovir 400 mg PO TID ×5 d, valacyclovir 500 mg PO BID ×3 d (unless primary outbreak: acyclovir 400 mg PO TID ×7–10 d, valacyclovir 1 g PO BID ×7–10 d) |
| *Chlamydia trachomatis* serovars D-K | Urethritis: dysuria, urethral pruritis, urinary frequency, penile discharge Cervicitis: dyspareunia, postcoital bleeding, vulvovaginal irritation, cervical discharge, dysuria, urinary frequency Proctitis: bleeding (particularly with bowel movements), tenesmus, anal discharge, perianal pruritis | Azithromycin 1 g PO ×1 dose Doxycycline 100 mg PO BID ×7 d |
| Gonorrhea (*Nessieria gonorrhoeae*) | Similar spectrum of disease as anogenital chlamydial infections | Ceftriaxone 250 mg IM ×1 dose + azithromycin 1 g PO × 1 dose Treatment failure on follow-up: consider antibiotic resistance in addition to reinfection |
| Lymphogranuloma venereum (*Chlamydia trachomatis* serovars L1, L2, L2a, L3) | Painless genital ulcer that progresses to painful lymphadenopathy, late-stage disease associated with permanent lymphatic stricture | Doxycycline 100 mg PO BID × 21 d |
| Syphilis (*Treponema pallidum*) | Primary syphilis: painless, non-purulent genital ulcer (i.e. chancre) Secondary syphilis: maculopapular rash involving the palms/soles, condyloma lata (raised, large, white-grey lesions on mucous membranes), systemic lymphadenopathy, constitutional symptoms Latent syphilis: asymptomatic Tertiary syphilis: cutaneous gummas (granulomatous lesions with central necrosis), tabes dorsalis and other neurological manifestations, cardiovascular disease | Primary, secondary, early-latent syphilis: Benzathine penicillin G 2.4 million units IM single dose Late-latent syphilis, latent syphilis of unknown duration, non-neurological tertiary syphilis: Benzathine penicillin G 7.2 million units in 3 divided doses of 2.4 million units given a week apart Neurosyphilis: Aqueous crystalline penicillin G 18–24 million units per day, administered as 3–4 million units IV every 4 h or continuous infusion, for 10–14 days |
| Bacterial vaginosis | Malodorous ("fishy") clear vaginal discharge, mild vaginal pruritis | Metronidazole 500 mg PO BID × 7 d |
| Vulvovaginal candidiasis (Candida spp.) | Vaginal pruritis, vaginal soreness, dyspareunia, dysuria, white/curd-like ("cottage cheese") vaginal discharge | Fluconazole 150 mg PO × 1 dose Various topical azole therapies |

(continued)

**Table 14.3**  (continued)

| Pathogen/Disease | Classic patient complaint(s) | Treatment recommendations |
|---|---|---|
| Trichomoniasis (Trichomonas vaginalis) | Malodorous yellow-green vaginal discharge, vulvar pruritis<br>Consider as possible etiology of urethritis (see above for symptoms) in men if refractory to empiric GC/CT therapy | Metronidazole 2 g PO × 1 dose |
| Pubic lice (*Pediculosis pubis*) | Anogenital pruritis, visible organisms in pubic hair | 1 % Permethrin cream rinse applied and washed off after 10 min<br>Pyrethrins + piperonyl butoxide applied and washed off after 10 min |
| Scabies (*Sarcoptes scabiei*) | Crusted linear/serpentine cutaneous lesions with associated pruritis | 5 % Permethrin cream applied to body from neck down, washed off after 8–14 h (i.e. overnight)<br>Ivermectin 200 μg/kg with repeated dose at 2 weeks |

*Note:* Viable alternative therapies are available, see 2015 CDC Treatment Guidelines for more information

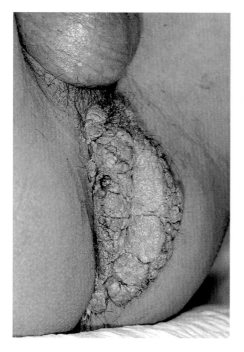

**Fig. 14.8**  This image shows a severe case of anorectal genital warts, also known as condylomata acuminata (singular: condyloma acuminata). These lesions are associated with an infection with human papilloma virus (HPV)

specific. In immunocompromised patients, those who lesions are growing or large in size, or with atypical features such as induration or ulceration it is prudent to biopsy for potential pre-malignant or malignant lesions.

## Treatment

Treatment can generally be classified as chemical/physical ablation, immunomodulation, or surgical removal. The type of treatment initiated should be selected based on extent of the disease and patient follow-up. Podophyllin, tricholroacetic acid (TCA), and 5-fluorouracil (5-FU)/epinephrine gel have all been used as chemical agents. Imiquimod and interferon alpha are two immunomodulating agents used for treatment. Cryotherapy, laser ablation, and surgical excision are also options for removal.

## Prevention

The quadrivalent HPV vaccine provides protection from the two most common HPV strains causing anogenital warts. For more information about the HPV vaccines please see Chap. 17.

## Bacterial Vaginosis

### Epidemiology

Bacterial vaginosis (BV) is a common infection in women caused by the loss of normal vaginal flora of lactobacilli and the overgrowth of polymicrobial facultative anaerobes. This infection is of particular importance to sexual health providers of WSW, as multiple studies have shown an association between female sexual partners and BV. During 2001–2004, the NHANES found the

**Fig. 14.9** This image shows a HPV-related genital wart on the cervix. Note the associated inflammation and bleeding

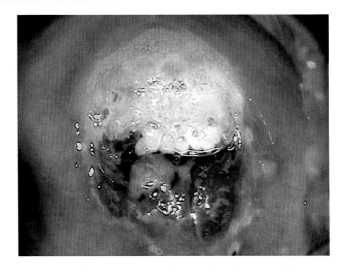

**Fig. 14.10** This image shows the appearance of clue cells typical of bacterial vaginosis on light microscopy. Note the numerous bacteria coating the sloughed epithelial cells from the female genital tract

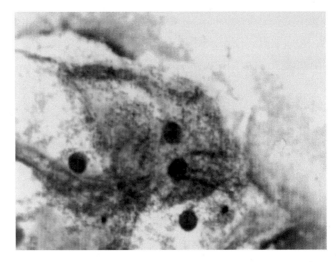

prevalence of BV in women who reported sex with a woman was significantly higher at 45.2 % than the overall prevalence of 29.2 % [61]. Additionally, self-identified lesbian women in an age-matched study in the UK showed an increased odds (of 2.5) for BV [62]. There is some evidence that a monogamous, long-term same-sex relationship is protective against BV, while more partners promote a disruption in the vaginal microbiota and increase BV rates [63]. Providers should be aware of this increased risk when treating and counseling WSW.

## Clinical Presentation

BV can present with urethritis and vaginitis, though patients more often complain of increased vaginal discharge and of a "fishy" odor. This odor classically worsens with sexual intercourse and menstruation. Many patients will be asymptomatic. The diagnosis of BV is made when they meet 3 of 4 Amsel's Criteria: abnormal gray discharge, vaginal pH of greater than 4.5, a positive amine "whiff" test, and clue cells on wet prep (see Fig. 14.10).

## Diagnosis

Common bacterial pathogens identified include *Gardnerella vaginalis*, *Mycoplasma hominis*, *Bacteroides* species, *Peptostreptococcus* species, *Fusobacterium* species, *Prevotella* species, and *Atopobium vaginae*. These can also be normal vaginal flora but become pathogenic when an as yet unidentified change in the vaginal microenvironment allows overgrowth of these species. The diagnosis of BV is clinical. Given the normal presence of these bacterial species in healthy vaginal flora, a positive culture for does not diagnose BV without corresponding clinical symptoms. The exception to this is in research wherein the Nugent criteria use gram stain to diagnose.

### Treatment

Current treatment recommendations include metronidazole and clindamycin, with the former preferred. These come in both topical and oral administrations. Typically the oral regimens are more expensive, though many patients prefer the oral route. Often BV is recurrent and may require multiple or extended courses of antiobiotics. Additionally, patients who smoke cigarettes should be counseled on cessation as smoking has been linked to this infection [63]. BV should be treated regardless of symptoms due to increased risk for other pelvic and post-operative infections. Extra consideration of this diagnosis should be given to pregnant patients or those seeking to become pregnant as BV has been associated with low birth weight, premature rupture of membranes, and prematurity [64].

Though not classically considered a sexually transmitted infection, there may be a case for partner testing and treatment of BV in the case of WSW. In the aforementioned UK study, a significantly higher correspondence rate of 87 % was seen in lesbian-identified couples [63]. While this was not associated with sexual practices that increase the risk of exchange of vaginal secretions (such as toys) or with receptive oral sex, this significant concordance may necessitate partner testing and treatment. This is an especially important consideration in refractory cases.

### Vulvovaginal Candidiasis

*Candida* infections are one of the three leading causes of vaginitis. This common infection happens in up to 75 % women and up to 5 % of these patients will experience recurrent episodes [65]. This is not traditionally considered in a sexually transmitted infection but has been associated with higher numbers of female partners in WSW

[66]. This is similar to heterosexual studies linking a higher number of male partners to increased risk for vulvovaginal candidiasis (VVC). There is no established link between any particular sexual practice, such as use of toys, and the development of VVC.

Symptoms of infection include a thick, white, curd-like discharge as well as accompanying pruritus, burning, dysuria, and dyspareunia. Candida spp. are considered part of the natural vaginal flora and symptomatic candidiasis is typically caused by an overgrowth of these organisms. The diagnosis requires both clinical symptoms and evidence of the yeast on either probe testing or microscopic visualization on wet prep with 10 % KOH (see Fig. 14.11).

VVC can be defined as either uncomplicated or complicated. Complicated infections are those that present with severe symptoms, infections with non-*albicans* spp., four or more recurrent infections in 1 year, or infections in high-risk patient groups such as women with diabetes, other vulvovaginal pathology, immunosuppression, or pregnancy. Patients with complicated VCC may require more extended treatment and are more likely to fail standard treatment [67]. In patients presenting with complicated VVC with otherwise normal risk factors it is prudent to test for an underlying risks such as diabetes or an immunocompromised state, such as previously unknown HIV infection.

There are many treatment regimens and antifungal agents available for VVC. Many patients prefer oral fluconazole and the standard regimen of a one-time dose of 150 mg. For recurrent infections a more intensive regimen with a second dose of 150 mg fluconazole 3 days after the first has been shown to increase cure rates. In infections that fail -azole therapy, a 2-week regimen of 600-mg capsule boric acid intravaginally daily for 2 weeks is effective.

### *Trichomonas vaginalis* (Trichomoniasis)

*Trichomonas vaginalis* is a protozoan parasite that is largely sexually transmitted. Though principally transmitted through intercourse, there

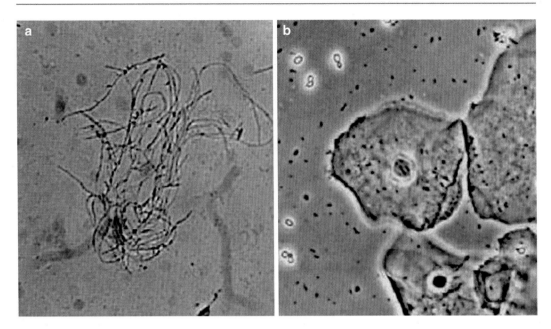

**Fig. 14.11** This image shows the hyphae and associated budding typical of vaginal candidiasis seen on light microscopy

have been reports of trichomonads spread through passive transmission through vectors such as shared damp washcloths or towels. In one study of lesbian couples with trichomoniasis, this was the suggested route of transmission in one concordant couple [68]. This infection may be present along with other causes of vaginitis, especially BV. Treatment of this condition is important to reduce partner transmission as well as reduction of transmission of HIV. In a recent study of trichomoniasis in HIV positive women, trichomoniasis was associated with higher HIV-1 viral shedding [69]. In the same study, trichomoniasis synergistically increased HIV viral shedding in patients who also had BV.

Typically these infections are asymptomatic; however, it is one of the three most common causes of vaginitis in female patients. Rarely, it has been a cause of urethritis in male patients. Signs of infection with *Trichomonas* are typical vaginitis symptoms of odor, discharge, dyspareunia, and itching. The discharge of trichomoniasis tends to be copious, frothy, and often has a yellow-green tinge. Discharge of this quality should raise suspicion for this disease. Diagnosis can often be accomplished with microscopic

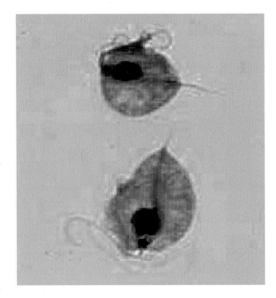

**Fig. 14.12** This image shows trichomoniasis as seen on light microscopy. These organisms are often confused with cervical squamous cells on Pap smear analysis

examination of vaginal discharge (wet mount), on which trichomonads can be seen as motile flagellated organisms (see Fig. 14.12). There are also DNA probes for *T. vaginalis*, which may be of use if organisms are not found on wet mount

**Fig. 14.13** This image depicts the dome-shaped, pearly lesions typical of an infection with molluscum contagiosum virus

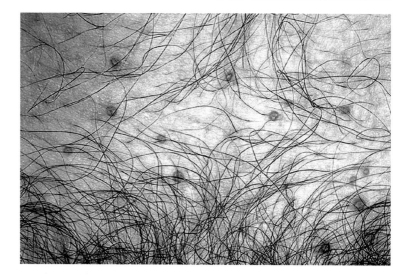

but diagnosis seems probable. Treatment of trichomoniasis is usually metronidazole as a one-time 2 g oral dose, though metronidazole at 500 mg given orally three times daily for 7 days is an alternative. There is evidence of metronidazole-resistant *T. vaginalis*, including a case report in a lesbian couple [70]. Tinidazole is a reasonable first option in the case of metronidazole-resistant infections.

### *Pediculosis pubis*: Pubic Lice

Pubic Lice (or "crabs") is an infestation with the louse *Pedculosis pubis* and characterized by pruritus in the genital and perianal region. The adult organism and nits are visible to the naked eye and are diagnostic of this infection. Spread through sexual contact, the lice are predominant in the genital area. Though rarely infesting the scalp, any region of hair is a potential site of infection, especially the axilla. Treatment is with topical drugs such as malathion 0.05 % or permethrin 5 %. Oral ivermectin 200 mcg/kg in two doses a week apart is a systemic option. Additionally, nit-combs can be used to aid in decontamination. Sexual partners should also be examined and treated. Patients should be instructed to wash all bedding and towels and dry on high heat. Anything that cannot be washed should be bagged for 72 h or longer to kill remaining lice.

Infection with *Pediculosis pubis* should prompt testing for other sexually transmitted infections, as up to 30 % of patients with pubic lice are found to have another sexually transmitted infection [71].

### Molluscum Contagiosum

Molluscum contagiosum is a poxvirus spread by skin-to-skin contact. Traditionally thought of as a disease of children, these lesions are also a sexually transmitted infection and, when spread in this manner, are found in the anogenital region, inner thighs, and lower abdomen. Typically the virus manifests as 2–5 mm diameter flesh-toned, papular lesions with central umbilication (see Fig. 14.13). Most often the disease is self-limited, and lesions are cleared within a few months, though rarely they may persist for years. In the immunocompromised patient, a more severe infection can occur with confluence of multiple lesions. These can mimic other infections and biopsy may be required for diagnosis.

Diagnosis is usually made by visual inspection with the classic lesions; however, when performed, biopsy shows intracellular pox inclusion bodies. While the disease is most often self-limited, treatment may be warranted for faster clearance and to prevent further spread via autoinoculation or to others via sexual contact.

There is no standard of care for treatment of the lesions, though most first-line therapies are ablative (such as cryotherapy, curettage or electrocautery). Podophyllotoxin and, to a lesser extent, imiquimod have also been used for treatment. In immunocompromised patients with disseminated infection, trichloroacetic acid and cidofovir have been studied as possible treatment options.

Infection with molluscum contagiosum should prompt further testing for other sexually transmitted infections.

## Scabies

*Sarcoptes scabiei* (var. *hominis*) is a human parasitic mite that burrows into the epidermis and lays eggs therein. In an immunocompetent host this typically results in a strong immunologic response characterized by intense pruritus and raised, scaled lesions that follow the burrowed path of individual mites. Transmission of mites is almost completely through skin-to-skin contact and, with a predilection for intertriginous and genital regions, often can be transmitted during sexual activity. The burden of scabies infections varies widely across the globe, being as high as 43 % of persons in some developing-world communities, though the prevalence in developed countries has been reported around 2–3 per 1000 [72].

The typical presentation of scabies is crusted linear or serpentine lesions with intense itching; often these are located in the hands, wrists, ankles, elbows, and genitals and intertriginous regions. Crusted, or Norwegian, scabies is a superinfection of thousands to millions of mites and has been described in immunocompromised hosts such as patients with advanced HIV infection [73]. Unlike the typical presentation of scabies, these patients present with non-pruritic, hyperkeratotic, scaled plaques typically with an acral distribution and resembling psoriasis. Diagnosis in either case is made through skin scrapings demonstrating mites, ovum, or feces. Identification of burrows may be aided by application and subsequent removal of washable marker as a means of highlighting the lesions.

If infection is suspected highly and no mites are seen, it is prudent to treat empirically as diagnostic tests for scabies are not sensitive, and mites are often difficult to isolate.

Scabies infestations require medical and environmental measures. Medical management of the infestation can be accomplished with 5 % permethrin cream overnight. This may require two treatments 1 week apart. An oral option is two doses of oral ivermectin (200 mcg/kg each, 1 week apart). Both may be required for patients with crusted scabies. Sexual partners should be examined for scabies and treated appropriately. The hypersensitivity reaction to scabies infestations can last for weeks after the mites have been killed, so continued itching does not necessarily imply treatment failure. Patients may respond to sedating antihistamines, while corticosteroids should largely be avoided to prevent missed treatment failure. In addition to medical management, patients should be advised to machine wash and dry on high heat any items with which they have come into contact. Non-washable items should be bagged and stored for 72 h to kill remaining mites.

## Other Pathogens

While this chapter has discussed some of the major pathogens causing STI in the US (LGBT) population(s), there are others that are of interest, and which should be kept in mind in the appropriate clinical context.

It is important to note that human herpesviruses (HHV) can be spread through sexual contact (specifically, the exchange of body fluids). While not considered classic STI, both Epstein-Barr virus (the etiologic agent of mononucleosis) and cytomegalovirus can cause a mononucleosis-like syndrome, with fever and adenopathy (including inguinal adenopathy). There are case reports of Kaposi sarcoma (KS) in MSM who are not HIV+ [74]. Human herpesvirus-8, the etiologic agent of KS, can be spread sexually, and should be considered in immunocompromised MSM who present with the characteristic skin/mucous membrane findings of KS.

The hepatitis viruses can also be spread by sexual contact. With case reports in the late 1990s, hepatitis A was noted to be increasingly common epidemiologically in MSM, and shortly after, was added to the list of vaccines to be considered in special populations (specifically, MSM) [75]. More recently, sexual activity has been appreciated as an important mode of transmission of hepatitis C, and the cause of several clusters of cases [76]. Both hepatitis C and hepatitis B are relatively highly prevalent and incident in MSM populations, especially those who are co-infected with HIV, and this remains the case despite the universal recommendation for hepatitis B vaccination [77, 78].

In addition to these sexually transmitted pathogens, some pathogens may be spread by intimate (not necessarily sexual) contact and may travel along networks. As LGB populations are, in part, defined by their sexual activity, and sexual activity often occurs within the context of a network, some pathogens may be encountered disproportionately in LGB populations (as well as T populations) or subpopulations regardless of sexual contact.

For example, methicillin-resistant *Staphylococcus aureus* (MRSA), which can be spread by any form of intimate or close contact (amongst other modes of transmission), has been reported in clusters of MSM whose only exposure was sexual contact [79]. Not all cases of transmission of MRSA lead to identifiable disease; some lead to colonization, though the two are correlated. Some studies have not shown higher rates of carriage of MRSA in MSM when compared to the general population [80], lending support to the hypothesis that the increase in MRSA infections seen in MSM may be due to spread along (sexual) networks, or in some other more limited way, rather than by higher colonization rates of the MSM population in general.

Recently, an outbreak of invasive meningococcal disease has been reported in MSM in certain urban areas [81]. In these cases, it is unclear that sexual contact has played a role in transmission. Regardless, many have advocated immunization of MSM against meningococcus,

and recently some public health departments have started immunization campaigns in select cities [82].

Thus, it is important for those who provide care for LGBT populations to be attuned to both traditional STI and non-traditional pathogens that may be transmitted along the networks of our LGBT patients.

# A Brief Discussion of Clinical Syndromes

## Genital Ulcerative Lesions

Patients presenting with ulcerative lesions of the genitals almost immediately raise concern for sexually transmitted infection. Though other non-infectious etiologies (Behcet's disease, Crohn's disease, drug reactions) may be the culprit, in sexually active adults a sexually transmitted infection is the most common etiology. HSV and primary/secondary syphilis, respectively, make up the vast majority of these cases. In 2012 HSV was the cause of about 240,000 office visits [15]. 15,667 cases of primary and secondary Syphilis cases were reported to the CDC in 2012 [15]. Chancroid (caused by the bacterium *Haemophilus ducreyi*) is the other most common cause, and in comparison had 15 reported cases in 2012 [15]. Other sexually transmitted infections that cause ulcerative lesions are lymphogranuloma venereum (*C. trachomatis*) and granuloma iguinale (*Klebsiella granulomatia*). Though these are both rarer, of note LGV when seen in more developed countries was associated with MSM sexual activity [83].

History and physical exam are the most useful in determining the etiologic agent of ulcerative genital disease. The typical HSV presentation is multiple, painful and burning vesicular lesions with occasional bilateral lymphadenopathy. Primary syphilitic lesions are classically painless, indurated, and with clean bases. Chancroid often presents with multiple, painful, ragged-edged ulcerations with classically unilateral, suppurative lymphadenopathy. In contrast, the ulcerative lesion of LGV is less commonly seen, while bilateral, suppurative adenopathy raises suspicion for this etiology. Finally granuloma iguinale has a classic beefy, granular ulceration without true adenopathy.

Given the potential overlap in presentation, and the possibility of atypical presentation, diagnostic testing becomes critical. The most useful tests are HSV PCR of a swab of the lesion (though culture and/or Tzanck smear may be useful in certain circumstances), RPR (or treponemal antibody test), and Gram stain from the edge of the ulcer (if chancroid is suspected). In the MSM population, especially those with recent international travel, LGV PCR or serology may be considered. When the etiology remains unclear with the above means, biopsy is warranted. For more information on HSV, Syphilis, and LGV please see the respective pathogen sections above.

## Urethritis

Symptomatic urethritis in men is classically characterized by mucopurulent or purulent urethral discharge, dysuria (pain on urination), and/or urethral pruritus. Infectious urethritis as a syndrome is classically divided by etiology into gonococcal urethritis and non-gonococcal urethritis (NGU). Gonococcal urethritis is caused by *Neisseria gonorrhoeae* as its name suggests. NGU most commonly results from infection with *Chlamydia trachomatis*, but *Mycoplasma genitalium*, *Trichomonas vaginalis*, HSV-1 and -2, and adenovirus may also be responsible [84]. Many cases of NGU may not have an identifiable etiology upon comprehensive laboratory analysis [85]. Empiric therapy is thus recommended regardless of the outcome of diagnostic studies when treating men with symptoms of urethritis.

A health care provider's first step in assessing a patient with possible urethritis should be to establish clinical evidence of disease. Providers should look for urethral discharge when examining a patient. If available, Gram stain of discharge can detect elevated white blood cell counts ($\geq 5$ WBC per oil immersion field, suggestive of urethritis) and/or Gram-negative intracellular diplococci (diagnostic for gonococcal urethritis).

First-void urinalysis can be used to look for presence of leukocyte esterase (a nonspecific indicator of urogenital tract infection) or white blood cells on microscopy ($\geq 10$ WBC per high-power field). Once a diagnosis of urethritis is made (or heavily suspected), further etiological testing is indicated to ensure proper treatment. This primarily includes NAAT for GC and CT.

Treatment should be started immediately upon diagnosis. Specific therapy for GC and CT are discussed in their respective sections above. It is important to note that, although azithromycin and doxycycline are approved antibiotic regimens for the treatment of NGU, azithromycin has proved superior in the treatment of *M. genitalium* urethritis [85]. If a patient fails initial therapy and noncompliance and pathogen reexposure are ruled out, further diagnostic testing for HSV or *T. vaginalis* may be indicated. HSV diagnosis and treatment is discussed above. Of note, MSM are at low-risk for *T. vaginalis* unless they also participate in sexual intercourse with women [22].

## Proctitis

Clinically, proctitis in men is characterized by inflammation of the distal 10–12 cm of the anorectum and is associated with anorectal pain, anorectal discharge, and/or tenesmus (a persistent sensation of needing to pass stool despite an empty rectal vault). This syndrome must be differentiated from proctocolitis and enteritis, which involve more proximal regions of the gastrointestinal tract and are caused by different pathogens despite possible overlapping clinical pictures. As mentioned above, the majority of cases of gonococcal and chlamydial proctitis in MSM are asymptomatic, highlighting the need for effective screening strategies. Besides CT and GC, *Treponema pallidum* (i.e. syphilis) and HSV-1 and -2 must also be considered as possible etiologies of infectious proctitis [22].

Providers should ensure they are completing effective sexual histories to screen for men who may participate in receptive anal intercourse as this is the sexual behavior that primarily puts patients at risk for infectious proctitis. Patients should be examined for rectal discharge or any external ulcerative lesions. Anoscopy may be necessary to visualize more proximal areas of the distal rectal mucosa. Diagnostic and therapeutic information for the pathogens mentioned above (i.e. GC, CT, HSV-1 and -2, syphilis) are discussed in their respective sections.

## Cervicitis

Inflammation of the uterine cervix is often an asymptomatic condition discovered on routine health maintenance. When patients present with symptoms, typical complaints include mucopurulent discharge, post-coital bleeding or intermenstrual spotting, dysuria, dyspareunia, or vulvovaginal irritation. The most common causes of this condition are gonorrhea and *chlamydia*, which are discussed in detail earlier in the chapter.

Patients with the above symptoms warrant a pelvic exam. If cervical motion or adnexal tenderness is elicited, NAAT for gonorrhea and chlamydia should be performed. There are no prominent reports of transmission of the aforementioned pathogens between female partners, though male partners of WSW should be tested and treated for these infections. Empiric treatment should cover both pathogens. Untreated cervicitis may progress to pelvic inflammatory disease, tubo-ovarian abscess, and salpingitis. It is important to test regularly for these infections in WSMW, as untreated cervicitis may progress to these more serious infectious as well as infertility.

## Vaginitis

Vaginitis is a common clinical complaint of female patients characterized by vaginal burning, itching, odor, and abnormal discharge. The vast majority of these cases are caused by three etiologies: bacterial vaginosis, candidiasis, and trichomoniasis. Of note WSW patients are at equal—and in the case of BV, increased—risk for these infections. These three causes are each elaborated within the specific pathogen sections

above. Though inflammatory and atrophic changes can also be to blame, these are not discussed here.

This clinical syndrome should raise concern for an infectious cause as over 90 % of cases are due to an infection or overgrowth of natural flora. When seeing a patient with these complaints a pelvic exam with careful examination of the vulvar skin for evidence of infection is warranted. Samples for wet mount, potassium hydroxide testing, the amine whiff test, and pH testing are advisable in almost all cases. These should be taken from the mid-portion of the vagina to avoid contamination with cervical mucus. Specific DNA probes for the most common causes may be warranted if the above testing and physical exam are non-diagnostic. Finally, depending upon the risk factors of the patient, remembering that identity does not determine sexual behavior, DNA amplification testing for gonorrhea and *Chlamydia* may also be a consideration.

**Acknowledgement** Figures used with permission from: Gross G and Tyring SK, eds. Sexually Transmitted Infections and Sexually Transmitted Diseases. Heidelberg: Springer, 2011.

## References

1. Center for Disease Control and Prevention. HIV Surveillance Report, vol. 23; 2011. http://www.cdc.gov/hiv/topics/surveillance/resources/reports/. Published February 2012. Accessed 22 Aug 2014.
2. Centers for Disease Control and Prevention. Sexually transmitted disease surveillance 2011. Atlanta: U.S. Department of Health and Human Services; 2012.
3. Pathela P, Blank S, Sell RL, Schillinger JA. The importance of both sexual behavior and identity. Am J Public Health. 2006;96(5):765. author reply 766.
4. Young RM, Meyer IH. The trouble with "MSM" and "WSW": erasure of the sexual minority person in public health discourse. Am J Public Health. 2005; 95(7):1144–9.
5. World Health Organization. HIV/AIDS; Online Q&A. Online at http://who.int/features/qa/71/en. Accessed 01 May 2014.
6. Centers for Disease Control and Prevention. HIV/AIDS; Basic Statistics. Online at http://www.cdc.gov/hiv/basics/statistics.html. Accessed 01 May 2014.
7. Centers for Disease Control and Prevention. HIV among gay, bisexual, and other men who have sex

with men. Online at http://www.cdc.gov/hiv/risk/gender/msm/facts/index.html. Accessed 01 May 2014.

8. Centers for Disease Control and Prevention. HIV among African Americans. Online at http://www.cdc.gov/hiv/risk/racialethnic/aa/facts/index.html. Accessed 01 May 2014.

9. Zelota NM, Pilcher CD. Diagnosis and management of acute HIV infection. Infect Dis Clin N Am. 2007; 21(1):19–48.

10. United States Preventive Services Task Force (USPSTF). Screening for HIV. Online at http://www.uspreventiveservicestaskforce.org/uspstf13/hiv/hiv-summ.pdf. Accessed 29 June 2014. Also available as Moyer VA. Screening for HIV: U.S. preventive services task force recommendation statement. Ann Intern Med. 2013;159(1):51–60.

11. Panel on Antiretroviral Guidelines for Adults and Adolescents. Guidelines for the Use of Antiretroviral Agents in HIV-1-Infected Adults and Adolescents. Available at http://aidsinfo.nih.gov/ContentFiles/AdultandAdolescentGL.pdf

12. Panel on opportunistic infections in HIV-infected adults and adolescents. Guidelines for the prevention and treatment of opportunistic infections in HIV-infected adults and adolescents: recommendations from the Centers for Disease Control and Prevention, the National Institutes of Health, and the HIV Medicine Association of the Infectious Diseases Society of America. Available at http://aidsinfo.nih.gov/contentfiles/lvguidelines/adult_oi.pdf

13. Aberg JA, Gallant JE, Ghanem KG, Emmanuel P, Zingman BS, Horberg MA. Primary care guidelines for the management of persons infected with HIV: 2013 update by the HIV medicine association of the infectious diseases society of America. Clin Inf Dis. 2014;58(1):e1–e34. Also available online at http://www.hivma.org/HIV_Guidelines/.

14. Grant RM, et al. Preexposure chemoprophylaxis for HIV prevention in men who have sex with men. N Engl J Med. 2010;363(27):2587–99.

15. Centers for Disease Control and Prevention. Sexually transmitted disease surveillance 2012. Atlanta: U.S. Department of Health and Human Services; 2013.

16. Detels R, Green AM, Klausner JD, et al. The incidence and correlates of symptomatic and asymptomatic Chlamydia trachomatis and Neisseria gonorrhoeae infections in selected populations in five countries. Sex Transm Dis. 2011;38(6):503–9.

17. Cecil JA, Howell MR, Tawes JJ, et al. Features of Chlamydia trachomatis and Neisseria gonorrhoeae infection in male Army recruits. J Infect Dis. 2001;184(9):1216–9.

18. Kent CK, Chaw JK, Wong W, et al. Prevalence of rectal, urethral, and pharyngeal chlamydia and gonorrhea detected in 2 clinical settings among men who have sex with men: San Francisco, California, 2003. Clin Infect Dis. 2005;41(1):67–74.

19. Turner AN, Reese PC, Ervin M, Davis JA, Fields KS, Bazan JA. HIV, rectal chlamydia, and rectal gonorrhea

in men who have sex with men attending a sexually transmitted disease clinic in a midwestern US city. Sex Transm Dis. 2013;40(6):433–8.

20. Stamm WE. Chlamydia trachomatis Infections of the Adult. In Holmes KK, Sparling PF, Stamm WE, et al., editors. Sexually transmitted diseases. 4th ed. New York: McGraw-Hill; 2008.

21. Schachter J, Chernesky MA, Willis DE, et al. Vaginal swabs are the specimens of choice when screening for Chlamydia trachomatis and Neisseria gonorrhoeae: results from a multicenter evaluation of the APTIMA assays for both infections. Sex Transm Dis. 2005;32(12):725–8.

22. Centers for Disease Control and Prevention. Sexually Transmitted Diseases Treatment Guidelines, 2015. MMWR Recomm Rep 2015;64(No. RR-3): 1–137.

23. Scott HM, Bernstein KT, Raymond HF, Kohn R, Klausner JD. Racial/ethnic and sexual behavior disparities in rates of sexually transmitted infections, San Francisco, 1999-2008. BMC Public Health. 2010;10:315.

24. Sherrard J, Barlow D. Gonorrhoea in men: clinical and diagnostic aspects. Genitourin Med. 1996;72(6):422–6.

25. Walker CK, Sweet RL. Gonorrhea infection in women: prevalence, effects, screening, and management. Int J Womens Health. 2011;3:197–206.

26. Soper DE. Pelvic inflammatory disease. Obstet Gynecol. 2010;116(2 Pt 1):419–28.

27. Kinghorn GR, Rashid S. Prevalence of rectal and pharyngeal infection in women with gonorrhea in Sheffield. Br J Vener Dis. 1979;55(6):408–10.

28. CDC MMWR report. Vol. 61(31). 2012.

29. Kirkcaldy RD, Zaidi A, Hook III EW, et al. Neisseria gonorrhoeae antimicrobial resistance among men who have sex with men and men who have sex exclusively with women: the Gonococcal Isolate Surveillance Project, 2005-2010. Ann Intern Med. 2013;158(5 Pt 1):321–8.

30. Bradley H, Markowitz LE, Gibson T, McQuillan GM. Seroprevalence of Herpes Simplex Virus Types 1 and 2—United States, 1999–2010. J Infect Dis. 2014;209(3):325–33.

31. Copen CE, Chandra A, Martinez G. Prevalence and timing of oral sex with opposite-sex partners among females and males aged 15–24 years: United States, 2007–2010. National Health Statistics Reports; 2012; No. 56. Hyattsville, MD: National Center for Health Statistics.

32. Xu F, Sternberg MR, Markowitz LE. Men who have sex with men in the United States: demographic and behavioral characteristics and prevalence of HIV and HSV-2 infection results from national health and nutrition examination survey 2001–2006. Sex Transm Dis. 2010;37(6):399–405.

33. Schillinger JA, McKinney CM, Garg R, et al. Seroprevalence of herpes simplex virus type 2 and characteristics associated with undiagnosed infection: New York City, 2004. Sex Transm Dis. 2008; 35(6):599–606.

34. Ryder N, Jin F, McNulty AM, Grulich AE, Donovan B. Increasing role of herpes simplex virus type 1 in

first-episode anogenital herpes in heterosexual women and younger men who have sex with men, 1992-2006. Sex Transm Infect. 2009;85(6):416–9.

35. Marrazzo JM, Stine K, Wald A. Prevalence and risk factors for infection with herpes simplex virus type-1 and -2 among lesbians. Sex Transm Dis. 2003; 30(12):890–5.

36. Mark HD, Sifakis F, Hylton JB, et al. Sex with women as a risk factor for herpes simplex virus type 2 among young men who have sex with men in Baltimore. Sex Transm Dis. 2005;32(11):691–5.

37. Gupta R, Warren T, Wald A. Genital herpes. Lancet. 2007;370(9605):2127–37.

38. Tronstein E, Johnston C, Huang ML, et al. Genital shedding of herpes simplex virus among symptomatic and asymptomatic persons with HSV-2 infection. JAMA. 2011;305(14):1441–9.

39. Mertz GJ, Benedetti J, Ashley R, Selke SA, Corey L. Risk factors for the sexual transmission of genital herpes. Ann Intern Med. 1992;116(3):197–202.

40. Lafferty WE, Coombs RW, Benedetti J, Critchlow C, Corey L. Recurrences after oral and genital herpes simplex virus infections. N Engl J Med. 1987; 316(23):1444–9.

41. Engelberg R, Carrell D, Krantz E, Corey L, Wald A. Natural history of genital herpes simplex virus type 1 infection. Sex Transm Dis. 2003;30(2):174–7.

42. Martin ET, Krantz E, Gottlieb SL, et al. A pooled analysis of the effect of condoms in preventing acquisition of HSV-2 infection. Arch Intern Med. 2009;169(13):1233–40.

43. Socato G, Wald A, Wakabayashi E, Vieira J, Corey L. Evidence of latency and reactivation of both herpes simplex virus (HSV)-1 and HSV-2 in the genital region. J Infect Dis. 1998;177(4):1069–72.

44. Filen F, Strand A, Allard A, Blomberg J, Herrmann B. Duplex real-time polymerase chain reaction assay for detection and quantification of herpes simplex virus type 1 and herpes simplex virus type 2 in genital and cutaneous lesions. Sex Transm Dis. 2004;31(6): 331–6.

45. Ramaswamy M, McDonald C, Smith M, et al. Diagnosis of genital herpes by real time PCR in routine clinical practice. Sex Transm Infect. 2004;80(5): 406–10.

46. Corey L, Wald A, Patel R, et al. Once-daily valacyclovir to reduce the risk of transmission of genital herpes. N Engl J Med. 2004;350(1):11–20.

47. Fife KH, Crumpacker CS, Mertz GJ, Hill EL, Boone GS. Recurrence and resistance patterns of herpes simplex virus following cessation of > or = 6 years of chronic suppression with acyclovir. Acyclovir Study Group. J Infect Dis. 1994;169(6):1338–41.

48. The Centers for Disease Control, Primary and Secondary Syphilis – United States, 1998. CDC.gov. Web. Accessed 11 Apr 2014.

49. Stephenson J. Syphilis outbreak sparks concerns. JAMA. 2003;289(8):974. JAMA. Web. Accessed 28 Mar 2014.

50. Heffelfinger J, et al. Trends in primary and secondary syphilis among men who have sex with men in the

United States. Am J Public Health. 2007;97(6):1076–83. Alpha Publications. Web. Accessed 28 Mar 2014.

51. Klausner J, et al. Tracing a syphilis outbreak through cyberspace. JAMA. 2000;284(4):447–9. JAMA Web. Accessed 28 Mar 2014.

52. Su J, et al. Primary and secondary syphilis among black and hispanic men who have sex with men: case report data from 27 states. Ann Intern Med. 2011;155(3):145–51. Annals.org. Web. Accessed 28 Mar 2014.

53. Campos-Outcalt D, Hurwitz S. Female-to-female transmission of syphilis: a case report. Sex Transm Dis. 2002;29:119–20. Accessed 28 Mar 2014, at Journals.lww.com.

54. Ghanem KG. Neurosyphilis: a historical perspective and review. CNS Neurosci Ther. 2010;16:157–68.

55. Leslie DE, Azzato F, Karapanagiotidis T, Letdon J, Fyfe J. Development of a real-time PCR assay to detect Treponema Pallidum in clinical specimens and assessment of the assay's comparison with serological testing. J Clin Microbiol. 2007;45:93–6. Accessed May 22, 2014, at jcm.asm.org.

56. Harding AS, Ghanam KG. The performance of cerebrospinal fluid treponemal-specific antibody tests in neurosyphilis: a systematic review. Sex Transm Dis. 2012;39:291–7.

57. O'Hanlan KA, Crum CP. Human papillomavirus-associated cervical intraepithelial neoplasia following lesbian sex. Obstet Gynecol. 1996;88:702–3. Accessed on 22 May 2014, at ovidsp.tx.ovid.com.

58. Anderson TA, Schick V, Herbenick D, Dodge B, Fortenberry JD. A study of human papillomavirus on vaginally inserted sex toys, before and after cleaning, among women who have sex with women. Sex Transm Infect. 2014;90(7):529–31.

59. Goldstone S, Palefsky JM, Giuliano AR, et al. Prevalence of and risk factors for human papillomavirus (HPV) infection among HIV-seronegative men who have sex with men. J Infect Dis. 2011;203:66. Accessed 22 May 2014, at jid.oxfordjournals.org.

60. Goldie SJ, Kuntz KM, Weinstein MC, Freedberg KA, Palefsky JM. Cost-effectiveness of screening for anal squamous intraepithelial lesions and anal cancer in human immunodeficiency virus-negative homosexual and bisexual men. Am J Med. 2000;108:634–41. Accessed 22 May 2014, at sciencedirect.com.

61. Koumans EH, Sternberg M, Bruce C, et al. The prevalence of bacterial vaginosis in the United States 2001-2004; Associations with symptoms, sexual behaviors, and reproductive health. Sex Transm Dis. 2007;34(11):864–9. Accessed 11 Apr 2014, at journals.lww.com.

62. Bailey JV, Farquhar C, Owen C. Bacterial vaginosis in lesbians and bisexual women. Sex Transm Dis. 2004;31:691–4. Accessed 11 Apr 2014, at journals.lww.com.

63. Bradshaw CS, Walker SM, Vodstrcil LA, et al. The influence of behaviors and relationships on the vaginal microbiota of women and their female partners: The WOW Health Study. J Infect Dis. 2014;209:1562–72. Accessed 22 May 2014 at jid.oxfordjournals.org.

64. Hillier SL, Nugent RP, Eschenbach DA, et al. Association between bacterial vaginosis and preterm delivery of low-birth-weight infant. The Vaginal Infections and Prematurity Study Group. N Engl J Med. 1995;333:1737–42. Accessed 22 May 2014, at nejm.org.

65. Monif GR. Classification and pathogenesis of vulvovaginal candidiasis. Am J Obstet Gynecol. 1985;152: 935–9.

66. Bailey J, et al. Vulvovaginal candidiasis in women who have sex with women. Sex Transm Dis. 2008;35(6):533–6. Journals.LWW.com. Web. Accessed 11 Apr 2014.

67. Sobel JD, Kapernick PS, Zervos M, et al. Treatment of complicated Candida vaginitis: comparison of single and sequential doses of fluconazole. Am J Obstet Gynecol. 2001;185:363–9. Accessed 22 May 2014, at sciencedirect.com.

68. Muzny C, et al. Genotypic characterization of Trichomonas vaginalis isolates among women who have sex with women in sexual partnerships. Sex Transm Dis. 2012;39(7):556–8. Journals.LWW.com. Web. Accessed 26 Mar 2014.

69. Fastring D, et al. Co-occurrence of Trichomonas vaginalis and Bacterial Vaginosis and Vaginal Shedding of HIV-1 RNA. Sex Transm Dis. 2014;41(3):173–9. Journals.LWW.com. Web. Accessed 26 Mar 2014.

70. Kellock DJ, O'Mahoney CP. Sexually acquired metronidazole-resistant trichomoniasis in a lesbian couple. Geniutourin Med. 1996;72:60–1. PMC. Web. Accessed 26 Mar 2014.

71. Chapel T, et al. Pediculosis pubis in a clinic for treatment of sexually transmitted diseases. Sex Transm Dis. 1979;6(4):257.

72. Fuller CL. Epidemiology of scabies. Curr Opin Infect Dis. 2013;26:123–6. Journals.LWW.com. Web. Accessed 27 Mar 2014.

73. Schlesinger I, Oelrich DM, Tyring SK. Crusted (Norwegian) scabies in patients with AIDS: the range of clinical presentations. South Med J. 1994;87(3):352–6. MEDLINE with Full Text. Web. 27 March 2014.

74. Lanternier F, et al. Kaposi's sarcoma in HIV-negative men having sex with men. AIDS. 2008;22(10):1163–8.

75. Advisory Committee on Immunization Practices. Adult immunization schedules. MMWR. 2014;63(5): 110–2.

76. Bradshaw D, Matthews G, Danta M. Sexually transmitted hepatitis C infection: the new epidemic in MSM? Curr Opin Infect Dis. 2013;26(1):66–72.

77. Kingsley LA, Rinaldo CR, Lyter DW, Valdiserri RO, Belle SH, Ho M. Sexual transmission efficiency of hepatitis B virus and human immunodeficiency virus among homosexual men. JAMA. 1990;264(2): 230–4.

78. Gough E, Kempf MC, Graham L, Manzanero M, Hook EW, Bartolucci A, Chamot E. HIV and Hepatitis B and C incidence rates in US correctional populations and high risk groups: a systematic review and meta-analysis. BMC Public Health. 2010;10:777–91.

79. Diep BA, et al. Emergence of multidrug-resistant, community-associated, methicillin-resistant Staphylococcus aureus clone USA 300 in men who have sex with men. Ann Intern Med. 2008;148(4):249–57.

80. Antoniou T, et al. Community-associated methicillin-resistant Staphylococcus aureus colonization in men who have sex with men. Int J STD AIDS. 2009;20(3):180–3.

81. Centers for Disease Control and Prevention. Notes from the field: serogroup C invasive meningococcal disease among men who have sex with men – New York City, 2010-2012. MMWR. 2013;61(51):1048.

82. County of Los Angeles Public Health Department. Public health issues new vaccination recommendations for men who have sex with men (MSM) at-risk for invasive meningococcal disease. Public Health News. April 2, 2014.

83. Pathela P, Blank S, Schillinger JA. Lymphogranuloma venereum: old pathogen, new story. Curr Infect Dis Rep. 2007;9(2):143.

84. Bradshaw CS, Tabrizi SN, Read TR, et al. Etiologies of nongonococcal urethritis: bacteria, viruses, and the association with orogenital exposure. J Infect Dis. 2006;193(3):336–45.

85. Schwebke JR, Rompalo A, Taylor S, et al. Re-evaluating the treatment of nongonococcal urethritis: emphasizing emerging pathogens – a randomized clinical trial. Clin Infect Dis. 2011;52(2):163–70.

# Dermatology

# 15

## Brian Ginsberg

## Purpose

The purpose of this chapter is to explore the dermatologic needs of and services available to the LGBTI community.

## Learning Objectives

- Describe differences in dermatologic disease presentation and frequency within LGBT patients, reflecting the community's diverse sexual practices *(PC5)*
- Define the three major ways that HIV can affect the skin *(PC5)*
- Describe the work-up and various presentations of common sexually transmitted infections (STIs), including HPV, herpes, and syphilis *(PC1, PC2, PC6)*
- Identify at least 3 ways how cosmetic dermatology can play a role in the transitioning process, providing non-invasive options for facial transformation *(PC3, PC4)*

## Overview

Dermatology is more than just skin deep. It is the study of the skin, hair, nails and mucosa. Findings may represent primary diseases, manifestations of an internal insult, or consequences of an external event. Of the thousands of dermatologic conditions, those affecting most LGBT patients will be equivalent to that of the general population, with the same most-common conditions being acne, eczema, seborrheic dermatitis, psoriasis, infections and skin cancer. Explored in this chapter are these and other conditions, with attention to how their rates, causes and presentations may differ in this population. In addition, the roles of a dermatologist in the care of the LGBT individual are examined, such as in treating these conditions, uncovering systemic disorders, encountering behavioral and environmental effects, and providing cosmetic options for the transitioning transgender patient.

Dermatology has its own unique language, and it may therefore be helpful to browse the following list of definitions of commonly used terms that will be encountered in this chapter:

- Alopecia—hair loss
- Atrophy—thinning of the skin
- Blanching—loss of redness with pressure
- Bulla—a raised lesion greater than 1 cm in diameter filled with clear fluid
- Crust—dried blood, serum, or pus

B. Ginsberg, M.D. (✉)
The Ronald O. Perelman Department of
Dermatology, NYU Langone Medical Center,
New York, NY, USA
e-mail: brian.ginsberg.md@gmail.com

© Springer International Publishing Switzerland 2016
K.L. Eckstrand, J.M. Ehrenfeld (eds.), *Lesbian, Gay, Bisexual, and Transgender Healthcare*,
DOI 10.1007/978-3-319-19752-4_15

- Ecchymosis—bruise from extravasated red blood cells
- Erosion—loss of part of the epidermis
- Erythema—redness
- Exanthem—a rash in the setting of a viral illness
- Excoriation—skin injury due to scratching
- Fissure—linear cut into the skin
- Glabrous—hairless
- Hyperkeratosis—thickened stratum corneum; scale
- Hypertrophic—thickening of the dermis; skin lines are not accentuated
- Lichenification—thickening of the epidermis; skin lines are accentuated
- Macule—a flat lesion less than 1 cm in diameter
- Morbilliform—measles-likes; generalized coalescing red macules and/or papules
- Nodule—a rounded lesion with a prominent deep component
- Papule—a raised lesion less than 1 cm in diameter
- Patch—a flat lesion greater than 1 cm in diameter
- Paronychia—inflammation of the nail unit
- Petechiae—small, non-blanching, red macules from extravasated blood
- Plaque—a raised lesion greater than 1 cm in diameter
- Pruritus—itch
- Purpura—large, non-blanching, red patches from extravasated blood
- Pustule—a raised lesion less than 1 cm in diameter filled with purulent fluid
- Ulcer—loss of the full epidermis or deeper
- Xerosis—dryness

## Sexually Transmitted Infections

Sexual practice has long been a focus of LGBT healthcare, and is one of the major factors that contribute to the spectrum of the community's dermatologic concerns. While the disease entities are not unique, their presentations and frequen-

cies vary when compared to the general population. Men who have sex with men (MSM) and transgender women have an increased prevalence of most sexually transmitted infections (STIs), not limited to HIV, anogenital warts, herpes simplex, syphilis, gonorrhea, chlamydia and infectious hepatitis [1]. Women who have sex with women (WSW), on the other hand, have reduced rates of most STIs, but it should not be assumed that this risk is zero [2]. Many STIs are transmissible by oral sex, vaginal-vaginal intercourse, and sex-toy use. Furthermore, a significant percentage of WSW is currently having or has at one point also had sex with men [3].

Another factor affecting the diverse STI patterns in the LGBT community is the manner in which the infections are obtained. Aside from common presentations on genitalia, diseases may present perianally if the patient engaged in receptive anal sex or oral-anal contact, the latter also attributing to perioral presentations as does oral-genital sexual activity. For post-operative transgender patients, the presentation and prevalence of an STI may reflect the donor tissue used for the neogenitalia. All of the above reflects the imperative to take a thorough sexual and, in the case of transgender patients, surgical history. Furthermore, non-infectious etiologies should always remain in the differential diagnosis (Table 15.1) (Fig. 15.1a–f).

## HIV and AIDS

Nearly 1.1 million people in the United States are currently living with HIV infection. Of the 50,000 new cases each year, approximately 75 % are in MSM, with a disproportionately elevated rate in young African American men [4]. The Center for Disease Control estimates an even higher prevalence amongst transgender women, with data from outside of the United States showing HIV rates as high as 50 times that of the general population [5].

There are three principle ways that HIV affects the skin: primary infection, secondary disease prevalence, and medication side effects.

**Table 15.1** Common non-infectious causes of anogenital disease

| Inflammatory diseases | Benign growths | Malignant growths |
|---|---|---|
| • Psoriasis<br>• Lichen planus<br>• Lichen sclerosis et atrophicus<br>• Lichen simplex chronicus<br>• Contact dermatitis [from condoms, lubricants, wipes]<br>• Fixed drug eruption<br>• Zoon's balanitis | • Epidermoid cysts<br>• Angiokeratomas<br>• Acrochordons (skin tags)<br>• Pearly penile papules *(penis only)*<br>• Vestibular papillomatosis *(vulva only)* | • Erythroplasia of Queyrat<br>• Bowenoid papulosis<br>• Squamous cell carcinoma<br>• Extramammary Paget's disease<br>• Melanoma |

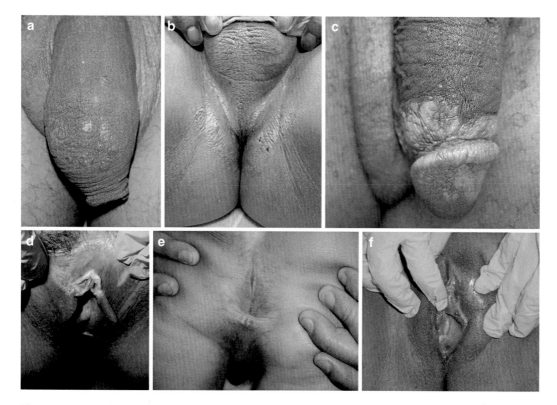

**Fig. 15.1** Non-infectious anogenital diseases: (**a**) Psoriasis, (**b**) Inverse psoriasis, (**c**) Lichen planus, (**d**) Lichen sclerosus et atrophicus, (**e**) Eczema, (**f**) Skin tags

## Primary HIV Infection (Acute Retroviral Syndrome)

Primary HIV infection is defined by HIV viral presence in the blood prior to antibody formation. While many patients are completely asymptomatic, up to 80 % experience a viral syndrome that can include fever, sore throat, lymphadenopathy, and a morbilliform rash. This occurs 2–4 weeks after exposure and, while the systemic syndrome may last from days to over 10 weeks, the rash typically persists only 4–5 days. Blanching, red macules and papules coalesce centrally on the trunk and proximal extremities and progress caudally, reminiscent of other viral exanthems or drug eruptions (Fig. 15.2). Oral and anogenital ulcerations sometimes develop. Being that this occurs prior to antibody formation, serologic testing is often negative, and direct DNA or RNA detection may be indicated if HIV is suspected [6].

**Fig. 15.2** Primary HIV
infection—morbilliform
eruption

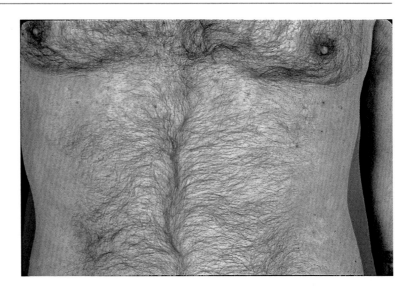

sarcoma (Fig. 15.3b). Eruptive atypical nevi
(moles) may develop, and melanoma risk is
increased. CD4 counts below 250 cells/mm$^2$ are
associated with less common infectious processes,
including disseminated or resistant herpes and
molluscum, extrapulmonary tuberculosis, bacil-
lary angiomatosis, and deep fungal infections (Fig.
15.3c). A patient with extremely low CD4 counts,
below 50 cells/mm$^2$, may have abnormal presentations of common infections, such as giant mol-
lusca and CMV-induced perianal ulcers, or unique
infectious etiologies, including cutaneous
*Mycobacterium avium* complex (Fig. 15.3d) [8].

## Diseases with Increased Incidence in HIV-Positive Patients

While some skin conditions are AIDS-defining,
numerous common dermatoses are more prevalent
in HIV-positive patients even with normal CD4
T-cell levels. These include inflammatory disorders, such as psoriasis, and common infections,
including tinea and warts. The most common condition affecting HIV-positive patients is folliculitis, followed by condyloma, seborrheic dermatitis,
and generalized xerosis (Fig. 15.3a). As counts
drop below 500 cells/mm$^2$, cutaneous malignancy
risk begins to increase, including basal and squamous cell carcinomas, cutaneous non-Hodgkin
lymphoma, Merkel cell carcinoma, and Kaposi

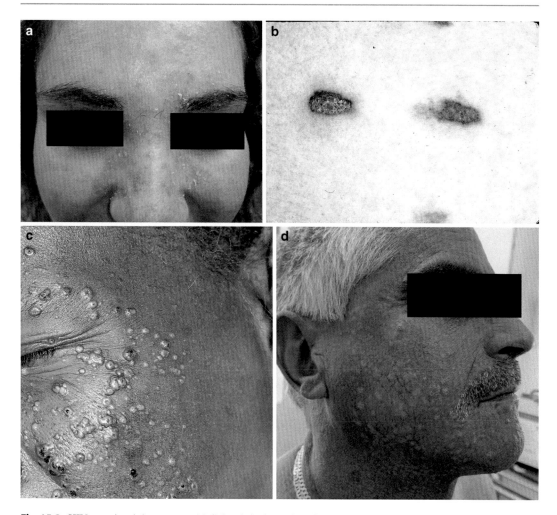

**Fig. 15.3** HIV-associated dermatoses: (**a**) Seborrheic dermatitis, (**b**) Kaposi's sarcoma, (**c**) Histoplasmosis, (**d**) Giant molluscum contagiosum

## Treatment-Associated Dermatoses

The advent of highly active antiretroviral therapy (HAART) revolutionized the care of HIV-positive patients, but not without cutaneous effects. The initiation of treatment may result in the Immune Reconstitution Inflammatory Syndrome (IRIS), with worsening of an infectious, inflammatory, or even neoplastic etiology [10]. Individual HAART medications have their own toxicities, ranging from non-specific rashes and other mild effects (nail darkening, alopecia) to severe presentations, not limited to hypersensitivity syndromes, Stevens-Johnson syndrome, and Toxic Epidermal Necrosis (Table 15.2) (Fig. 15.4) [11]. These potentially fatal eruptions may also be caused by non-HAART medications frequently used by HIV-positive patients, especially trimethoprim-sulfamethoxazole, a common prophylaxis against *Pneumocystis jiroveci* pneumonia [12].

One notable side effect of protease inhibitors and nucleoside reverse-transcriptase inhibitors is lipodystrophy [13]. It manifests as a loss of fat in the face and extremities, with a gain of fat in the upper back, breasts, and viscera. There is no known method to reverse HAART-induced lipodystrophy. However, Sculptra® (poly-L-lactic acid) is an injectable synthetic filler that is FDA-approved for the correction of facial lipoatrophy, providing up to 2 years of dramatic cosmetic improvement via volume replacement (Fig. 15.5a, b) [14].

**Table 15.2** Dermatologic manifestations of commonly used HAART medications

| Medication | Dermatosis |
|---|---|
| Abacavir | Hypersensitivity syndrome/DRESS |
| Emtricitabine | Xerosis, rash, palmoplantar hyperpigmentation |
| Lamivudine | Paronychia, alopecia, rash, pruritus |
| NNRTIs (i.e. Efavirenz, Nevirapine, Rilpivirine) | Morbilliform eruption, SJS/TEN, DRESS |
| Protease Inhibitors (i.e. Atazanavir, Darunavir, Ritonavir) | Morbilliform eruption, SJS/TEN, lipodystrophy, paronychia, periungual pyogenic granulomas, pruritus, xerosis |
| Raltegravir | Rash, SJS/TEN, DRESS |
| Tenofovir | Rash |
| Zidovudine | Pigmentation (nails, skin, mucosa), rash, vasculitis, lipodystrophy, acral erythema |

*Note:* "Rash" includes morbilliform, pustular, and urticarial eruptions
*SJS* Stevens-Johnson syndrome, *TEN* toxic epidermal necrosis, *DRESS* drug reaction with eosinophilia and systemic symptoms

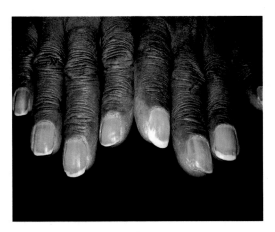

**Fig. 15.4** Zidovudine-induced nail hyperpigmentation

## Human Papillomavirus

There are approximately 120 genotypes of Human Papillomavirus (HPV) affecting the skin and mucosa with differing clinical appearances, most typically in the form of warts (papilloma, condyloma, verruca) [15]. The most common subtypes associated with sexual transmission are HPV-6 and -11 and portend no malignant potential. However, infection with oncogenic subtypes, most commonly HPV-16 and -18, is clinically indistinguishable [16].

Clinical presentation of HPV infection reflects its mode of acquisition. Condyloma accuminata (anogenital warts) are obtained during either penetrative or receptive intercourse. Appearance can range from skin-colored to hyperpigmented and from flat papules to fungating masses. They develop on the penis, vulva, perineum, perianal skin, or associated folds, and may proceed intraorificially, including intravaginally and intra-anally (Fig. 15.6a, b). They have also been described on the neovaginas of post-operative transgender women, including one case of condyloma gigantea, a rapidly growing, locally destructive, but non-malignant variant [17, 18]. Oral sex can also transmit HPV and lead to perioral and intraoral manifestations (Fig. 15.6c).

Malignant subtypes must be considered with an HPV diagnosis, given the concern for squamous cell carcinoma. HPV is responsible for 5 % of all cancers, notably penile, vulvar, vaginal, cervical, anal, and oropharyngeal carcinomatosis [19]. Perivaginal and perianal condyloma may warrant an internal exam with Papanicolaou smear to assess mucosal involvement, including condyloma of neovaginas, given the many reported cases of neovaginal HPV-associated malignancy. Other less common HPV-induced malignancy-associated lesions include bowenoid papulosis and erythroplasia of Queyrat.

Diagnosis of benign variants is usually made clinically. The differential diagnosis includes molluscum contagiosum, another viral STI appearing as umbilicated, dome-shaped papules (Fig. 15.6d). If the lesions are uncharacteristic, resistant to treatment, or with any concern for malignancy, a biopsy can be taken for histopathologic examination for atypia. In addition, HPV typing is obtainable for these samples to assess malignant potential.

Prevention is essential for HPV given its oncogenicity, with condoms being first-line. Several studies have shown that sex toys, even after washing, carry HPV at high rates; therefore,

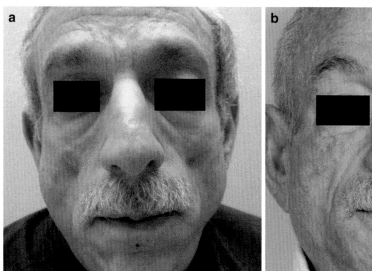
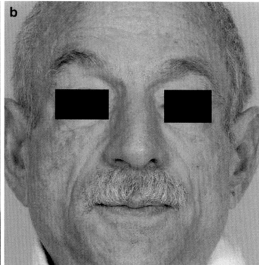

**Fig. 15.5** HIV-associated lipoatrophy: (**a**) before, and (**b**) after a series of Sculptra injections (10 vials). *Credit to Dr. Linda Franks

counseling about condom use on dildos and vibrators should be considered [20]. Another way of HPV prevention is through vaccination. Gardasil® is a quadrivalent vaccine protecting against HPV subtypes 6, 11, 16, and 18, accounting for the majority of benign and malignant lesions [21]. If already infected, treatment options include destructive therapies (liquid nitrogen, trichloroacetic acid, electrodessication), cytotoxic agents (podophyllotoxin), local immunoregulation (interferon, imiquimod), or if large or malignant, surgery [22].

> **Helpful Hint**
> While perianal papules should be suspicious for sexually transmitted diseases, including condyloma or molluscum, the diagnosis of hemorrhoids must be considered prior to biopsy or treatment to avoid vascular compromise.

## Herpes Simplex Virus (HSV)

The Herpesvirus family comprises 8 major genotypes, with HSV-1 and -2 producing all forms of herpes simplex, or more colloquially, herpes. Herpes is very common in the general population, with one third of people experiencing a symptomatic oral or anogenital infection, and one in six people between the ages of 14 to 49 having genital herpes, many of which are asymptomatic [23]. Rates in both MSM and/or HIV-positive patients are even higher [24]. While HSV-1 accounts for most cases of oral herpes (gingivostomatitis, cold sores) and HSV-2 induces the majority of anogenital herpes, both genotypes may cause either entity. In fact, HSV-1 now accounts for the majority of cases of anogenital herpes in young adults in many developed countries, including the United States, Canada, and the United Kingdom [25].

Regardless of anatomic site or genotype, herpes simplex presents as grouped vesicles, preceded or accompanied by pain, and lasts for approximately 1 week (Fig. 15.7a, b). Some cases present as non-healing ulcers, especially on perianal skin or in HIV-positive patients with low CD4 counts (Fig. 15.7c). In many cases, active disease is clinically asymptomatic and yet still contagious to sexual partners, including the majority of anogenital infections [26]. Herpes can also affect non-orogenital mucocutaneous surfaces, including the fingers (herpetic whitlow), torso (herpes gladiatorum), eyes (herpes keratoconjunc-

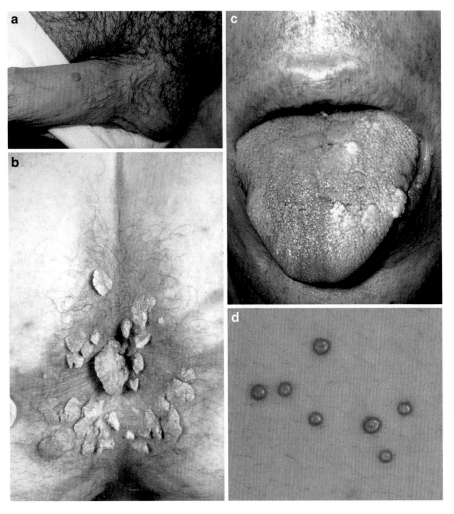

**Fig. 15.6** (**a**) Condyloma accuminata (penis). (**b**) Condyloma accuminata (perianal). (**b**) Condyloma accuminata (tongue). (**d**) Molluscum contagiosum

tivitis), central nervous system (herpes meningitis), or pre-existing patches of eczema (eczema herpeticum) (Fig. 15.7d) [27].

Diagnosis is usually made clinically. Vesicle fluid can be sent for viral DNA PCR, directly visualized for cytopathic change with a Tzanck smear, or stained for immunofluorescence with an HSV-specific antibody. Serologic testing is available, and, less commonly, a lesional biopsy can be performed for histopathologic confirmation [28]. While herpes usually persists for a lifetime, attributing to its latency in local dorsal root ganglia, treatment is with antiviral therapies and

can be taken either as needed for outbreaks or as chronic suppressive therapy [29].

## Syphilis

Syphilis is a bacterial infection caused by the spirochete *Treponema pallidum*. It is obtained through sexual contact, with the primary chancre occurring almost exclusively on anogenital skin. Approximately 5 % of cases of primary syphilis occur on extragenital locations, including the lips, perianal skin, and several documented cases

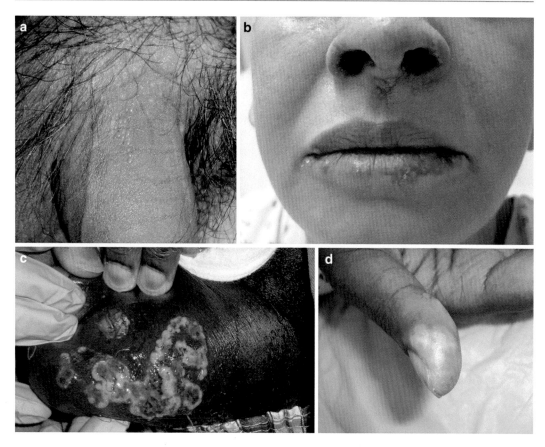

**Fig. 15.7** (**a**) Herpes simplex (genital). (**b**) Herpes simplex (labialis). (**c**) Herpes simplex (genital) in an immunocompromised HIV-positive patient. (**d**) Herpetic whitlow

on the finger acquired through mutual masturbation and digital-anal acts [30, 31].

Primary syphilis presents approximately 3 weeks after infection (ranging from 10 to 90 days). It begins as a solitary papule that develops into a painless, well-circumscribed, firm ulcer (chancre), usually accompanied by local lymphadenopathy (Fig. 15.8a). As this lesion is painless, many cases often go undiagnosed [32].

If untreated, the primary lesion regresses within weeks and dissemination will occur simultaneously or up to 6 months later, resulting in secondary syphilis in almost all cases. There are a variety of mucocutaneous manifestations of secondary syphilis, with most people presenting with generalized, non-pruritic, copper-colored, scaly papules, notably also present on the palms and soles, and sometimes with involvement of the hairline (corona veneris) (Fig. 15.8b–d). Other

features may include oral mucous patches and perléche, moth-eaten alopecia, and anogenital condylomata lata. This stage is also frequently preceded or accompanied by systemic symptoms, including fever, malaise, lymphadenopathy, and other flu-like symptoms. Ocular involvement should also be ruled out. Secondary syphilis will spontaneously resolve in 3–12 weeks even if untreated. The large variety of presentations of secondary syphilis has given it the reputation of being the great imitator in dermatology [33].

Untreated cases of secondary syphilis then enter a latency phase, which may persist indefinitely as in 70 % of cases, or progress to tertiary (or "late") syphilis after months to years. At this stage, organisms may invade and cause symptoms to major organs, including the cardiovascular, musculoskeletal, and central nervous systems.

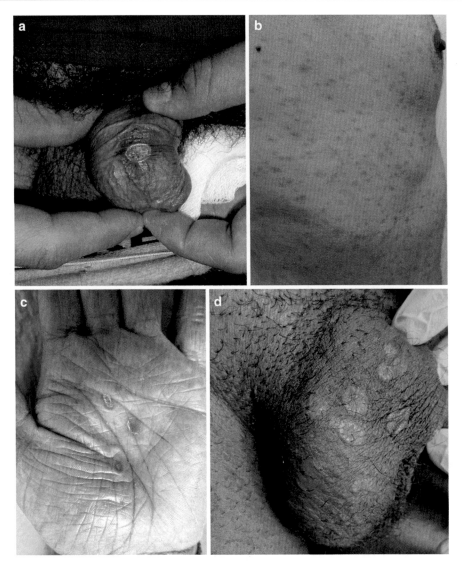

**Fig. 15.8** (**a**) Primary syphilis chancre. (**b**) Secondary syphilis eruption. (**c**) Secondary syphilis—palmar involvement. (**d**) Secondary syphilis—condylomata lata

The most sensitive and specific diagnostic method for detecting primary syphilis is by direct spirochete visualization with darkfield microscopy, although this is typically not available to most providers. All stages of syphilis can be detected with serologic testing for cardiolipin, a non-specific membrane lipid present in 80 % of cases [as measured by the rapid plasma reagin (RPR) and Venereal Disease Research Laboratory (VDRL) assays]. Confirmation is by treponemal-specific tests [the microhemagglutination assay

for antibodies to *T. pallidum* (MHA-TP) or the fluorescent treponemal antibody absorption assay (FTA-ABS)] [34].

Treatment for syphilis is with antibiotics, with dosing, course and antibiotic choice varying by stage. Penicillin is the preferred first-line treatment for all stages if not allergic. The treatment regimen does not vary based on HIV status. After treatment, the CDC recommends clinical and laboratory evaluation with non-treponemal serologies at 6 and 12 months, with

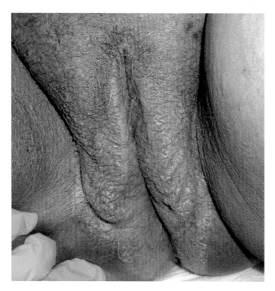

**Fig. 15.9** Lichen simplex chronicus of the vulva

more frequent evaluations in HIV-positive patients at 3, 9, and 24 months as well. Treponemal-specific testing will remain positive despite treatment, so should only be used diagnostically. Sexual partners may also be considered for testing [35].

---

**Helpful Hint**

Any generalized eruption with involvement of the palms or soles is highly suspicious for secondary syphillis

---

## Gonorrhea and Chlamydia

Gonorrhea and chlamydia are bacterial STIs caused by *Neisseria gonorrhea* and *Chlamydia trachomatis*, respectively. They most commonly cause urethritis, presenting as dysuria and urgency, and don't directly cause cutaneous manifestations other than pruritus. Therefore, they should be considered in the differential diagnosis of pruritus without rash of the genitals or anus, depending on sexual practice [36]. Cases have also been documented in the neovaginas of postoperative transgender women [37]. In WSW,

vaginal infection with *Trichomonas vaginalis* should also be considered when there is itch without rash.

Chronic pruritus and associated scratching may induce various skin changes, including lichen simplex chronicus, which should be recognized as a secondary phenomenon (Fig. 15.9). Diagnosis is made by culture, DNA hybridization or PCR [38]. Treatment is often directed at both organisms, given the high rates of co-infection, and tailored to sensitivities if available [39]. Lichen simplex chronicus, if present, is treated with topical corticosteroids.

Of note, disseminated *Neisseria gonorrhea* may present as an arthritis-dermatosis syndrome, with hemorrhagic pustules on distal extremities, often over joints. Non-dermatologic manifestations of both diseases include pelvic inflammatory disease, from direct spread, or involvement of internal organs if disseminated [40].

## Candida

While *Candida* spp., a common yeast commensal in many women, is not classically felt to be an STI, it may be spread through sexual contact, including vaginal-vaginal actions [41]. It can affect any aspect of the anogenital region. The skin becomes beefy red with discrete satellite lesions and, sometimes, pustules. When only affecting the penis, it presents as balanitis or balanoposthitis, could become eroded, and the associated edema in an uncircumcised man may prevent foreskin retraction. In male groin infection, the scrotum may be involved, helping to distinguish it from tinea cruris (jock itch), which spares this area (Fig. 15.10a, b). Vulvar infections frequently are associated with curdy, white vaginal discharge (Fig. 15.10c). Fissures often accompany perianal infection [42].

Diagnosis is made with a fungal swab and culture. Treatment is with topical antifungals alone when only cutaneous involvement is present, but may require systemic treatment if severe or refractory. Vaginal involvement requires either intravaginal suppositories or oral antifungal therapy [43].

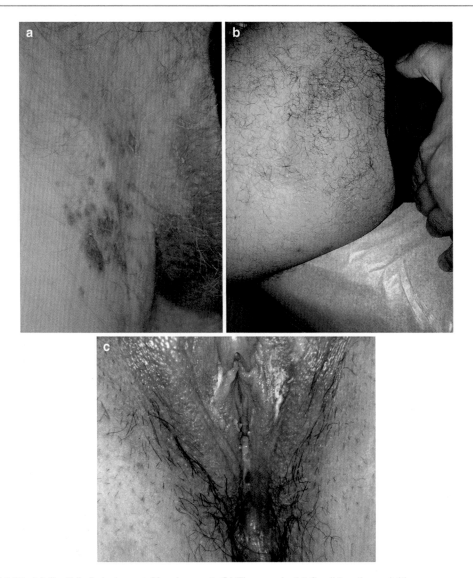

**Fig. 15.10** (**a**) Candidiasis (note scrotal involvement). (**b**) Tinea cruris. (**c**) Candida vulvovaginitis

## Hepatitis B & C

The hepatitis B virus (HBV) is a double-stranded DNA hepadnavirus spread through sexual activity or other contact with blood. Acute infection with HBV may cause serum sickness: urticaria or, less commonly, urticarial vasculitis accompanied by flu-like symptoms (Fig. 15.11a). This often precedes clinically apparent liver disease by up to 6 weeks [44]. Longer standing HBV infection has been associated with polyarteritis nodosa (PAN), a small- and medium-vessel vasculitis presenting cutaneously as tender, ulcerating, subcutaneous nodules along vascular tracts, usually of the distal lower extremities. The other skin presentation of PAN is livedo racemosa, a net-like purpura, which may occur in conjunction with or irrespective of the tender nodules. Severe systemic involvement may be present and should be assessed, especially renal, cardiovascular and neurologic. Skin-limited PAN is more typically associated with hepatitis C [45, 46].

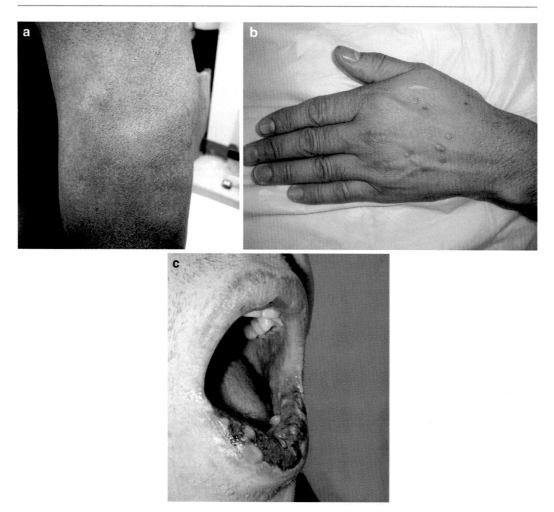

**Fig. 15.11** (**a**) Urticaria in the setting of serum sickness. (**b**) Lichen planus. (**c**) Lichen planus, oral-ulcerative subtype

The hepatitis C virus (HCV) is a single-stranded RNA flavivirus spread primarily through blood exposure and less commonly through sexual activity, although still presenting at increased rates in the MSM and HIV-positive populations. Associated with HCV and not HBV is lichen planus, which presents as pruritic, pink-purple, polygonal papules with scale [47] (Fig. 15.11b). Many cases also have oral involvement, and when ulcerative, is the most suspicious subtype for HCV infection (Fig. 15.11c). HCV has also been linked to porphyria cutanea tarda, a photodermatosis in which blisters develop in areas of sun exposure, classically the dorsal hands [48]. As opposed to PAN, the vasculitis associated with HCV is a small-vessel leukocytoclastic vasculitis due to circulating cryoglobulin, presenting as palpable purpura of the lower extremities [49] Approximately 84 % of cases of type II cryoglobulinemia are associated with HCV infection. Finally, a rare dermatosis called necrolytic acral erythema is almost universally linked to HCV and manifests as painful, well-demarcated, annular plaques with raised, red, crusted borders on the distal extremities [50]. In all of the above conditions, treatment of the underlying infectious hepatitis may improve the cutaneous pathologies.

## Methicillin-Resistant *Staphylococcus aureus*

*Staphylococcus aureus* is a common bacterial pathogen of the skin. Methicillin-resistant strains have been documented since the early 1960s, initially spread nosocomially, which emerged to be a community-acquired threat in the new millennium. Currently, Methicillin-Resistant *Staphylococcus aureus* (MRSA) may be the most common cause of purulent skin and soft tissue infections in the United States, with a disproportionally higher rate in MSM and/or HIV-positive individuals [51, 52].

The most common presentation of *S. aureus* skin infection, including MRSA, is as an abscess (furuncle). These may be very large and even necrotic, often causing a surrounding cellulitis (Fig. 15.12). Other types of pathologies may be mild, such as folliculitis or impetigo, or rarely more severe, including staphylococcal scalded skin syndrome, necrotizing fasciitis or toxic shock [53].

Diagnosis is made by wound culture, and treatment is with antibiotics tailored to the sensitivities. If warranted, empiric antibiotic therapy is often started before sensitivities return, and should be chosen based on patient demographics, community MRSA prevalence, and local antibiograms. Topical or oral antibiotics are used in mild infections, with severe cases requiring intravenous therapy. For a simple abscess, an incision and drainage (I&D) is the only necessary treatment. Antibiotics do not provide additional benefit, and should only be used if the abscess is associated with cellulitis or phlebitis, there are signs of systemic involvement, the patient has relevant comorbidities or immunosuppression, or an I&D has already failed. Oral antibiotics should also be prescribed for abscesses on difficult-to-drain sites, including the face, hands, and genitalia [54].

> **Helpful Hint**
> Local antibiograms can be obtained from nearby hospitals and microbiology laboratories.

## Skin as a Sign of Behaviors and Comorbidities

The LGBT population has an increased prevalence of psychiatric comorbidities and high-risk behaviors. As many of these entities carry a stigma, the patient may be unlikely to disclose important information that could substantially affect their health. It is therefore the physician's responsibility to recognize clues that reveal these hidden practices. Even without a history, the skin can provide significant insight into underlying pathologies and actions.

### Substance Abuse

LGBT individuals have an increased rate of substance abuse compared to the general population, especially in the youth demographics [55]. Substance abuse directly impacts the health of the individual, and further increases the likelihood of participating in other high-risk behaviors, including unprotected sexual intercourse [56].

Skin manifestations of alcohol abuse have been shown to occur in 43 % and 33 % of affected men and women, respectively [57]. Non-specific changes include photodistributed grey-brown hyperpigmentation, nail changes, and increased

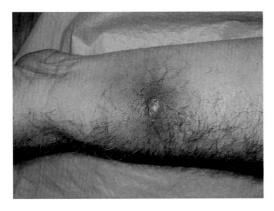

**Fig. 15.12** MRSA

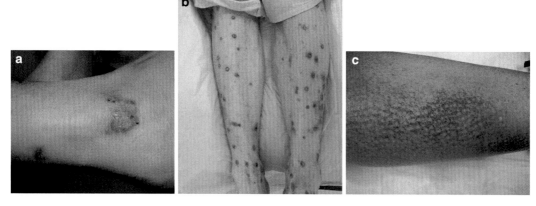

**Fig. 15.13** (**a**) Lichen simplex chronicus. (**b**) Prurigo nodularis. (**c**) Macular amyloidosis

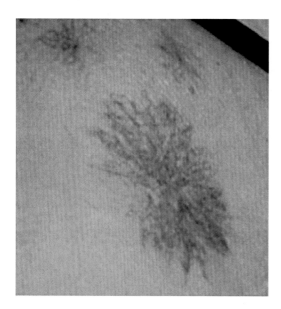

**Fig. 15.14** Spider telangiectasia

pruritus, with possible associated secondary changes from scratching (Fig. 15.13a–c). Vascular changes include spider telangiectasia, cherry angiomas, flushing, palmar erythema, and prominent abdominal vasculature (caput medusae) (Fig. 15.14). This is particularly relevant as increased spider telangiectases in alcohol abusers are associated with higher rates of esophageal varicosities [58]. Skin signs of visceral disease may be apparent, including jaundice, reflecting concomitant hyperbilirubinemia. Common dermatoses, including psoriasis, seborrheic dermati-

tis, and nummular eczema, all have increased prevalence in alcohol abusers. Oral mucosal changes include an atrophic red tongue, a sign of vitamin $B_{12}$ deficiency, or chronic gingival inflammation. Finally, many types of cutaneous malignancy are increased, including aggressive, infiltrative basal cell carcinomas and oral squamous cell carcinomas [59].

Mucocutaneous signs of drug abuse vary based on the offending substance (Table 15.3). All types of substance abuse portend to increased infection rates. Polymicrobial infections involving bacteria and yeast are common and antibody-resistant strains may predominate. Infections often present locally at the place of drug entry, such as cellulitis, abscess, pyomyositis or necrotizing fasciitis. Systemic infections have cutaneous manifestations, including palmar Janeway lesions, digital Osler nodes and nail splinter hemorrhages of bacterial endocarditis. Furthermore, there is an increased transmission of HIV and viral hepatitis, each with their associated dermatoses detailed earlier in this chapter.

## Body Image Concerns

Members of the LGBT population have diverse body image issues given the differing social pressures within their individual communities. Gay men are at a greater risk than their heterosexual counterparts for wanting to either be thinner or

**Table 15.3** Mucocutaneous signs of drug abuse

| Drug | Skin manifestation |
|------|--------------------|
| Cocaine | Vasculitis<br>Raynaud's phenomenon<br>Acute generalized exanthematous pustulosis<br>*Snorting: warts, nasal irritant dermatitis*<br>*Crack: palmar/digital hyperkeratosis* |
| Methamphetamine | Excoriations (from pruritus/formication)<br>Xerosis |
| Heroin | Flushing<br>Excoriations (from pruritus/formication)<br>Pseudoacanthosis nigricans |
| MDMA/Ecstasy | Acne-like eruption |
| Inhalants | Perinasal irritant dermatitis |
| Injectable drugs | Tracts<br>Ulcers<br>Pseudoaneurysm<br>Local and systemic infection<br>*Skin popping: depressed, round scars* |
| Adulterants | Levamisole: retiform purpura with ulceration<br>Talc, Starch: granulomas<br>Sclerosant: lymphedema |

have a more muscular physique [60]. This is demonstrated by the increased rates of body dysmorphic disorder, eating disorders and anabolic steroid abuse. On the opposite end of the spectrum, obesity has proven to be a significant health problem amongst lesbians, and a leading cause of increased morbidity and mortality [61].

## Body Dysmorphic Disorder

Dermatologists encounter individuals with body dysmorphic disorder (BDD, dysmorphophobia) at an elevated level compared to many other medical specialties, affecting 9–14 % of all dermatologic clinic patients [62]. BDD is defined as the feeling of being deformed or misshapen, even with all evidence of the contrary [63]. Individuals become fixated on certain aspects of their body, most commonly the face, breasts, genitalia or hair. Patients present with complaints beyond what is evident on exam and are often unable to perceive the alternative even after being told by the physician. They often desire unnecessary or extreme amounts of products and procedures, and frequently are not satisfied with the outcomes.

BDD can be classified as either a delusional disorder, a variant of obsessive-compulsive disorder, or on a spectrum in between. Treatment should be targeted based on which component is felt to drive the patient's thoughts and behaviors. Any patient exhibiting signs of BDD should be steered away from unnecessary products and procedures and screened for referral to psychiatric management.

## Eating Disorders

The social pressures that induce body dysmorphic disorder in gay subcultures may also be responsible for the development of eating disorders. Approximately 10–25 % of people with eating disorders are men, with 10–42 % identifying as gay or bisexual, above the rate of homosexuality and bisexuality within the male population (3.6 %) [64–66]. Many cases of transgender women with eating disorders have also been reported [67].

Early malnutrition presents with scalp hair loss (telogen effluvium), lanugo hair formation, xerosis, pruritus, and/or poor wound healing. More significant nutrient deficiencies lead to associated deficiency syndromes, not limited to pellagra (niacin), scurvy (vitamin C), acrodermatitis enteropathica (zinc), or frequently a combination. These conditions often don't respond to standard dermatologic remedies, and regress only with the re-institution of that which was deficient [68].

Bulimia nervosa may be more difficult to clinically appreciate than anorexia nervosa as not all patients develop significant weight loss. One study found that gay men were two and a half times more likely to engage in binging and purging activity than heterosexual men [69]. Cutaneous signs of these activities include facial petechiae from retching, interdigital intertrigo, paronychia, and the development of calluses and scars on the dorsal knuckles of fingers used to purge (Russell's sign). Mucosal signs include erosions, poor dentition, and salivary gland enlargement.

## Anabolic Steroid Abuse

Anabolic steroids may be considered a drug of abuse in the gay male population. While not used to induce euphoria, there are two principle reasons why gay men take advantage of the muscle-building property of corticosteroids. Social pressures have lead to a culture in which men desire the perfect, stronger body. In addition, individuals with AIDS may utilize these chemicals to counteract their disease-associated muscle wasting [70].

Abuse of anabolic corticosteroids leads to an increased prevalence of acne vulgaris. Steroid-acne, contrary to classic acne vulgaris, has a stronger predilection for the torso in addition to affecting the face (Fig. 15.15). Other dermatologic manifestations include male-patterned hair loss of the scalp (androgenetic alopecia) with an increase in quantity and coarseness of hair on the body (hirsuitism). This is in conjunction with other physical findings, not limited to gynecomastia and testicular atrophy [71].

> **Helpful Hint**
> Any muscular patient with significant acne on their trunk without much facial involvement should raise suspicion for anabolic steroid use.

## Obesity

As opposed to gay and bisexual men and transgender women who show increased rates of psychopathology with the goal of weight loss or toning, lesbians experience elevated rates of obesity. Obesity alone is associated with various skin pathologies, including skin tags, striae distensae (stretch marks), and hyperhidrosis (increased sweating). The physical burden of excess mass may lead to pressure-induced plantar hyperkeratosis, friction-induced dyspigmentation, and the growth of polymicrobial intertrigo within semi-occlusive skinfolds. Impairment in lymphatic and venous flow may lead to lymphedema, stasis dermatitis, lipodermatosclerosis, and leg ulcers, some of which are irreversible [72].

Obesity is associated with elevated rates of insulin resistance and diabetes mellitus. Dermatologic signs range from the minor but common symptoms of acanthosis nigricans and non-scarring bullae to less commonly occurring eruptive xanthomas and widespread granuloma annulare (Fig. 15.16). Even more infrequent but severe dermatoses may develop, including scleredema and necrobiosis lipoidica diabeticorum [73].

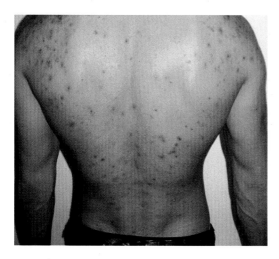

**Fig. 15.15**  Steroid acne

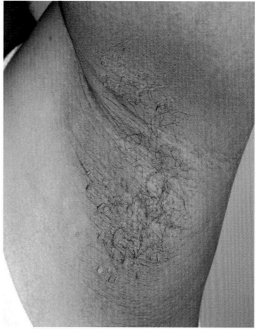

**Fig. 15.16**  Acanthosis nigricans and skin tags

## Skin Signs of Depression and Anxiety

Depression and anxiety affect members of the LGBT community at rates higher than the general population, and often exist concomitantly. On the skin, signs of scratching or picking without an underlying cause for itch are often the first signal. Such neurotic excoriations occur in the setting of depression and anxiety, and the actions are frequently unbeknownst to the patient and thus difficult to stop. Repeated manipulation can induce secondary changes or even traumatic ulcerations that in turn can itch and lead to a difficult to manage itch-scratch cycle (Fig. 15.17a). Patients may also scratch at pre-existing lesions, including acne (acne excoriée) [74].

Self-manipulation can also be directed at one's hair and nails. Trichotillomania (hair plucking) presents as hair loss of varying sizes in irregularly shaped patches or on atypical sites, frequently affecting the eyebrows (Fig. 15.17b). Nail changes include irregularly frayed and shortened edges from nail biting, or median nail dystrophy from a habit tic, appearing like a thin Christmas tree down the center of bilateral thumb nails. Treatment of all of the above is directed at the underlying psychiatric comorbidity, with skin care focused on symptomatic relief of itch and open wounds.

> **Helpful Hint**
>
> It is mindful to always pay attention to the patient as a whole, even during history taking, as they may unconsciously perform the automatisms that have induced their dermatologic condition.

## Intimate Partner Violence

Intimate partner violence (IPV) is a large problem in the LGBT community. It is has been credited as the third most severe health issue for gay men, following AIDS and substance abuse, and is thought to affect 15–20 % of gay and lesbian relationships [75]. The prevalence among transgender individuals may be more than double that of lesbian and gay people [76].

The most frequent sign of physical abuse on the skin is ecchymoses. While a common entity, evidence of a non-accidental cause includes unusually high numbers, abnormal shapes, and locations in areas not prone to injury, most commonly the head, neck, buttock and genitalia. Other signs of abuse include bite marks or multiple burns. Significant anogenital trauma should raise suspicion for sexual abuse. Any suspected

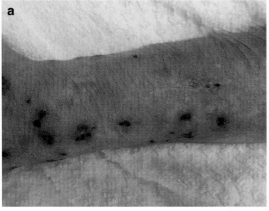
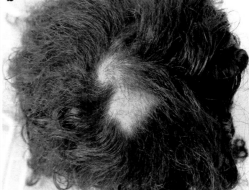

**Fig. 15.17** (**a**) Neurotic excoriations. (**b**) Trichotillomania

case of IPV should be discussed with the patient, and every care facility should have information regarding where to go and who to contact if the patient desires to do so [77].

## Transgender-Specific Dermatology

To the transgender individual, the body's exterior proves to be an area of focus from the moment they realize that it is incongruent from their true gender. A person often undergoes a variety of processes to eliminate or improve upon this discordance, which may directly or indirectly impact their skin. This section outlines dermatologic considerations that result from these effects, both intentional and unexpected, and provides information about how a dermatologist may aid in the transitioning process.

> **Helpful Hint**
> Some transgender patients may be reluctant to show their chest/breast or genitalia to a practitioner if they are not made to feel comfortable. As examining these areas are often critical for disease diagnosis and cancer screening, they should not be automatically dismissed, but rather care should be taken to establish a level of comfort with the patient, discussing the manner and importance of the exam before beginning it.

## Hormone-Associated Changes

Often the first step in the medical management of transitioning is via hormone therapy. Transgender men most commonly take testosterone, available in many forms. Transgender women most commonly take a combination of estrogen with an anti-androgen, including spironolactone, cyproterone acetate, a GnRH agonist, or a 5-alpha reductase inhibitor. In their endogenous forms, these hormones are well known to have an impact on sebum production and hair growth. It is therefore no surprise that similar changes have been observed with exogenous preparations [78, 79].

## Sebum Production

Sebum is the triglyceride-rich oil produced by the skin's sebaceous glands and functions as a natural emollient. One study examined the effects of hormones on sebum production in both transgender men and women. Transgender women taking estrogens and anti-androgens had a rapid and sustained reduction in sebum production, where as transgender men taking testosterone had a gradual but significant increased production. In this study, all transgender women had improvement in acne. Given the reduction in the skin's natural moisturizer, another anecdotally reported but unmeasured affect would be increased xerosis, pruritus, and even eczema. To combat dryness and eczema, a gentle skin care regimen would be advised, limiting bathing to once a day, to be done with warm water and a moisturizing soap, in conjunction with liberal emollient use throughout the day. A topical steroid may have to be added if the eczematous changes are not controlled by these measures alone.

In the above and similar studies, transgender men almost universally developed acne, a majority of which affected both the face and the back. For many people, this is only temporary, starting to improve by 2 years after initiating the testosterone. Many over-the-counter products may be tried for mild acne, including benzoyl peroxide and salicylic acid washes. Some cases require the addition of a topical antibiotic or retinoid, and for more moderate-to-severe cases, an oral antibiotic. Oral retinoids are standardly used for severe or recalcitrant nodulocystic acne, which while not seen in any subjects of the aforementioned studies, have been anecdotally observed in many patients.

## Hair Growth

The effects of hormones on hair are very evident in the general population, with at least 80 % of cisgender men experiencing androgenetic hair loss by age 70. Transgender men, while experiencing minimal-to-no hair loss in the first few years of treatment, have been shown to have mild frontotemporal hair loss in one third of cases and moderate-to-severe alopecia in another third after long-term testosterone supplementation. As opposed to testosterone's effect on scalp hair, it causes beard and body hair to increase, both in number and diameter, which is an often-desired consequence. Primary management of androgenetic hair loss in transgender men is with topical minoxidil (Rogaine®). The use of the oral anti-androgen finasteride (Propecia®) in transgender men has not been directly studied. Anecdotal reports note efficacy, however caution should be had with taking finasteride within the first few years of taking testosterone, as it may paradoxically inhibit secondary hair growth elsewhere and reduce clitoral/penile enlargement. A more definitive approach to hair restoration is with hair transplantation, with topical and oral regimens continued afterwards to stop further hair loss in non-transplanted scalp areas.

Transgender women taking estrogens and anti-androgens experience hair loss on both the beard and body. While the hair loss on the body is often complete, substantial facial hair may remain even after a year of treatment, although typically fewer and smaller in diameter. Various depilatory techniques are now available to eliminate the need for shaving, an undesirable daily routine for transgender women. For limited areas, topical eflornithine may be used twice daily, with results only sustainable during use. More permanent hair removal can be achieved with a series of four-to-six laser treatments tailored to the patient's hair and skin color, which today provides lasting results and requires only occasional maintenance treatments. Electrolysis is a more time-consuming and sometimes more painful procedure, being that each hair is targeted individually, but serves as an option for patients not eligible for laser treatment, including people with white or gray hair.

## Post-operative Scarring

While the performance of gender confirmation surgery (sex reassignment surgery) is not by dermatologists, understanding the procedures is essential for managing post-operative patients. Surgery may result in scarring that could be aesthetically unpleasing or have associated pruritus. Scars may be red and atrophic or, in some individuals, hypertrophic or keloidal. Over-the-counter treatments, including onion extract gel, topical vitamin E, and silicone gel sheeting have demonstrated limited to no efficacy in scar prevention or treatment [80]. Hypertrophic scars and keloids can be reduced in size and firmness with intralesional glucocorticoid injections, a very effective treatment introduced over 50 years ago [81]. Larger keloids may require surgical repair. Laser therapy has revolutionized scar treatment, with different lasers used to improve the redness and contour of flat or atrophic scars [82].

## Facial Transformation

For many transgender individuals, one of the most sought-out goals is to be able to pass as one's true rather than natal gender. While hormones play an important role in reshaping one's face and body, the resulting effects may not be satisfactory for the patient. If the patient so desires, there are many options available for facial transformation, both non-invasive and surgical. This section presents the non-invasive, surgery-sparing options performed by many dermatologists and plastic surgeons.

### Assessing the Masculinity or Femininity of the Face

In order to make a face appear more masculine or feminine, it is best to understand the differences between the classic male and female facial structure. Many studies have explored these differences, noting varied position, shapes and sizes of certain facial features (Table 15.4) [83].

### Non-invasive Techniques for Facial Transformation

Surgical implants and cranioplasty are the predominant methods to permanently alter the shape of the face. Non-permanent and non-invasive techniques may be preferred, used adjunctive to surgery, or could be the only options available for

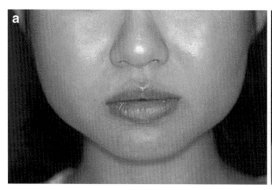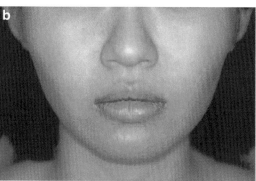

**Fig. 15.18** (**a**) Before, and (**b**) after botulinum toxin injection into the masseter muscles for facial contouring. *Credit to Dr. Woffles Wu, Singapore as obtained from "Aesthetic Surgery of the Facial Mosaic" (Panfilov)—Figures 72.10 a and b

**Table 15.4** Gender-associated differences in facial structures

|  | Masculine | Feminine |
|---|---|---|
| Supraorbital ridge | Protruded | Flat |
| Eyebrows | Flat, thick | Peaked, thin |
| Eyes | Squinted | Open |
| Nose | Large, wide | Small, concave |
| Cheeks (Zygoma) | Large, flat | Thin, pronounced |
| Lips (Vermillion) | Thin | Full |
| Jaw (Mandibular angle) | Squared, narrow | Smooth, obtuse |
| Chin | Wide, rectangular | Narrow, trapezoidal |

the patient who is not a surgical candidate. Cosmetic injectables can be used to either reshape the face or help give the illusion of certain gender-identifying facial features.

Botulinum toxin, derived from the bacteria *Clostridium botulinum*, is an exotoxin that produces muscular denervation via pre-synaptic acetylcholine blockade. Injections into the forehead and glabella can be used to give the appearance of a flatter forehead, and strategic distribution in these areas and periorbitally can lift, peak, or flatten the eyebrow. Botulinum toxin can also be injected laterally to the orbit, eliminating "crow's feet," and giving the illusion of a more open and feminine eye. Injection into the nasal columella may provide some lift to the tip of the nose.

Masseter injections are used to smooth the angle of the jaw (Fig. 15.18a, b). All effects typically last 3–4 months, and sustained responses have been noted with repeated treatments [84].

Cosmetic filler is used to lift or add volume to areas of the face. For transgender patients, this could be used to make cheeks more prominent, lips more full, or reshape the chin to being either wider or more pointed. Non-permanent filler may last from 6 months to 2 years depending on its components, most frequently hyaluronic acid, calcium hydroxyapatite, or poly-L-lactic acid. Permanent fillers include Silicone and Artefill©, and are used much less frequently due to the risk of granulomatous side effects [85].

## Non-physician Administration of Permanent Filler

It is estimated that 16–29 % of transgender women have had permanent filler injections by unlicensed, nonmedical personnel, who promise desired outcomes at significantly reduced prices [86, 87]. Furthermore, pumping parties allow for large groups to undergo these injections simultaneously, leading to the sharing of equipment and injectables. The products are often not medical-grade and may be admixed with other substances. Aside from silicone, there have been reports of injections with paraffin, lanolin, beeswax, petroleum jelly, tire sealant, and various oils [88–90]. In addition, sterility is limited and organisms may reside in the equipment or filler itself.

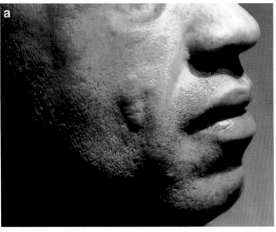
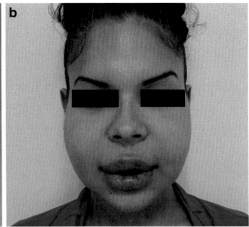

**Fig. 15.19** (a) Granuloma from silicone injection. *Credit to Dr. Derek Jones as obtained from "Facial rejuvination" (Goldberg)—Figure 5.14. (b) Silicone gran- ulomas and angioedema from non-medical injections into the lips and cheeks

With silicone injection, the most common complication is granuloma formation at the site of injection, appearing as a firm, sometimes red, nodule. Granulomatous reactions have occurred from other injected materials, some at distant sites due to filler migration [91]. Angioedema can develop, felt to be from a protein contaminant rather than the silicone itself [92]. Large volume injection into breasts or hips may occlude vasculature, leading to lymphedema and venous compromise [93]. Due to the lack of sterility, infection is not uncommon, and cases of atypical mycobacterial infection have been seen [94]. Sadly, there have been several documented cases of multisystem organ failure and death with large volume injection for body contouring (Fig. 15.19a, b).

Treatment is based on the resultant reaction, with multiple approaches frequently required [95]. Infection must always be suspected, ruled-out, and even empirically treated, with broad-coverage that includes atypical mycobacteria. Other treatments for cutaneous disease include glucocorticoid injections and surgical excision for granulomas, antihistamines for angioedema, and a variety of anecdotal systemic agents for more severe disease. Patients often necessitate chronic treatment and have poor cosmetic outcomes.

> **Helpful Hint**
> Always rule-out or treat a concomitant bacterial infection, including atypical mycobacteria, before initiating immunosuppressive therapies for the management of filler complications.

## Ethical and Legal Considerations

There are no laws that govern when and how physicians perform gender confirmation procedures on their patients. However, most practitioners operate based on the standards of care as set forth by the World Professional Association for Transgender Health [96]. The criteria for all chest surgeries are that the patient be the age of consent and have mental health professional documentation of persistant gender dysphoria, with additional guidelines for genital surgery. Although facial surgeries do not require any of the above criteria, mental health professionals may aid in helping the patient to make an informed and well-timed decision about any facial procedure, even for those that are not permanent.

# References

1. Katz KA, Furnish TJ. Dermatology-related epidemiologic and clinical concerns of men who have sex with men, women who have sex with women, and transgender individuals. Arch Dermatol. 2005;141(10):1303–10.
2. Gorgos LM, Marrazzo JM. Sexually transmitted infections among women who have sex with women. Clin Infect Dis. 2011;53 Suppl 3:S84–91.
3. Diamant AL, Schuster MA, McGuigan K, Lever J. Lesbians' sexual history with men: implications for taking a sexual history. Arch Intern Med. 1999;159(22):2730–6.
4. Centers for Disease Control and Prevention (CDC). HIV among gay and bisexual men. Atlanta: CDC; 2014 May. Available from: http://www.cdc.gov/hiv/risk/gender/msm/facts/index.html
5. Centers for Disease Control and Prevention (CDC). HIV among transgender people. Atlanta: CDC; 2013 Dec. Available from: http://www.cdc.gov/hiv/risk/transgender/index.html
6. Lapins J, Gaines H, Lindback S, Lidbrink P, Emtestam L. Skin and mucosal characteristics of symptomatic primary HIV-1 infection. AIDS Patient Care STDS. 1997;11(2):67–70.
7. Mays SR, Kunishige JH, Truong E, Kontoyiannis DP, Hymes SR. Approach to the morbilliform eruption in the hematopoietic transplant patient. Semin Cutan Med Surg. 2007;26(3):155–62.
8. Zancanaro PC, McGirt LY, Mamelak AJ, Nguyen RH, Martins CR. Cutaneous manifestations of HIV in the era of highly active antiretroviral therapy: an institutional urban clinic experience. J Am Acad Dermatol. 2006;54(4):581–8.
9. Rashidghamat E, Bunker CB, Bower M, Banerjee P. Kaposi Sarcoma in HIV-negative men who have sex with men. Br J Dermatol. 2014;171(5):1267–8.
10. Lehloenya R, Meintjes G. Dermatologic manifestations of the immune reconstitution inflammatory syndrome. Dermatol Clin. 2006;24(4):549–70. vii.
11. Kong HH, Myers SA. Cutaneous effects of highly active antiretroviral therapy in HIV-infected patients. Dermatol Ther. 2005;18(1):58–66.
12. Taqi SA, Zaki SA, Nilofer AR, Sami LB. Trimethoprim-sulfamethoxazole-induced Steven Johnson syndrome in an HIV-infected patient. Indian J Pharmacol. 2012;44(4):533–5.
13. James J, Carruthers A, Carruthers J. HIV-associated facial lipoatrophy. Dermatol Surg. 2002;28(11):979–86.
14. Burgess CM, Quiroga RM. Assessment of the safety and efficacy of poly-L-lactic acid for the treatment of HIV-associated facial lipoatrophy. J Am Acad Dermatol. 2005;52(2):233–9.
15. Cardoso JC, Calonje E. Cutaneous manifestations of human papillomaviruses: a review. Acta Dermatovenerol Alp Pannonica Adriat. 2011;20(3):145–54.
16. Baseman JG, Koutsky LA. The epidemiology of human papillomavirus infections. J Clin Virol. 2005;32 Suppl 1:S16–24.
17. Wasef W, Sugunendran H, Alawattegama A. Genital warts in a transsexual. Int J STD AIDS. 2005;16(5):388–9.
18. Yang C, Liu S, Xu K, Xiang Q, Yang S, Zhang X. Condylomata gigantea in a male transsexual. Int J STD AIDS. 2009;20(3):211–2.
19. Parkin DM. The global health burden of infection-associated cancers in the year 2002. Int J Cancer. 2006;118(12):3030–44.
20. Anderson TA, Schick V, Herbenick D, Dodge B, Fortenberry JD. A study of human papillomavirus on vaginally inserted sex toys, before and after cleaning, among women who have sex with women and men. Sex Transm Infect. 2014;90(7):529–31.
21. Ribeiro-Muller L, Muller M. Prophylactic papillomavirus vaccines. Clin Dermatol. 2014;32(2):235–47.
22. Hathaway JK. HPV: diagnosis, prevention, and treatment. Clin Obstet Gynecol. 2012;55(3):671–80.
23. Xu F, Sternberg MR, Kottiri BJ, McQuillan GM, Lee FK, Nahmias AJ, Berman SM, Markowitz LE. Trends in herpes simplex virus type 1 and type 2 seroprevalence in the United States. JAMA. 2006;296(8):964–73.
24. Bohl DD, Katz KA, Bernstein K, Wong E, Raymond HF, Klausner JD, McFarland W. Prevalence and correlates of herpes simplex virus type-2 infection among men who have sex with men, san francisco, 2008. Sex Transm Dis. 2011;38(7):617–21.
25. Gupta R, Warren T, Wald A. Genital herpes. Lancet. 2007;370(9605):2127–37.
26. Mertz GJ. Asymptomatic shedding of herpes simplex virus 1 and 2: implications for prevention of transmission. J Infect Dis. 2008;198(8):1098–100.
27. Simmons A. Clinical manifestations and treatment considerations of herpes simplex virus infection. J Infect Dis. 2002;186 Suppl 1:S71–7.
28. LeGoff J, Pere H, Belec L. Diagnosis of genital herpes simplex virus infection in the clinical laboratory. Virol J. 2014;11(1):83.
29. Cernik C, Gallina K, Brodell RT. The treatment of herpes simplex infections: an evidence-based review. Arch Intern Med. 2008;168(11):1137–44.
30. Allison SD. Extragenital syphilitic chancres. J Am Acad Dermatol. 1986;14(6):1094–5.
31. Streit E, Hartschuh W, Flux K. Solitary lesion on finger. Primary syphilitic lesion on finger. Acta Derm Venereol. 2013;93(2):251–2.
32. Lautenschlager S. Cutaneous manifestations of syphilis : recognition and management. Am J Clin Dermatol. 2006;7(5):291–304.
33. Domantay-Apostol GP, Handog EB, Gabriel MT. Syphilis: the international challenge of the great imitator. Dermatol Clin. 2008;26(2):191–202. v.
34. Shockman S, Buescher LS, Stone SP. Syphilis in the United States. Clin Dermatol. 2014;32(2):213–8.

35. Centers for Disease Control and Prevention (CDC). Syphilis treatment and care. Atlanta: CDC; 2013 Aug. Available from: http://www.cdc.gov/std/syphilis/treatment.htm

36. de Vries HJ. Skin as an indicator for sexually transmitted infections. Clin Dermatol. 2014;32(2):196–208.

37. Haustein UF. Pruritus of the artificial vagina of a transsexual patient caused by gonococcal infection. Hautarzt. 1995;46(12):858–9.

38. van Liere GA, Hoebe CJ, Dukers-Muijrers NH. Evaluation of the anatomical site distribution of chlamydia and gonorrhoea in men who have sex with men and in high-risk women by routine testing: cross-sectional study revealing missed opportunities for treatment strategies. Sex Transm Infect. 2014;90(1):58–60.

39. Mehta SD. Gonorrhea and Chlamydia in emergency departments: screening, diagnosis, and treatment. Curr Infect Dis Rep. 2007;9(2):134–42.

40. Skerlev M, Culav-Koscak I. Gonorrhea: new challenges. Clin Dermatol. 2014;32(2):275–81.

41. Bailey JV, Benato R, Owen C, Kavanagh J. Vulvovaginal candidiasis in women who have sex with women. Sex Transm Dis. 2008;35(6):533–6.

42. Hay RJ. The management of superficial candidiasis. J Am Acad Dermatol. 1999;40(6 Pt 2):S35–42.

43. Martins N, Ferreira IC, Barros L, Silva S, Henriques M. Candidiasis: predisposing factors, prevention, diagnosis and alternative treatment. Mycopathologia. 2014;177(5-6):223–40.

44. Cribier B. Urticaria and hepatitis. Clin Rev Allergy Immunol. 2006;30(1):25–9.

45. Janssen HL, van Zonneveld M, van Nunen AB, Niesters HG, Schalm SW, de Man RA. Polyarteritis nodosa associated with hepatitis B virus infection. The role of antiviral treatment and mutations in the hepatitis B virus genome. Eur J Gastroenterol Hepatol. 2004;16(8):801–7.

46. Saadoun D, Terrier B, Semoun O, Sene D, Maisonobe T, Musset L, Amoura Z, Rigon MR, Cacoub P. Hepatitis C virus-associated polyarteritis nodosa. Arthritis Care Res (Hoboken). 2011;63(3):427–35.

47. Mahboobi N, Agha-Hosseini F, Lankarani KB. Hepatitis C virus and lichen planus: the real association. Hepat Mon. 2010;10(3):161–4.

48. Ryan Caballes F, Sendi H, Bonkovsky HL. Hepatitis C, porphyria cutanea tarda and liver iron: an update. Liver Int. 2012;32(6):880–93.

49. Lauletta G, Russi S, Conteduca V, Sansonno L. Hepatitis C virus infection and mixed cryoglobulinemia. Clin Dev Immunol. 2012;2012:502156.

50. Raphael BA, Dorey-Stein ZL, Lott J, Amorosa V, Lo Re III V, Kovarik C. Low prevalence of necrolytic acral erythema in patients with chronic hepatitis C virus infection. J Am Acad Dermatol. 2012;67(5):962–8.

51. Gorwitz RJ. A review of community-associated methicillin-resistant Staphylococcus aureus skin and soft tissue infections. Pediatr Infect Dis J. 2008;27(1):1–7.

52. Antoniou T, Devlin R, Gough K, Mulvey M, Katz KC, Zehtabchi M, Polsky J, Tilley D, Brunetta J, Arbess G, Guiang C, Chang B, Kovacs C, Ghavam-Rassoul A, Cavacuiti C, Corneslon B, Berger P, Loutfy MR. Prevalence of community-associated methicillin-resistant Staphylococcus aureus colonization in men who have sex with men. Int J STD AIDS. 2009;20(3):180–3.

53. Hansra NK, Shinkai K. Cutaneous community-acquired and hospital-acquired methicillin-resistant Staphylococcus aureus. Dermatol Ther. 2011;24(2):263–72.

54. Liu C, Bayer A, Cosgrove SE, Daum RS, Fridkin SK, Gorwitz RJ, Kaplan SL, Karchmer AW, Levine DP, Murray BE, Rybak MJ, Talan DA, Chambers HF. Infectious Diseases Society of A. Clinical practice guidelines by the infectious diseases society of America for the treatment of methicillin-resistant Staphylococcus aureus infections in adults and children. Clin Infect Dis. 2011;52(3):e18–55.

55. Marshal MP, Friedman MS, Stall R, Thompson AL. Individual trajectories of substance use in lesbian, gay and bisexual youth and heterosexual youth. Addiction. 2009;104(6):974–81.

56. Ploeg RJ, Goossens D, Sollinger HW, Southard JH, Belzer FO. The Belzer-UW solution for effective long-term preservation in canine pancreas transplantation. Transplant Proc. 1989;21(1 Pt 2):1378–80.

57. Rosset M, Oki G. Skin diseases in alcoholics. Q J Stud Alcohol. 1971;32(4):1017–24.

58. Foutch PG, Sullivan JA, Gaines JA, Sanowski RA. Cutaneous vascular spiders in cirrhotic patients: correlation with hemorrhage from esophageal varices. Am J Gastroenterol. 1988;83(7):723–6.

59. Liu SW, Lien MH, Fenske NA. The effects of alcohol and drug abuse on the skin. Clin Dermatol. 2010;28(4):391–9.

60. Morrison MA, Morrison TG, Sager CL. Does body satisfaction differ between gay men and lesbian women and heterosexual men and women? A meta-analytic review. Body Image. 2004;1(2):127–38.

61. Fredriksen-Goldsen KI, Kim HJ, Barkan SE, Muraco A, Hoy-Ellis CP. Health disparities among lesbian, gay, and bisexual older adults: results from a population-based study. Am J Public Health. 2013;103(10):1802–9.

62. Mufaddel A, Osman OT, Almugaddam F, Jafferany M. A review of body dysmorphic disorder and its presentation in different clinical settings. Prim Care Companion CNS Disord. 2013;15(4).

63. American Psychiatric Association. Diagnostic and statistical manual of mental disorders. 5th edn. Washington, DC; 2013.

64. Hudson JI, Hiripi E, Pope Jr HG, Kessler RC. The prevalence and correlates of eating disorders in the National Comorbidity Survey Replication. Biol Psychiatry. 2007;61(3):348–58.

65. Carlat DJ, Camargo Jr CA, Herzog DB. Eating disorders in males: a report on 135 patients. Am J Psychiatry. 1997;154(8):1127–32.

66. Russell CJ, Keel PK. Homosexuality as a specific risk factor for eating disorders in men. Int J Eat Disord. 2002;31(3):300–6.
67. Ewan LA, Middleman AB, Feldmann J. Treatment of anorexia nervosa in the context of transsexuality: a case report. Int J Eat Disord. 2014;47(1):112–5.
68. Strumia R. Eating disorders and the skin. Clin Dermatol. 2013;31(1):80–5.
69. French SA, Story M, Remafedi G, Resnick MD, Blum RW. Sexual orientation and prevalence of body dissatisfaction and eating disordered behaviors: a population-based study of adolescents. Int J Eat Disord. 1996;19(2):119–26.
70. Bolding G, Sherr L, Elford J. Use of anabolic steroids and associated health risks among gay men attending London gyms. Addiction. 2002;97(2):195–203.
71. Walker J, Adams B. Cutaneous manifestations of anabolic-androgenic steroid use in athletes. Int J Dermatol. 2009;48(10):1044–8. quiz 1048.
72. Boza JC, Trindade EN, Peruzzo J, Sachett L, Rech L, Cestari TF. Skin manifestations of obesity: a comparative study. J Eur Acad Dermatol Venereol. 2012;26(10):1220–3.
73. Murphy-Chutorian B, Han G, Cohen SR. Dermatologic manifestations of diabetes mellitus: a review. Endocrinol Metab Clin North Am. 2013;42(4):869–98.
74. Koblenzer CS. Cutaneous manifestations of psychiatric disease that commonly present to the dermatologist--diagnosis and treatment. Int J Psychiatry Med. 1992;22(1):47–63.
75. Houston E, McKirnan DJ. Intimate partner abuse among gay and bisexual men: risk correlates and health outcomes. J Urban Health. 2007;84(5): 681–90.
76. Ard KL, Makadon HJ. Addressing intimate partner violence in lesbian, gay, bisexual, and transgender patients. J Gen Intern Med. 2011;26(8):930–3.
77. Reddy K, Lowenstein EJ. Forensics in dermatology: part II. J Am Acad Dermatol. 2011;64(5):811–24. quiz 825–6.
78. Giltay EJ, Gooren LJ. Effects of sex steroid deprivation/administration on hair growth and skin sebum production in transsexual males and females. J Clin Endocrinol Metab. 2000;85(8):2913–21.
79. Wierckx K, Van de Peer F, Verhaeghe E, Dedecker D, Van Caenegem E, Toye K, Kaufman JM, T'Sjoen G. Short- and long-term clinical skin effects of testosterone treatment in trans men. J Sex Med. 2014;11(1):222–9.
80. Morganroth P, Wilmot AC, Miller C. JAAD online. Over-the-counter scar products for postsurgical patients: disparities between online advertised benefits and evidence regarding efficacy. J Am Acad Dermatol. 2009;61(6):e31–47.
81. Ledon JA, Savas J, Franca K, Chacon A, Nouri K. Intralesional treatment for keloids and hypertrophic scars: a review. Dermatol Surg. 2013;39(12):1745–57.
82. Oliaei S, Nelson JS, Fitzpatrick R, Wong BJ. Laser treatment of scars. Facial Plast Surg. 2012;28(5):518–24.
83. Hennessy RJ, McLearie S, Kinsella A, Waddington JL. Facial surface analysis by 3D laser scanning and geometric morphometrics in relation to sexual dimorphism in cerebral--craniofacial morphogenesis and cognitive function. J Anat. 2005;207(3):283–95.
84. Maas C, Kane MA, Bucay VW, Allen S, Applebaum DJ, Baumann L, Cox SE, Few JW, Joseph JH, Lorenc ZP, Moradi A, Nestor MS, Schlessinger J, Wortzman M, Lawrence I, Lin X, Nelson D. Current aesthetic use of abobotulinumtoxinA in clinical practice: an evidence-based consensus review. Aesthet Surg J. 2012;32(1 Suppl):8S–29.
85. Kontis TC. Contemporary review of injectable facial fillers. JAMA Facial Plast Surg. 2013;15(1):58–64.
86. Wilson E, Rapues J, Jin H, Raymond HF. The Use and Correlates of Illicit Silicone or "Fillers" in a Population-Based Sample of Transwomen, San Francisco, 2013. J Sex Med. 2014;11(7):1717–24.
87. Garofalo R, Deleon J, Osmer E, Doll M, Harper GW. Overlooked, misunderstood and at-risk: exploring the lives and HIV risk of ethnic minority male-to-female transgender youth. J Adolesc Health. 2006;38(3):230–6.
88. Behar TA, Anderson EE, Barwick WJ, Mohler JL. Sclerosing lipogranulomatosis: a case report of scrotal injection of automobile transmission fluid and literature review of subcutaneous injection of oils. Plast Reconstr Surg. 1993;91(2):352–61.
89. Hage JJ, Kanhai RC, Oen AL, van Diest PJ, Karim RB. The devastating outcome of massive subcutaneous injection of highly viscous fluids in male-to-female transsexuals. Plast Reconstr Surg. 2001;107(3): 734–41.
90. Murray R. Transgender woman arrested after injecting Fix-AFlat into patient's rear end. 2011. http://www.nydailynews.com/news/crime/transgender-woman-arrested-injecting-fix-a-flat-patient-rear-article-1.980273. Accessed on 15 June 2014.
91. Farina LA, Palacio V, Salles M, Fernandez-Villanueva D, Vidal B, Menendez P. Scrotal granuloma caused by oil migrating from the hip in 2 transsexual males (scrotal sclerosing lipogranuloma). Arch Esp Urol. 1997;50(1):51–3.
92. Sclafani AP, Fagien S. Treatment of injectable soft tissue filler complications. Dermatol Surg. 2009;35 Suppl 2:1672–80.
93. Gaber Y. Secondary lymphoedema of the lower leg as an unusual side-effect of a liquid silicone injection in the hips and buttocks. Dermatology. 2004;208(4):342–4.
94. Fox LP, Geyer AS, Husain S, Della-Latta P, Grossman ME. Mycobacterium abscessus cellulitis and multifocal abscesses of the breasts in a transsexual from illicit intramammary injections of silicone. J Am Acad Dermatol. 2004;50(3):450–4.
95. Styperek A, Bayers S, Beer M, Beer K. Nonmedical-grade injections of permanent fillers: medical and medicolegal considerations. J Clin Aesthet Dermatol. 2013;6(4):22–9.
96. WPATH. Standards of care for the health of transsexual, transgender and gender nonconforming people. WPATH, 7th version 2012. Available at www.wpath.org

# Urologic Issues in LGBT Health

# 16

Matthew D. Truesdale, Benjamin N. Breyer, and Alan W. Shindel

## Purpose

In this chapter we will provide a brief primer on urologic care with a focus on the particular needs of LGBT persons. It is our hope that this manuscript will be of use to primary care physicians who will see LGBT persons with urologic issues and to urologists who may not be familiar with issues germane to the LGBT community. We will address general urologic issues but will focus on urologic issues for which there is evidence of significant differences between LGBT and non-LGBT patients.

## Learning Objectives

- Identify at least three ways in which urologic healthcare is sensitive for LGBT patients (PC2, PBLI1, PBLI1, ICS2)

M.D. Truesdale, M.D. (✉)
B.N. Breyer, M.D., M.S.
Department of Urology, University of California, San Francisco, San Francisco, CA, USA
e-mail: matthew.truesdale@ucsf.edu; bbreyer@urology.ucsf.edu

A. W. Shindel, M.D., M.A.S.
Department of Urology, University of California, Davis, Sacramento, CA, USA
e-mail: alan.shindel@ucdmc.ucdavis.edu

- Describe lower urinary tract symptoms and how they may manifest in LGBT patients (PC5)
- Describe sexual function and dysfunction in LGBT patients (PC5)
- Discuss opportunities for screening for urologic malignancy in LGBT patients (PC3, PC4)

## Urologic Healthcare for the LGBT Patient

A safe and welcoming environment is the foundation of productive encounters between health care providers and patients. In Western societies, heterosexuality and gender identity concordant with genital sex is the presumed norm. Individuals who are sexually attracted to members of the same sex (e.g. lesbian, gay, bisexual) and persons whose biological sex differs from their gender identity (transgender) are often collectively referred to as members of the LGBT (lesbian/gay/bisexual/transgender) community. A few key issues must be addressed when considering the "LGBT community":

1. While sexual expression is a key difference between LGBT and non-LGBT persons, LGBT persons may differ from their heterosexual peers in non-sexual ways (e.g. social support structures). Holistic assessment of the particular needs of an LGBT person includes

© Springer International Publishing Switzerland 2016
K.L. Eckstrand, J.M. Ehrenfeld (eds.), *Lesbian, Gay, Bisexual, and Transgender Healthcare*,
DOI 10.1007/978-3-319-19752-4_16

understanding of LGBT issues that may not specifically relate to sexual activity.

2. Although many refer to the "LGBT community", it is important to recognize that there is no single unified LGBT community; rather, there are diverse communities of lesbian, gay, bisexual, and transgender persons who frequently have a common interest in advocacy and education of the public at large about sexual and gender diversity.

3. LGBT is the most familiar acronym to most individuals. The terms "queer" or "questioning" have been adopted by some individuals who do not identify as heterosexual nor as lesbian, gay, bisexual, or transgender. The acronym LGBT is sometimes extended to read LGBTQ; for the sake of convenience we will restrict use in this manuscript to LGBT while acknowledging that some gender/sexuality variant persons may not identify with the term "LGBT". Medical concerns related to patients affected by differences of sex development are discussed in Chap. 22.

## Talking to LGBT Patients

Personal issues and potentially embarrassing issue regarding sexuality and urinary function) are routinely discussed during urologic consultation. During the urologic visit, it is critical for a patient to feel empowered to share important aspects of his/her history without fear of judgment or alienation from the provider. The intrinsic sensitivity of urologic issues is compounded when they must be discussed in the context of a patient with a non-normative sexual or gender identity. It is thus imperative that the provider strive to create an open and judgment-free environment so that key pieces of the patient's history can be incorporated into the evaluation and plan of treatment.

Because patients who do not disclose their sexual orientation and/or gender identity are at risk of worse health outcomes, health care providers must elicit these issues with sensitivity to ensure optimal patient care [1]. The provider should facilitate an environment where the patient is able to share this information without fear of recrimination [2]. Openness between patient and provider is critical to building of rapport and trust, which is fundamental to the therapeutic relationship [3]. Information on sexuality and gender is of particular relevance to urology as this specialty is concerned with medical issues germane to the genitals and sexual activity.

In establishing rapport with patients it is critical to use inclusive language and to avoid assumptions in eliciting the medical and sexual history. Specific examples include avoidance of gender-specific pronouns when referring to a patient's sexual partner(s) and not presuming that an individual is heterosexual. Conversely, a practitioner should not presume that an individual's professed identity is concordant with their behavior. Up to 7 % of American women 18–59 years of age report a sexual history with another women; over half of these women identify as heterosexual [4]. Similarly, estimates indicate that over 70 % of self-identified lesbians have a history of sexual relationships with men; as many as 6 % of lesbians in one study reported sex with a male partner within the past year [5]. In a similar fashion, there exist a population of men who report heterosexual orientation but engage in sexual activities with other men [6]. Because there is often discrepancy between professed orientation and behavior (historical or current), some researchers favor the descriptive terms "men who have sex with men" (MSM) and "women who have sex with women" (WSW) to terms such as gay or lesbian, respectively.

## Urologic Issues

### Urinary Function

Normal urine production, storage and transport depend on the functioning and coordination of the kidneys, ureters, bladder, and urethra (Fig. 16.1).

The kidneys continuously filter the blood, producing urine as the excretory byproduct. Urine is transported by peristalsis of the ureters from the kidneys to the urinary bladder, where it is stored until it can be conveniently evacuated [7].

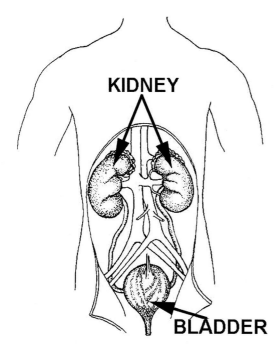

**Fig. 16.1** This coronal view of the urinary tract shows the kidneys, which filter blood to create urine. Urine drains out through the ureters to be stored in the bladder, prior to evacuation (Image Courtesy, J. Ehrenfeld)

The bladder is a compliant hollow organ lined with mucosa overlaid on a muscular layer (the detrusor). The healthy bladder is compliant, meaning it can fill at low pressures and accommodate a large volume of fluid. The urethra is the tube which urine passes from the urinary bladder during micturition. In men, the urethra passes through the prostate, which is a gland responsible for the production of seminal fluid [7].

In both men and women urine is held in the bladder by action of the internal and external urethral sphincters. The internal sphincter is located in the vicinity of the bladder neck and consists of involuntary smooth muscle under the control of the autonomic nervous system. The external urinary sphincter is located in the proximal portion of the urethra; this sphincter is contracted to prevent unwanted leakage. The external urethral sphincter is under voluntary control. Normal storage of urine depends on compliance of the bladder, relaxation of the detrusor muscle, and adequate capacity to coapt the urethra. Failure of any of these mechanisms leads to incontinence (involuntary loss of urine). Incontinence is subdi-

vided into urgency incontinence (loss of urine with sudden overpowering urge) and stress incontinence (loss of urine with ValSalva or other increase in intraabdominal pressure) [7].

During urination, the brain receives sensory input that the bladder is full, triggering the cascade of events leading to micturition. The brain sends a signal to the urethral sphincters to relax followed by contraction of the detrusor muscle, which surrounds the bladder. Squeezing of the detrusor muscle forces urine out of the bladder and through the urethra. Normal voiding depends on detrusor contraction, simultaneous relaxation of both urinary sphincters, and a low resistance urethra allowing for unobstructed urine flow. Failure of any of these mechanisms may lead to a variety of lower urinary tract symptoms (LUTS). LUTS are common in both men and women and can lead to significant impairment in quality of life [8, 9]. LUTS are commonly divided into "obstructive" or "irritative" categories [2, 10].

**Obstructive**
1. Weak urinary stream.
2. Need to strain (Valsalva maneuver) with urination.
3. Incomplete emptying, or a sensation of urine remaining in the bladder at the completion of a void.

**Irritative**
1. Urinary urgency or the strong and immediate need to urinate without delay or warning.
2. Urinary frequency defined as the need to void multiple times in an excessive and bothersome way without a normal time interval generally <1–2 h.
3. Nocturia or voiding multiple times during the night.
4. Post Void Dribbling

The most common cause of obstructive symptoms is increased urinary outflow resistance along the urethra. For men, this often is the result of an enlarged prostate or a urethral stricture (i.e. a scar of the urethral lumen from past injury or infection). In women obstructive symptoms can be due to kinking of the urethra, which can result from prolapse of the bladder or other organs through the vagina, displacing the path of the urethra and increasing outflow urinary resistance. In severe cases obstructive LUTS can produce a form of incontinence called "overflow incontinence" in which the bladder does not completely empty and urine dribbles out from the urethra when intravesical pressure becomes high enough to exceed urethral closure pressure [11].

Irritative symptoms often have a more complicated pathophysiology but are generally due to an over-activity of the detrusor muscle; this stimulates a spasm-like sensation that triggers a sensation of needing to void. Detrusor overactivity may be secondary to spinal injury, neurodegenerative conditions, bladder irritation from inflammation or infection, or it may be idiopathic.

> **Helpful Hint**
>
> It is important to recognize that there is often significant overlap between obstructive and irritative symptoms; the etiology of a patient's LUTS may be multifactorial and may require urologic investigation to accurately diagnose [10].

LUTS are a significant impediment to overall quality of life and represent a substantial cost in terms of healthcare expenditures and loss of productivity [12]. Loss of urinary control may also contribute to social isolation and depression [13]. Aside from symptomatic bother, inability to adequately void predisposes patients to urinary tract infection, urolithiasis, and in extreme cases renal failure due to back pressure on the kidneys.

## LUTS in Men

The prostate is the organ most commonly associated with LUTS in men, primarily due to benign prostate hypertrophy (BPH, also referred to as Benign Prostate Enlargement BPE). In BPH there is enlargement of the prostate gland, leading to compression of the urethra and narrowing of urethral caliber (Fig. 16.2). This tends to restrict urine outflow. BPH is strongly associated with age although the degree of bother from BPH does not always correlate with the degree of glandular enlargement. While enlargement of the prostate plays an important role, local and systemic inflammation may also contribute to symp-

**Fig. 16.2** Sagittal Section of the male pelvis. The prostate surrounds the urethra but does not protrude into the urethral lumen. In the setting of BPE or BPH (not shown) the urethra is compressed by the enlarged prostate and urine flow is restricted (Image Courtesy, J. Ehrenfeld)

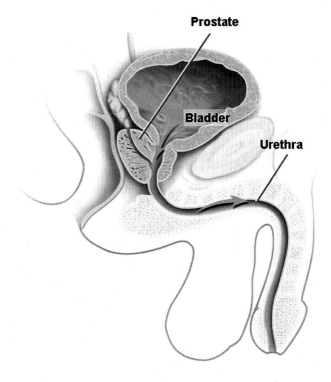

toms [14] and possibly even to hypertrophy by inducing cells to multiply and grow [15]. This synergistic effect may accelerate prostate growth and progression of LUTS in men.

The most common inflammatory triggers in the prostate include pathogens like viruses and bacteria. Men with a history of urinary tract infections and/or sexually transmitted infections (STI) are more likely to develop LUTS [16]. Progressive growth in the size of the prostate is also a contributing factor to LUTS in men. Diabetes, obesity and the metabolic syndrome have all been linked to an increase risk of LUTS [17].

HIV infection is another important risk factor for LUTS. In a urodynamic study of HIV infected men with LUTS it was determined that the underlying cause of LUTS in 61 % of these men was neurological (e.g. cerebral toxoplasmosis and HIV encephalitis [18]. These data are from an era before the introduction of Highly Active Retroviral Therapy (HART) and hence these neurologic entities are much less common in contemporary HIV infected persons. In contemporary series HIV associated LUTS are thought to be related to pro-inflammatory nature of the disease process, increased risk of UTI, and/or neuropathic injury to the detrusor nerves [19, 20].

Major depression is common in men with LUTS. Depression has been shown to increase inflammatory markers in patients and it is thought that these effects contribute to the pathophysiology of LUTS [21, 22]. A study by Johnson et al. in 2010 found that men suffering from depression had higher urinary symptom scores (worse voiding symptoms) as compared to healthy controls [23]. Breyer et al. also found a significant association between depression and suicidal ideation and lower urinary tract symptoms [24]. In addition to the inflammatory response induced by the depressive state, it is also hypothesized that the pathologic synthesis and regulation of serotonin observed in depressed individuals may place these same individuals at risk for developing idiopathic detrusor overactivity [25]. Since the detrusor muscle contraction is responsible for normal voiding, instability of this muscle could lead to increased urinary symptoms.

Although the physiology of LUTS is similar amongst all men regardless of sexual behavior, specific risks have been identified in MSM. MSM have a higher rate of STI compared to the general population [26, 27]. Breyer et al. reported that MSM with a history of gonorrhea, urinary tract infections, and prostatitis were more likely to report LUTS compared to their MSM peers [28]. In a related study Breyer et al. reported that men with AIDS were more likely to report moderate to severe lower urinary tract symptoms as compared to non-HIV infected men as well as men with HIV but not AIDS (Fig. 16.3) [28].

Similarly, depression is more prevalent in the LGBT community and has been identified as a predictor of LUTS in MSM [28]. For these reasons, MSM should be screened for LUTS and counseled accordingly [29]. A common screening tool for urinary symptoms in men is the International Prostate Symptom Score (IPSS) (also known as the American Urologic Association Symptom Score) [30].

> **Helpful Hint**
> While LUTS in men are commonly attributed to prostate pathology, bladder instability may occur in men. Potential etiologies include neurologic lesions, chronic obstruction from BPH, urinary tract infections, and idiopathic causes. These possibilities should be considered when evaluating a male patient with LUTS.

## LUTS in Women

Symptoms and etiologies for LUTS and incontinence in women differ markedly from what is observed in men, largely due to anatomic differences between genders. Obstructive LUTS are relatively infrequent in women but irritative symptoms occur at a high rate and women are at a much higher risk of incontinence than men due to markedly lower urethral resistance. Symptoms

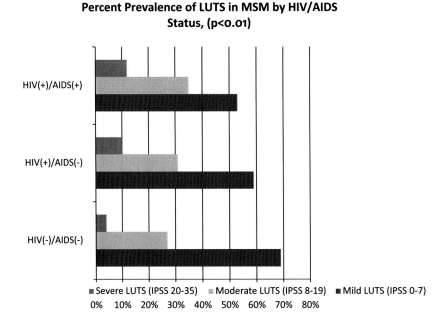

**Fig. 16.3** Prevalence of LUTS in MSM by HIV/AIDS Status

are often a result of changes in the pelvic floor musculature, which can occur after childbirth. These changes can cause kinking of the urethra resulting in obstructive symptoms, which can then evolve to include overactive symptoms from incomplete emptying of the bladder.

In addition, following menopause, changes in estrogen levels can result in the vaginal mucosa to become thinner and more friable. For, some women this can be manifested in irritation with voiding and result in increased urinary frequency and even recurrent urinary tract infections.

Lesbian and bisexual women have higher rates of obesity compared to heterosexual women [31], a condition that has been associated with greater risk of LUTS [32]. At the same time, lesbian women are less likely to have a history of pregnancy, which is a risk factor for incontinence. Whether WSW have a significantly different prevalence for LUTS/incontinence compared to their heterosexual peers is unclear; unpublished data from our group indicate that the prevalence of LUTS and incontinence in WSW is generally similar to what is observed in non-WSW females

(Shindel, unpublished data). However, the high prevalence of LUTS/incontinence in women in general dictates that WSW be screened and appropriately treated for LUTS/incontinence.

## Treatment of LUTS

Treatment options for lower urinary tract symptoms range from behavioral modification to medications to surgical interventions. Picking the appropriate therapy depends on the individual needs of the patient and should be based on the patient's reported symptoms. Treatment should be initiated if symptoms are bothersome or if symptoms are presenting a risk to a patient's health (e.g. worsening renal function, recurrent urinary tract infections, urolithiasis).

Behavioral interventions are often the first line of therapy for LUTS. Men or women with bothersome LUTS can try to void regularly (i.e. every 3 h) or perform double voiding which means voiding to presumed completed, waiting, and then attempt to void again immediately to excrete any remaining urine from the bladder. Such behaviors can improve bladder emptying and decrease LUTS. Other interventions include decreasing oral fluid intake in the evening and at night to decrease the severity of nocturia. Changing the dosing of diuretics to earlier in the day can also improve nighttime urinary symptoms. Finally, avoiding bladder irritants like caffeine, citrus, alcohol, carbonated beverages, and spicy foods can help to decrease bladder over activity.

**Helpful Hint**
Behavioral interventions can often improve urinary symptoms without the potential risks of medication or surgery.

For LUTS refractory to behavioral modification, three classes of medications are frequently prescribed. **The first three categories are specifically indicated for natal men and are not FDA approved for use in natal women.**

**Alpha-blockers** (e.g. terazosin, doxazosin, tamsulosin, sildosin, alfuzosin, etc.) block adrenergic nerve endings which are responsible for contraction of smooth muscle in the vicinity of the internal urethral sphincter and prostate; this has the effect of increasing the luminal diameter of the prostatic urethra during voiding and improving urinary flow. Symptoms can improve immediately but generally take 2–3 weeks for noticeable relief. Side effects including weakness, orthostatic hypotension and anejaculation. The rates of orthostatsis/weakness are markedly lower in modern selective alpha blockers. However, alpha blockers may have a synergistic hypotensive effect when taking with inhibitors of phosphodiesterase type 5 (PDE5I) that are used to promote penile erection (e.g. sildenafil, vardenafil, tadalafil, avanafil); patients should be cautioned about this potential drug interaction and advised to take these classes of medications at least 4 h apart in time. Although orthostatic symptoms are markedly less with

modern alpha blockers anejaculation is more common (~14–35 %) [33, 34]. Ejaculatory disturbance may be of great significant to MSM as ejaculation has been shown to be an important sign of sexual gratification in this population [35].

**5-alpha reductase inhibitors** (5ARI, e.g. finasteride, dutasteride) inhibit the enzyme 5-alpha reductase which converts testosterone to dihydrotestosterone, the primary active androgen in the prostate. This results in decreased growth of the prostate and can even cause the prostate to shrink in size up to about 20 %. 5ARI are most effective in men with very large prostates. 5ARI have also been shown in a randomized controlled trial to significantly reduce the risk of BPH progression (e.g. urinary retention, requirement for surgery, UTI, renal failure) when used as monotherapy or in combination with an alpha blocker. Men on this medication generally will have a halving of serum PSA (prostate specific antigen) so this must be taken into consideration when interpreting the screening test for prostate cancer. This medication does not work immediately and may need to be taken regularly for 6 months before noticeable improvements are seen. Reported side effects include decreased sex drive, smaller amount of ejaculate, erectile dysfunction, and gynecomastia [36].

**Tadalafil** is a selective inhibitor of the enzyme phosphodiesterase type 5. This drug was initially approved for management of erectile dysfunction (ED) in men but has also established efficacy in the management of LUTS in men with BPH when taken as a daily dose. While the subjective benefit of tadalafil for LUTS is established, treatment with this drug has not been shown to improve objective measures such as urine flow rate and post void residual urine. Side effects of tadalafil include congestion, stuffy nose, headache, and myalgias [37].

**Anticholinergics** (e.g. oxybutynin, tolterodine, solfenacin, darifenacin, trospium) block cholinergic nerve endings which are responsible for initiation of bladder contraction and can be helpful for patients with overactive bladder symptoms. By decreasing the intensity of bladder contractions, patients with irritative LUTS may be able to postpone voiding and decrease urinary frequency. The medication works quickly and its effects are generally noticed in the first days to weeks of stable dosage. Side effects include dry mouth, dizziness, constipation and drowsiness. There is some concern that these drugs may precipitate urinary retention in patients with pronounced urethral obstruction. Anti-cholinergics should not be used in persons with narrow angle glaucoma and should be used with caution in elderly persons using other anti-cholinergic or nervous system active drugs due to increased risk of mental status change [38].

For some patients, medications and behavioral changes are not sufficient to treat LUTS. These patients should be referred to a urologist for counseling and discussion of surgical treatment options. Examples of surgical treatments include Transurethral Resection of the Prostate (TURP) in men with BPH, urethral sling surgery for incontinence (primarily in women but useful in some cases for men), and intravesical injection of botulinum toxin in patients of any gender who have refractory bladder overactivity [39].

## Sexual Behavior and Health

Clear and important differences exist regarding sexual behavior between heterosexual and LGBT patients. Perhaps most important for clinicians is understanding the important and unique differences in sexual dysfunction among these populations in order to properly screen and treat LGBT persons. Data regarding same-sex sexual behavior has been dominated by the role sexual behavior and dysfunction on the impact of HIV transmission in MSM [40, 41]. Existing studies on sexual function/satisfaction are often qualitative in nature, include small populations, and utilize non-validated metrics or single item questions to elucidate information. This last limitation stems from the fact that the majority of validated instruments for assessment of sexual function use language geared towards heterosexuals and have not been validated in the LGBT population [42, 43].

Taking an appropriate sexual history is fundamental to promoting sexual wellness and the fundamental skills relevant to taking a sexual health history in cis-gendered heterosexual persons apply to sexual health history in LGBT persons. However, normalizing statements (e.g. "Many of my patients…", "Some people have sex with women, some with men, some with both, and others with neither.") and open ended questions (e.g. "What questions do you have about your sexual health?") are of particular importance in comfortable sexual health inquiry for LGBT persons. "Yes/no" questions can still be useful in initiating the conversation (e.g. "Do you have any concerns or questions about sexuality that you would like to address during this visit?") Further questioning as to the type of sexual activity the patient engages can be important for many aspects of the urologic assessment ranging from risks for sexually transmitted infections to counseling for treatment of prostate cancer. Asking the patient if they engage in oral, anal, or vaginal sex and clarifying if the behavior is receptive or insertive can accurately characterize the patient's sexual activity.

> **Helpful Hint**
> There is great variability in sexual expression amongst LGBT persons; it if helpful to understand the exact sort of sexual activity the patient engages in.

## The Sexual Response Cycle

Williams Masters and Virginia Johnson are credited with the first large scale systematic investigation of sexual response in men and women. From their observations Masters and Johnson developed a four phase sexual response cycle consisting of Arousal, Plateau, Orgasm, and Resolution [44]. The sex therapist Helen Singer Kaplan modified this linear response cycle to incorporate a desire phase which precedes arousal [45].

Alternative models for sexual response in women that are more circular in nature have been proposed by several experts [46]. While these newer models have some merit the linear response models remain very useful for classification of sexual disruptions. An outline of the physiological events associated with difference phases of the sexual response cycle (omitting plateau) and classification of specific disruptions of these phases is presented in Table 16.1.

> **Helpful Hint**
> In virtually all cases of sexual problem/dysfunction there are both biological and psychological factors at play.

## Sexual Function in Natal Men

Much has been uncovered in recent years regarding the complexities involved in male sexual behavior. From arousal to erection to ejaculation, sexual function requires a complex coordination of incoming and outgoing stimuli all presided over by the brain. Brain imaging studies of men during sexual activity have identified the mesodiencephalic transition zone (an area in the center of the brain) as the area which receives sensory information from the genitals, anus, rectum and prostate during sexual activity that is carried to

the brain by the spinal cord during ejaculation [47]. This area contains dopaminergic nerve cells controlled by dopamine—a neurotransmitter linked with rewarding behaviors—and may explain why genital and anal stimulation is so strongly pleasurable and rewarding [48].

Penile erection is the best understood aspect of male sexuality and the issue most amenable to treatment. Erection of the penis occurs via dilation of the cavernous arteries, which supply blood to the corpora cavernosa of the penis. The vascular events that drive penile erection are mediated by a complex interplay of the cavernous nerves which innervate the cavernous arteries. Release of nitric oxide from these nerves activates vascular guanylate cyclase, which in turns produces downstream molecular events that trigger muscular smooth relaxation in the arteries supplying the penis. With vasodilation, penile blood flow increases and the erectile tissue of the penis becomes engorged. As this tissue expands and becomes tumescent the emissary veins which drain the corpora cavernosa are compressed against the tunica albuginea of the corpora cavernosa; this has the effect of restricting blood flow out of the penis and leads to rigid penile erection [49].

Due to variation in sexual practice patterns the anus, prostate, and rectum are relevant to MSM as many (but not all) MSM engage in anal sex. The prostate is clearly a "sexual" erogenous zone and one that can provide sexual pleasure following digital stimulation or through anal receptive

**Table 16.1**  The sexual response cycle in biologically female and male persons and common nomenclature for sexual issues of each phase

|  | Biologically male | | Biologically female | |
|---|---|---|---|---|
|  | Physiological signs | Disruption classified as: | Physiological signs | Disruption classified as: |
| Desire | Pupillary dilation, tachycardia, tachypnea | Hypoactive sexual desire disorder | Pupillary dilation, tachycardia, tachypnea | Hypoactive sexual desire disorder |
| Arousal | Penile erection, scrotal contraction, nipple erection | Erectile dysfunction | Vulvar and clitoral swelling, vaginal lubrication and lengthening, nipple erection | Sexual arousal disorder (genital or subjective) |
| Orgasm | Ejaculation, muscular contractions, satisfaction, pleasure | Premature ejaculation, delayed ejaculation, anorgasmia | Muscular contractions in vagina, uterus, anus, satisfaction/pleasure | Female orgasmic disorder |
| Resolution | Detumescence of the penis, return to resting state | Priapism | Cessation of vaginal lubrication and lengthening, return to resting state | Persistent genital arousal disorder |

intercourse though researchers know little on the innervation pathways involved. It is important that patients be educated about the critical role that the prostate plays in sexual activity especially if the patient engages in anal receptive intercourse.

The neurologic and vascular systems are essential components of erectile response; hence, vascular diseases (e.g. diabetes, hypertension, hypercholesterolemia, tobacco use, obesity, lack of exercise) and nervous system lesions (e.g. spinal cord transaction, cavernous nerve injury during pelvic surgery) are major risk factors for ED. Other common causes of trouble with erections include medication side effects (particularly beta blockers, thiazide diuretics, and antidepressants), testosterone deficiency, and psychosocial issues within the patient or between patient and partner(s) [49].

## Sexual Dysfunction in MSM

### Erectile Dysfunction

Existing data suggest that rates of erectile dysfunction (ED) are higher in gay/bisexual men compared to their heterosexual peers. Bancroft et al. reported on a sample of 2937 men and found that only 42 % of gay identified men "never" experienced ED as compared to 54 % of heterosexual men [50]. An internet study investigated sexual wellness in osteopathic and allopathic medical schools in North America and compared rates of self reported sexual dysfunction. It was determined that ED was more prevalent amongst gay or bisexual identified men as compared to heterosexual men [51]. This finding of increased ED among MSM was also echoed in a study by Vansintejan et al. out of Belgian. The authors found that almost half of MSM sampled reported some difficulty with getting an erection. Factors associated with ED included increased age, single relationship status, versatile or passive sex role, and decreased libido [52]. Because gay men have a higher prevalence for tobacco and drug use compared to heterosexual men, their risk of ED is likely to be greater [53].

One major difficulty in studying erectile dysfunction in MSM is the fact that the standardized questionnaires commonly used in contemporary ED research are validated for use in heterosexual encounters only. Coyne et al. did validate a version of the International Index of Erectile Function (IIEF) in a population of HIV infected men who have sex with men. This instrument was used by Shindel et al. in an internet survey of sexual function in MSM. It was determined that ED was associated with increasing age (Fig. 16.4), AIDS, and LUTS [54]. LUTS and younger age were associated with greater risk of PE [54].

## Premature Ejaculation and Other Sexual Concerns

A number of other sexual problems may occur in men, including premature ejaculation (PE, defined most recently by the International Society for Sexual Medicine as ejaculation occurring in 1 min or less of penetration and associated with loss of sense of control and distress) [55]. It is noted that the definition applicable only to coital intercourse. The intent of these authors was not be to exclusionary; however, it was concluded that there was currently insufficient objective evidence to incorporate non-coital intercourse into the definition of PE. Until data on clinically relevant PE in MSM is available it is advised that clinicians and researchers use the same ISSM criteria for the diagnosis of PE in MSM [55].

Most contemporary reports suggest that the prevalence of early ejaculation is similar to slightly less in MSM compared to their heterosexual peers [50, 51, 56, 57]. Early ejaculation associated with bother is reported by between 15 and 34 % of MSM [54, 58, 59]. Controversy persists on the true burden of clinically relevant early ejaculation in general, let along in MSM. Most studies suggesting a ~30 % prevalence are based on single item reporting of subjective experiences rather than the most stringent criteria and hence it is likely that the true prevalence of clinical PE is less than 5 % [55, 60].

MSM with severe voiding symptoms, HIV infection, and who experience social recrimination

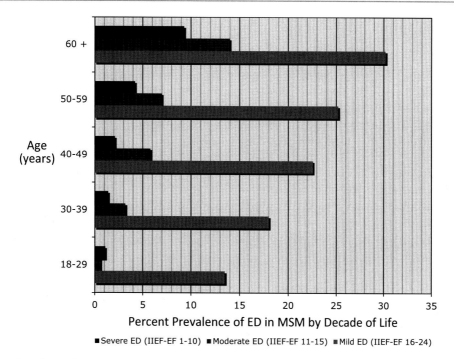

**Fig. 16.4** Prevalence of ED in MSM by decade of life

appear to have lower risk of early ejaculation compared to their MSM peers [59, 61, 62].

Aside from ED and PE, men may experience bothersome declines in sexual desire (aka hypoactive sexual desires disorder or low libido), difficulty attaining orgasm (anorgasmia), disruption of ejaculation (retrograde ejaculation or anejaculation), and Peyronie's Disease (an acquire deformity of the penis). These issues are less well understood but can pose a significant impediment to sexual satisfaction. A careful history can help elucidate the exact nature of sexual complaints in men; it should be borne in mind that many sexual concerns may be comorbid.

## Sexual Dysfunction, HIV, and AIDS

AIDS has been identified as significant risk factor for developing ED and/or premature ejaculation amongst MSM. Hypotheses for the etiology of this connection range from prolonged use of HART, exposure to opportunistic infections and, low CD4 counts although these associations have been inconsistently demonstrated to increase the prevalence of HIV [63–65]. Research by Hart attempted to identify differential risk factors for ED comparing HIV negative and positive MSM. The authors found an increased risk of ED among HIV(+) men (21 %) as compared to HIV (−) (16 %) despite the HIV (+) cohort having a younger median age. Risk factors for ED in HIV (−) men were older age (age 55+ versus age ≤40; 112 % increase), Black race (88 % increase), and cumulative years of cigarette smoking in pack-years (9 % increase). In HIV (+) men, risk factors were years of antihypertensive use and cumulative years of antidepressant use. Interestingly, HAART adherence years and CD4+ cell count were not found to significantly predict likelihood of ED [53]. The authors suggested that it the HIV—related medical comorbidities which may explain the increased prevalence of ED as opposed to a direct effect of the virus. Additional potential factors Testosterone deficiency is common in HIV positive persons and this may predispose to declines in libido and erectile capacity [66, 67]. Finally, the substantial psychosocial stressors of HIV infection (stigma, concern about infecting others, etc) may contribute to sexual issues in HIV positive persons [68].

In a study by Shindel, greater prevalence of erectile dysfunction was identified in men with progressive HIV infection 40–59 years of age as compared to HIV-negative men of similar age. When the authors controlled for other variables including age, number of sexual partners, and condom use they found that HIV alone was not a risk for ED but HIV with AIDS was associated with greater odds of ED [69].

Neither HIV nor AIDS was associated with an increased prevalence of early ejaculation in this study. Interestingly, use of phosphodiesterase 5 (PDE5) inhibitor drugs was found to be more common among HIV-infected men. In addition, HIV (+) men were more likely to have sought medical attention for sexual dysfunction as compared to HIV (−) MSM [69].

## Management of Sexual Concerns in Gay Men

Medical therapies for ED include oral phosphodiereterase type 5 inhibitors (PDE5I), vacuum erection devices (VED), intracavernosal injection therapy (ICI), intraurethral prostaglandin suppositories, and surgical implantation of inflatable or malleable penile prostheses [69].

PDE5I drugs are the first line agents of choice in medical management of ED. In the United States four PDE5I are currently available; sildenafil (Viagra®), vardenafil (Levitra® or Staxyn®), tadalafil (Cialis®), and avanafil (Stendra®). Other PDE5I are approved for use in other regions of the world. These drugs are highly effective but must be taken at least 1–2 h before planned intercourse. Potential side effects include congestion, headache, flushing, visual disturbance, and myalgia. Side effects are typically mild and self-limited. PDE5I should not be used in patients taking nitrate based therapy for angina and should not be taken within 4 h of alpha blocker medications [70].

Second and third line therapies for ED are often effective in cases where oral pharmacotherapy fails [70]. A complete discussion of these modalities is beyond the scope of this chapter but interested readers are referred to recent publications on management of ED in men [70] and to national and international organizations dedicated to sexual wellness in men such as the Sexual Medicine Society of North America (www.smsna.org) and the International Society for Sexual Medicine (www.ISSM.info)

## ED in HIV Positive Men

The issue of ED in HIV positive men is one of marked public health consequence as ED has been associated with failure to utilize safer sex practices (i.e. condoms) [68]. The treatment of ED in HIV positive persons has been controversial in the past due to concerns that this might promote sexual transmission of the virus [71]. A pilot study by Goltz attempted to identify any possible increased risk for contracting STIs amongst MSM receiving therapy for erectile dysfunction. The authors found that 1/3 of the sample had engaged in unprotected anal sex at the last erectile dysfunction medication use. Risks for engaging in unprotected sex were younger age and receiving the medication from the sexual partner [72].

While counseling on safer sex practices should accompany provision of erectogenic therapy in all contexts, there are no data suggesting that treatment of ED in and of itself increases risk of HIV infection. Treatment of ED may help some men with marginal erectile capacity retain erections despite condom use, thus facilitating safer sex [73]. Respect for persons and social justice are fundamental tenets of medical practice and indicate that HIV positive men with ED receive appropriate counseling and treatment for sexual issues, including ED [74].

## Management of Other Sexual Problems in Men

Hypoactive sexual desire disorder, orgasmic dysfunction, and Peyronie's Disease (a condition of acquired deformity of the penis) are present in gay men but are poorly characterized. Management of these concerns in gay men should follow established treatment protocols, including attention to general health, relationship status, and medications that may contribute to sexual issues (e.g. beta blockers, thiazide diuretics, antidepressants, anti-androgens, etc). It should be borne in mind that there is only one FDA approved medical therapy for Peyronie's Disease (injectable collagenase) and no approved pharmacotherapy for any other sexual concern in men.

## Sexual Function in Natal Women

Scientific understanding of female sexual response lags far behind where we stand with respect to understanding of male sexual response. In general the same molecular and vascular events occur during female sexual arousal although the end result is markedly different from what is observed in men [75]. The clitoris becomes erect in a fashion similar to the penis but does not become as rigid due to size and the relative thinness of the clitoral tunica. Vasodilation also plays an important role in promoting vaginal engorgement, lengthening, and lubrication [75]. There are no glandular elements within the vagina that produce lubrication. However, with increased vascular engorgement of the vaginal submucosa oncotic pressure leads to production of a transudative fluid that is passed through aquaporins on the vaginal mucosa into the vaginal lumen [76, 77].

Vascular and neurologic health factors in women have not been clearly and universally linked to sexual distress/dissatisfaction as they have been in men although women with severe injuries (e.g. spinal cord injury) do have marked impairments of sexual function [78].

## Sexual Dysfunction in WSW

Public health concerns about HIV spawned interest from the research community on sexual wellness in gay men; sexual wellness in lesbian and bisexual WSW remains very poorly studied in the mainstream biomedical literature. There is a dearth of validated tools for the quantitative assessment of sexual function in lesbian women.

Tracy and Junginger developed a version of the Female Sexual Function Index (FSFI) for use in lesbian women. The FSFI explores six domains relevant to female sexuality; Desire, Arousal, Lubrication, Orgasm, Satisfaction, and Pain. Women with lower scores on this index were identified to have "higher risk for sexual dysfunction." In the initial validation study, older age was associated with decreased sexual desire and overall sexual function. Stress was associated with worse sexual function whereas satisfying relationship with a partner were associated with better sexual function [79].

Shindel et al. utilized a version of this FSFI in an internet study of sexual function in 1566 WSW. Risk of distress sexual problems was calculated using previously established cut-off scores for the FSFI which were shown to approximate endorsement of sexual dissatisfaction in this cohort. After multivariable adjustment nulligravid women, women with OAB, and women with no partners or non-female partners were found to be at greatest risk of distress sexual issues [61].

There is a common perception among both providers and patients that STI risk is low in same-sex encounters between women. This may predispose WSW to entirely preventable STI. A study on barrier use in WSW was derived from this same data set and indicated that many WSW do not use barriers during sexual encounters, even outside the context of a monogamous relationship [80]. These data speak to the need for education on safer sex practices for WSW [5, 81, 82].

Shindel et al. found that while almost a quarter of the WSW sample reported symptoms of sexual dysfunction, only 11 % had actually sought help from a physician for these problems [61]. This highlights the importance of sexual health screening by physicians to help identify at risk patients and provide intervention to help improve sexual health in general but particularly in WSW.

Biomedical treatment options for sexual dysfunction in women in general are very limited; a selective estrogen receptor modulator has been approved for management of dyspareunia from vaginal penetration [83]. Other pharmaceuticals are used off label by some experts. A discussion of these medical treatment modalities is beyond the scope of this chapter but interested readers are referred to recent publication on this topic and the International Society for the Study of Women's Sexual Health (www.ISSWSH.org) for more information. Attention to psychosocial factors and relationship context remains an important consideration for sexual concerns in women.

## Genitourinary Malignancy

### Prostate Cancer in MSM

Prostate cancer is the number one noncutaneous cancer in men with a lifetime risk of the malignancy of almost 17 % [84]. No study has ever demonstrated an increased risk or incidence of prostate cancer in MSM. However, MSM are known to be less aware of the pathophysiology of prostate cancer and the impacts of its treatment as compared to their heterosexual counterparts [85]. Many factors contribute to this knowledge gap between MSM and heterosexual patients regarding prostate cancer and the effects of its treatment. The aforementioned concerns about disclosure of gay identity to a provider may dissuade some MSM from mentioning their particular concerns about sexual function to their provider [86]. Furthermore, the vast majority of survey tools for assessment of treatment response after prostate cancer have a heterosexist focus (e.g. questionnaires that ask if erection is sufficient for vaginal penetration) [87].

> **Helpful Hint**
>
> All men (including gay and bisexual men) are at risk for prostate cancer. Screening for prostate cancer is controversial but should be discussed with all men regardless of sexual orientation.

Given recent trends towards early treatment of prostate cancer the majority of the negative effects of the disease arise from treatment and not the malignancy itself. Treatments for prostate cancer include prostatectomy, external beam radiation therapy, brachytherapy and hormone deprivation therapy. Although these interventions can result in excellent disease free survival benefit, they also can result in significant comorbidities. The most common side effects resulting from prostate cancer treatment include ED, loss of ejaculation, painful anal receptive intercourse, urinary incontinence, and penile shortening. These side effects can have important consequences on quality of life for all men.

Although MSM and heterosexual men have similar concerns regarding prostate cancer and desire for cure, there are several unique differences regarding sexual behavior, which can impact the experience of the potential side effects. Although anal intercourse is not an exclusively gay male practice nor is it practiced by all MSM, it is more frequent in MSM. Anal penetration requires a more rigid erection than vaginal penetration due to anal muscle tone. Hence, even a small decrease in the firmness of the erection may have a greater impact on sexual performance for MSM who penetrate their partner anally (tops) as compared to heterosexual men engaging in vaginal intercourse. Anal receptive partners (bottoms) may experience pleasure from stimulation of the prostate gland. Loss of the prostate to surgery, rectal wall fibrosis from radiation, or anatomical changes in the pelvis which predispose men to anodyspareunia may exert a disproportionate influence on sexual enjoyment for MSM who bottom.

Despite an obvious impact of prostate cancer treatment on anal intercourse the paucity of research on this behavior makes counseling extremely difficult. Clinicians should ask patients (particularly MSM) preoperatively about the importance of insertive and receptive anal intercourse to their sexual expression. Pending the results of this revelation, clinicians can at least introduce the possibility of side effects following treatment and may even use this clinically relevant data to inform the type of intervention recommended.

The importance of ejaculation has also been demonstrated to be higher amongst MSM as compared to heterosexual men. It has been hypothesized that ejaculation is an important sign of sexual gratification among MSM. Furthermore, Wassersug hypothesized that the impact of the HIV epidemic changed the act of ejaculation making a visible ejaculation important from a disease transmission standpoint [35]. Given that ejaculation is dependent on an intact prostate, it is very important to counsel patients on the likelihood of ejaculation loss after surgery or radiation for prostate cancer.

Research also suggests that penis size plays a more important role in the psychosexual health of MSM, in that men with larger penises report improved health. A study by Grov et al. found that men with "below average" penis size fared significantly worse on a multifaceted score of psychosocial adjustment [88]. Given the incidence of penile shortening has been shown to be as high as 68–71 % of men following radical prostatectomy with a mean decrease of 1.1–4.0 cm [89, 90], it is important that MSM be informed of this potential side effect.

Qualitative research performed by Hartman et al. of same sex couples impacted by sexual dysfunction following radical prostatectomy highlight important differences between heterosexual and same sex relationships [91]. For example, navigating changing sexual roles following surgery is a unique challenge faced by same sex couples. For some couples, sexual roles may include one partner preferring anal receptive intercourse and the other anal insertive. Following surgery, these roles can evolve and impact the pre-surgical dynamic. Furthermore, the study identified the use of open relationship as a coping strategy for maintaining sexual satisfaction that has not been identified previously among heterosexual couples [91]. Such studies, illustrate the importance of tailored pre and postoperative counseling for same sex couples focusing on their unique dynamics and needs.

## Transgender Patients and Prostate Cancer

In male to female gender affirming surgery (GAS), the prostate is normally left in place given its intimate relationship with the urethra and the neuro-vascular bundles involved in sexual arousal and orgasm. Prostatectomy also carries substantial potential for urinary and sexual morbidity so there is little motivation to remove it in GAS. Despite this fact, the rates of prostate cancer in male to female transgender patients are extremely low. The exact numbers are unknown but there have been a few case reports of transgender patients on hormone therapy presenting with prostate cancer [92, 93]. By definition, these patients have castrate resistant prostate cancer and are treated as such. It is thought that the lower rate of prostate cancer among transgender patients is the deprivation of testosterone. For this reason, transgender patients who are not on hormonal supplementation or on incomplete blockade carry a risk of developing prostate cancer and should be screened similarly to men. Although controversial, this screening should include shared decision making with a discussion of risks of screening based on family history. Following this conversation, prostate cancer screening can include a PSA serum level and digital rectal exam. The most important concept is that transgender patients still have a prostate and therefore carry a risk for prostate cancer which varies based on the duration of hormone therapy.

## Bladder Cancer in LGBT Patients

The number one risk factor for developing urothelial cell carcinoma of the bladder is cigarette smoking [94–97]. Given the increased incidence of smoking among LGBT persons as compared to heterosexuals [98], there is a resultant increase in risk for developing bladder cancer. For this reason, screening LGBT patients for smoking is critical, so smoking cessation counseling can be appropriately initiated.

## References

1. Rothman EF, Sullivan M, Keyes S, Boehmer U. Parents' supportive reactions to sexual orientation disclosure associated with better health: results from a population-based survey of LGB adults in Massachusetts. J Homosex. 2012;59(2):186–200. doi: 10.1080/00918369.2012.648878.

2. Makadon HJ. Ending LGBT invisibility in health care: the first step in ensuring equitable care. Cleve Clin J Med. 2011;78(4):220–4. doi:10.3949/ccjm.78gr.10006. Review.

3. Stewart M, Brown JB, Donner A, et al. The impact of patient-centered care on outcomes. J Fam Pract. 2000;49:796–804.

4. Xu F, Sternberg MR, Markowitz LE. Women who have sex with women in the United States: prevalence, sexual behavior and prevalence of herpes simplex virus type 2 infection-results from national health and nutrition examination survey 2001-2006. Sex Transm Dis. 2010;37(7):407–13. doi:10.1097/OLQ.0b013e3181db2e18.

5. Diamant AL, Schuster MA, McGuigan K, Lever J. Lesbians' sexual history with men: implications for taking a sexual history. Arch Intern Med. 1999; 159(22):2730–6.

6. Goparaju L, Warren-Jeanpiere L. African American women's perspectives on 'down low/DL' men: implications for HIV prevention. Cult Health Sex. 2012;14(8):879–93. doi:10.1080/13691058.2012.703 328. Epub 2012 Jul 18.

7. Chung B, Sommer G, Brooks J. Anatomy of the lower urinary tract and male genitalia. In: Wein AJ, editor. Campbell-Walsh urology. 10th ed. Philadelphia, PA: Saunders; 2012. p. 33–70.

8. Milsom I, Kaplan SA, Coyne KS, Sexton CC, Kopp ZS. Effect of bothersome overactive bladder symptoms on health-related quality of life, anxiety, depression, and treatment seeking in the United States: results from EpiLUTS. Urology. 2012;80:90–6.

9. Coyne KS, Matza LS, Kopp ZS, et al. Examining lower urinary tract symptom constellations using cluster analysis. BJU Int. 2008;101:1267–73.

10. Abrams P, Chapple C, Khoury S, Roehrborn C, de la Rosette J. International Consultation on New Developments in Prostate Cancer and Prostate Diseases. Evaluation and treatment of lower urinary tract symptoms in older men. J Urol. 2013;189(1 Suppl):S93–101. doi:10.1016/j.juro.2012.11.021.

11. Roehrborn C. Benign prostatic hyperplasia: etiology, pathophysiology, epidemiology, and natural history. In: Wein AJ, editor. Campbell-Walsh urology. 10th ed. Philadelphia, PA: Saunders; 2012. p. 2570–610.

12. Coyne KS, Payne C, Bhattacharyya SK, et al. The impact of urinary urgency and frequency on health-related quality of life in overactive bladder: results from a national community survey. Value Health. 2004;7:455–63.

13. Breyer BN, Shindel AW, Erickson BA, Blaschko SD, Steers WD, Rosen RC. The association of depression, anxiety and nocturia: a systematic review. J Urol. 2013;190:953–7.

14. St Sauver JL, Sarma AV, Jacobson DJ, et al. Associations between C-reactive protein and benign prostatic hyperplasia/lower urinary tract symptom outcomes in a population-based cohort. Am J Epidemiol. 2009;169:1281–90.

15. Kessler OJ, Keisari Y, Servadio C, et al. Role of chronic inflammation in the promotion of prostatic hyperplasia in rats. J Urol. 1998;159:1049–53.

16. Sutcliffe S, Rohrmann S, Giovannucci E, et al. Viral infections and lower urinary tract symptoms in the third national health and nutrition examination survey. J Urol. 2007;178:2181–5.

17. Hammarsten J, Hogstedt B. Clinical, anthropometric, metabolic and insulin profile of men with fast annual growth rates of benign prostatic hyperplasia. Blood Press. 1999;8:29–36.

18. Hermieu JF, Delmas V, Boccon-Gibod L. Micturition disturbances and human immunodeficiency virus infection. J Urol. 1996;156:157.

19. Kuller LH, Tracy R, Belloso W, et al. Inflammatory and coagulation biomarkers and mortality in patients with HIV infection. PLoS Med. 2008;5, e203.

20. De Pinho AM, Lopes GS, Ramos-Filho CF, et al. Urinary tract infection in men with AIDS. Genitourin Med. 1994;70:30.

21. Miller AH, Maletic V, Raison CL. Inflammation and its discontents: the role of cytokines in the pathophysiology of major depression. Biol Psychiatry. 2009; 65:732–41.

22. Howren MB, Lamkin DM, Suls J. Associations of depression with C-reactive protein, IL-1, and IL-6: a meta-analysis. Psychosom Med. 2009;71:171–86.

23. Johnson TV, Abbasi A, Ehrlich SS, et al. Major depression drives severity of American Urological Association Symptom Index. Urology. 2010;76: 1317–20.

24. Breyer BN, Kenfield SA, Blaschko SD, Erickson BA. The Association of lower urinary tract symptoms, depression and suicidal ideation: data from the 2005-2006 and 2007-2008 National Health and Nutrition Examination Survey. J Urol. 2013. pii: S0022-5347(13)06106-5. doi:10.1016/j.juro.2013.12.012.

25. Steers WD, Litman HJ, Rosen RC. Overactive bladder, urge incontinence and emotional disorders. AUA Update Series, 27 (2008) lesson 4.

26. Centers for Disease Control and Prevention. Trends in HIV/AIDS diagnoses among men who have sex with men – 33 States, 2000–2006. MMWR Morb Mortal Wkly Rep. 2008; 57:681–6.

27. Kirkcaldy RD, Zaidi A, Hook III EW, Holmes KK, Soge O, del Rio C, et al. Neisseria gonorrhoeae antimicrobial resistance among men who have sex with men and men who have sex exclusively with women: The Gonococcal Isolate Surveillance Project, 2005–2010. Ann Intern Med. 2013;158(5 Pt 1):321–8.

28. Breyer BN, Vittinghoff E, Van Den Eeden SK, Erickson BA, Shindel AW. Effect of sexually transmitted infections, lifetime sexual partner count, and recreational drug use on lower urinary tract symptoms in men who have sex with men. Urology. 2012;79(1):188–93. doi:10.1016/j.urology.2011.07.1412. Epub 2011 Oct 2.

29. Breyer BN, Kenfield SA, Blaschko SD, Erickson BA. The association of lower urinary tract symptoms,

depression and suicidal ideation: data from the 2005-2006 and 2007-2008 National Health and Nutrition Examination Survey. J Urol. 2014;191(5):1333–9. doi:10.1016/j.juro.2013.12.012. Epub 2013 Dec 14.

30. Barry MJ, Fowler Jr FJ, O'Leary MP, et al. The American Urological Association symptom index for benign prostatic hyperplasia. The Measurement Committee of the American Urological Association. J Urol. 1992;148:1549–57. discussion 64.

31. Fredriksen-Goldsen KI, Kim HJ, Barkan SE, Muraco A, Hoy-Ellis CP. Health disparities among lesbian, gay, and bisexual older adults: results from a population-based study. Am J Public Health. 2013;103(10):1802–9. doi:10.2105/AJPH.2012.301110. Epub 2013 Jun 13.

32. Morandi A, Maffeis C. Urogenital complications of obesity. Best Pract Res Clin Endocrinol Metab. 2013;27(2):209–18. doi:10.1016/j.beem.2013.04.002. Epub 2013 May 4.

33. Chapple CR, Montorsi F, Tammela TL, Wirth M, Koldewijn E, Fernández Fernández E, European Silodosin Study Group. Silodosin therapy for lower urinary tract symptoms in men with suspected benign prostatic hyperplasia: results of an international, randomized, double-blind, placebo- and active-controlled clinical trial performed in Europe. Eur Urol. 2011;59(3):342–52. doi:10.1016/j.eururo.2010.10.046. Epub 2010 Nov 10.

34. Hellstrom WJ, Sikka SC. Effects of acute treatment with tamsulosin versus alfuzosin on ejaculatory function in normal volunteers. J Urol. 2006;176(4 Pt 1):1529–33.

35. Wassersug RJ, Lyons A, Duncan D, Dowsett GW, Pitts M. Diagnostic and outcome differences between heterosexual and nonheterosexual men treated for prostate cancer. Urology. 2013;82(3):565–71. doi:10.1016/j.urology.2013.04.022. Epub 2013 Jun 14.

36. Corona G, Rastrelli G, Maseroli E, Balercia G, Sforza A, Forti G, Mannucci E, Maggi M. Inhibitors of 5α-reductase-related side effects in patients seeking medical care for sexual dysfunction. J Endocrinol Invest. 2012;35(10):915–20. doi:10.3275/8510. Epub 2012 Jul 9.

37. Seftel AD, Farber J, Fletcher J, Deeley MC, Elion-Mboussa A, Hoover A, Yu A, Fredlund P. A three-part study to investigate the incidence and potential etiologies of tadalafil-associated back pain or myalgia. Int J Impot Res. 2005;17(5):455–61.

38. Cetinel B, Onal B. Rationale for the use of anticholinergic agents in overactive bladder with regard to central nervous system and cardiovascular system side effects. Korean J Urol. 2013;54(12):806–15. Epub 2013 Dec 10.

39. Soljanik I. Efficacy and safety of botulinum toxin A intradetrusor injections in adults with neurogenic detrusor overactivity/neurogenic overactive bladder: a systematic review. Drugs. 2013;73(10):1055–66. doi:10.1007/s40265-013-0068-5. Review.

40. Schwarcz S, Scheer S, McFarland W, Katz M, Valleroy L, Chen S, Catania J. Prevalence of HIV infection and predictors of high-transmission sexual risk behaviors among men who have sex with men. Am J Public Health. 2007;97:1067–75.

41. Lallemand F, Salhi Y, Linard F, Giami A, Rozenbaum W. Sexual dysfunction in 156 ambulatory HIV-infected men receiving highly active antiretroviral therapy combinations with and without protease inhibitors. J Acquir Immune Defic Syndr. 2002;30:187–90.

42. Rosen RC, Riley A, Wagner G, Osterloh IH, Kirkpatrick J, Mishra A. The international index of erectile function (IIEF): a multidimensional scale for assessment of erectile dysfunction. Urology. 1997;49:822–30.

43. Coyne K, Mandalia S, McCullough S, Catalan J, Noestlinger C, Colebunders R, Asboe D. The international index of erectile function: development of an adapted tool for use in HIV-positive men who have sex with men. J Sex Med. 2010;7:769–74.

44. Masters WH, Johnson VE. Human sexual response. Boston: Little, Brown; 1966.

45. Kaplan HS. Disorders of sexual desire. New York: Brunner/Mazel; 1979.

46. Basson R. A model of women's sexual arousal. J Sex Marital Ther. 2002;28:1–10.

47. Holstege G, Georgiadis JR, Paans AM, Meiners LC, van der Graaf FH, Reinders AA. Brain activation during human male ejaculation. J Neurosci. 2003;23:9185–93.

48. McBride WJ, Murphy JM, Ikemoto S. Localization of brain reinforcement mechanisms: intracranial self-administration and intracranial place-conditioning studies. Behav Brain Res. 1999;101:129–52.

49. Dean RC, Lue TF. Physiology of penile erection and pathophysiology of erectile dysfunction. Urol Clin North Am. 2005;32(4):379–95, v.

50. Bancroft J, Carnes L, Janssen E, Goodrich D, Long JS. Erectile and ejaculatory problems in gay and heterosexual men. Arch Sex Behav. 2005;34:285–97.

51. Breyer BN, Smith JF, Eisenberg ML, Ando KA, Rowen TS, Shindel AW. The impact of sexual orientation on sexuality and sexual practices in North American medical students. J Sex Med. 2010;7:2391–400.

52. Vansintejan J, Vandevoorde J, Devroey D. The GAy MEn Sex StudieS: erectile dysfunction among Belgian gay men. Int J Gen Med. 2013;6:527-34. doi:10.2147/IJGM.S45783. Print 2013.

53. Hart TA, Moskowitz D, Cox C, Li X, Ostrow DG, Stall RD, Gorbach PM, Plankey M. The cumulative effects of medication use, drug use, and smoking on erectile dysfunction among men who have sex with men. J Sex Med. 2012;9(4):1106–13.

54. Shindel AW, Vittinghoff E, Breyer BN. Erectile dysfunction and premature ejaculation in men who have sex with men. J Sex Med. 2012;9:576–84.

55. Serefoglu EC, McMahon CG, Waldinger MD, Althof SE, Shindel A, Adaikan G, Becher EF, Dean J, Giuliano F, Hellstrom WJ, Giraldi A, Glina S, Incrocci L, Jannini E, McCabe M, Parish S, Rowland D, Segraves RT, Sharlip I, Torres LO. An evidence-based

unified definition of lifelong and acquired premature ejaculation: report of the second international society for sexual medicine ad hoc committee for the definition of premature ejaculation. J Sex Med. 2014. doi:10.1111/jsm.12524.

56. Son H, Song SH, Kim SW, Paick JS. Self-reported premature ejaculation prevalence and characteristics in Korean young males: community-based data from an internet survey. J Androl. 2010;31(6):540–6. doi:10.2164/jandrol.110.010355. Epub 2010 Jul 29.

57. Jern P, Santtila P, Johansson A, Alanko K, Salo B, Sandnabba NK. Is there an association between same-sex sexual experience and ejaculatory dysfunction? J Sex Marital Ther. 2010;36(4):303–12. doi:10.1080/0092623X.2010.488102.

58. Sandfort TG, de Keizer M. Sexual problems in gay men: an overview of empirical research. Annu Rev Sex Res. 2001;12:93–120.

59. Hirshfield S, Chiasson MA, Wagmiller Jr RL, Remien RH, Humberstone M, Scheinmann R, Grov C. Sexual dysfunction in an internet sample of U.S. men who have sex with men. J Sex Med. 2009;7:3104–14.

60. Althof SE, McMahon CG, Waldinger MD, Serefoglu EC, Shindel AW, Adaikan PG, Becher E, Dean J, Giuliano F, Hellstrom WJ, Giraldi A, Glina S, Incrocci L, Jannini E, McCabe M, Parish S, Rowland D, Segraves RT, Sharlip I, Torres LO. An Update of the International Society of Sexual Medicine's Guidelines for the Diagnosis and Treatment of Premature Ejaculation (PE). J Sex Med. 2014 May 22. doi: 10.1111/jsm.12504.

61. Shindel AW, Rowen TS, Lin T-C, Li C-S, Robertson PA, Breyer BN. An internet survey of demographic and health factors associated with risk of sexual dysfunction in women who have sex with women. J Sex Med. 2012;9:1261–71.

62. Lau JT, Kim JH, Tsui HY. Prevalence and sociocultural predictors of sexual dysfunction among Chinese men who have sex with men in Hong Kong. J Sex Med. 2008;5(12):2766–79. doi:10.1111/j.1743-6109.2008.00892.x. Epub 2008 Jun 10. Erratum in: J Sex Med. 2009;6(8):2344.

63. Asboe D, Catalan J, Mandalia S, Dedes N, Florence E, Schrooten W, Noestlinger C, Colebunders R. Sexual dysfunction in HIV-positive men is multifactorial: a study of prevalence and associated factors. AIDS Care. 2007;19(8):955–65.

64. Crum-Cianflone NF, Bavaro M, Hale B, Amling C, Truett A, Brandt C, Pope B, Furtek K, Medina S, Wallace MR. Erectile dysfunction and hypogonadism among men with HIV. AIDS Patient Care STDs. 2007;21(1):9–19.

65. Ende AR, Lo Re III V, DiNubile MJ, Mounzer K. Erectile dysfunction in an urban HIV-positive population. AIDS Patient Care ST. 2006;20(2):75–8.

66. Ashby J, Goldmeier D, Sadeghi-Nejad H. Hypogonadism in human immunodeficiency virus-positive men. Korean J Urol. 2014;55(1):9–16. Epub 2014 Jan 15. Review.

67. Claramonte M, García-Cruz E, Luque P, Alcaraz A. Prevalence and risk factors of erectile dysfunction and testosterone deficiency symptoms in a rural population in Uganda. Arch Esp Urol. 2012;65(7):689–97. English, Spanish.

68. Santi D, Brigante G, Zona S, Guaraldi G, Rochira V. Male sexual dysfunction and HIV--a clinical perspective. Nat Rev Urol. 2014;11(2):99–109. doi:10.1038/nrurol.2013.314. Epub 2014 Jan 7.

69. Shindel AW, Horberg MA, Smith JF, Breyer BN. Sexual dysfunction, HIV, and AIDS in men who have sex with men. AIDS Patient Care STDS. 2011;25(6):341–9. doi:10.1089/apc.2011.0059. Epub 2011 Apr 18.

70. Porst H, Burnett A, Brock G, Ghanem H, Giuliano F, Glina S, Hellstrom W, Martin-Morales A, Salonia A, Sharlip I, ISSM Standards Committee for Sexual Medicine. SOP conservative (medical and mechanical) treatment of erectile dysfunction. J Sex Med. 2013;10(1):130–71.

71. Kell P, Sadeghi-Nejad H, Price D. An ethical dilemma: erectile dysfunction in the HIV-positive patient: to treat or not to treat. Int J STD AIDS. 2002;13(6):355–7.

72. Goltz HH, Coon DW, Catania JA, Latini DM. A pilot study of HIV/STI risk among men having sex with men using erectile dysfunction medications: challenges and opportunities for sexual medicine physicians. J Sex Med. 2012;9(12):3189–97. doi:10.1111/j.1743-6109.2012.02943.x. Epub 2012 Oct 4.

73. Sanders SA, Milhausen RR, Crosby RA, Graham CA, Yarber WL. Do phosphodiesterase type 5 inhibitors protect against condom-associated erection loss and condom slippage? J Sex Med. 2009;6(5):1451–6. doi:10.1111/j.1743-6109.2009.01267.x.

74. Rosen RC, Catania JA, Ehrhardt AA, Burnett AL, Lue TF, McKenna K, Heiman JR, Schwarcz S, Ostrow DG, Hirshfield S, Purcell DW, Fisher WA, Stall R, Halkitis PN, Latini DM, Elford J, Laumann EO, Sonenstein FL, Greenblatt DJ, Kloner RA, Lee J, Malebranche D, Janssen E, Diaz R, Klausner JD, Caplan AL, Jackson G, Shabsigh R, Khalsa JH, Stoff DM, Goldmeier D, Lamba H, Richardson D, Sadeghi-Nejad H. The Bolger conference on PDE-5 inhibition and HIV risk: implications for health policy and prevention. J Sex Med. 2006;3(6):960–75. discussion 973–5.

75. Yang CC, Cold CJ, Yilmaz U, Maravilla KR. Sexually responsive vascular tissue of the vulva. BJU Int. 2006;97(4):766–72.

76. Martin-Alguacil N, Schober J, Kow LM, Pfaff D. Arousing properties of the vulvar epithelium. J Urol. 2006;176(2):456–62. Review.

77. Munarriz R, Kim NN, Goldstein I, Traish AM. Biology of female sexual function. Urol Clin North Am. 2002;29(3):685–93. Review.

78. Kreuter M, Taft C, Siösteen A, Biering-Sørensen F. Women's sexual functioning and sex life after spinal cord injury. Spinal Cord. 2010;49:154–60.

79. Tracy JK, Junginger J. Correlates of lesbian sexual functioning. J Womens Health (Larchmt). 2007; 16(4):499–509.

80. Rowen TS, Breyer BN, Lin TC, Li CS, Robertson PA, Shindel AW. Use of barrier protection for sexual activity among women who have sex with women. Int J Gynaecol Obstet. 2013;120(1):42–5. doi:10.1016/j.ijgo.2012.08.011. Epub 2012 Oct 26.

81. Marrazzo JM, Coffey P, Bingham A. Sexual practices, risk perception and knowledge of sexually transmitted disease risk among lesbian and bisexual women. Perspect Sex Reprod Health. 2005;37(1):6–12.

82. Matthews AK, Brandenburg DL, Johnson TP, Hughes TL. Correlates of underutilization of gynecological cancer screening among lesbian and heterosexual women. Prev Med. 2004;38(1):105–13.

83. Goldstein SR, Bachmann GA, Koninckx PR, Lin VH, Portman DJ, Ylikorkala O, Ospemifene Study Group. Ospemifene 12-month safety and efficacy in postmenopausal women with vulvar and vaginal atrophy. Climacteric. 2014;17(2):173–82. doi:10.3109/136971 37.2013.834493. Epub 2013 Nov 23.

84. American Cancer Society: Cancer facts and figures 2008. http://www.cancer.org/acs/groups/content/@nho/documents/document/2008cafffinalsecuredpdf.pdf; 2008.

85. Asencio M, Blank T, Descartes L. The prospect of prostate cancer: a challenge for gay men's sexualities as they age. Sex Res Social Policy. 2009;6:38–51.

86. Thompson Jr EH. Expressions of manhood: reconciling sexualities, masculinities, and aging. Gerontologist. 2004;44:714–8.

87. Blank TO. Gay men and prostate cancer: invisible diversity. J Clin Oncol. 2005;23:2593–6.

88. Grov C, Parsons JT, Bimbi DS. The association between penis size and sexual health among men who have sex with men. Arch Sex Behav. 2010;39(3):788–97. doi:10.1007/s10508-008-9439-5. Epub 2009 Jan 13.

89. McCullough A. Penile change following radical prostatectomy: size, smooth muscle atrophy, and curve. Curr Urol Rep. 2008;9:492–9.

90. Benson JS, Abern MR, Levine LA. Penile shortening after radical prostatectomy and Peyronie's surgery. Curr Urol Rep. 2009;10(6):468–74. Review.

91. Hartman ME, Irvine J, Currie KL, Ritvo P, Trachtenberg L, Louis A, Trachtenberg J, Jamnicky L, Matthew AG. Exploring gay couples' experience with sexual dysfunction after radical prostatectomy: a qualitative study. J Sex Marital Ther. 2014;40(3):233–53.

92. Turo R, Jallad S, Prescott S, Cross WR. Metastatic prostate cancer in transsexual diagnosed after three decades of estrogen therapy. Can Urol Assoc J. 2013;7(7-8):E544–6. doi:10.5489/cuaj.175.

93. Miksad RA, Bubley G, Church P, Sanda M, Rofsky N, Kaplan I, Cooper A. Prostate cancer in a transgender woman 41 years after initiation of feminization. JAMA. 2006;296(19):2316–7.

94. Brennan P, Bogillot O, Cordier S, et al. Cigarette smoking and bladder cancer in men: a pooled analysis of 11 case-control studies. Int J Cancer. 2000; 86(2):289–94.

95. Brennan P, Bogillot O, Greiser E, et al. The contribution of cigarette smoking to bladder cancer in women (pooled European data). Cancer Causes Control. 2001;12(5):411–7.

96. Boffetta P. Tobacco smoking and risk of bladder cancer. Scand J Urol Nephrol Suppl. 2008;218:45–54.

97. Gandini S, Botteri E, Iodice S, et al. Tobacco smoking and cancer: a meta-analysis. Int J Cancer. 2008;122(1):155–64.

98. Cochran SD, Bandiera FC, Mays VM. Sexual orientation-related differences in tobacco use and secondhand smoke exposure among US adults aged 20 to 59 years: 2003-2010 National Health and Nutrition Examination Surveys. Am J Public Health. 2013;103(10):1837–44. doi:10.2105/AJPH.2013. 301423. Epub 2013 Aug 15.

# Obstetric and Gynecologic Care for Individuals Who Are LGBT

17

Kristen L. Eckstrand, Jennifer Potter, and E. Kale Edmiston

## Purpose

The purpose of this chapter is to provide an overview of obstetric and gynecologic care for LGBT individuals, understanding the unique differences between each of these communities, and how to optimize delivery of care in evolving political and healthcare landscapes.

## Learning Objectives

- Discuss the barriers in accessing and receiving OB/GYN care for LGBT individuals

K.L. Eckstrand, M.D., Ph.D. (✉)
Vanderbilt Program for LGBTI Health, Vanderbilt University Medical Center, Nashville, TN 37232, USA

Department of Psychiatry, University of Pittsburgh, Pittsburgh, PA, USA
e-mail: eckstrandkl@upmc.edu

J. Potter, M.D.
Harvard Medical School, Boston, MA, USA

Beth Israel Deaconess Medical Center, Boston, MA, USA

The Fenway Institute, Boston, MA, USA
e-mail: jpotter@bidmc.harvard.edu

E.K. Edmiston, PhD
Vanderbilt Program for LGBTI Health, Vanderbilt University Medical Center, Nashville, TN 37232, USA
e-mail: kale.edmiston@vanderbilt.edu

- Discuss the preventive, sexual health, surgical, and family-building OB/GYN health needs of individuals across the LGBT spectrum
- Discuss the social, economic, and political aspects of sexual, reproductive, and family planning care for LGBT communities

## Introduction

Obstetrics and gynecology (OB/GYN) has historically been defined as the provision of care to women, specifically their reproductive organs, across the lifespan and during pregnancy. This definition alienates certain individuals from care typically provided by OB/GYN practitioners, specifically cisgender men and transgender individuals. In actuality, OB/GYN encompasses the provision of care irrespective of sex, sexual orientation, gender identity, and natal pelvic anatomy. In addition to cisgender women, OB/GYN practitioners can care for:

- Transgender men (FTM) who retain natal pelvic structures and require routine OB/GYN care or select surgical procedures
- Transgender women (MTF) who may be candidates for breast cancer screening, STI screening, evaluation of postsurgical pelvic symptoms, and Pap testing of neovaginal tissue if there is potential of HPV infection

© Springer International Publishing Switzerland 2016
K.L. Eckstrand, J.M. Ehrenfeld (eds.), *Lesbian, Gay, Bisexual, and Transgender Healthcare*,
DOI 10.1007/978-3-319-19752-4_17

- All individuals seeking family planning support and prenatal and obstetrical care, including individuals who are partners and/or prospective parents
- All individuals who are eligible for anal Pap tests based on risk for anal HPV infection

Indeed, OB/GYN practitioners provide care to all individuals.

> **Helpful Hint**
> OB/GYN practitioners can provide care to all patients, regardless of sex, sexual orientation, gender identity, or natal pelvic anatomy.

Another important facet of OB/GYN is that the care provided requires exquisite sensitivity on the part of providers. As discussed in Chap. 13, gender dysphoria refers to the distress that some people, often transgender and gender nonconforming individuals, may experience when their body does not align with their gender identity. Distress in this context can manifest in many ways, including disgust or discontent with one's own body. Negative body image can also occur in individuals who have experienced interpersonal trauma [1], and LGBT individuals experience high rates of violence and interpersonal trauma [2]. For individuals living with trauma and/or experiencing gender dysphoria, the patient history and physical exam can be re-traumatizing. The context for what may be traumatic varies by individual but common re-traumatizing experiences in healthcare can include use of certain words or phrases to describe parts of the body, referring to exam findings as "normal", referencing the patient's physical appearance, exposure or touching of parts of the body, and the insertion of specula, swabs, or fingers in the vagina or anus. The potential for trauma or re-traumatization should prompt OB/GYN providers to approach LGBT patients with the utmost sensitivity and compassion (see section "Performing A Sensitive History and Physical"). Despite this, the strong association between OB/GYN and provision of care to cisgender women with natal female pelvic

**Table 17.1** Common biases and assumptions when caring for LGBT and gender nonconforming patients

| |
|---|
| • Heterosexuality |
| • All patients use traditional labels related to sexual orientation or gender identity |
| • Sexual orientation is based on appearance |
| • Sexual orientation is based on sexual practices |
| • Choice of sexual partners is always based on sexual orientation |
| • Sexual engagement is always a matter of choice |
| • Identity, attraction, and behavior don't change across the lifespan |
| • Gender identity is equivalent to sexual orientation |
| • Gender identity is based on natal sex or pelvic anatomy |
| • Gender identity depends on what interventions a patient has chosen in transitioning |
| • Transgender people must also be gay, lesbian, or bisexual |

organs often leads to heteronormative assumptions promoting bias, and even trauma, within healthcare.

While all healthcare providers carry some bias towards certain patients or diagnoses, it is important for all providers to recognize and mitigate their biases in order to provide compassionate and comprehensive healthcare to all patients. Key to mitigating bias for LGBT patients is to first be aware of common biases and assumptions that manifest in the OB/GYN context (see Table 17.1).

While the terminology is discussed in detail in Chap. 1, here *gender identity* refers to a person's innate, deeply-felt identification as a man, woman, or another gender which may or may not correspond to the person's external body or assigned sex at birth. *Sexual orientation* refers to a person's enduring physical, romantic, emotional, and/or spiritual attraction towards certain sexes/genders. It is important to distinguish sexual orientation and gender identity from one another, as well as from natal sex, sexuality, and sexual practices. Regardless of sexual orientation and gender identity, individuals may express their *attraction* or desires toward others through a variety of sexual practices, or *behaviors*. Attraction may be towards a certain sex (ex. male), body type (ex. masculine), or gender expression (ex. gender nonconforming). This summation of sexual orientation, attraction, and behavior influence the overall construct of sexuality. Importantly, each of these constructs can change over time [3, 4], requiring that providers continually assess these items to maintain patient rapport, evaluate risk, and support health.

Gender identity can also be expressed through *behavior,* from modifying gender expression to seeking medical or surgical interventions. Unlike aspects of sexuality that may change over adulthood, gender identity tends to be stable after childhood [5]; however, one's understanding of their own gender identity and gender expression may change as norms within societies and cultures evolve. Figure 17.1 describes some of the complex language and interplay between identity, attraction, and behavior as it relates to sexual orientation and gender identity.

The diversity of identity, attraction, and behavior across sexual orientations and gender identities thus requires a patient- and family-centered approach to care that takes each of these dimensions into account. Depending on a patient's motivations for accessing the healthcare system, the relative importance of these items to the patient and/or their immediate care may vary. Adept practitioners will not only understand these dimensions, but also be able to apply them seamlessly in the healthcare setting.

This chapter aims to support this level of competence among all health professions providing OB/GYN related care to LGBT patients, including understanding the barriers to OB/GYN care and health disparities faced by LGBT patients, recommendations for preventive screening, routine gynecologic care, fertility, and reproduction.

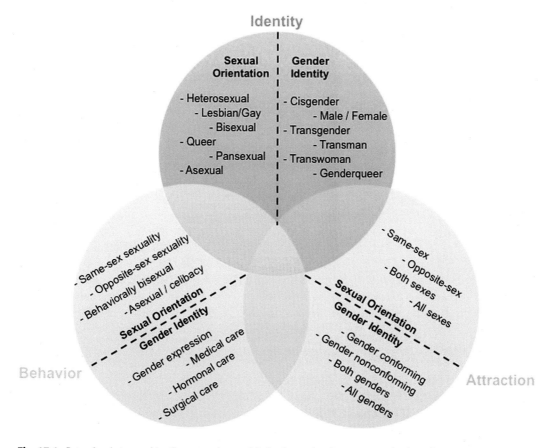

**Fig. 17.1** Interplay between identity, attraction, and behavior as it relates to sexual orientation and gender identity. *Figure provided by K. Eckstrand*

## Barriers to OB/GYN Care

While the general barriers to accessing and receiving healthcare for LGBT communities are discussed in Chap. 2, understanding barriers pertinent to OB/GYN care in particular will support improved provision of care to LGBT patients in this context. In general, LGBT individuals are more likely to delay emergent, primary, and preventive care [6–8]. This is due to significant barriers to care that include felt or perceived stigma and discrimination, prior negative experiences within health care, unequal access to health insurance, difficulty finding a provider competent in addressing the unique needs of LGBT patients, misperceptions about risk, and general health systems challenges in providing care for LGBT patients.

Because of OB/GYN's focus on sexual and reproductive health, conversations and elements of the physical examination may make patients feel particularly vulnerable, and when an interaction does not go well, this outcome will pose an additional barrier to receiving state-of-the-art health care. Understanding the nature and impact of interpersonal stigma is crucial in order to achieve truly supportive and productive provider-patient relationships. Interpersonal stigma describes interactions between individuals whereby one person is stigmatized [9]; this can include explicit discrimination such as abuse or violence, or implicit biases that can unconsciously shape attitudes or behaviors. The felt experience of interpersonal stigma when receiving OB/GYN care promotes patient reluctance to access care. For example, LGB women who felt they were discriminated against when receiving healthcare were less likely to have had a Pap test in the prior year [10]; this kind of reaction to stigma is especially pronounced among androgynous/gender nonconforming LGB women [11]. Indeed, the relationship that gender nonconforming or transgender patients have with their bodies can pose a significant barrier to care—especially if a provider is unaware or dismissive of this relationship during any part of the clinical encounter. For many LGBT people, a history of negative experiences with healthcare providers can evoke re-traumatization when accessing care, resulting in an avoidance of care. Even if LGBT individuals have not been discriminated against in healthcare but have experienced discrimination in other settings, fear of potential discrimination or a general sense of distrust of the healthcare system can also lead to avoidance of care.

When accessing care, implicit biases or assumptions (see Table 17.1) can cause challenges in provider-patient interactions that contribute to patient discomfort or distrust. Biases and assumptions leading to distrust or felt disrespect can occur at any point during the patient-provider encounter:

- *Intake & Waiting Room:* clinic forms not allowing for disclosure of sexual orientation or gender identity, or negative encounters with front desk or clinical support staff
- *Introductions:* not ascertaining or applying appropriate terminology for gender identity, pronouns, name, sexual orientation, and/or partner status
- *Patient History:* assumptions conflating identity, attraction, and/or behavior (i.e., provider asks a patient who identifies as lesbian about contraception before inquiring about sexual orientation and sexual behavior) or not trusting a patient's response to questions
- *Physical Examination:* not using the language that a patient has used for themselves or assuming the exam may not be traumatic

Clinicians need to be able to mitigate their own biases and assumptions within patient-provider encounters such that when errors occur, they are able to re-establish rapport rather than continuing to alienate patients from engaging fully in care. Clinicians also serve as role models for clinic staff; modeling appropriate, respectful behavior—including apologizing and mitigating bias—is a critical component of leading an interprofessional team to support patient care.

Even when providers have a professional and compassionate bedside manner, the lack of provider training can still result in inequitable care. From the time of enrollment in undergraduate medical education through postgraduate (residency) and continuing education years, a dearth of instructional materials are available to support clinician competence in providing care to LGBT patients [12, 13]. This training deficit is also present in other health professions [14, 15]. The lack of training encompasses clinical knowledge, the facts and information necessary to provide competent patient care to LGBT patients within health systems; addressing negative attitudes or unconscious bias that may affect a provider's behaviors towards an LGBT patient; and facilitating the development of a broad spectrum of skills that are necessary to provide competent care for an LGBT patient. This lack of training is apparent across specialties, including OB/GYN, however improved training itself can support a healthcare infrastructure welcoming of all LGBT individuals in healthcare, from patients to providers [16, 17].

Improved training itself can further address the barrier of misperception of risk among patients and providers. Misperception of risk can be understood through the discrepancies between (1) what patients believe, (2) what providers believe, and (3) what evidence demonstrates. Within OB/GYN, one example of risk misperception is HPV infection and cervical cancer among lesbian, gay, and bisexual (LGB) women. Studies have demonstrated that LGB women are less likely than heterosexual women to believe they can be infected by HPV, which leads to a decrease in HPV vaccination uptake and receipt of Pap tests [18]. Most providers do not ask about sexual orientation, thereby failing to apply orientation as a useful marker in identifying risk, despite evidence that LGB women are at increased risk for breast cancer [19–21]. Indeed, one small study among women diagnosed with breast cancer demonstrated that no providers asked about sexual orientation [22]. Other misperceptions about risk in the LGBT community commonly held between patients and providers can include:

- LGB women do not need preventive vaccines such as HPV, hepatitis A/B
- LGB women do not need to be screened for STIs
- LGB women and transgender men do not need to be screened for cervical cancer
- Transgender women and transgender men are not at risk for developing breast cancer
- Transgender men are not at risk for developing ovarian or endometrial cancer

- Transgender women are not at risk for developing prostate cancer
- Intimate partner violence between partners identifying as LGBT does not occur or is rare
- Transgender men taking cross-gender hormone therapy cannot get pregnant
- LGB women do not need contraception

Structural concerns further contribute to the disparities in care. For example, while access to comprehensive health insurance is improving for LGBT individuals, significant barriers still remain that adversely affect LGBT patients, particularly those requiring OB/GYN care. These barriers center on the fact that insurance covers sex-specific, rather than person-specific, health maintenance and disease. For example, insurance may cover Pap tests for a transgender man with natal female pelvic organs while he is insured as female, but not if he is insured as male. Similarly, transwomen taking long term cross-gender hormone therapy may not be able to get coverage for mammography. Gender-affirming surgical procedures are variably excluded, largely based on societal bias that these procedures are not medically necessary and represent unnecessary expenditures. However, preliminary evidence suggests gender transition is helpful in improving mental health [23] and presumably, other aspects of quality of life. Beyond transgender-specific exclusions, many insurance companies don't cover certain assisted reproductive technologies—which can be the primary roadblock to same-sex couples building families.

Electronic health records (EHRs) can be used to support continuity of care and clinical decision making when caring for LGBT patients. There is substantial controversy regarding documentation of sexual orientation and gender identity (see Chap. 7); however, EHRs can be used to record gender identity, pronouns, name, sexual orientation, and/or partner status, which can remind all team members participating in a patient's care how to best establish and/or maintain rapport. Further, EHRs can support evidence-based clinical decision-making to address the above misperceptions about risk by integrating screening protocols appropriate for each individual's unique circumstance into the EHR. Disclosure and improved care are integrally linked: for example, women—even younger women [24]—who disclose their sexual orientation are 2–3× more likely than women who do not disclose their orientation to adhere to cervical cancer screening recommendations [25–27]. Asking about and documenting sexual orientation and gender identity in EHRs in a systematic way can support improved preventive care.

## Performing a Sensitive History and Physical Exam

Performing a sensitive history and physical exam should be a priority for all patients. This is particularly true when working with patients who are likely to have experienced trauma and/or who may be uncomfortable with their bodies, and when the chief complaint is related to a sensitive topic (e.g. pain during sex, abnormal bleeding, galactorrhea, etc.). Of utmost importance during both the history and physical is for the patient to feel they are in control of the encounter. This locus of control can include environmental factors, interpersonal factors, and personal factors (see Table 17.2)—each of which can be facilitated with a sensitive history and physical exam.

## History

When beginning a clinical encounter, particularly with new patients, it is helpful to begin with introductions, informing patients of the scope of practice, a statement affirming their presence, and empowering patients to begin the encounter. For example, *"Good morning, my name is Dr. Smith and I am one of the gynecologists here. I know we haven't met before, but I understand you have some concerns you'd like to discuss so I'm glad you came in. How can I help you today?"* It can also be helpful to ask patients in advance if there are ways that the experience can be made more comfortable (ex. not standing between the patient and the door), and to request that they inform you if they feel uncomfortable during any part of the encounter.

Based on the patient's response to this initial inquiry, further conversation can explore concerns that the patient voices. It is important to keep the past medical history relevant to the patient's presenting concerns, rather than asking questions purely out of curiosity. If patients appear confused, explaining why certain questions are being asked can facilitate disclosure of sensitive information. As some patients may feel disgust or shame around certain words used to describe parts of the body, asking what terminology they would like to have used can help patients talk more openly about their concerns. For example, some patients may want to say "chest" rather than "breasts" or front or back "hole" when referring to the vagina or anus. Using the patient's language throughout the encounter is not only supportive, but reduces confusion and helps to elucidate a more thorough history.

As the patient is telling their story, pay attention to their body language and responsiveness. Do they become restless or cross their arms? Do they break eye contact or look at the ground?

**Table 17.2** Factors contributing to patient locus of control

| Environmental | Interactional | Internal |
|---|---|---|
| • Door open or closed<br>• Location of provider relative to self<br>• Presence of a support person of one's own choosing<br>• Visibility of exam equipment (ex. specula)<br>• Temperature of the room and equipment (e.g., warming of speculum and/or lubricant)<br>• Degree of physical vulnerability (e.g., appropriate draping, patient position on exam table, etc.)<br>• Time spent in clinical encounter | • Nonverbal communication (e.g., eye contact)<br>• Choice of language (e.g., use of pronouns, anatomical terms)<br>• Provider listening/responsiveness<br>• Physical touch (e.g., obtaining permission before proceeding) | • Self-acceptance<br>• Agency, decision-making capacity |

Do they become withdrawn or avoid answering questions? Does the tone of their voice change? These can all be signs that the patient is uncomfortable. In these circumstances, it can be helpful to reflect back to the patient that it looks like they are having a difficult time and ask what is causing distress. Offering tissues or a glass of water, asking if they need a moment alone or what else they think might be helpful can all be ways to help establish trust.

### Physical Exam

The physical exam—and the pelvic exam in particular—can be extremely difficult, even traumatic, experiences. If there is no urgent need to perform an exam based on the patient's chief complaint, deferring it until a later time is appropriate. Performing physical exams only when clearly needed and always with the express permission of the patient is crucial in building trust.

Before beginning an exam, explain to patients what procedures will be performed and why, and what to expect in terms of how and where parts of the body will be touched. Remember to continue using patients' preferred anatomical terminology throughout this explanation. After outlining the exam, ask patients if there are parts of the exam that they are concerned about, and whether there are things that would make the exam easier. Some patients may have had a similar exam before and if so, ask what made the experience comfortable for them. For other patients, offering options to ease the exam can be helpful. For example, some patients may prefer to have the exam completed as quickly as possible whereas others may want the exam to be done slowly. In certain circumstances, patients can be offered an antianxiety medication (e.g., short-acting benzodiazepine) in order to perform the exam most comfortably. If a speculum exam is required, ask patients if they would prefer to insert the speculum themselves. Some patients may also wish to observe the exam; offering a hand mirror for the patient to hold and rest on the inside of their leg so that they can observe may help to relieve anxiety about the

procedure. It may be helpful for some patients to be able to make eye contact with the provider during the exam. Anal Pap tests can be performed with a patient lying on their side or in the same position as the speculum exam, so allow patients to choose what they prefer. Some patients may want a support person to join them in the room. Finally, before beginning the exam, emphasize to the patient that they will be in control throughout the experience and can ask to stop the exam at any time.

When performing the exam itself, unless explicitly requested otherwise by the patient, always explain what you propose to do next and give ample warning about the next part of the body to be touched. If the patient becomes visibly distressed during any part of the exam, ask what you can change to make the exam more comfortable. Some patients may not be able to articulate how to improve the exam, so asking a more directed question such as, "Do you want me to stop the exam?" can provide the patient an option that they can answer non-verbally. Once the exam has been completed, offer patients the opportunity to debrief about the experience.

## OB/GYN-Related Health Disparities and Screening Recommendations among LGBT Populations

OB/GYN practitioners can address many of the health disparities faced by LGBT individuals. While the disparities affecting LGBT individuals vary by sexual orientation and gender identity, they also depend on natal and current sex anatomy, sexual and behavioral risk factors, use of exogenous sex steroids, and many other factors. Based on the available literature, this section will focus on population-level disparities affecting LGB cisgender women and transgender men and women, while acknowledging the research caveats arising from not accounting for gender nonconformity among LGB cisgender women and sexual orientation among transgender individuals. Other influencing factors will be discussed relative to the specific disparities below.

## Lifestyle Factors

Throughout this section, lifestyle factors influencing heightened risk among LGBT populations for certain OB/GYN-related health conditions are discussed. Briefly, these include:

- LGBT individuals are more likely to smoke [28, 29]
- LGB cisgender individuals are more likely to drink heavily or have had difficulties with alcohol in the past [28, 29]
- Cisgender lesbians are more likely to be overweight [28]
- LGB cisgender women have higher rates of nulliparity, more sexual partners, older age at first childbirth, and fewer pregnancies [19–21]

Why these risk factors may be present for individual patients is complex. For example, the explanations for LGB cisgender women being overweight include that they may be "protected from pervasive cultural messages about the ideal female body by lesbian cultural values" [30], an overweight appearance may affirm certain aspects of gender expression, and/or overeating may be a coping mechanism. Similarly alcohol and tobacco use among LGBT communities may be coping mechanisms used to manage minority stress (see Chaps. 2, 4, and 13), or they may be part of community culture in a certain geographic location. It is important to determine an individual's motivations for engaging in lifestyle behaviors despite negative health consequences. Discussing this information with patients provides information that is crucial for devising successful intervention strategies and educational approaches.

Lifestyle modification can be helpful in reducing risk for certain health conditions, however supporting behavioral risk modification as a practitioner requires understanding how patients are and are not able to change, their own expectations of themselves, how to best support their change and, most importantly, how to be an ally during the change process. Motivational interviewing is one strategy for understanding and engaging patient-centered change. It is a nonjudgmental practice using open-ended questions, reflective listening, and affirmation to engage patients in evaluating specific behaviors relative to their personal values, the potential benefits of change, and structuring goals for change. Among gay and bisexual men, motivational interviewing has been shown to reduce sexual-risk taking and substance use [31]. More generally, motivational interviewing has been shown to be effective to reduce tobacco, alcohol, and illicit substance use, support weight loss, and increase physical activity—all behaviors that reduce risk for chronic disease [32]. As discussed previously, "outness" to providers has the potential to help reduce risk and keel patients' engaged in care. However, irrespective of the preferred outcome from a risk reduction standpoint (ex. healthy weight, tobacco cessation), supporting patient control in goal setting and healthcare is extremely important for the clinical encounter among LGBT individuals [33, 34].

## Cancer

### Breast Cancer

While some studies have not found elevated risk [35, 36], increasing evidence over the past decade suggests that LGB cisgender women are at increased 5-year [28] and lifetime risk for breast cancer due to higher rates of nulliparity, lower rates of abortion, fewer pregnancies, lower rates of breastfeeding, and older age at first childbirth, as well as higher rates of obesity, smoking, and alcohol use [19–21] (see Table 17.3). Indeed, according to the National Health Interview Survey, women cohabitating with other women had greater age-adjusted risk for fatal breast cancer [37]. While studies on the actual incidence and prevalence of breast cancer among LGB cisgender women are limited, preliminary research does show that 1-year incidence rates for breast cancer in premenopausal women are slightly elevated in both lesbian and bisexual women compared with heterosexual women [38].

Despite this heightened risk, evidence suggests that LGB cisgender women are less likely than heterosexual women to have health insurance or to have had regular screening with mammography

**Table 17.3** Cancer incidence, prevalence, and screening recommendations in LGBT populations receiving OB/GYN care

| | Community | Research (compared to general population) | Screening recommendations |
|---|---|---|---|
| Breast cancer | LGB women | • Increased 5-year [28] and lifetime [19–21] risk for breast cancer<br>• Greater age-adjusted risk for fatal breast cancer (HR = 3.2, CI 1.01–10.21) [37]<br>• Decreased receipt of regular mammography [19, 29]<br>• One-year incidence rates of breast cancer elevated in both lesbian (IRR, 1.06; 95 % CI, 1.06–1.06) and bisexual (IRR, 1.10; 95 % CI, 1.10–1.10) women [38] | • Biennial screening mammography for women 50–74 years (USPSTF Grade B [39])<br>• Screening mammography before age 50 should take into account genetic mutation (BRCA1/2) and patient values (USPSTF Grade C [39]) |
| | Transmen | • No studies of risk/screening<br>• No increased risk of cancer [40, 41] | • Biennial mammography is recommended in MTF transgender individuals if additional risk factors (BRCA2 mutation, positive family history, etc.) are present (AJR [42]; UCSF [43])<br>• FTM should receive annual chest wall/axillary exam and mammography as for natal females (UCSF [43]) |
| | Transwomen | • No studies of risk/screening<br>• No increased risk of breast cancer [40, 41]<br>• Cases more likely to be diagnosed at a later stage and fatal [40, 41] | |
| Ovarian cancer[a] | LGB women | • LGB women are at higher risk [44]<br>• No studies available on incidence/prevalence | • Do not screen as there are no effective screening modalities (USPSTF Grade D [45]) |
| | Transmen | • No studies on risk, incidence/prevalence | |
| Cervical cancer[a] | LGB women | • LGB women have lower rates of HPV vaccine uptake [18]<br>• Lesbian women have lower receipt of Pap tests compared with bisexual or heterosexual women [24, 46–48]<br>• No studies on incidence/prevalence of cervical cancer | • HPV vaccine for all genders (CDC [49, 50])<br>• For all individuals with a cervix: Pap test every 3 years for people ages 21–65 OR Pap test plus HPV test every 5 years for people ages 30–65 (USPSTF Grade A [51, 52])<br>• Primary HPV screening in people ages 25–29 [53] |
| | Transmen | • Lower rates of Pap tests [54]<br>• Greater odds of having a lifetime Pap test with unsatisfactory cytology [55]<br>• No studies on incidence/prevalence of cervical cancer | |
| Vulvar/Vaginal cancer[b] | LGB women | • No studies on risk, incidence/prevalence | • HPV vaccine for all genders (CDC [49, 50])<br>• Regular visual inspection of the vaginal vault in patients who have had gender-affirming surgery with penile inversion technique [43] |
| | Transmen | • No studies on risk, incidence/prevalence | |
| | Transwomen | • No studies on risk, incidence/prevalence | |

(continued)

**Table 17.3** (continued)

| | Community | Research (compared to general population) | Screening recommendations |
|---|---|---|---|
| Endometrial cancer[a] | LGB women | • No studies on risk, incidence/prevalence, however theoretical increased risk to increased smoking/alcohol use [28, 29, 56], obesity [28], higher rates of nulliparity and polycystic ovarian syndrome [57, 58] (PCOS), and decreased use of oral contraceptives [59] | • No available screening test / screening recommendations<br>• Educate patients to report any abnormal or post-menopausal bleeding to a healthcare provider |
| | Transmen | • No studies on risk, incidence/prevalence | |
| Anal cancer | LGB women | • 17.2 % of lesbians have engaged in lifetime anal receptive intercourse [60]<br>• Bisexual women are 2.5 times more likely to engage in anal receptive intercourse than heterosexual or lesbian women [61]<br>• No studies on incidence/prevalence | • HPV vaccine for all genders (CDC [49, 50])<br>• Anal Pap test based on risk and patient preference for screening |
| | Transmen | • 25 % of transgender men have engaged in unprotected anal intercourse [62, 63]<br>• No studies on incidence/prevalence | |
| | Transwomen | • 80 % of transgender women have engaged in unprotected anal intercourse [62, 63]<br>• No studies on incidence/prevalence | |

*USPSTF* United States Preventive Services Task Force, *AJR* American Journal of Roentgenology

[a]Transwomen are not at risk for ovarian cancer, cervical cancer, endometrial cancer, and unwanted pregnancies due to the absence of natal pelvic structures that these conditions affect

[b]Neovaginal cancer is rare, but may occur in transwomen depending on the surgical technique used for construction of the neovagina

in accordance with ACS guidelines [19, 29, 64]. While systemic barriers to care may contribute to this disparity, misperception of risk may also influence the decreased rates of screening. In one small sample ($n = 150$ LGB cisgender women, 400 heterosexual cisgender women), LGB cisgender women, compared with their heterosexual counterparts, had lower intentions to obtain mammography (OR 0.40, CI 0.21–0.75) [65]. In this sample, the relationship between sexual orientation and intent to obtain screening was mediated by the beliefs that they are less likely to ever get breast cancer and perceived greater disadvantages of mammography [65]. This finding has yet to be replicated and thus may also be an effect of the specific sample size and population. One study found that a targeted intervention of 2 h sessions once per week for a month that promoted breast cancer prevention among LGB cisgender women significantly increased rates of mammography screening (OR 2.13, CI 1.9–2.40) [66]. However, even in the absence of such an intervention, LGB women who report more trust in their medical provider are more likely to report intention to receive mammography, suggesting provider trust is an important component of supporting breast cancer prevention among LGB cisgender women [65].

Breast cancer screening recommendations [39] for average-risk LGB cisgender women are equivalent to those for their heterosexual counterparts (see Table 17.3):

- Biennial screening mammography for women 50–74 years (USPSTF Grade B)
- Biennial screening mammography before age 50 years should be an individual patient's decision informed by discussion of risk assessment and careful consideration of the patient's values regarding specific benefits and harms (USPSTF Grade C)
- The USPSTF recommends against clinicians teaching women how to perform breast self-examination (Grade D)
- The family history should be regularly updated and patients with histories suggestive of a genetic predisposition to breast cancer should be referred for genetic counseling (NCCN [67]).

> **Helpful Hint**
> All LGB cisgender women should receive mammography screening in accordance with guidelines from the United States Preventive Services Task Force (USPSTF).

Less information is known about the contribution of risk factors, incidence, and prevalence of breast cancer in individuals who are transgender. The first report of breast cancer in a transgender individual was published in 1988, presenting the case of a transgender woman who had been receiving cross-gender hormone therapy (CGHT) [68]—subsequently causing controversy over the ethical implications of providing estrogen in the context of increasing risk for estrogen dependent cancers. Since that publication, others have reported cases of breast cancer in both transgender men [69, 70] and transgender women [22, 23, 25, 26]. While no studies have systematically looked at risk for breast cancer, two studies examining incidence of breast cancer have been published. The first study examined the electronic health records of 3,102 transgender individuals, finding that risk for breast cancer was lower in transgender men (5.9 per 100,000 person-years) and transgender women (4.1 per 100,000 person-years) compared with cisgender women, but within expected norms for cisgender men [40]. The second study of 5,135 transgender individuals similarly did not find an increased incidence of breast cancer, but did report that all cases in transwomen were identified at a late stage and were fatal [41]. Another study found that among transwomen, breast cancer occurs at a younger age and is more commonly estrogen receptor negative than in cisgender males [42].

Because of the paucity of data on the incidence and prevalence of breast cancer among transgender individuals and the long-term effects of any masculinizing or feminizing cross-gender hormone therapy, there are limited recommendations for breast cancer screening for transgender individuals. The UCSF Center for Transgender Excellence and the American College of Roentgenology (ACR) address mammography screening for transgender women, recommending that transwomen who have received feminizing hormone therapy for 5 or more years and have additional risk factors, such as a BRCA mutation or positive family history, undergo routine mammography screening [39, 42, 43, 71]. Fortunately, it has been demonstrated that both mammography and breast sonography are easily performed in transwomen even if they have received breast implants [72], so presence of implants should not deter regular screening. Among transmen, the UCSF Center for Transgender Excellence recommends annual chest wall/axillary exam and mammography as for natal females [43]. This is recommended for several reasons: transmen may have chest tissue that may have been exposed to estrogen during a typical feminizing puberty; transmen may not be able to afford, or even want, breast reduction surgeries or cross gender hormone therapy and therefore may still have breast tissue; and breast tissue, particularly in the axilla and around the nipple-areola complex, can still be present even after top surgery. Risk assessment tools such as the Gail Model [73] have only been validated in cisgender women and should not be used to estimate risk in transgender individuals. Therefore, the best approach currently is for providers to engage transgender patients in a discussion of breast cancer risk and allow patients to participate in decision-making about whether or not and how often to undergo mammography screening.

> **Helpful Hint**
> All individuals retaining breast tissue with any lifetime estrogen exposure should be screened for breast cancer based on risk.

Among women who have been diagnosed with breast cancer, coping mechanisms for LGB cisgender women (and likely transgender individuals) are consistent with those of their heterosexual counterparts, including the importance of social support for positive coping [74] and support from partners [75]. Social support in this context includes providers, where disclosure of sexual orientation to providers is related to greater perceived social support [74]. This is important not only for medical providers, but also surgical providers. For example, when discussing reconstructive surgery of the breast, LGB women may voice different aspects of decision-making other than aesthetic appearance that are integral to their sexual orientation, including body strength and physical functioning. Similarly, transgender individuals may have a unique relationship with their bodies that requires personalized decision-making and care regarding type of reconstruction procedure elected or whether to even undergo reconstruction at all. Surgeons who focus on the aesthetic appearance of the breast, without discussing other aspects of reconstruction important to patients, may "other" LGBT individuals [76].

## Cervical Cancer

Similar to breast cancer, LGB cisgender women are at elevated risk for cervical cancer compared to heterosexual cisgender women due to certain risk factors. These include cervical infection by the human papilloma virus (HPV), multiple past or current sexual partners, early age at first coitus, history of sexually transmitted infections (STIs), and decreased use of safer sex techniques [10, 19, 20, 29, 77], as well as other factors that may weaken the immune system over time including obesity and cigarette smoking [9]. Two common assumptions among patients and providers influence the perception of risk for cervical cancer: that cisgender lesbian women have not, or do not currently, engage in vaginal intercourse with men, and that penile-vaginal intercourse is required to transmit HPV. Contrary to these beliefs, 75–80 % of lesbian women have had sexual intercourse with a cisgender male in their lifetime [60, 78]. Lesbian women can also partner with transwomen, who may have a penis. Furthermore, HPV can be transmitted between female sex partners who have never had penile-vaginal intercourse with men [79–81]. Ten percent of WPW who have never had prior penile-vaginal intercourse with men have cervical cytological abnormalities [82, 83]. Research on risk for cervical cancer in transgender men retaining a cervix is limited, although some studies report higher levels of tobacco use and history of sexual violence [6, 56].

Because of these risks, all individuals who retain a cervix should follow current cervical cancer screening guidelines:

- Screen women aged 21–65 years with cytology alone (Pap test) every 3 years or, for women aged 30–65 years who want to lengthen the screening interval, screen with a combination of cytology and human papillomavirus (HPV) testing every 5 years [51] (USPSTF Grade A)
- All natal females between the ages of 9 and 26 and all natal males between ages 9 and 21 should receive the three dose series of the 9-valent HPV vaccine (if available, otherwise use the quadravalent HPV vaccine); all natal males between ages 22 and 26 may also be vaccinated [50].
- Primary HPV screening can be considered as an alternative to the aforementioned screening methods [53]

While it is beyond the scope of this chapter to discuss the details of management after an abnormal Pap test or positive HPV test, all individuals with a cervix should receive care as recommended by the American Society for Colposcopy and Cervical Pathology [84].

> **Helpful Hint**
> All individuals retaining a cervix should be screened for cervical cancer according to current US population guidelines

Despite these recommendations, there is disparate utilization of Pap tests and HPV vaccination among LGBT communities. Lesbian cisgender women are less likely to receive annual and routine Pap tests [47, 48, 77] compared with their bisexual and heterosexual counterparts.

This may be in part due to age and education, as some studies demonstrate that Pap test screening is lower among younger women [24, 46] while the screening gap is less pronounced among older, well-educated LGB cisgender women [25, 26]. And, while 45 % of LGB women ages 18–26 have initiated HPV vaccination and 70 % of those starting the vaccine series have finished [85], uptake of the HPV vaccine is lower among lesbian cisgender women [18].

Similarly, transgender men retaining a cervix have a 37 % lower odds of receiving routine Pap tests compared with cisgender women [54]. Further, when Pap tests are obtained, transgender men have a 10 times higher odds of having a Pap test with unsatisfactory cytology [55]. Length of time on testosterone is associated with an unsatisfactory Pap test result [55], and testosterone can cause atrophy of epithelial cells in the cervix that can histologically mimic cervical dysplasia [86], suggesting that the effects of testosterone may produce the histological changes. However, patient and/or provider discomfort with the exam may also influence the ability to obtain a technically optimal specimen [55]. Irrespective of the cause, an abnormal Pap test may result in the need for repeat screening. Because of the invasive nature of a Pap test, particularly among individuals who may have a different relationship with their body than cisgender females, providers should take extra sensitivity and care when explaining the necessity for, and performing, a repeat Pap test.

> **Helpful Hint**
> All natal females between the ages of 9 and 26 and all natal males between ages 9 and 21 should receive the HPV-9 vaccine; all natal males between ages 22 and 26 may also be vaccinated.

To date, no studies have reported the incidence/prevalence of cervical cancer, responses to treatment, or experiences of survivorship among LBGT individuals.

## Other Gynecologic Cancers

Little is known about ovarian, endometrial, and vaginal/vulvar cancer in LGBT individuals. Due to heightened risk factors as discussed in the sections on breast and cervical cancer, it is believed that LGB cisgender women are at increased risk for ovarian cancer [44]. Cases of ovarian cancer in transgender men taking testosterone as part of cross-gender hormone therapy have been reported [87, 88], leading some to hypothesize that androgens may increase risk for ovarian cancer in transgender men [89]. No studies have addressed risk, incidence and/or prevalence; however, such studies would probably not change management as current recommendations recommend against screening for ovarian cancer as no screening method has yet been found to be effective. Similarly, no studies have evaluated response to treatment for ovarian cancer or survivorship experience in these populations.

Similarly, the increased incidence of smoking and alcohol use [28, 29, 56] and obesity [28], higher rates of nulliparity and polycystic ovarian syndrome (PCOS) [57, 58], and decreased use of oral contraceptives [59] may increase the risk for endometrial cancer in LGB cisgender women and transgender men. No studies to date have discussed the risk, incidence, prevalence, treatment, or survivorship. As a result, until there is a better understanding of endometrial cancer in LGBT communities, any vaginal/genital bleeding after menopause or testosterone-induced cessation of menstruation should be evaluated by a healthcare provider. Patients experiencing any abnormal bleeding (e.g. after menopause, during perimenopause, after testosterone-induced cessation of menstruation, heavy/prolonged bleeding, irregular bleeding cycles, etc.) should be encouraged to contact their healthcare provider immediately.

> **Helpful Hint**
> Change to any abnormal bleeding should be evaluated at any time. Abnormal bleeding includes bleeding occurring more often than every 21 days, bleeding lasting longer than 8 days, very heavy bleeding, bleeding occurring between menses in premenopausal women, and any bleeding after menopause.

Risk, incidence, prevalence treatment, and survivorship experiences for vaginal and vulvar cancer in LGBT communities are unknown. As most vulvar and vaginal cancers are due to HPV infection, providers should follow the aforementioned recommendations for HPV vaccination. In transgender women who have had genital gender affirming surgery using the penile inversion technique (see Chap. 20), the majority of the neovagina is keratinized epithelium but some urethral tissue may be present. As a result, there is still a small risk for cancer of the neovaginal vault [90]. Pap tests of the neovaginal vault are not recommended due to the low risk; however, periodic visual inspection for lesions is recommended [43]. Similar to other cancers, HIV infection can increase risk for cancer of penile tissue [91]; as transwomen are at increased risk for HIV infection [92], HIV status may prompt the desire for more routine visual inspection. Conversations with patients to understand risk and desire for screening of the vaginal vault in the absence of evidence showing that such screening is of any proven value should be used to help guide preventive care.

## Gynecologic Cancer Survivorship

Survivorship concerns following gynecologic cancer are incredibly important to address, and little research is available discussing survivorship concerns in LGB women and transgender men. In general, survivors of gynecologic cancer face an overall reduced health status, including concerns related to physical, sexual, psychosocial, and structural health [93–97]. While these symptoms typically improve over time, improvements may not be seen until 5–10 years after treatment. Further, the severity of these symptoms varies with type of treatment, with surgical and radiotherapeutic interventions each causing dysfunction. For example, radiotherapeutic interventions are associated with long-term bowel, bladder, and sexual dysfunction [93] whereas more radical surgical interventions are associated with decreased sexual activity, function, and satisfaction [98]. Early age of diagnosis, lower socioeconomic status, and disease comorbidity also decrease quality of life. A completed review of survivorship is beyond the scope of this

**Table 17.4** Permission, limited information, specific suggestions, and intensive therapy (PLISSIT) model conversations about sexuality and intimacy

| Step | Purpose | Example questions |
|---|---|---|
| Permission | Invite patient to discuss sexual health | • "I would like to check in to see how you are doing with respect to sexuality and intimacy. Is that okay with you?" |
| Limited information | Normalize sexual health and any concerns | • "After cancer treatment, many people are concerned about sex and intimacy. How has your experience been?" |
| Specific suggestions | Provide easy, action-oriented methods to incorporate | • "Vaginal dryness can often be helped with lubricant before and during sex" |
| Intensive therapy | Offer referral or resources if the patient is not comfortable or more expert advise is required | • "It sounds like it might help to talk with an expert in sexual health. May I provide a referral?" |

chapter; however survivorship concerns that may differ between LGBT and heterosexual cisgender populations will be discussed.

Long-term physical symptoms that can affect quality of life following gynecologic cancer include bladder and bowel dysfunction, fatigue, neuropathy, early menopause, ovarian failure and infertility. Ovarian failure and infertility, particularly in younger individuals and those who have not yet had children, can cause distress, depression, and decreased sexual functioning [99]. LGB cisgender women often have children at a later age than heterosexual cisgender women, and therefore may be less likely to have children or have had fewer children at the time of infertility. For transmen, the loss of fertility may be a concern, however what may be most challenging is the potential for long-term dysfunction to be a constant reminder of a part of their body that they may cause distress/dysphoria.

Sexual health is an important part of many people's lives, including individuals who are LGBT, and should continue to be so after surviving cancer [96]. However, sexual function can be impaired across all stages of the sexual response cycle after cancer treatment. Decreased lubrication, inability to achieve orgasm, and pain or discomfort during receptive sexual activity, are common among gynecologic cancer survivors. Radiotherapy and surgical interventions (e.g. hysterectomy, salpingo-ophorectomy, etc.) can produce dimensional changes of the vaginal vault, and can result in complications such as fibrosis or fistula development that impact certain sexual practices. It is recommended that providers working with survivors of gynecologic cancers discuss

these concerns [97]. One such model for addressing these concerns is the PLISSIT model, where providers use the framework of "Permission, Limited Information, Specific Suggestions, and Intensive Therapy" for discussion (see Table 17.4). Based on the concern, endocrine therapies (e.g. vaginal estrogen for vaginal dryness, transdermal testosterone for libido), lubricants, or other treatment options can be discussed.

There is a range of psychosocial concerns that can occur after gynecologic cancer, including depressive or anxiety disorders, worry or fear of recurrence, body image concerns, coping with the invasiveness of treatment, and difficulty returning to a sense of normalcy. Body image concerns may be more common in people who have previously experienced gender dysphoria or other body-related concerns. Similarly, the invasiveness of procedures can themselves be traumatic and re-traumatizing in individuals with a history of trauma. As discussed in previous sections, these experiences are more common among transgender individuals and LGB cisgender women. These experiences are compounded by financial difficulties, access to caregivers, and employment concerns. Older LGB women, and likely transgender individuals, are more likely to experience poverty when compared with heterosexual cisgender individuals and even cisgender gay men [100]. Further, LGBT individuals as a whole are less likely to have a partner, children, or an identifiable close relative to call for help [101] and are thus less likely to have a stable caregiver.

Social support and partner support are incredibly important components of survivorship for individuals recovering from gynecologic cancer

[102]. As discussed previously, older LGBT individuals are less likely to have a partner, but may have good social support networks. Social and partner support are particularly beneficial if the support network is stable across diagnosis, treatment, and recovery, if support is focused on emotional support rather than financial or practical support, and if patients do not feel as though they are a burden to those around them [93]. Certain patients also find support in their chosen faith or in the ability to engage in activities that provide a sense of accomplishment [95]. Survivorship planning that includes these factors is important, particularly among LGBT patients who may not have the same support networks as heterosexual or cisgender individuals.

## Anal Cancer

Risk for anal cancer is similar to other HPV-associated cancers, where unprotected receptive anal intercourse, multiple sex partners, smoking, and immunosuppression increase the likelihood of anal cancer. In addition, a history of chronic local inflammation and pelvic radiation increase risk. It is important to remember that lesbian and bisexual cisgender women are at risk for anal cancer if they have engaged in anal intercourse. Twenty-six percent of young WSW have engaged in anal intercourse [103] and 17.2 % of lesbian cisgender women have engaged in at least one lifetime act of anal intercourse [60]; bisexual cisgender women are 2.5 times more likely than heterosexual or lesbian women to have engaged in anal intercourse [61]. HPV anogenital co-infection is common, even in the absence of anal intercourse, where 42.4 % of women who present with high-grade cervical intraepithelial lesion (CIN2+) also have concurrent HPV infection [104]. Even among cisgender women without a known gynecologic neoplastic process, 8 % of women have concurrent cervical and anal HPV infections [105]. Transgender individuals engaging in receptive anal intercourse are also at risk for anal cancer. Approximately 80 % of transgender women and 25 % of transgender men have engaged in unprotected anal intercourse [62, 63].

While the incidence/prevalence of anal cancer in LGB cisgender women and transgender individuals is unknown, and no consensus statements have been made, HPV vaccination is recommended. There are no screening recommendations regarding the use of anal Pap smears; however, for patients at higher risk, providers can discuss risk and the available screening options with patients. If screening is desired or strongly recommended based on risk, HPV-associated anal dysplasia or intraepithelial neoplasia (AIN) can be detected using an anal Pap test. Anal pap tests are easily performed:

1. Request that the patient refrain from anal receptive intercourse for 24 hours prior to the test
2. Place the patient in the lateral recumbent position or dorsal lithotomy position if also performing a cervical Pap test
3. Moisten a Dacron swab with sterilized or non-sterilized water
4. Spread the area around the anus the with the index and thumb of the non-dominant hand
5. Insert the Dacron swab into the anus until it hits the wall of the rectum, approximately 5-6 cm
6. Rotate the swab several times, placing firm lateral pressure on the swab handle
7. Slowly withdraw the swab from the anal canal, being sure to sample the squamocolumnar (transition) area
8. Place the swab in methanol-based preservative-transport solution and agitate for 60 s
9. Preserve the specimen until time of interpretation

The interpretation of anal cytology is less sensitive and specific than that of cervical cytology [106]; however it is recommended that all patients with any form of anal dysplasia, including atypical squamous cells of undetermined significance, undergo high resolution anoscopy [107]. Therefore, it is important for providers who perform anal Pap tests have the ability to perform or refer to providers trained in HRA should the test reveal atypical results.

## Sexually Transmitted Infections

The details of STI transmission, epidemiology, and treatment are discussed in detail in Chap. 14; however, they will be discussed briefly here as they relate to OB/GYN care. When discussing STIs, it is important to distinguish sexual orientation and gender identity from sexual practices. Sexual orientation and gender identity develop across the lifespan, and sexual practices vary widely even among women who partner exclusively with women [108], thus assumptions about sexual practices based on identity are inadequate to assess risk. Further, social determinants of health also influence STI risk and acquisition in LGBT communities. A thorough and sensitive sexual history, as discussed in Chap. 6, will help guide and support risk assessment, diagnosis, treatment, and prevention.

Among women who partner with women, 75–80 % have had sex with cisgender men [60, 78, 108]. Of that 80 %, approximately 40 % first had sex with cisgender men before the age of 16, and 38 % have had more than 6 male sexual partners. Further, among WPW, 57 % have had more than 6 female sexual partners [108]. This suggests that young WPW are at high risk for STIs due to early sexual debut and number of sexual partners [109]. Specifically, young women who identify as bisexual or are unsure of their sexual orientation have 40 % higher odds for STIs [46]. This risk is partially explained by high rates of sexual coercion, emotional distress, and substance use [110]. Interventions to promote safe sex practices, self-acceptance and acceptance by friends and family, as well as reduction in substance abuse can be helpful in reducing STI risk and promoting healthy development in young women questioning their sexual orientation.

Across all age ranges, LGB cisgender women have higher rates of bacterial vaginosis [108, 111], which is not universally considered to be an STI. Sexual practices transmitting vaginal fluid (ex. a sexual partner with BV, vaginal lubricant use, sharing vaginal sex toys) and receptive oral-vulvovaginal sex increase transmission of BV [111, 112]. However, transmission is multifactorial and also depends on an individual's BV-associated bacteria profile (ex. *G. vaginalis*, *A. vaginae*, *Leptotrichia* spp., *Megasphaera-1*, *Lactobacillus crispatus*) and current smoking status [112, 113]. Despite this, one targeted intervention on safe sex practices did not change the

prevalence of BV among WPW even among women who participated in safe sex practices, suggesting the multifactorial nature of BV is a larger driver of infection [114]. Treatment is recommended in women who are experiencing symptomatic infection and up to date treatment recommendations can be found on through the CDC [115]. Additional management should focus primarily on early identification of symptomatic infection through patient education, smoking cessation, and discussions with sexual partner(s) about seeking testing and practices reducing risk for BV.

**Helpful Hint**

Risk for STIs and subsequent counseling is based on sexual behavior, however this information should be obtained in a manner respectful of sexual orientation and gender identity

LGB cisgender women are also at risk for other STIs. Herpes virus (HSV) infections differ by the gender of sexual partners. Among women who identify as heterosexual, the rate of HSV-2 infection is 23.8 % compared with 3 % of women who have no history of male sexual partners [116]. When contrasting by self-identified sexual orientation, HSV-2 seropositivity occurred in 8.2 % of women who identify as gay or lesbian, 35.9 % in women who identify as bisexual, and 45.6 % of women who identify as heterosexual but who have had a lifetime sexual encounter with another woman [116]. In contrast, HSV-1 seropositivity is common across sexual orientations, often due to oral transmission of the virus in early childhood. Among WPW, HSV-2 seropositivity is associated with increasing number of male partners, whereas HSV-1 is associated with increasing number of female sexual partners [117]. HSV seropositivity does not indicate the location of infection, however, as both HSV-1 and HSV-2 can infect the oral and genital regions. Clinically, it can be important to identify the viral subtype of genital HSV as it affects patient counseling and management. HSV-1 infection is likely to be more severe during the first episode but have fewer recurrences, and is less likely to be shed asymptomatically. In contrast, HSV-2 is more likely to recur and be shed asymptomatically—which is believed to be the primary mode of transmission [118]. First-time clinical episodes of genital herpes can be treated with antiviral agents, although patients should be informed that even though the infection may not recur, it could still be spread to partners through asymptomatic shedding. For patients who have recurrent infections, antiviral agents can be taken daily to prevent symptom recurrence and lower risk of transmission to partners. However, all patients should be aware of their capacity to spread the virus through oral or genital contact, even in the absence of active lesions.

Rates and infection patterns of gonorrhea and chlamydia in LGB cisgender women are largely unknown. While one large study suggests that lesbian women have slightly higher rates of chlamydia than bisexual or heterosexual women [119], this finding has not been consistent across other studies [108]. Samples in these studies were geographically limited, suggesting that rates of disease may be due to geographic location, socioeconomic status, and sexual networks. However, in patients who acquire an STI, there is a greater likelihood of HIV acquisition. All patients who present with symptoms consistent with an STI should also be offered testing for other STIs, including HIV.

Less is known about STI risk in individuals who identify as transgender, as most of the research has focused on the increased incidence of HIV/AIDS among transgender women (see Chap. 14). Engagement in commercial sex work, male preference in sexual partners, unemployment, disclosure of gender identity, abuse based on gender identity, and depressive symptoms are all associated with higher risk of HIV, and therefore likely other STIs [120, 121]. Because of the similarity in natal pelvic anatomy, risk and management for STIs in transgender men is similar to that of cisgender women and, as discussed previously, the sensitivity of the physical exam should be of utmost importance.

## Barrier Protection, Contraception, and Unwanted Pregnancy

Barrier protection methods (e.g. "male" and "female" condoms, dental dams, latex gloves, etc.) can reduce STI transmission. Among an international sample of women who partner with women ($n = 1557$ participants), 87.3 % reported never using barrier protection when receiving oral sex, 63.4 % when receiving sex toy stimulation, and 88.1 % when receiving digital sex [122]. In a larger sample ($n = 3116$ participants), approximately 60 % of women who partner with women reported using shared sex toys with a partner and 25–30 % did not clean the sex toys before sharing [123]. These studies suggest that misperception of risk and lack of education can play a role in non-use of barrier protection; however, additional obstacles include the cost of dental dams and reduction in sexual pleasure often associated with barrier methods.

The diversity of sexual behaviors and lack of use of barrier protection within the LGBT community, combined with the elevated risk for sexual coercion, assault, and commercial sex work, make unwanted pregnancy and contraception highly relevant topics for OB/GYN practitioners. Moreover, evidence suggests that these topics are increasingly important among younger LGBT individuals. Whereas cisgender lesbian women over 40 are less likely to have been pregnant, given birth, had a miscarriage, and/or had an abortion [28] compared with their heterosexual counterparts, LGB cisgender adolescents are more likely to have sex under the influence of alcohol, have multiple sexual partners, have unprotected sex, and experience unwanted pregnancy [110]. This is particularly true among bisexual cisgender women, who have the earliest sexual debut, highest numbers of male partners, greatest use of emergency contraception, and highest frequency of pregnancy termination [109]. However, behaviorally bisexual LGB adolescent females are also more likely to use hormonal contraception compared with lesbian and gay female teens [59].

To date, there have been no studies on unwanted pregnancy among transgender men.

However, the high rates of sexual assault among transgender individuals [124] suggest that there is a significant likelihood for unwanted pregnancy. Patient misperception about the contraceptive effects of testosterone may also result in unwanted or unplanned pregnancy. Irrespective of the outcome of the pregnancy, navigating pregnancy as a pregnant male can be a challenging experience both psychologically and socially. In this setting, clinicians can provide an affirming environment, particularly if patients can be engaged in care throughout the pregnancy.

Among all LGBT individuals, sensitive sexual history taking (see Chap. 6) can be used to discuss pregnancy risk and desire to prevent unwanted pregnancy. If patients are interested in pregnancy prevention, contraceptive methods and their effectiveness should be discussed. For transgender men who do not want to carry a pregnancy, hysterectomies are a viable option to discuss [125], but barrier methods should still be used for STI protection.

Contraception options and their effectiveness should be discussed with all eligible patients. For transmen, discussion can include the fact that contraception can affirm gender identity.

## Polycystic Ovarian Syndrome

Polycystic ovarian syndrome is a common endocrine disorder that can affect individuals who have ovaries. While there is a genetic component, obesity is the most highly recognized lifestyle factor associated with the development and symptom severity of PCOS [126]. The higher rates of obesity in LGB cisgender women have led some to believe that the incidence of PCOS is higher in LGB cisgender women. To date, only one study ($n = 618$; 254 lesbian women, 364 heterosexual women) has examined this hypothesis, finding higher rates of PCOS in lesbian-identified women [57]. Interestingly, lesbian women with PCOS had higher androgen levels compared with heterosexual women with PCOS, which also may be due to differences in obesity and insulin resistance observed among lesbian women.

While the pathogenesis of PCOS is beyond the scope of this text, both androgen and estrogen excess are characteristic of the disease process. As a result, some studies have hypothesized that the incidence of PCOS might be increased among transgender men taking testosterone; this has been supported by several [58, 89, 127] but not all studies [128].

Irrespective of incidence, it is important for providers to understand how sexual orientation and gender identity may impact PCOS treatment. While diet and reduction of insulin resistance are mainstays of treatment, many individuals also take oral contraceptive pills (OCPs) to regulate their periods. For individuals whose sexual practices are unlikely to result in pregnancy or who may not be sexually active with men or who do not wish to have a period because of male gender identity, the idea of OCPs may be stigmatizing or personally challenging. Providers should engage patients in a thorough discussion of the patient's expectations of treatment and how to include consideration of their identity to optimize treatment at an individual level.

## Trauma

While interpersonal violence is discussed in detail in Chap. 10, OB/GYN providers should be familiar with the high rates of emotional, physical, and sexual trauma faced by LGB cisgender women and transgender individuals. Beginning at a young age, women under the age of 18 who identify as bisexual or have sexual partners of multiple genders are more likely to experience parental physical abuse, physical dating violence, and emotional victimization [129]. LGB cisgender female youth are also more likely to have been forced to have sex by a male partner [109, 129]. Beyond trauma in family and relationship spaces, there is a strong likelihood that younger LGBT individuals having difficulty at school, with 81.9 % of LGBT youth reporting verbal harassment at school [130]. Among adults, 46 % of bisexual women report having been raped in their lifetime and greater than 50% of transgender individuals report being assaulted or raped by an intimate partner [124, 131]. Even when seeking support, transgender men are more likely than cisgender people to experience violence in domestic violence shelters [132].

For individuals who have a history of trauma, the health care environment can be triggering. Events such as sitting in a waiting room with strangers, to disclosing sexual orientation and/or gender identity, to exposing and having areas of the body examined can cause a heightened state of anxiety or even the re-experiencing of trauma. The manifestations of anxiety may be misinterpreted by providers as unfriendly, defensive, withdrawn, or threatening. Reacting to these perceived emotions can exacerbate the experience of trauma in a way that can be detrimental to the patient-provider relationship and subsequent provision of healthcare. Approaching patients in a non-threatening way, using a calm but compassionate demeanor, and understanding how to de-escalate challenging situations are crucial to engaging patients with a trauma history in their own healthcare. Providers can also support resilience, the ability to adapt to adversity and recover from trauma, in a variety of ways above and beyond creating a welcoming environment. Providers can empower patients to take ownership of their own healthcare, creating an internal locus of control that supports patients to feel in control of their health [33]. Finally, normalizing identities and experiences to promote patient self-acceptance and a positive LGBT identity can empower patients in their own lives outside of the healthcare system [34].

## Sexual Health and Satisfaction

While previous sections of this chapter have discussed risky sexual encounters and disease prevention, management, and treatment, a full discussion of sexual health includes positive sexuality and sexual relationships. Providers may not always feel comfortable discussing concerns about sexuality, often citing lack of training [133], fear of being intrusive, concern about how to respond to divulged information,

discomfort with the topic, and clinical time constraints [134]; however, patients do want to talk to their providers about sex, but often don't because they fear a judgmental reaction [135], and prefer their provider to initiate the conversation [136]. Patient support begins with the understanding that sex and sexuality are important aspects of personhood for many individuals, and sexual health is an integral aspect of holistic care.

The sexual response cycle, which comprises the physical and emotional changes that occur during sexual stimulation and arousal, is a key aspect of the conversation when discussing sexual health with patients. The sexual response cycle consists of four phases:

- Excitement (Phase 1) results from arousing mental, emotional, or physical stimuli that in turn result in an increase in heart rate, respiratory rate, and blood pressure; an accompanying increase in blood flow to erectile tissue (clitoris, penis); lubrication of the vagina; and upward movement of the testicles toward the perineum
- Plateau (Phase 2) refers to an intensification of the sensations that build during Phase 1, and is often accompanied by an increasing sense of pleasure during ongoing sexual stimulation; contraction of the pubococcygeus muscle; contraction of the urethral sphincter of the penis; secretion of pre-ejaculatory fluid from the penis; increased lubrication of the vagina; and swelling of the outer vagina
- Orgasm (Phase 3) represents the culmination of the plateau phase, with the occurrence of peak sexual pleasure accompanied by rapid muscle contractions of muscles in the pelvis, including the vagina, uterus, and anus; ejaculation from the penis
- Resolution (Phase 4) occurs after orgasm and is the return of the body to it's pre-excitation state, including the detumescence of the penis

The stimuli promoting this response cycle, the experience during each phase, and the transition between phases vary widely across individuals irrespective of sexual orientation and gender identity.

This latter point is important for patients, in that sexual behaviors don't define one's sexual orientation and sexual orientation doesn't define what sexual acts are pleasurable. For example, some individuals may enjoy penetrative sexual practices whereas others may primarily prefer other forms of stimulation (e.g. clitoral stimulation). Some individuals choose to use sexual aids (vibrators, dildos, prostate stimulators, etc.) or engage in certain sexual practices (BDSM, kink, etc.). From a clinical standpoint, it is important to not only educate patients in how to minimize risk in these practices, but also to be supportive of consensual sexual practices that patients find enjoyable.

Using validated sexual health scales can be helpful in understanding and determining sexual health concerns. For example, the Female Sexual Function Index [137] evaluates certain aspects of the sexual response cycle (desire, arousal, lubrication, orgasm pain, satisfaction) whereas the Female Sexual Distress Scale [138] evaluates patient distress from sexual complaints. Other scales can be used to look at relationship cohesion (Dyadic Adjustment Scale [139]) and intimacy (Personal Assessment of Intimacy in Relationships [140]). While the names of these questionnaires presume female gender identity and a monogamous, two-partner relationship structure, they can apply to anyone with natal female pelvic structures and interpersonal relationships. As previously introduced, the PLISSIT scale (see Table 17.4) is a simple way of initiating a patient-centered dialogue about sexuality.

## Fertility and Reproduction

Family building is an incredibly important part of the lives of many individuals. External support for family building is often required, irrespective of sexual orientation and gender identity. Some individuals may object to LGBT family building, including providers. One study, published in 2010, demonstrated that 14 % of OB/GYN providers would discourage assisted reproductive technologies in LGB women partnered with women. While this is more common among male and religiously-affiliated providers [141], these may be the only providers in certain areas of the country. The American Academy of Child and Adolescent Psychiatry, American Academy of Family Physicians, American Academy of Pediatrics, American Psychiatric Association, American Medical Association, and American Society for Reproductive Medicine have all affirmed policies in support of LGBT families. The present section discusses the medical aspects of LGBT family building as it relates to OB/GYN care, whereas the medico-legal concerns of LGBT family building are discussed in Chap. 9.

It is important for providers to support LGBT individuals seeking medical support during family building not only in accessing reproductive services but also in validating family composition.

This validation is important throughout pregnancy and during birth, as many LGBT individuals may fear engaging in the birth process or intimacy that heterosexual couples can enjoy without discrimination [142]. This is particularly true for transgender men, where there is generally a lack of resources for transgender men desiring and/or carrying a pregnancy. The experience of pregnancy as a male can be incredibly challenging, as there are difficult gender stereotypes to overcome both internally and externally [143, 144].

## Foster Parenting/Adoption

Briefly, the process of foster parenting and adoption is state and jurisdiction dependent, and may restrict adoption based on marital status and sexual orientation. Currently, all states allow a single LGBT individual to petition to adopt or foster a child, however not all states allow joint adoption by same sex couples. Sometimes adoption or foster agencies require letters of recommendation, which can be an easy way for providers to support LGBT families.

## Alternative Insemination

Alternative insemination (AI) can be used to support a pregnancy in any person with the natal anatomy to carry a pregnancy, including cisgender women and transgender men. Individuals electing to receive alternative insemination will decide whether to receive sperm from a known or unknown donor. Selection of donor sperm may be done through licensed sperm bank, where individuals may choose sperm based on donor criteria (eye color, racial/ethnic background, educational attainment, etc.). Sperm can then be frozen and stored until the time of insemination. Donor insemination is typically performed via one of several techniques beyond the scope of this chapter, but typically during the natural menstrual cycle hours before the ovum is released. However some individuals may opt to enhance ovulation and likelihood of pregnancy success with the selective estrogen receptor modulator, clomiphene.

Transgender women can also be sperm donors if gametes are stored prior to the initiation of cross gender hormone therapy [145]. Transgender men can carry pregnancies, even after having received cross-gender hormone therapy [143]. Unlike transgender women, transgender men can initiate hormone therapy and then cease hormones in order to become pregnant, and oocytes do not have to be stored in advance. Testosterone treatments are usually delayed until after delivery in order to carry a healthy pregnancy to term.

The success of AI depends on the type of insemination procedure, age of patient, presence and degree of endometriosis, egg quality, and/or damage to the fallopian tubes. Importantly, while some have suggested that risk factors such as obesity and tobacco use may challenge the success of alternative insemination, studies have shown that there is no difference in pregnancy rate, live birth rate, or miscarriages between LGB cisgender women and heterosexual cisgender women [146]. As with all individuals who are relying on alternative insemination to conceive, the loss of a pregnancy can result in a heightened sense of grief for LGBT families due to the increased time/resources necessary for conception and the degree of planning required [147]. Furthermore, AI can be quite costly (between $300 and $700 per cycle, with numerous cycles usually required) and individuals may not have the resources to attempt AI multiple times.

## Surrogacy

Gay or bisexual cisgender men may opt to become fathers using surrogacy, where an individual with the capacity to carry a child carries the pregnancy for the intended parents. This can include gestational surrogacy, where the pregnancy can result from the transfer of a fertilized embryo, often with the sperm of one of the intended fathers, created through in vitro fertilization (IVF) to the intended surrogates. Traditional surrogacy, where the surrogate is inseminated artificially or naturally, can also be used. Surrogacy is typically a more costly endeavor, and thus can be unattainable for many same-sex male couples [148, 149].

## Conclusion

OB/GYN clinicians have a host of opportunities to enhance care and promote the health of individuals of diverse sexual orientations, gender identities and gender expressions. As discussed above, LGBT individuals are at increased risk for numerous OB/GYN related concerns and disparities in health outcomes, which should prompt providers to consider how to modify their own practice to support the health of patients identifying as LGBT. This care begins with learning how to empower patients to be in control of their own healthcare throughout the healthcare experience, to reduce the potential for re-traumatization, and to create a safe environment that supports patients to return for future evidence-based care. OB/GYN providers also have a unique opportunity to support LGBT individuals in building families. In addition, the breadth of health concerns encountered in OB/GYN practice allows providers to serve as a bridge to help patients in need connect to other key health care specialties, such as mental health (Chap. 13) and primary care and prevention (Chap. 8). Comprehensive OB/GYN care that is sensitive to sexual orientation, gender identity, and gender expression can therefore be pivotal in promoting the overall health of LGBT individuals.

# References

1. Weaver TL, Griffin MG, Mitchell ER. Symptoms of posttraumatic stress, depression, and body image distress in female victims of physical and sexual assault: exploring integrated responses. Health Care Women Int. 2014;35(4):458–75.

2. Eckstrand KL, Sciolla AF, Potter J. Trauma and resilience in the lives of people who are or may be LGBT, gender nonconforming, and/or born with DSD: Implications for clinical care and health outcomes. In: Hollenbach A, Eckstrand KL, Dreger AD, editors. Implementing curricular and institutional climate changes to improve health care for individuals who are LGBT, gender nonconforming, or born with DSD: a resource for medical educators. Washington, DC: Association of American Medical Colleges; 2014.

3. Mock SE, Eibach RP. Stability and change in sexual orientation identity over a 10-year period in adulthood. Arch Sex Behav. 2012;41(3):641–8.

4. Savin-Williams RC, Joyner K, Rieger G. Prevalence and stability of self-reported sexual orientation identity during young adulthood. Arch Sex Behav. 2012;41(1):103–10.

5. Hidalgo MA, Ehrensaft D, Tishelman AC, et al. The gender affirmative model: what we know and what we aim to learn. Hum Dev. 2013;56:285–90.

6. Grant JM, Mottet LA, Tanis J, Herman JL, Harrison J, Keisling M. Injustice at every turn: a report of the National Transgender Discrimination Survey. Washington, DC: National Center for Transgender Equality; 2011.

7. When health care isn't caring: lambda legal's survey of discrimination against LGBT people and people with HIV. New York: Lambda Legal; 2010.

8. (IOM) IoM. The health of lesbian, gay, bisexual, and transgender people: building a foundation for better understanding. Washington, DC; 2011.

9. Hatzenbuehler ML, Link BG. Introduction to the special issue on structural stigma and health. Social Sci Med (1982). 2014;103:1–6.

10. Rankow EJ, Tessaro I. Cervical cancer risk and Papanicolaou screening in a sample of lesbian and bisexual women. J Fam Pract. 1998;47(2):139–43.

11. Clark MA, Bonacore L, Wright SJ, Armstrong G, Rakowski W. The cancer screening project for women: experiences of women who partner with women and women who partner with men. Women Health. 2003;38(2):19–33.

12. Obedin-Maliver J, Goldsmith ES, Stewart L, et al. Lesbian, gay, bisexual, and transgender–related content in undergraduate medical education. JAMA. 2011;306(9):971–7.

13. Hollenbach A, Eckstrand KL, Dreger AD. Implementing curricular and climate changes to improve health care for individuals who are LGBT, gender nonconforming, or born with

DSD. Washington, DC: Association of American Medical Colleges; 2014.

14. Lim FA, Bernstein I. Promoting awareness of LGBT issues in aging in a baccalaureate nursing program. Nurs Educ Perspect. 2012;33(3):170–5.

15. McCabe PC, Rubinson F. Committing to social justice: The behavioral intention of school psychology and education trainees to advocate for lesbian, gay, bisexual, and transgendered youth. Sch Psychol Rev. 2008;37:469–86.

16. Kelley L, Chou CL, Dibble SL, Robertson PA. A critical intervention in lesbian, gay, bisexual, and transgender health: knowledge and attitude outcomes among second-year medical students. Teach Learn Med. 2008;20(3):248–53.

17. Sanchez NF, Rabatin J, Sanchez JP, Hubbard S, Kalet A. Medical students' ability to care for lesbian, gay, bisexual, and transgendered patients. Fam Med. 2006;38(1):21–7.

18. Agenor M, Peitzmeier SM, Gordon AR, Haneuse S, Potter J, Austin SB. Sexual orientation identity disparities in HPV knowledge and uptake in a national probability sample of young U.S. women. Ann Intern Med. 2015.

19. Cochran SD, Mays VM, Bowen D, et al. Cancer-related risk indicators and preventive screening behaviors among lesbians and bisexual women. Am J Public Health. 2001;91(4):591–7.

20. Case P, Austin SB, Hunter DJ, et al. Sexual orientation, health risk factors, and physical functioning in the Nurses' Health Study II. J Women's Health. 2004;13(9):1033–47.

21. Brandenburg DL, Matthews AK, Johnson TP, Hughes TL. Breast cancer risk and screening: a comparison of lesbian and heterosexual women. Women Health. 2007;45(4):109–30.

22. Boehmer U, Case P. Physicians don't ask, sometimes patients tell: disclosure of sexual orientation among women with breast carcinoma. Cancer. 2004;101(8):1882–9.

23. Bailey L, Ellis SJ, McNeil J. Suicide risk in the UK trans population and the role of gender transition in decreasing suicidal ideation and suicide attempt. Ment Health Rev J. 2014;19(4):209–20.

24. Reiter PL, McRee AL. Cervical cancer screening (Pap testing) behaviours and acceptability of human papillomavirus self-testing among lesbian and bisexual women aged 21-26 years in the USA. J Fam Plann Reprod Health Care. 2014.

25. Diamant AL, Schuster MA, Lever J. Receipt of preventive health care services by lesbians. Am J Prev Med. 2000;19(3):141–8.

26. Tracy JK, Lydecker AD, Ireland L. Barriers to cervical cancer screening among lesbians. J Women's Health. 2010;19(2):229–37.

27. Tracy JK, Schluterman NH, Greenberg DR. Understanding cervical cancer screening among lesbians: a national survey. BMC Public Health. 2013;13:442.

28. Dibble SL, Roberts SA, Nussey B. Comparing breast cancer risk between lesbians and their heterosexual sisters. Womens Health Issues. 2004;14(2):60–8.

29. Roberts SJ, Patsdaughter CA, Grindel CG, Tarmina MS. Health related behaviors and cancer screening of lesbians: results of the Boston Lesbian Health Project II. Women Health. 2004;39(4):41–55.

30. Pitman GE. Body image, compulsory heterosexuality, and internalized homophobia. J Lesbian Stud. 1999;3(4):129–39.

31. Parsons JT, Lelutiu-Weinberger C, Botsko M, Golub SA. A randomized controlled trial utilizing motivational interviewing to reduce HIV risk and drug use in young gay and bisexual men. J Consult Clin Psychol. 2014;82(1):9.

32. Rubak S, Sandbæk A, Lauritzen T, Christensen B. Motivational interviewing: a systematic review and meta-analysis. Br J Gen Pract. 2005;55(513):305–12.

33. Carter II LW, Mollen D, Smith NG. Locus of control, minority stress, and psychological distress among lesbian, gay, and bisexual individuals. J Couns Psychol. 2014;61(1):169.

34. Stitt AL. The cat and the cloud: ACT for LGBT locus of control, responsibility, and acceptance. J LGBT Issues Couns. 2014;8(3):282–97.

35. Boehmer U, Miao X, Ozonoff A. Cancer survivorship and sexual orientation. Cancer. 2011;117(16): 3796–804.

36. Frisch M, Smith E, Grulich A, Johansen C. Cancer in a population-based cohort of men and women in registered homosexual partnerships. Am J Epidemiol. 2003;157(11):966–72.

37. Cochran SD, Mays VM. Risk of breast cancer mortality among women cohabiting with same sex partners: findings from the National Health Interview Survey, 1997-2003. J Womens Health. 2012;21(5):528–33.

38. Austin SB, Pazaris MJ, Rosner B, Bowen D, Rich-Edwards J, Spiegelman D. Application of the Rosner-Colditz risk prediction model to estimate sexual orientation group disparities in breast cancer risk in a U.S. cohort of premenopausal women. Cancer Epidemiol Biomarkers Prev. 2012;21(12):2201–8.

39. Force USPST. Screening for breast cancer: U.S. Preventive Services Task Force recommendation statement. Ann Intern Med. 2009;151(10):716–26. W-236.

40. Gooren LJ, van Trotsenburg MA, Giltay EJ, van Diest PJ. Breast cancer development in transsexual subjects receiving cross-sex hormone treatment. J Sex Med. 2013;10(12):3129–34.

41. Brown GR, Jones KT. Incidence of breast cancer in a cohort of 5,135 transgender veterans. Breast Cancer Res Treat. 2015;149(1):191–8.

42. Maglione KD, Margolies L, Jaffer S, et al. Breast cancer in male-to-female transsexuals: use of breast imaging for detection. Am J Roentgenol. 2014; 203(6):W735–40.

43. Excellence UCfT. General prevention and screening. http://transhealth.ucsf.edu/trans?page=protocol-screening-S1X. Accessed March 26, 2015.

44. Dibble SL, Roberts SA, Robertson PA, Paul SM. Risk factors for ovarian cancer: lesbian and heterosexual women. Oncol Nurs Forum. 2002;29(1): E1–7.

45. Danforth KN, Im TM, Whitlock EP. Addendum to screening for ovarian cancer: evidence update for the US preventive services task force reaffirmation recommendation statement.

46. Charlton BM, Corliss HL, Missmer SA, et al. Reproductive health screening disparities and sexual orientation in a cohort study of U.S. adolescent and young adult females. J Adolesc Health. 2011; 49(5):505–10.

47. Agenor M, Krieger N, Austin SB, Haneuse S, Gottlieb BR. At the intersection of sexual orientation, race/ethnicity, and cervical cancer screening: assessing Pap test use disparities by sex of sexual partners among black, Latina, and white U.S. women. Soc Sci Med. 2014;116:110–8.

48. Agenor M, Krieger N, Austin SB, Haneuse S, Gottlieb BR. Sexual orientation disparities in Papanicolaou test use among US women: the role of sexual and reproductive health services. Am J Public Health. 2014;104(2):e68–73.

49. Prevention CfDCa. HPV Vaccines.

50. Petrosky E, Bocchini JA, Jr., Hariri S, et al. Use of 9-Valent Human Papillomavirus (HPV) Vaccine: Updated HPV Vaccination Recommendations of the Advisory Committee on Immunization Practices. Morbidity and Mortality Weekly Report 2015; 64(11):300–304.

51. Force USPST. Final Recommendation Statement Cervical Cancer: Screening; 2008.

52. Saslow D, Solomon D, Lawson HW, et al. American Cancer Society, American Society for Colposcopy and Cervical Pathology, and American Society for Clinical Pathology screening guidelines for the prevention and early detection of cervical cancer. CA Cancer J Clin. 2012;62(3):147–72.

53. Huh WK, Ault KA, Chelmow D, et al. Use of primary high-risk human papillomavirus testing for cervical cancer screening: interim clinical guidance. Gynecol Oncol. 2015;136:178–82.

54. Peitzmeier SM, Khullar K, Reisner SL, Potter J. Pap test use is lower among female-to-male patients than non-transgender women. Am J Prev Med. 2014; 47(6):808–12.

55. Peitzmeier SM, Reisner SL, Harigopal P, Potter J. Female-to-male patients have high prevalence of unsatisfactory Paps compared to non-transgender females: implications for cervical cancer screening. J Gen Intern Med. 2014;29(5):778–84.

56. Conron KJ, Scott G, Stowell GS, Landers SJ. Transgender health in Massachusetts: results from a household probability sample of adults. Am J Public Health. 2012;102(1):118–22.

57. Agrawal R, Sharma S, Bekir J, et al. Prevalence of polycystic ovaries and polycystic ovary syndrome in lesbian women compared with heterosexual women. Fertil Steril. 2004;82(5):1352–7.

58. Baba T, Endo T, Ikeda K, et al. Distinctive features of female-to-male transsexualism and prevalence of gender identity disorder in Japan. J Sex Med. 2011;8(6):1686–93.

59. Charlton BM, Corliss HL, Missmer SA, Rosario M, Spiegelman D, Austin SB. Sexual orientation differences in teen pregnancy and hormonal contraceptive use: an examination across 2 generations. Am J Obstet Gynecol. 2013;209(3):204.e1–8.

60. Diamant AL, Schuster MA, McGuigan K, Lever J. Lesbians' sexual history with men: implications for taking a sexual history. Arch Intern Med. 1999;159(22):2730–6.

61. Kerr DL, Ding K, Thompson AJ. A comparison of lesbian, bisexual, and heterosexual female college undergraduate students on selected reproductive health screenings and sexual behaviors. Womens Health Issues. 2013;23(6):e347–55.

62. Clements-Nolle K, Marx R, Guzman R, Katz M. HIV prevalence, risk behaviors, health care use, and mental health status of transgender persons: Implications for public health intervention. Am J Public Health. 2001;91(6):915.

63. Nemoto T, Operario D, Keatley J, Han L, Soma T. HIV risk behaviors among male-to-female transgender persons of color in San Francisco. Am J Public Health. 2004;94(7):1193–9.

64. Fredriksen-Goldsen KI, Kim HJ, Barkan SE, Muraco A, Hoy-Ellis CP. Health disparities among lesbian, gay, and bisexual older adults: results from a population-based study. Am J Public Health. 2013;103(10):1802–9.

65. Hart SL, Bowen DJ. Sexual orientation and intentions to obtain breast cancer screening. J Womens Health. 2009;18(2):177–85.

66. Bowen DJ, Bradford J, Powers D. Comparing sexual minority status across sampling methods and populations. Women Health. 2006;44(2):121–34.

67. Network NCC. Clinical practice guidelines in oncology http://www.nccn.org/professionals/physician_gls/f_guidelines.asp. Accessed March 24, 2015.

68. Pritchard TJ, Pankowsky DA, Crowe JP, Abdul-Karim FW. Breast cancer in a male-to-female transsexual. A case report. JAMA. 1988;259(15):2278–80.

69. Shao T, Grossbard ML, Klein P. Breast cancer in female-to-male transsexuals: two cases with a review of physiology and management. Clin Breast Cancer. 2011;11(6):417–9.

70. Burcombe RJ, Makris A, Pittam M, Finer N. Breast cancer after bilateral subcutaneous mastectomy in a female-to-male trans-sexual. Breast. 2003;12(4):290–3.

71. Hembree WC, Cohen-Kettenis P, Delemarre-van de Waal HA, et al. Endocrine treatment of transsexual persons: an Endocrine Society clinical practice guideline. J Clin Endocrinol Metab. 2009;94(9):3132–54.

72. Weyers S, Villeirs G, Vanherreweghe E, et al. Mammography and breast sonography in transsexual women. Eur J Radiol. 2010;74(3):508–13.

73. Chen J, Pee D, Ayyagari R, et al. Projecting absolute invasive breast cancer risk in white women with a model that includes mammographic density. J Natl Cancer Inst. 2006;98(17):1215–26.

74. Boehmer U, Linde R, Freund KM. Sexual minority women's coping and psychological adjustment after a diagnosis of breast cancer. J Womens Health. 2005;14(3):214–24.

75. White JL, Boehmer U. Long-term breast cancer survivors' perceptions of support from female partners: an exploratory study. Oncol Nurs Forum. 2012;39(2):210–7.

76. Boehmer U, Linde R, Freund KM. Breast reconstruction following mastectomy for breast cancer: the decisions of sexual minority women. Plast Reconstr Surg. 2007;119(2):464–72.

77. Matthews AK, Brandenburg DL, Johnson TP, Hughes TL. Correlates of underutilization of gynecological cancer screening among lesbian and heterosexual women. Prev Med. 2004;38(1):105–13.

78. Price JH, Easton AN, Telljohann SK, Wallace PB. Perceptions of cervical cancer and Pap smear screening behavior by women's sexual orientation. J Community Health. 1996;21(2):89–105.

79. O'Hanlan KA, Crum CP. Human papillomavirus-associated cervical intraepithelial neoplasia following lesbian sex. Obstet Gynecol. 1996;88(4 Pt 2):702–3.

80. Bailey JV, Kavanagh J, Owen C, McLean KA, Skinner CJ. Lesbians and cervical screening. Br J Gen Pract. 2000;50(455):481–2.

81. Marrazzo JM, Gorgos LM. Emerging sexual health issues among women who have sex with women. Curr Infect Dis Rep. 2012;14(2):204–11.

82. Marrazzo JM. Genital human papillomavirus infection in women who have sex with women: a concern for patients and providers. AIDS Patient Care STDs. 2000;14(8):447–51.

83. Marrazzo JM, Koutsky LA, Stine KL, et al. Genital human papillomavirus infection in women who have sex with women. J Infect Dis. 1998;178(6):1604–9.

84. Massad LS, Einstein MH, Huh WK, et al. 2012 updated consensus guidelines for the management of abnormal cervical cancer screening tests and cancer precursors. J Low Genit Tract Dis. 2013;17(5 Suppl 1):S1–27.

85. McRee AL, Katz ML, Paskett ED, Reiter PL. HPV vaccination among lesbian and bisexual women: findings from a national survey of young adults. Vaccine. 2014;32(37):4736–42.

86. Miller N, Bedard Y, Cooter N, Shaul D. Histological changes in the genital tract in transsexual women following androgen therapy. Histopathology. 1986;10(7):661–9.

87. Dizon DS, Tejada-Berges T, Koelliker S, Steinhoff M, Granai CO. Ovarian cancer associated with testosterone supplementation in a female-to-male transsexual patient. Gynecol Obstet Investig. 2006;62(4):226–8.

88. Hage JJ, Dekker JJ, Karim RB, Verheijen RH, Bloemena E. Ovarian cancer in female-to-male

transsexuals: report of two cases. Gynecol Oncol. 2000;76(3):413–5.

89. Spinder T, Spijkstra JJ, van den Tweel JG, et al. The effects of long term testosterone administration on pulsatile luteinizing hormone secretion and on ovarian histology in eugonadal female to male transsexual subjects. J Clin Endocrinol Metab. 1989;69(1):151–7.

90. Weyers S, Lambein K, Sturtewagen Y, Verstraelen H, Gerris J, Praet M. Cytology of the 'penile' neovagina in transsexual women. Cytopathology. 2010;21(2):111–5.

91. Bleeker MC, Heideman DA, Snijders PJ, Horenblas S, Meijer CJ. Epidemiology and etiology of penile cancer. In: Muneer A, Arya M, Horenblas S, editors. Textbook of penile cancer: Springer; 2012. pp. 1–11.

92. Baral SD, Poteat T, Strömdahl S, Wirtz AL, Guadamuz TE, Beyrer C. Worldwide burden of HIV in transgender women: a systematic review and meta-analysis. Lancet Infect Dis. 2013;13(3):214–22.

93. Pfaendler KS, Wenzel L, Mechanic MB, Penner KR. Cervical cancer survivorship: long-term quality of life and social support. Clin Ther. 2015;37(1):39–48.

94. Wu H-S, Harden JK. Symptom burden and quality of life in survivorship: a review of the literature. Cancer Nurs. 2015;38(1):E29–54.

95. Frazier LM, Miller VA, Horbelt DV, Delmore JE, Miller BE, Averett EP. Employment and quality of survivorship among women with cancer: domains not captured by quality of life instruments. Cancer Control. 2009;16(1):57.

96. Dizon DS, Suzin D, McIlvenna S. Sexual health as a survivorship issue for female cancer survivors. Oncologist. 2014;19(2):202–10.

97. Duska L, Fader A, Dizon D. Survivorship in gynecologic cancer: enduring the treatment toward a new normal. Paper presented at: American Society of Clinical Oncology educational book/ASCO. American Society of Clinical Oncology. Meeting; 2013.

98. Plotti F, Nelaj E, Sansone M, et al. Sexual function after modified radical hysterectomy (Piver II/Type B) vs. classic radical hysterectomy (Piver III/Type C2) for early stage cervical cancer. A prospective study. J Sex Med. 2012;9(3):909–17.

99. Carter J, Chi DS, Brown CL, et al. Cancer-related infertility in survivorship. Int J Gynecol Cancer. 2010;20(1):2–8.

100. Goldberg NG. The impact of inequality for same-sex partners in employer-sponsored retirement plans. Los Angeles, CA: The Williams Institute; 2009.

101. Improving the lives of LGBT older adults. LGBT Movement Advancement Project Services and Advocacy for Gay, Lesbian, Bisexual and Transgender Elders; 2010.

102. Salani R. Survivorship planning in gynecologic cancer patients. Gynecol Oncol. 2013;130(2):389–97.

103. Herrick AL, Matthews AK, Garofalo R. Health risk behaviors in an urban sample of young women who have sex with women. J Lesbian Stud. 2010;14(1):80–92.

104. Sehnal B, Dusek L, Cibula D, et al. The relationship between the cervical and anal HPV infection in women with cervical intraepithelial neoplasia. J Clin Virol. 2014;59(1):18–23.

105. Slama J, Sehnal B, Dusek L, Zima T, Cibula D. Impact of risk factors on prevalence of anal HPV infection in women with simultaneous cervical lesion. Neoplasma. 2015;62(2):308–14.

106. Roberts JM, Thurloe JK. Comparison of the performance of anal cytology and cervical cytology as screening tests. Sex Health. 2012;9(6):568–73.

107. Arain S, Walts AE, Thomas P, Bose S. The anal Pap smear: cytomorphology of squamous intraepithelial lesions. CytoJournal. 2005;2(1):4.

108. Bailey J, Farquhar C, Owen C, Mangtani P. Sexually transmitted infections in women who have sex with women. Sex Transm Infect. 2004;80(3):244–6.

109. Tornello SL, Riskind RG, Patterson CJ. Sexual orientation and sexual and reproductive health among adolescent young women in the United States. J Adolesc Health. 2014;54(2):160–8.

110. Herrick A, Kuhns L, Kinsky S, Johnson A, Garofalo R. Demographic, psychosocial, and contextual factors associated with sexual risk behaviors among young sexual minority women. J Am Psychiatr Nurses Assoc. 2013;19(6):345–55.

111. Marrazzo JM, Thomas KK, Agnew K, Ringwood K. Prevalence and risks for bacterial vaginosis in women who have sex with women. Sex Transm Dis. 2010;37(5):335.

112. Marrazzo JM, Thomas KK, Fiedler TL, Ringwood K, Fredricks DN. Risks for acquisition of bacterial vaginosis among women who report sex with women: a cohort study. PLoS One. 2010;5(6), e11139.

113. Evans AL, Scally AJ, Wellard SJ, Wilson JD. Prevalence of bacterial vaginosis in lesbians and heterosexual women in a community setting. Sex Transm Infect. 2007;83(6):470–5.

114. Marrazzo JM, Thomas KK, Ringwood K. A behavioural intervention to reduce persistence of bacterial vaginosis among women who report sex with women: results of a randomised trial. Sex Transm Infect. 2011;87(5):399–405.

115. Workowski KA, Bolan G. Sexually transmitted diseases treatment guidelines. Centers for Disease Control and Prevention; 2014.

116. Xu F, Sternberg MR, Markowitz LE. Women who have sex with women in the United States: prevalence, sexual behavior and prevalence of herpes simplex virus type 2 infection—Results from National Health and Nutrition Examination Survey 2001–2006. Sex Transm Dis. 2010;37(7):407–13.

117. Marrazzo JM, Stine K, Wald A. Prevalence and risk factors for infection with herpes simplex virus type-1

and-2 among lesbians. Sex Transm Dis. 2003; 30(12):890–5.

118. Wald A, Zeh J, Selke S, Ashley RL, Corey L. Virologic characteristics of subclinical and symptomatic genital herpes infections. N Engl J Med. 1995;333(12):770–5.

119. Singh D, Fine DN, Marrazzo JM. Chlamydia trachomatis infection among women reporting sexual activity with women screened in family planning clinics in the Pacific Northwest, 1997 to 2005. Am J Public Health. 2011;101(7):1284–90.

120. Nuttbrock L, Bockting W, Rosenblum A, et al. Gender abuse, depressive symptoms, and HIV and other sexually transmitted infections among male-to-female transgender persons: a three-year prospective study. Am J Public Health. 2013;103(2):300–7.

121. Nuttbrock L, Hwahng S, Bockting W, et al. Lifetime risk factors for HIV/STI infections among male-to-female transgender persons. J Acquir Immune Defic Syndr (1999). 2009;52(3):417.

122. Rowen TS, Breyer BN, Lin T-C, Li C-S, Robertson PA, Shindel AW. Use of barrier protection for sexual activity among women who have sex with women. Int J Gynecol Obstet. 2013;120(1):42–5.

123. Schick V, Rosenberger JG, Herbenick D, Reece M. Sexual behaviour and risk reduction strategies among a multinational sample of women who have sex with women. Sex Transm Infect. 2012; 88(6):407–12.

124. Kenagy GP. Transgender health: findings from two needs assessment studies in Philadelphia. Health Social Work. 2005;30(1):19–26.

125. Obedin-Maliver J, Light A, DeHaan G, Steinauer J, Jackson R. Vaginal hysterectomy as a viable option for female-to-male transgender men. Obstet Gynecol. 2014;123:126S–7.

126. Teede H, Deeks A, Moran L. Polycystic ovary syndrome: a complex condition with psychological, reproductive and metabolic manifestations that impacts on health across the lifespan. BMC Med. 2010;8(1):41.

127. Grynberg M, Fanchin R, Dubost G, et al. Histology of genital tract and breast tissue after long-term testosterone administration in a female-to-male transsexual population. Reprod Biomed Online. 2010;20(4):553–8.

128. Ikeda K, Baba T, Noguchi H, et al. Excessive androgen exposure in female-to-male transsexual persons of reproductive age induces hyperplasia of the ovarian cortex and stroma but not polycystic ovary morphology. Hum Reprod. 2012:des385.

129. Friedman MS, Marshal MP, Guadamuz TE, et al. A meta-analysis of disparities in childhood sexual abuse, parental physical abuse, and peer victimization among sexual minority and sexual nonminority individuals. Am J Public Health. 2011;101(8): 1481–94.

130. Kosciw JG, Greytak EA, Bartkiewicz MJ, Boesen MJ, Palmer NA. The 2011 National School Climate Survey: The Experiences of Lesbian, Gay, Bisexual and Transgender Youth in Our Nation's Schools. ERIC; 2012.

131. Chestnut S, Dixon E, Jindasurat C. Lesbian, gay, bisexual, transgender, queer, and HIV-affected hate violence in 2012. New York: A report from the National Coalition of Anti-Violence Programs (NCAVP). 2013.

132. Hate Violence Against Lesbian, Gay, Bisexual, Transgender, Queer and HIV-Affected Communities in the United States in 2013. New York, NY: National Coalition of Anti-Violence Programs; 2014.

133. Parish SJ, Clayton AH. Continuing medical education: sexual medicine education: review and commentary (CME). J Sex Med. 2007;4(2):259–68.

134. McGarvey E, Peterson C, Pinkerton R, Keller A, Clayton A. Medical students' perceptions of sexual health issues prior to a curriculum enhancement. Int J Impot Res. 2003;15(5):S58.

135. Marwick C. Survey says patients expect little physician help on sex. JAMA. 1999;281(23):2173–4.

136. Wittenberg A, Gerber J. Recommendations for improving sexual health curricula in medical schools: results from a two-arm study collecting data from patients and medical students. J Sex Med. 2009;6(2):362–8.

137. Baser RE, Li Y, Carter J. Psychometric validation of the Female Sexual Function Index (FSFI) in cancer survivors. Cancer. 2012;118(18):4606–18.

138. DeRogatis L, Clayton A, Lewis-D'Agostino D, Wunderlich G, Fu Y. Validation of the Female Sexual Distress Scale-Revised for assessing distress in women with hypoactive sexual desire disorder. J Sex Med. 2008;5(2):357–64.

139. Spanier GB. The measurement of marital quality. J Sex Marital Ther. 1979;5(3):288–300.

140. Schaefer MT, Olson DH. Assessing intimacy: the pair inventory. J Marital Fam Ther. 1981;7(1): 47–60.

141. Lawrence RE, Rasinski KA, Yoon JD, Curlin FA. Obstetrician–gynecologists' beliefs about assisted reproductive technologies. Obstet Gynecol. 2010;116(1):127–35.

142. Dahl B, Fylkesnes AM, Sørlie V, Malterud K. Lesbian women's experiences with healthcare providers in the birthing context: a meta-ethnography. Midwifery. 2013;29(6):674–81.

143. Light AD, Obedin-Maliver J, Sevelius JM, Kerns JL. Transgender men who experienced pregnancy after female-to-male gender transitioning. Obstet Gynecol. 2014;124(6):1120–7.

144. Ellis SA, Wojnar DM, Pettinato M. Conception, pregnancy, and birth experiences of male and gender variant gestational parents: it's how we could have a family. J Midwifery Womens Health. 2014; 60(1):62–9.

145. T'Sjoen G, Van Caenegem E, Wierckx K. Transgenderism and reproduction. Curr Opin Endocrinol Diabetes Obes. 2013;20(6):575–9.

146. Nordqvist S, Sydsjö G, Lampic C, Åkerud H, Elenis E, Svanberg AS. Sexual orientation of women does not affect outcome of fertility treatment with donated sperm. Hum Reprod. 2014:det445.

147. Peel E. Pregnancy loss in lesbian and bisexual women: an online survey of experiences. Hum Reprod. 2009:dep441.

148. Norton W, Hudson N, Culley L. Gay men seeking surrogacy to achieve parenthood. Reprod Biomed Online. 2013;27(3):271–9.

149. Riggs DW, Due C. Gay fathers' reproductive journeys and parenting experiences: a review of research. J Fam Plann Reprod Health Care. 2014;40(4): 289–93.

# Part V

## Transgender Health

# Interdisciplinary Care for Transgender Patients

# 18

Christopher A. McIntosh

## Learning Objectives

- Describe the importance of communication between providers in transgender care *(KP1, ICS1, ICS2, ICS3, Pr1, Pr2)*
- Discuss strategies to respectfully engage with transgender patients and provide an environment for optimal care *(ICS1, ICS4, PR1, Pr2)*
- Identify at least three strengths each interdisciplinary team role brings to comprehensive holistic health care for transgender patients *(IPC1, Pr3)*

## Introduction

Interdisciplinary care for transgender patients is advocated by every major health body that has published comprehensive care guidelines [1–3]. Some reasons for this are obvious and some are not. In modern health care we value interdisciplinary care in general, and have evidence for it's effectiveness in a number of areas (rehabilitation: [4]; primary care: [5]; geriatrics: [6]; mental health: [7–9]) and so in thinking equitably, we would want such care for transgender people as well.

C.A. McIntosh, M.Sc., M.D., F.R.C.P.C. (✉)
Centre for Addiction and Mental Health, University
of Toronto, Toronto, ON, Canada
e-mail: chris.mcintosh@utoronto.ca

Nevertheless, there is good reason to consider specifically why interdisciplinary care for transgender people is important. For this chapter, the term "interdisciplinary" as opposed to "multidisciplinary" will be used because the former implies communication between the providers [4]. Such communication is important because the interventions sought by some transgender people to relieve gender dysphoria by necessity cross disciplines. Subsequent chapters in this section of the book will address in detail hormone and surgery treatments for gender dysphoria. Often the physicians providing such treatments may have only very basic, if any, training in the behavioral sciences. The latter is necessary in order to assess for gender dysphoria and to look for mental health issues that ought to be addressed prior to or concurrently with the gender concerns [1]. This chapter will look first at some basic principles of care for the transgender patient, then explore the roles of the individual disciplines in their care.

## The Basics: What All Providers Need to Know

### Language and Terminology

A first step in the engagement of transgender people in care is to understand the importance of language. Gender is built into the grammar of the English language, and an individual crossing or

© Springer International Publishing Switzerland 2016
K.L. Eckstrand, J.M. Ehrenfeld (eds.), *Lesbian, Gay, Bisexual, and Transgender Healthcare*,
DOI 10.1007/978-3-319-19752-4_18

blurring societal gender lines will run into pitfalls related to language, as will the health care provider working to build a therapeutic relationship [10].

How an individual feels about their name is important to determine. Many transgender individuals dislike their birth name because most first names evoke an associated gender (e.g., Robert, Tiffany) though some do not (Robin, Leslie). Growing up, they may have preferred a shortened version of their birth name, or a nickname. Ask a patient about their preferred name of address and have a clear place for indicating this preferred name on the medical record.

> **Helpful Hint**
> Administrative staff should be given clear instructions to use the preferred name. If a person does legally change their name, make sure you promptly update your documentation to reflect this.

Pronouns are another area of attention. At some point in their transition process, a transgender individual will usually ask to be referred to by the pronouns, titles and gendered nouns associated with the preferred gender role (he, she, Ms, Mr, man, woman, daughter, son). This is a significant and important step for the individual, and for individuals seeking certain gender change surgical interventions, is a required part of eligibility requirements for their treatment (see below). As such it is important that these requests be acknowledged and respected. It is understood that doing so is not meant to be a denial on the part of the health care provider of medically significant information about the patient's biological sex. Nevertheless a respectful therapeutic relationship that acknowledges these language issues is key to earning the patient's trust. At times, individuals who identify with an alternative gender may ask to be referred to by a gender neutral pronoun (e.g. the singular "they") or a pronoun of their own invention. Trying one's best to accommodate these requests can go a long way in developing and maintaining the therapeutic relationship.

Sometimes transgender individuals who suffer from gender dysphoria (see below) will try to partially alleviate this by using alternative language for their sexed body parts, (e.g. FTM individuals who refer to their "chest" rather then breasts). If this is noticed in early discussions, it can improve the relationship for the provider to follow their lead. Primary care providers in particular should pay attention to this and ask about preferred language, as it may facilitate a patient's comfort with breast and genital examination. (This is frequently deferred by many transgender patients [11].) This guideline obviously is meant for patient communication; standards of medical documentation will require conventional terminology.

> **Helpful Hint**
> Preferred terms used to refer to transgender people do evolve over time. For example, the "-ed" suffix on the term "transgendered" is now by convention dropped. For this chapter the terms "trans woman" will describe a person wishing to transition from male to female (MTF), and "trans man" will describe a person wishing to transition from female to male (FTM).

## Distress Associated with the Transgender Experience

Broadly speaking the unique distress that many transgender people have relates to both body experience and environmental experience. These two kinds of experience are distinct, but they interact (Fig. 18.1). One important kind of distress associated with body experience is called gender dysphoria. This is the distress that generally motivates transgender people to seek out hormone and surgery interventions to more closely align their sense of their psychological gender with their experience of their body. Dysphoria can occur for the typical *gender role* socioculturally associated with one's sex, for one's *genitals*, or for one's *secondary sex characteristics* (body hair, body shape, pitch of voice), and for individuals seeking hormones and surgery, typically all three.

# Environmental Experience

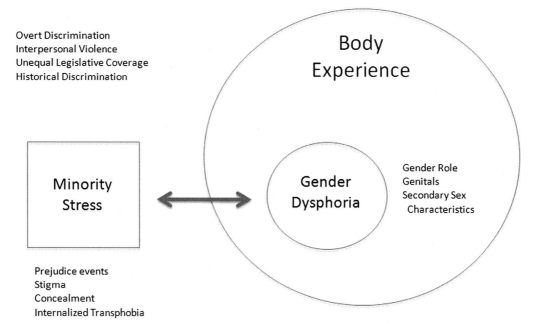

Overt Discrimination
Interpersonal Violence
Unequal Legislative Coverage
Historical Discrimination

Body Experience

Minority Stress

Gender Dysphoria

Gender Role
Genitals
Secondary Sex
  Characteristics

Prejudice events
Stigma
Concealment
Internalized Transphobia

**Fig. 18.1** Two types of distress associated with the transgender experience

**Helpful Hint**
Gender Dysphoria as a diagnosis is described by the fifth edition of the Diagnostic and Statistical Manual (DSM-5 [12]; see American Psychiatric Association 2013 for criteria). It should be noted that the DSM-5 explicitly states that having a transgender identity itself is not a mental disorder, it is the psychological distress of gender dysphoria that is considered a matter for clinical attention.

One important kind of environmental experience is minority stress. Transgender people experience chronic minority stress as they try to make their way in a world that enforces rigid gender roles and that often views them with hostility and scorn. Meyer [13] has conceptualized a minority stress model for lesbian, gay and bisexual individuals, and there has been considerable

interest in applying the model as well to transgender people. Meyer and other researchers have identified a number of mechanisms of minority stress experience including *prejudice events* (outright discrimination, abuse and violence) [14], *stigma* [15, 16], *concealment* of one's minority status, and *internalized homophobia and transphobia* [17, 18]; (see Fig. 18.1).

Minority stress theory postulates that the higher rates of certain mental health disorders in the LGBT population [19]) compared the general population are not a result of any innate psychopathology associated with being lesbian, gay, bisexual or transgender (as wrongly argued in past debates, see Drescher [20] for a review) but due to the psychological effects of discrimination.

Both minority stress and gender dysphoria can adversely affect health and wellness in transgender people. Interventions such as socially transitioning, or treatment with hormones or surgery to masculinize or feminize the body alleviate gender dysphoria in most cases. Minority stress, as well as other environmental stressors such as issues with relationships, financial hardships, and general life satisfaction may improve somewhat as the gender dysphoria improves, but often more assistance is needed in these areas, and sometimes patients may be disappointed that gender interventions did not ameliorate these other stressors, and may have made some worse.

Achieving the best possible outcome from transitioning is a primary goal of interdisciplinary care for the transgender patient, and one where mental health professionals in particular can be very helpful (see below).

## Members of the Interdisciplinary Team

In this section, a description of the clinical role of the team member is followed by an illustrative clinical vignette. For brevity's sake I have limited the number of professionals though one could easily include others.

### The Nurse

Nursing professionals play a crucial role in providing an optimal environment for culturally competent health care for the transgender patient. In many health care settings, nurses are the first and most frequent professional contact during an episode of care. Nurses can set the tone for professional, respectful care standards on a clinical team which can go a long way to improving a patient's experience of the health care system [21]. Home care nurses and nurses at long-term care facilities with training in culturally competent care can ensure that the transgender individual has a positive experience in accessing these services.

*Maria, an inpatient mental health nurse assesses Penny, a trans woman admitted from the emergency department with a several week history of profound depression. Later at the nursing station, a team member makes an unflattering comment about Penny's growth of facial hair. Maria reminds the team member that lack of*

*motivation to groom oneself is a common symptom among their depressed patients, and that there is a responsibility to treat patients equitably. As Penny recovers, Maria ensures safe and appropriate grooming materials are available and provides Penny with privacy.*

## The Primary Care Physician or Nurse Practitioner

The primary care physician (PCP) or nurse practitioner (NP) will often be the health care provider charged with coordinating the care of the transgender patient by referring to appropriate providers. As such they are the control center of the interdisciplinary team and other professionals involved in the care of the transgender individual should maintain open lines of communication with them. An important role of the PCP or NP is to maintain a holistic picture of the transgender patient's overall health, so that preventative health considerations like cancer screening, smoking cessation, and metabolic issues are not lost in the patient's drive to move forward with a transition process.

*Jerome, a young trans man is following up with his nurse practioner Charles about the progress of his transition. He has been doing very well on weekly intramuscular injections of testosterone, which have caused cessation of menses and the development of facial hair and a vocal pitch in a tenor range, all of which are much appreciated by Jerome. Charles indicates that he has received a copy of the letter from Jennifer, the clinical psychologist who recently assessed his readiness to proceed with chest surgery, and it is very positive. The only issue to be addressed is Jerome's half pack per day smoking habit. Both Charles and Jennifer have worked with Jerome's preferred surgeon, Eleanor, and know that she will want him to quit, to reduce risks related to intubation during the surgery and healing of the incisions. Jerome agrees and mentions that he and a new friend he met at a trans youth support group have decided to quit together. Charles offers nicotine replacement therapy but Jerome declines.*

## The Internist, Endocrinologist or Other Hormone Prescribing Physician

There are a number of good guidelines published regarding the endocrine care of transgender individuals, and Chapter __ in this volume is also devoted to this topic. One significant challenge for the endocrinologist is to identify gender dysphoria diagnostically and assess readiness issues that ought to be addressed prior to or concurrently with treatment. The ability to do so with confidence is aided by having ready access to a mental health practitioner. The importance of having confidence in the diagnosis and readiness is counter-balanced by the understanding that substantive delays in care can be agonizing for the patient experiencing severe gender dysphoria. There may also be harm reduction considerations if, for example, a patient is obtaining hormones from another non-medical source. Antiandrogens such as cyproterone and spironolactone (for trans women) or peptide gonadotropin releasing hormone agonists (GnRH-A) such as leuprolide and buserelin (for both trans men and trans women), which reduce the ongoing effects of endogenous sex hormones, can be considered as a bridging treatment if there are readiness and/or diagnostic issues that need to be clarified.

Interdisciplinary communication is important on a number of issues related to hormones that may cross discipline lines, such as smoking cessation and estrogen, and mental health side effects of hormones (which, if they occur at all, are usually transient and mild, though may be more significant in individuals with certain pre-existing mental health diagnoses, especially if not stabilized). As well, liaising with the surgeon on the issue of presurgical hormones may be important, depending on the type of surgery.

*Rebecca, a married trans woman in her late thirties is seeing Lesley, an endocrinologist, for the first visit to discuss hormone therapy. Lesley takes a careful history and finds out that Rebecca and her wife of 15 years remain committed to staying in their marriage and plan to remain sexually active. In discussing the benefits, risks and side effects of hormones Lesley mentions decreased libido and erections. Rebecca realizes that she may have to discuss the issue of sex further with her wife and discloses that she feels intensely dysphoric during intercourse, but fears her wife will leave if she cannot maintain their sexual intimacy adequately. Lesley sends Rebecca to get baseline bloodwork and books a follow-up to discuss things further, as well as providing a referral to a family therapist.*

## The Surgeon

Surgeons who perform gender confirming surgery may have been trained in a number of surgical disciplines. Plastic surgeons typically perform breast augmentation for trans women, mastectomy and male chest reconstruction for trans men, and genital operations for both trans men and trans women. Gynecologists perform hysterectomy for trans men. Urologists may provide orchiectomy for trans women and be involved in urethral extension for genital surgeries for trans men.

[Chapter __ in this volume discusses surgical interventions in detail.]

Interdisciplinary communication is of considerable importance for surgical care. Most surgeons are not well trained in mental health, and it is recommended that they depend on mental health professionals for the diagnosis of gender dysphoria and assessment of eligibility and readiness. *Eligibility* criteria for surgery depend on the surgery being sought. Gonadal surgery (hysterectomy, orchiectomy) generally requires 1 year of prior treatment with exogenous hormones. Genital surgery requires a minimum of 1 year of full-time, continuous experience living in the new gender role. Surgical standards of the World Professional Association for Transgender Health (WPATH) stipulate that chest surgeries require one letter and gonadal and genital surgeries two letters from assessing behavioral health professionals [1].

Other important lines of interdisciplinary communication in surgical care are with the primary care physician or internist in preparing the patient medically for surgery and with the endocrinologist regarding the issue of hormone treatment or discontinuation prior to surgery.

*Ilan is a gynecologist who stops by to check on Joseph who is one day postoperative from a laparoscopically assisted vaginal hysterectomy and bilateral salpingo-oopherectomy. He is recovering very well and is suitable to be discharged home later today. Ilan dictates a discharge summary with copies sent to Joseph's primary care physician and endocrinologist.*

## The Mental Health Practitioner

The mental health practitioner plays an important and active role in interdisciplinary care of the transgender patient. Mental health practitioners can come from a variety of training backgrounds, such as psychology, psychiatry, and social work. The role of the mental health practitioner can include clinical assessment for gender dysphoria and/or mental health conditions that may also be a source of clinical attention. Other roles can include treatment of identified co-occurring conditions, family interventions to aid in discussing the issues with family, and supportive treatment through the process of transitioning.

Many transgender people have a negative view of mental health practitioners, who they may perceive as being hostile or pathologizing of their experience. This can present a challenge in developing a therapeutic relationship. It is important to recognize that historically the relationship between the mental health fields and transgender people has been characterized by misunderstanding and that individuals may indeed have good reason to be wary [22].

Issues that a mental health practitioner can help the patient to explore with psychotherapy include: self-esteem, past traumas and their effects on current functioning, anxiety about their gender role presentation, relationship issues with partners, coming out to family and friends, and other challenges [23].

The holistic approach that mental health practitioners employ in looking at the multifactorial sources of a patient's distress make them essential members of the treatment team. As identified previously in Fig. 18.1, distress associated with the transgender experience is not only the embodied experience of gender dysphoria, but also the environmental experience of minority stress and its psychological consequences.

Hormone and surgery interventions address the gender dysphoria, but what about factors related to minority stress, not to mention other psychosocial stressors?

Assessment of *readiness* to proceed with transition is a key role of the mental health provider and helps to identify collaboratively with the patient areas that ought to be addressed prior to or concurrently with transition. Patients often have good insight into these areas already, but sometimes do not. Insight may be hindered by a strong belief that transition will resolve these other issues, be they mental health issues, financial issues, discrimination from employers or family members, or other important concerns.

An important counterweight to minority stress is *resilience* or positive adaptation in the face of significant adversity [13, 24]. Development of resilience may be a necessary treatment goal for many patients. Resilience in transgender people is a relatively new area of study, but those studies published identify a few clinically noteworthy associations: Testa et al. [25] identified that prior awareness of the existence of other transgender people as well as actual engagement with them, were independently associated with measures of improved affect and psychological comfort, suggesting transgender community connection may be important in developing resilience. Other studies have identified supportive family [26, 27] and personal spiritual growth [27, 28] as resiliency factors, suggesting a role for family therapy and supportive chaplaincy on the interdisciplinary team.

*Robert is a psychiatrist assessing Karen, a trans woman referred by her family doctor due to a significant history of depression. Robert takes a careful history to identify the factors contributing to the depression, which Karen believes is related only to the gender dysphoria she has for her genitalia. From the interview, Robert formulates an understanding of Karen's depression as multifactorial, where the gender dysphoria is only one contributor. Together they come up with a comprehensive treatment plan that addresses biological, psychological, social and spiritual factors.*

## The Social Worker

Social workers may play the role of a mental health clinician on the interdisciplinary team (see above) and are also invaluable for their attention to social factors that may be exacerbating a client's distress. Because of discrimination, transgender people can be socially marginalized. Transgender people who are homeless or underhoused may face special challenges in accessing appropriate services, as shelters are frequently divided by gender [29]. Transgender people in abusive situations may be reluctant to access needed services such as police protection because of either perception or past experience that police officers will be discriminatory. Such marginalization may also lead transgender people to have a poor understanding of what their legal rights are in cases of eviction or family conflicts such as child custody disputes. Options for welfare and disability pension support may also be areas where clients need the assistance of a social worker.

Transgender people benefit from connection with other people in the trans community and a social worker can be extremely helpful to a client by being up to date on the latest community resources and support groups both in-person and online.

*Marjorie is a social worker in a women's shelter assessing Lucas, a young trans man who recently became homeless after his parents kicked him out of their house after he came out to them as trans. Lucas is devastated by their reaction and having difficulty figuring out what to do next. He initially went to a men's shelter but left because it was "scary". Marjorie welcomes Lucas and ensures other staff are aware of his preferred name and pronouns. She refers to a social work colleague who does counseling with trans youth, and works to help him access housing and vocational resources.*

## The Chaplain

As hypothesized by Follins, Walker and Lewis [24], religious affiliation for transgender individuals can be "bittersweet", with parallels to what is known about religious faith in LGB individuals (see Hamblin and Gross [30] for a review). While personal spiritual growth can promote resilience, and religious affiliation is associated with positive psychological functioning in the general population, this is clearly contextual when it comes to LGBT individuals. Doctrinaire teaching about the immorality of homosexuality (often conflated with gender identity) in some conservative religious communities can be a significant source of psychological distress.

As such transgender individuals with religious faith may be experiencing significant conflict about transition and what it means personally to them, as well as to their family and faith community. Having a supportive chaplain on the interdisciplinary team can be a great boon to these patients.

*Mark, a family therapist working with Julia, a trans woman, and her wife Ruby, refers to chaplaincy because the couple is trying to reconcile their conservative Christian upbringing with the client's need to transition to relieve her gender dysphoria. Sara, the chaplain, works with Julia and Ruby to explore what their core spiritual values are, how important (or not) doctrine is to their faith, and how they will address reaction from the other members of their congregation.*

## The Speech-Language Pathologist

Vocal changes can be a desired but involuntary consequence for trans men taking testosterone or an aspiration for trans women hoping to feminize their voices. In both cases the services of a speech language pathologist are valued. Voice may be overlooked by health care providers but is often of considerable importance to the patient. Improved satisfaction with voice can lead to significant gains in self-esteem, confidence, and comfort in the preferred gender role. Screening questions about use of the voice in the patient's occupation or hobbies can identify situations in which referral to a voice specialist is appropriate. Some advocate a modified approach to testosterone therapy in trans men who are professional singers. For such individuals a singing coach experienced in working with trans men or adolescent boys going through puberty may be very helpful. Trans women who use their voice occupationally (significant telephone work or vocal interaction with clients or colleagues) can suffer from vocal strain if they are attempting in a haphazard way to feminize their voices.

*Caitlin, a trans woman who has been on estrogen and spironolactone for 3 years, has been satisfied with many of the changes that hormones have wrought, but remains highly dissatisfied with her masculine sounding voice. She is referred to Gina, a speech language pathologist, who teaches her about the many factors that lead to a gender perception of voice, which is illuminating for Caitlin because she had always assumed pitch was the only factor. Gina puts together a number of vocal exercises for Caitlin to begin working on.*

## The Dietician

Healthy eating is of course a laudable goal for everyone, but there are specific areas in which attention to eating and nutrition in transgender care is important. The prevalence of eating disorders among transgender people is unknown, though Vocks et al. [31] did show that both the trans men and trans women in their sample had higher scores on some eating disorder symptoms scales compared to cisgender individuals.

In clinical practice it is not uncommon to hear how eating and body image interacts with issues of gender identity and gender dysphoria. For trans men, a lean build may be prized in order to emphasize musculature, reduce fat stores in breast tissue or hips, or to induce amenorrhea. On the other hand, some trans men recognize that obese males have gynecomastia and therefore such a build can support their appearance as male. Trans women may want to lose weight due to cultural pressures to be thin, to minimize muscle bulk or to fit better into women's clothing. Consultation with a registered dietician on these matters can help with identifying realistic goals and healthier behaviors.

As well, hormone interventions of both kinds have weight gain, hypertension, lipid abnormalities and Type II diabetes as potential conse-

quences so dietary interventions to prevent or manage these disorders may be advised.

Surgeons often have obesity limits for their patients in order to optimize the outcome of the intervention and minimize risk associated with the surgery and the anaesthesia. These guidelines may be more strict for surgeons operating at private plastic surgery centers compared to those operating at hospitals. It can be a frustrating experience for a patient to meet other criteria, but be limited by weight issues. Obese patients unable to lose sufficient weight with diet modification and exercise should be evaluated for possible bariatric interventions.

*Tom is a trans man who has begun testosterone therapy, which has been very helpful in relieving his gender dysphoria, but has led to significant weight gain, especially in his abdomen. He is referred to Allison, a dietician working on his primary care team. Allison works with Tom to examine his dietary patterns and to plan for some reasonable goals to work on, including increasing his level of physical activity. Tom reports that he had previously enjoyed going to the gym, but has felt awkward doing so since he has begun to appear more masculine, and has developed anxiety about change rooms.*

## The Occupational Health or Vocational Professional

Work issues come up frequently in transgender care. The interventions sought to relieve gender dysphoria, especially surgical interventions, are expensive and, unfortunately, often not covered by public or private health insurance (see below). As such earning enough money to cover living expenses as well as save for the future is a high priority for many. This goal can be undermined by the experience of discrimination in job interviews or the workplace. A vocational therapist can be very helpful in helping an unemployed transgender patient manage the challenges of finding work.

Professionals in a workplace's occupational health department can play a crucial and highly valued role in supporting their transgender employees by initiating educational interventions for colleagues and liaison with human resource professionals to ensure trans-positive workplace policies. It is important to recognize that working in the preferred gender role can be a component of *treatment* for gender dysphoria. For some individuals a social transition to the preferred gender role may be sufficient for relief of their distress. For many others who eventually seek genital surgery, a "full time, continuous, gender role experience" of at least 1 year is considered a minimal requirement for proceeding (WPATH Standards of Care, version 7: [1]). Documentation of this gender role experience from employers may be required by the patient seeking genital surgery, which may take the form of a brief letter indicating the employee presents to work in the preferred gender role and is addressed by their preferred name.

*Dora is an occupational therapist in the employee health office of an automobile manufacturing company. She is approached by a human resources officer about Sandy, who has informed the company she plans to present as female to the workplace after she gets back from a brief leave of absence. Dora invites Sandy to come in for a visit with her to plan for a smooth workplace transition.*

## The Insurance or Benefits Professional

Coverage of transition related medications and procedures is an ongoing challenge for transgender individuals. In the United States, many transgender people were denied *basic* health insurance based solely on being transgender, a practice now illegal under the Affordable Care Act. Even in countries that have publicly funded health insurance, like Canada, coverage can be vulnerable to political whims, as when coverage for gender reassignment surgery was delisted as a benefit in Ontario between 1998 and 2008 [32].

However, many employers now provide insurance coverage for transgender health and a recent report from the Williams Institute indicates that they can do so at little to no cost [33]. Transgender

inclusion in health insurance plans is also the subject of ongoing advocacy [34]. Insurance and benefits professionals can be a part of an interdisciplinary health team by examining their policies and supporting change toward greater transgender inclusion.

One area that is important to consider in this regard is the issue of cosmetic versus medically necessary procedures. Policies sometimes are restrictive with respect to procedures traditionally associated with cosmesis, such as electrolysis or chest/breast reconstruction procedures. It is important to recognize that when the medical goal is relief of gender dysphoria, then these procedures are indeed medically necessary.

Additionally, policy restrictions on travel outside of state, provincial or national jurisdictions for care should be modified for these procedures as the number of medical professionals who perform these procedures (especially the genital operations) are relatively few.

## Program Models of Interdisciplinary Teams

Because of the inherently interdisciplinary nature of transgender care, programs that emphasize the interdisciplinary team should be the gold standard of care. Patients should not be left with the burden of coordinating their care and convincing the various health professionals involved to communicate with each other.

There are several North American models of such care:

The University of California San Francisco (UCSF) Center of Excellence for Transgender Care is an interdisciplinary service where clinical coordination of care between medical, surgical and mental health services is modeled, and other advocacy and support services are readily available.
http://transhealth.ucsf.edu/

The Mazzoni Center in Philadelphia similarly offers clinical, mental health and support services for transgender individuals in a coordinated fashion.
http://mazzonicenter.org

The Sherbourne Health Centre in Toronto, Ontario, has been an innovator in the field of LGBT and particularly transgender health. It also has adapted a widely available interdisciplinary care model available in the Ontario called the Family Health Team (FHT) to the purposes of better coordinated transgender health [5].

http://sherbourne.on.ca/lgbt-health/health-services/

http://www.health.gov.on.ca/en/pro/programs/fht/

## Summary

Transgender care can be complex because issues of assessment, treatment and support necessarily cross the areas of expertise of different health care providers. Thus an interdisciplinary team, that is, a team made up of providers of different disciplines who also communicate well with each other, can make a tremendous difference to an individuals patient care experience and outcome. This chapter described a basic approach to engaging the transgender patient in care and explored types of distress associated with the transgender experience. The composition of an interdisciplinary team and the roles of team members was outlined, though an exhaustive list might include some members left out here for brevity's sake.

While work in this area can be challenging, it also has great rewards in being able to help an individual alleviate distress and improve their quality of life. It is also brings the great pleasure of working with talented colleagues.

## References

1. Coleman E, Bockting W, Botzer M, Cohen-Kettenis P, DeCuypere G, Feldman J, Fraser L, Green J, Knudson G, Meyer WJ, Monstrey S, Adler RK, Brown GR, Devor AH, Ehrbar R, Ettner R, Eyler E, Garofalo R, Karasic DH, Lev AI, Mayer G, Meyer-Bahlburg H, Hall BP, Pfäfflin F, Rachlin K, Robinson B, Schechter LS, Tangpricha V, van Trotsenburg M, Vitale A, Winter S, Whittle S, Wylie KR, Zucker K. Standards of care for the health of transsexual, transgender, and gender-nonconforming people, version 7. Int J Transgend. 2011;13:165–232.

2. Hembree WC, Cohen-Kettenis P, Delemarre-van de Waal HA, Gooren LJ, Meyer 3rd WJ, Spack NP, Tangpricha V, Montori VM. Endocrine treatment of transsexuals persons: an Endocrine Society clinical practice guideline. J Clin Endocrinol Metab. 2009;94:3132–54.

3. Royal College of Psychiatrists. Good practice guidelines for the assessment and treatment of adults with gender dysphoria; 2013. http://www.rcpsych.ac.uk/publications/collegereports.aspx

4. Momsen AM, Rasmussen JO, Nielsen CV, Iversen MD, Lund H. Multidisciplinary team care in rehabilitation: an overview of reviews. J Rehabil Med. 2012;44:901–12.

5. Rosser WW, Colwill JM, Kasperski J, Wilson L. Progress of Ontario's Family Health Team Model: A Patient-Centered Medical Home. Ann Fam Med. 2011;9:165–71.

6. Tinetti ME. Preventing falls in elderly persons. N Engl J Med. 2003;348(1):42–9.

7. Craven MA, Bland R. Better practices in collaborative mental health care: an analysis of the evidence base. Can J Psychiatry. 2006;51 Suppl 1:1S–72S.

8. Meadows GN, Harvey CA, Joubert L, Barton D, Bedi G. Best practices: the consultation–liaison in primary-care psychiatry program: a structured approach to long-term collaboration. Psychiatr Serv. 2007;58:1036–8.

9. Rubin AS, Littenberg B, Ross R, Wehry S, Jones M. Effects on processes and costs of care associated with the addition of an internist to an inpatient psychiatry team. Psychiatr Serv. 2005;56:463–7.

10. Langer SJ. Gender (dis)agreement: a dialogue on the clinical implications of gendered language. J Gay Lesbian Ment Health. 2011;15:300–7.

11. Feldman J, Spencer K. Gender dysphoria in a 39-year-old man. CMAJ. 2014;186:49–50.

12. American Psychiatric Association. Diagnostic and statistical manual of mental disorders. 5th ed. Arlington, VA: American Psychiatric Publishing; 2013.

13. Meyer IH. Prejudice, social stress, and mental health in lesbian, gay, and bisexual populations: conceptual issues and research evidence. Psychol Bull. 2003;129:674–97.

14. Garnets LD, Herek GM, Levy B. Violence and victimization of lesbians and gay men: mental health consequences. J Interpers Violence. 1990;5:366–83.

15. Crocker J. Social stigma and self-esteem: situational construction of self-worth. J Exp Soc Psychol. 1999;35:89–107.

16. Steele CM. A threat in the air: how stereotypes shape intellectual identity and performance. Am Psychol. 1997;52:613–29.

17. Meyer IH, Dean L. Internalized homophobia, intimacy, and sexual behavior among gay and bisexual men. In: Herek GM, editor. Stigma and sexual orien-

tation: understanding prejudice against lesbians, gay men, and bisexuals. Thousand Oaks, CA: Sage; 1998.

18. Hill DB, Willoughby BLB. The development and validation of the genderism and transphobia scale. Sex Roles. 2005;53:531–44.

19. Cochran SD, Mays VM. Lifetime prevalence of suicide symptoms and affective disorders among men reporting same-sex sexual partners: results from NHANES III. Am J Public Health. 2000;90:573–8.

20. Drescher J. I'm Your Handyman: a history of reparative therapies. J Homosex. 1998;36(1):19–42.

21. Beemer BR. Gender dysphoria update. J Psychosoc Nurs Ment Health Serv. 1996;34:12–9.

22. McIntosh CA. Psychotherapy and transgender and transsexual people: bridging the gap. Workshop presented at Annual Meeting of GLMA. San Juan, Puerto Rico; 2007.

23. Fraser L. Depth psychotherapy with transgender people. Sex Relatsh Ther. 2009;24:126–42.

24. Follins L, Walker J, Lewis MK. Resilience in Black lesbian, gay, bisexual, and transgender individuals: a critical review of the literature. J Gay Lesbian Ment Health. 2014;18:190–212.

25. Testa RJ, Jimenez CL, Rankin S. Risk and resilience during transgender identity development: the effects of awareness and engagement with other transgender people on affect. J Gay Lesbian Ment Health. 2014;18:31–46.

26. Koken JA, Bimbi DS, Parsons JT. Experiences of familial acceptance and rejection among transwomen of color. J Fam Psychol. 2009;23(6):853–60.

27. Singh AA, McKleroy VS. "Just getting out of bed is a revolutionary act": the resilience of transgender people of color who have survived traumatic life events. Traumatology. 2011;17:34–44.

28. Golub SA, Walker JJ, Longmire-Avital B, Bimbi DS, Parsons JT. The role of religiosity, social support, and stress-related growth in protecting against HIV risk among transgender women. J Health Psychol. 2010;15:1135–44.

29. Spicer SS. Healthcare needs of the transgender homeless population. J Gay Lesbian Ment Health. 2010;14:320–39.

30. Hamblin RJ, Gross AM. Religious faith, homosexuality and psychological well-being: a theoretical and empirical review. J Gay Lesbian Ment Health. 2014;18:67–82.

31. Vocks S, Stahn C, Loenser L, Tegenbauer U. Eating and body image disturbances in male-to-female and female-to-male transsexuals. Arch Sex Behav. 2009;38(3):364–77.

32. Ajandi J. Neoconservativism and health care: access and equity for people who are transgender, two-spirit, and intersex. J Res Women Gender [Digital Journal]. Accessed at: https://digital.library.txstate.edu/handle/10877/4429

33. Herman JL. Costs and benefits of providing transition-related health care coverage in employee health benefit plans: findings from a survey of employers. Los Angeles, CA: The Williams Institute; 2013. http://williamsinstitute.law.ucla.edu/research/transgender-issues/costs-benefits-providing-transition-related-health-care-coverage-herman-2013/.

34. Transgender Law Center. Organizing for transgender health care. San Francisco, CA; 2012. http://transgenderlawcenter.org/issues/health/orgguide

# Medical Transition for Transgender Individuals

# 19

Asa E. Radix

## Purpose

The purpose of this chapter is to provide an overview of medical transition (feminizing and masculinizing regimens) for transgender individuals

## Learning Objectives

- Describe the terminology, process, and consent challenges for cross-gender hormone therapy *(KP1, KP3, KP5, PC3, PC6)*
- Discuss the physiological changes, time frame associated with hormonal transition, and potential adverse outcomes *(PC4, PC6)*
- Define the appropriate clinical and laboratory monitoring while on transition regimens *(PC6)*
- Identify at least 3 insurance/reimbursement concerns and other structural barriers for medical transition *(SBP1, SBP4, SBP6)*

## Terminology

*Transition* refers to the process of affirming a gender identity that is different from the birth-assigned gender role. For some individuals this may be a social transition, involving changes in gender roles and expression without the need to medically feminize or masculinize their bodies. For others however transition includes the use of cross-gender hormone therapy and/or surgical procedures that fall under the umbrella of gender confirming surgeries [1].

*Social transition* may include items such as changing names, pronouns and appearance to align with the affirmed gender. Non-medical interventions for transgender men may include "binding" or compressing the breasts, and "packing" material in the groin area to create a more masculine appearance. For transgender women, non-medical interventions may include pushing the testicles into the inguinal canal area and placing the penis between the legs, held in place by tape or tight underwear, a process known as "tucking".

*Medical transition* is the use of cross-gender hormone therapy to induce the secondary sex characteristics of the affirmed gender while suppressing those of the natal sex. For transgender men this usually requires the use of testosterone. For transgender women, combinations of estrogens and androgen blockers are typically used. Although hormones have been used for medical

A.E. Radix, M.D., M.P.H. (✉)
Callen-Lorde Community Health Center,
356 West 18th Street, New York, NY 10011, USA
e-mail: aradix@callen-lorde.org

© Springer International Publishing Switzerland 2016
K.L. Eckstrand, J.M. Ehrenfeld (eds.), *Lesbian, Gay, Bisexual, and Transgender Healthcare*,
DOI 10.1007/978-3-319-19752-4_19

**Table 19.1** Surgical transition procedures

| Feminizing procedures | Masculinizing procedures |
|---|---|
| Hormones (estrogen) | Hormones (testosterone) |
| Androgen blockers | Androgen blockers |
| Breast augmentation | Chest masculinization |
| Vaginoplasty | Hysterectomy |
| Labiaplasty | Salpingo-oophorectomy |
| Orchiectomy | Phalloplasty |
| Tracheal shave | Metoidioplasty |
| Facial bone reduction | Vaginectomy |
| Rhinoplasty | Scrotoplasty |
| | Urethroplasty |
| | Testicular prostheses |

transition for over seven decades, these are considered "off label" use in the USA.

*Surgical transition* refers to a wide array of surgical procedures (Table 19.1). The most common surgery undertaken by transgender men is mastectomy, also known as "top surgery". Genital surgery ("bottom surgery") for transgender men includes creation of a phallus (phalloplasty or metoidioplasty) as well as hysterectomy and oophorectomy. Transgender women may undergo breast augmentation, facial feminization as well as genital surgery to create a neovagina using penile tissue (penile inversion vaginoplasty) or resected sigmoid colon tissue (colo-vaginoplasty).

## Barriers to Care

A recent national survey demonstrated that people of transgender experience are less likely to utilize both preventive and emergency medical care [2]. Reasons include high rates of discrimination in health care settings, including being denied care, being less likely to have medical insurance or afford care and encountering medical providers who are not knowledgeable about their unique health issues. The lack of gender appropriate identification may also limit access to medical services.

In the USA, transition-related health care is often excluded from commercial health insurance plans and Medicaid, the nation's largest public health plan for over 57 million low income persons [3, 4]. Transition related health costs were not tax deductible until 2010 as they were

deemed cosmetic procedures and not medically necessary [5]. A white paper produced by the Human Rights Campaign Foundation researched organizations that voluntarily completed questionnaires for the Corporate Equality Index. The Foundation identified only 206 private sector employers and 5 public entities (University of California and the University of Michigan, the cities of Minneapolis, New York, and San Francisco) that offer transition inclusive coverage [6]. A needs analysis among transgender persons revealed that 47 % were uninsured [7], much higher than the national average, and highlighted the difficulty both insured and uninsured participants had accessing health care services.

The U.S. Department of State changed their policy in 2011 allowing gender marker changes on passports without the need for surgical interventions. Medical providers can assist their transgender patients with obtaining vital gender appropriate and affirming identity documents, thereby improving access to health care, education and job opportunities. The medical provider need only confirm that the client has received appropriate clinical treatment for gender transition.

> **Helpful Hint**
> There are resources available to assist your clients locating trans-inclusive health insurance plans.
> https://www.hrc.org/resources/entry/finding-insurance-for-transgender-related-healthcare

## Utilization of Transition-Related Health Services

In a recent Behavioral Risk Factor Surveillance System survey conducted in Massachusetts, addition of a question on gender identity allowed researchers to estimate the prevalence of being transgender at 0.5 % [8], a far greater prevalence than previous studies that determined transgender identity based on undergoing surgical transition.

Community based surveys determine that over 60 % of transgender persons have taken cross-sex hormones [2], with highest rates among transgender women and those over age 50, however many transgender and gender nonconforming persons (up to 41 % of natal females) do not plan to initiate hormones [9].

> **Helpful Hint**
> Transgender people may not wish to undergo medical or surgical transition—be careful not to make assumptions

## Standards of Care for Medical Transition

Provision of cross-sex hormone therapy in the USA and other countries has usually followed the standards of care, first published by the Harry Benjamin International Gender Dysphoria Association (HBIGDA) in 1979 and its subsequent revisions. HBIGDA, now renamed The World Professional Association for Transgender Health (WPATH), recently released its seventh version of the Standards of Care for the Health of Transsexual, Transgender, and Gender Nonconforming People [1].

Early versions of the standards of care required a mental health evaluation to determine eligibility and readiness of transgender clients to initiate cross-sex hormones. In some instances family members were interviewed to verify that the client had gender dysphoria [10–12]. The process of transition was termed "triadic therapy" and required a period of "real life experience" and psychotherapy before proceeding to hormones and surgery. After a period of evaluation the mental health professional would provide a letter that stated the individual had met the eligibility criteria and could proceed with medical interventions. This letter became the necessary pathway for many transgender persons to access hormonal transition.

The requirements for psychotherapy presented particular challenges for transgender persons in the United States, especially for those who were uninsured and of limited income. Healthcare providers and advocates were also increasingly critical of the restrictive guidelines, stating that it negatively impacted on patient autonomy and held transgender patients to a different standard than non-transgender clients, even for comparable irreversible procedures [13].

The most recent version of the standards of care (WPATH version 7) allows for a more individualized and flexible approach to medical transition and has no mandatory eligibility or readiness criteria. These changes reflect new knowledge such as evidence highlighting positive clinical outcomes and low rates of adverse effects, including regret [1, 14].

## The Informed Consent Model

During the 1990s, several health centers and health care professionals in the United States, including the Callen-Lorde Community Health Center in New York City and Howard Brown Health Center in Chicago, questioned the need for the psychotherapy and the mental health letter before accessing cross-sex hormones. The centers believed that transgender identity was not pathological and that requirements for mental health evaluation and eligibility letters were unnecessary and created barriers to care. Policies that historically limited hormones and other medical therapies to those determined to be "real" transsexuals often resulted on patients employing autobiographical narratives that conformed to the heteronormative and gender binary biases of their healthcare providers [15]. Medical providers were justifiably concerned that these stringent requirements for mental health assessments could result in clients adjusting their stories to meet the eligibility and readiness criteria, an issue that has recently been described in the literature [16]. The philosophy of the informed consent model was based on patient autonomy, self-determination, informed decision making and harm reduction. Instead of a mental health provider determining eligibility for medical transition, the primary care provider is responsible for screening clients for serious mental and medical concerns and discussion the known risks and benefits of treatment.

If the client is able to make an informed decision regarding the treatment plan, then cross-sex hormone therapy is initiated. The informed consent model integrates transgender care firmly into a primary care and health promotion model instead of in a mental health framework.

The authors of the recently published WPATH standards of care specifically addressed the informed consent models implemented by Callen-Lorde and other centers such as The Fenway Health Center and The Tom Waddell Health Center. They stated that despite a greater emphasis on the roles of mental health providers in the standards of care, the informed consent models are "consistent with" the current version of the SOC. Furthermore, they acknowledge that although a mental health screening is indicated, psychotherapy is not an absolute requirement for hormones, and furthermore recognize that for some this may be an unnecessary hurdle [1].

## DSM-5

The conceptualization of gender identity has changed over time, with a move towards depathologization of transgender identity. The newly released Diagnostic and Statistical Manual of Mental Disorders, Fifth Edition (DSM-5) [17] that replaced the diagnosis of gender identity disorder with that of gender dysphoria, supported the concept that transgender identification could be regarded as part of human diversity without an automatic need for psychotherapeutic intervention.

## Adult and Adolescent Guidelines

The guidelines for medical transition usually differentiate between treatment of adolescents and adults [1, 18]. Medical transition for adolescents usually requires a team approach consisting of experienced psychotherapists, endocrinologists and pediatricians or adolescent specialists. Going through puberty may cause extreme suffering for the transgender adolescent. Treatment is initiated with puberty-suppressing medications, usually a gonadotropin releasing hormone (GnRH) analogue, e.g., leuprolide acetate, no sooner than Tanner stages 2–3 [18]. This has additional advantages of preventing the irreversible secondary sex characteristics of the natal sex to develop (e.g., beard growth and deepening of the voice in natal males and breast growth in natal females), making it easier for transgender youth to present socially in the affirmed gender. The treatment is also fully reversible, and puberty will resume if the puberty-suppressing medications are discontinued. When on treatment, close anthropometric monitoring, as well as evaluations of bone age, bone density and hormone levels are required. At approximately age 16, cross-sex hormone therapy can be initiated. Due to the complex medico-legal and psychological concerns regarding treatment of transgender adolescents, medical providers should seek assistance of clinical experts in this field. The discussion of medical transition below refers to hormone therapy for adults.

## Initiating Hormones

The goal of medical transition is to induce the secondary sex characteristics of the affirmed sex. This is done through a combination of reducing the endogenous hormone levels of the natal (genetic) sex and by replacing with those of the reassigned sex (see Fig. 19.1) [18].

## The Medical Intake

During the medical intake the medical provider should assess the transgender client for any medical conditions that may be exacerbated by the initiation of cross-sex hormones and evaluate their ability to make an informed decision about medical treatment.

- The medical history, ask about:
  - Coronary artery disease
  - Cerebrovascular disease
  - Hormone-related cancers, e.g. breast, uterine
  - Hepatitis
  - Thromboembolic disease

**Fig. 19.1**
Hypothalamic-
pituitary-gonadal (HPG)
axis (Source:
K. Eckstrand)

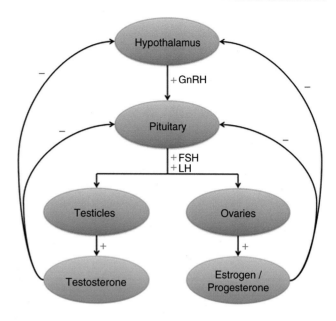

- Gallstones
- Erythrocytosis
- Migraine headaches
- Depression, anxiety, or psychosis
- Alcohol, tobacco, and other drug use
  (The presence of hormonally responsive cancers and/or active thromboembolic disease are considered contraindications to initiation of cross-sex hormones. Re-evaluate after the condition has stabilized).
• The physical exam should evaluate for the conditions noted above.
• Baseline laboratory testing:
  - Complete blood count
  - Lipid profile
  - Basic metabolic panel: BUN, creatinine, electrolytes
  - Prolactin level (for transgender women already on hormones)
  - Screening for HIV and sexually transmitted diseases
• Mental Health and Informed consent
  - Identify mental health issues that may negatively impact initiation of hormones
  - Discuss risks and benefits of hormonal regimens and confirm patient can provide informed consent to treatment
  - Discuss fertility and reproductive health (cross-sex hormones may negatively impact

fertility). Clients should be given advice about options, including cryopreservation of ova, and semen storage. Contraceptive needs should be discussed with transgender men.
  - Assess that the patient's goals and understanding of cross-sex hormone therapy matches the general nature and purpose of treatment
  - Assess and provide psychosocial support and referrals as needed
  - Explore patients' social transition needs such as peer support, psychotherapy, documentation needs e.g., identification documents

**Helpful Hint**
Transgender men who have sex with men should be counseled about the possibility of pregnancy when on testosterone. Discuss contraceptive options including condoms, depot-medroxyprogesterone acetate (DMPA) and Intrauterine Devices (IUDs).

**Documentation**
Many programs have created consent forms for clients to sign before initiating cross-sex hormones that lists all potential complications of

treatment. Regardless of whether a form is used, the medical provider should fully document all discussions held during the visit.

## Initiation of Cross-Sex Hormones (Feminizing Regimens)

For feminizing regimens, most published guidelines recommend a combination of estrogen with androgen blockers [1, 18]. Estrogen can be taken in different forms, including 17-beta-estradiol (transdermal, oral or intramuscular preparations). Conjugated equine estrogen and ethinyl estradiol (the main constituent in combined oral contraceptive pills) were previously used in feminizing regimens, however these are now discouraged due to increased risk of venous thromboembolism [19]. The androgen blocker used most frequently in the USA is spironolactone, however in Europe cyproterone acetate is predominantly used.

Transgender clients may obtain their hormones via the internet or through friends (so called "black market" or "street" hormones) and have access to drugs not commonly found in the USA. They may be unaware of correct dosing, potential drug interactions and adverse effects. A full inventory of all medications taken should be obtained during the intake.

Many guidelines allow for a range of estrogen to be used, e.g., for oral estradiol (Estrace®) a usual range of 2 mg/day to 6 mg/day is used. For intramuscular use e.g., estradiol valerate (Delestrogen®), the usual range is 5–20 mg im every 2 weeks (or 2–10 mg im every week). Spironolactone is usually dosed at 100–200 mg per day, however doses up to 300 mg per day may be used (Table 19.2).

**Initial Dosing**
- Initiate the lowest doses of estrogen and spironolactone with evaluation in 4 weeks. At this time the dose can be increased to the maintenance (average) dose.

**Follow-Up**
- Patients should be evaluated every 2–3 months in the first year and then every 6 months to monitor for adverse effects.
- If spironolactone is used as the androgen blocker, close attention should be paid to electrolytes (potassium) and blood pressure (assess for hypotension)
- Serum testosterone and estrogen levels should be maintained in the average female range (serum testosterone <55 ng/dl, serum estradiol 200 pg/ml). Measure levels every 3 months until stable
- Serum prolactin should be monitored once each year

**Effects of Therapy**
- Breast development starts within 3 months with maximum effect in 3 years
- Slowing of androgenic hair loss
- Fat redistribution (smaller waist, wider hips) starts within 3 months with full effect by 3 years

**Table 19.2** Feminizing regimens

|  | Starting dose | Average dose | Maximum dose |
|---|---|---|---|
| Estrogens |  |  |  |
| Estradiol oral | 2 mg/day | 4 mg/day | 8 mg/day |
| Estradiol valerate intramuscular | 5 mg IM every 2 week | 20 mg IM every 2 weeks | 20 mg IM every 2 weeks |
| Estradiol patch (preferred over age 45) | 25 mcg/day | 100 mcg/day | 200 mcg/day |
| Conjugated Estrogen Not recommended | 1.25–2.5 mg/day | 5 mg/day | 5 mg/day |
| Ethinyl estradiol Not recommended |  |  |  |
| Androgen blockers |  |  |  |
| Spironolactone oral | 50 mg/day | 200–300 mg/day | 400 mg/day |
| Finasteride oral | 1 mg/day | 1–5 mg/day | 5 mg/day |

Adapted from the Callen-Lorde Transgender Health Protocols, 2013

- Testicular atrophy starts within 3 months
- Decrease in erections starts within 3 months
- Reduction in muscle mass starts within 3 months
- No effect on voice pitch
- No effect on beard hair—electrolysis may be required

**After Orchiectomy**
- Lower doses of estrogens are recommended, usually half of the dose used before surgery.
- Anti-androgens (spironolactone) can be stopped.
- Clients may wish to continue dihydrotestosterone blockers if androgenic hair loss continues.

**HIV Infection**
- HIV disease is not a contraindication to feminizing hormone therapy. In fact, hormone therapy may improve engagement and retention in care [20]. There are no specific data on interactions between the doses of estrogens commonly used in feminizing regimens and antiretroviral regimens. Most of the available data is based on studies with oral contraceptives (ethinyl estradiol). Metabolism of estrogens occurs via the cytochrome P450 enzyme system, thus potential drug–drug interactions may exist between estrogens and Non-nucleoside reverse transcriptase inhibitors (NNRTIs) and the Protease inhibitors (PIs). Most boosted PIs decrease ethinyl estradiol levels. The effects of Non-nucleosides vary, e.g. nevirapine decreases estrogen levels, etravirine and rilpvirine increase ethinyl estradiol levels, whereas efavirenz appears to have no effect on levels. There are no known drug-drug interactions between ethinyl estradiol and the antiretroviral classes of NRTIs/NtRTIs, integrase inhibtors, CCR5 antagonists or fusion inhibitors. DHHS recommends that oral contraceptives and unboosted amprenavir (or fosamprenavir) not be co-administered due to a decrease in amprenavir serum concentrations; therefore, unboosted fosamprenavir should probably be avoided with estrogens in feminizing regimens. Consider monitoring estradiol levels when initiating or changing anti-retroviral therapy.

**Helpful Hint**
Although Finasteride is not very effective as an androgen blocker, it may be used if spironolactone is not tolerated or used together with spironolactone to slow androgenic hair loss

**Table 19.3** Masculinizing Regimens

| Hormone | Starting dose | Average dose | Maximum dose |
|---------|---------------|--------------|--------------|
| Testosterone (cypionate or enanthate) intramuscular | 100 mg every 2 weeks Or 50 mg every week IM | 200 mg every 2 weeks Or 100 mg every week IM | 200 mg every 2 weeks Or 100 mg every week IM |
| Transdermal Testosterone gel 1 % | 2.5 g daily | 5–10 g daily | 10 g daily |
| Testosterone patch | 2.5 mg/daily | 5 mg/daily | 7.5 mg/daily |

Adapted from the Callen-Lorde Transgender Health Protocols, 2013

## Initiation of Cross-Sex Hormones (Masculinizing Regimens)

Testosterone therapy is used for masculinization [1, 18]. Testosterone can be taken in different forms, including transdermal, oral or intramuscular preparations (Table 19.3).

### Initial Dosing
- Initiate the lowest dose of testosterone with evaluation in 4 weeks. At this time the dose can be titrated to the maintenance (average) dose
- Testosterone cypionate is usually suspended in cottonseed oil while Testosterone enanthate is suspended in sesame oil; enquire about allergies before initiating treatment

### Follow-Up
- Patients should be evaluated every 2–3 months in the first year and then every 6 months to monitor for adverse effects.
- Close attention should be paid to lipids and hemoglobin. For clients receiving oral testosterone, the liver (transaminases) should be closely monitored.
- Serum testosterone should be maintained in the average male range. Serum testosterone goal is 320–1000 ng/dL. Measure levels every 3 months until stable
- Measure serum testosterone level half-way between injections

### Effects of Therapy
- Acne and oily skin starts 1–6 months, usually resolved within 2 years
- Facial hair starts in 6–12 months
- Fat redistribution starts 1–6 months
- Menses cease within 2–6 months

- Vaginal atrophy 3–6 months
- Deepening of the voice within 6–12 months

## Adverse Effects of Cross-Sex Hormone Regimens

Cross-sex hormone therapy is usually well tolerated and has a low risk of adverse events.

### Cancer
Both short and long term follow-up of transgender persons receiving cross gender hormones demonstrate that there appear to be no increase in cancer outcomes, including breast, uterus or prostate cancer [14, 21–23]. Prostate cancer may be more aggressive when diagnosed in transgender women who have taken cross-sex hormones and androgen blockers, however data are limited. The PSA level is low when on androgen blockers and is not very useful for monitoring.

### Cardiovascular Risk
Several studies have shown that cardiovascular and cerebrovascular mortality is increased, particularly among transgender women on hormones [21, 24, 25]. The studies were not adjusted for risk factors (such as tobacco use and HIV) that are highly prevalence in this population. Ethinyl estradiol and conjugated equine estrogens are associated with higher rates of cardiovascular disease and are no longer recommended. Clients should be counseled about the risks of tobacco use and smoking cessation prioritized. Close monitoring and treatment of traditional risk factors, e.g., hyperlipidemia and hypertension. Transdermal estrogens may convey a lower risk of cardiovascular disease and are the preferred route for older clients or those with elevated cardiovascular risk.

## Venous Thromboembolism

Estrogen is a risk factor for venous thromboembolism, especially oral ethinyl estradiol. For women at increased risk e.g., due to mobility issues or tobacco use, transdermal estrogen is preferred.

## Hyperlipidemia

High triglycerides have been seen in transgender persons receiving testosterone or estrogen. Transgender men may experience a lowering of the HDL cholesterol [26].

## Erythrocytosis / Polycythemia

Elevated hematocrits have been seen in transgender men receiving testosterone, thus levels should be monitored at least every 6 months. The testosterone dose should be decreased or discontinued if the hematocrit increases above 50 %. Therapeutic phlebotomy has also been used to treat this condition however there are no guidelines for when and how often to perform phlebotomy. The usual goal is a hematocrit of 45 %.

## Skin

Testosterone increases skin oiliness and acne in transgender men, especially in the first year. Mild fronto-temporal androgenic hair loss may also occur with long term testosterone use [27].

## Hyperprolactinemia and Prolactinomas

Prolactin levels usually increase in transgender women receiving estrogen. Prolactin levels should be monitored at least yearly as there have been reports of prolactinomas occurring after long-term estrogen use. Serum prolactin levels over 50 ng/mL are uncommon and usually respond to reducing the estrogen. If persistent elevations occur, the possibility of a prolactinoma should be considered

## Ostoepenia and Osteoporosis

Bone density appears to be preserved in transgender men receiving testosterone, however transgender women have a higher prevalence of osteopenia, even before initiating hormones [28, 29]. The endocrine society guidelines recommend screening those at average risk starting at age 60. For those who have undergone gonadectomy (orchiectomy or oophorectomy), there is a high risk of osteoporosis if cross-sex hormones are discontinued [18].

## Cancer Screening

Transgender individuals should continue cancer screening following standard guidelines for their natal sex if organs exist.

## Breast and Cervical Cancer Screening

Transgender men who have a cervix should follow cervical cancer screening guidelines for natal females. Breast cancer screening should continue for those who have not undergone mastectomy. For those who have undergone mastectomy, the potential still exists for breast cancer occurring in remaining breast tissue. In addition, aromatization of testosterone to estrogen occurs and may be a risk for estrogen-receptor positive breast cancer. A recent study has revealed a lower risk of breast cancer among transgender men who have undergone mastectomy, in line with that for natal men [22]. Guidelines however still recommend that breast cancer screening continue as per natal females [30].

Although the risk of breast cancer does not appear to be elevated in transgender women with a history of estrogen therapy compared with natal males [22], some guidelines recommend following breast cancer screening recommendations for natal women due to concerns about long term estrogen use [18, 30].

There is no established role for cervical cancer screening in transgender women who have undergone vaginoplasty procedures, however annual visual inspection of the neovagina is recommended to evaluate for other issues, for example genital warts or ulcers.

Screening for other cancers, e.g. lung and colon, remain the same as for non-transgender persons.

---

**Helpful Hint**
- The Prostate specific antigen level (PSA) is falsely low among transgender women receiving androgen blockers and therefore is not useful for screening
- After vaginoplasty, the prostate is examined by palpation of the anterior neovaginal wall

## Summary

This section provided an overview of medical transition (feminizing and masculinizing therapy) whereas the following section will focus on options for those who undergo surgical transition. The following on-line resources are available to provide further information on provision of culturally competent healthcare to clients of transgender experience.

## Appendix

### Resources for Transgender Care

- Callen-Lorde Community Health Center: http://www.callen-lorde.org
- Fenway Community Health: www.fenway-health.org
- Howard Brown Health Center: http://www.howardbrown.org/hb_services.asp?id=37
- University of Minnesota, Center for Sexual Health: http://www.phs.umn.edu/clinic/transgender/home.html
- Tom Waddell Health Center: www.sfdph.org/dph/comupg/oservices/medSvs/hlthCtrs/TransgenderHlthCtr.asp
- UCSF Center of Excellence for Transgender Care: http://transhealth.ucsf.edu/trans?page=protocol-00-00

## References

1. Coleman E, Bockting W, Botzer M. Standards of care for the health of transsexual, transgender, and gender-nonconforming people, version 7. Int J Transgend. 2011;13:165. 13 SRC – GoogleScholar.
2. Grant JM, Mottet LA, Tanis J. National Transgender Discrimination Survey Report on Health and Health Care. Washington, DC: National Center for Transgender Equality and the National Gay and Lesbian Task Force; 2010.
3. Lombardi E. Enhancing transgender health care. Am J Public Health. 2001;91(6):869–72.
4. Gehi P, Arkles G. Unraveling injustice: race and class impact of medicaid exclusions of transition-related health care for transgender people. Sex Res Soc Policy. 2007;4(4):7–35.
5. O'Donnabhain RG. Rhiannon G. O'Donnabhain, Petitioner v. Commissioner of Internal Revenue; 2010.
6. Fidas D, Green J, Wilson A. Transgender-inclusive health care coverage and the corporate equality index. Washington, DC: Human Rights Campaign Foundation; 2012.
7. Xavier JM et al. A needs assessment of transgendered people of color living in Washington, DC. Int J Transgend. 2005;8(2–3):31–47.
8. Conron KJ et al. Transgender health in Massachusetts: results from a household probability sample of adults. Am J Public Health. 2012;102(1):118–22.
9. Kuper LE, Nussbaum R, Mustanski B. Exploring the diversity of gender and sexual orientation identities in an online sample of transgender individuals. J Sex Res. 2012;49(2–3):244–54.
10. Walker PAB, Jack C, Green R, Laub DR, Reynolds CL, Wollman L. Standards of care: the hormonal and surgical sex reassignment of gender dysphoric persons. Arch Sex Behav. 1985;14(1):79–90.
11. Levine SB, Brown GB, Coleman E, Cohen-Kettenis P, Hage JJ, Van Maasdam J, Petersen M, Pfäfflin F, Schaefer L. Harry Benjamin International Gender Dysphoria Association's The standards of care for gender identity disorders. Int J Transgend. 1998;2(2). http://web.archive.org/web/20070502001025/http://www.symposion.com/ijt/ijtc0405.htm
12. Meyer W, Bocting W, Cohen-Kettenis P, Coleman E, DiCeglie D, Devor H, Gooren L, Hage JJ, Kirk S, Kuiper B, Laub D, Lawrence A, Menard Y, Monstrey S, Patton J, Schaefer L, Webb A, Wheeler C. The Harry Benjamin International Gender Dysphoria Association's Standards of Care for Gender Identity Disorders, Sixth Version. Int J Transgend. 2001;5(1). http://www.symposion.com/ijt/soc_2001/index.htm
13. Hale CJ. Ethical problems with the mental health evaluation standards of care for adult gender variant prospective patients. Perspect Biol Med. 2007; 50(4):491–505.
14. Gooren LJ, Giltay EJ, Bunck MC. Long-term treatment of transsexuals with cross-sex hormones: extensive personal experience. J Clin Endocrinol Metab. 2008;93(1):19–25.
15. Nieder TO, Richter-Appelt H. Tertium non datur – either/or reactions to transsexualism amongst health care professionals: the situation past and present, and its relevance to the future. Psychol Sex. 2011; 2(3):224–43.
16. Pimenoff V, Pfäfflin F. Transsexualism: treatment outcome of compliant and noncompliant patients. Int J Transgend. 2011;13(1):37–44.
17. American Psychiatric Association, A.P.A.D.S.M.T.F. Diagnostic and statistical manual of mental disorders: DSM-5. 2013; Available from: http://dsm.psychiatryonline.org/book.aspx?bookid=556
18. Hembree WC et al. Endocrine treatment of transsexual persons: an Endocrine Society clinical practice guideline. J Clin Endocrinol Metab. 2009;94(9): 3132–54.

19. Asscheman H et al. Venous thrombo-embolism as a complication of cross-sex hormone treatment of male-to-female transsexual subjects: a review. Andrologia. 2014;46(7):791–5.
20. Yehia BR et al. Retention in care and health outcomes of transgender persons living with HIV. Clin Infect Dis. 2013;57(5):774–6.
21. Asscheman H et al. A long-term follow-up study of mortality in transsexuals receiving treatment with cross-sex hormones. Eur J Endocrinol. 2011; 164(4):635–42.
22. Gooren LJ et al. Breast cancer development in transsexual subjects receiving cross-sex hormone treatment. J Sex Med. 2013;10(12):3129–34.
23. Gooren L, Morgentaler A. Prostate cancer incidence in orchidectomised male-to-female transsexual persons treated with oestrogens. Andrologia. 2014; 46(10):1156–60.
24. Dhejne C et al. Long-term follow-up of transsexual persons undergoing sex reassignment surgery: cohort study in Sweden. PLoS One. 2011;6(2), e16885.
25. Wierckx K et al. Prevalence of cardiovascular disease and cancer during cross-sex hormone therapy in a large cohort of trans persons: a case-control study. Eur J Endocrinol. 2013;169(4):471–8.
26. Elamin MB et al. Effect of sex steroid use on cardiovascular risk in transsexual individuals: a systematic review and meta-analyses. Clin Endocrinol (Oxf). 2010;72(1):1–10.
27. Wierckx K et al. Short- and long-term clinical skin effects of testosterone treatment in trans men. J Sex Med. 2014;11(1):222–9.
28. Van Caenegem E et al. Low bone mass is prevalent in male-to-female transsexual persons before the start of cross-sex hormonal therapy and gonadectomy. Bone. 2013;54(1):92–7.
29. Van Caenegem E et al. Bone mass, bone geometry, and body composition in female-to-male transsexual persons after long-term cross-sex hormonal therapy. J Clin Endocrinol Metab. 2012;97(7):2503–11.
30. Unger CA. Care of the transgender patient: the role of the gynecologist. Am J Obstet Gynecol. 2014; 210(1):16–26.

# Surgical Treatments for the Transgender Population

**20**

Randi Ettner

## Purpose

The purpose of this chapter is to provide an overview of the various surgical interventions in the treatment of gender dysphoria, and what constitutes appropriate use of these protocols.

## Learning Objectives

- Identify at least five historical and contemporary medical, legal, religious and ethical objections to gender-confirming surgeries *(KP4, SBP1, SBP4)*
- List the surgical procedures specific to male-to-female patients and female-to-male patients and define the criteria for providing surgical interventions *(PC3, PC4)*
- Discuss the role of surgery in supporting transgender individuals, process for accessing surgery, and possible complications of surgery *(PC3, PC5)*
- Identify at least three strategies for collaborating with medical and mental health providers for comprehensive health care before, during, and after surgical treatment *(Pr3, IPC1)*

R. Ettner, Ph.D. (✉)
New Health Foundation Worldwide,
1214 Lake Street, Evanston, IL 60201, USA
e-mail: rettner@aol.com

## Introduction to Gender Affirming Surgery

The first recorded description of a surgical attempt to change an individual's sex was reported in Germany, in 1931. But the agony of severe gender dysphoria was frequently relieved by earlier, crude surgical attempts which often amounted to mutilation [1].

Ancient people witnessed the castration of animals, and the subsequent cessation of masculinization. This process, when applied to human males, resulted in the creation of Eunuchs—known to exist since Biblical times [2]. While many Eunuchs were individuals who intentionally underwent castration to relieve gender dysphoria, others were boys, involuntarily castrated to preserve voice quality [3].

Modern surgical sex reassignment surgery (also known as gender-affirming surgery) began, in earnest, in the twentieth century. The surgical treatment of wounds, necessitated by the traumatic injuries sustained in World War I, led to significant advances in soft tissue reconstructive surgical techniques. The simultaneous discovery of the synthesis of sex steroid hormones allowed for the previously impossible acquisition of secondary sex characteristics [2]. This aggregation of hormones and surgery gave hope to those struggling with gender dysphoria.

© Springer International Publishing Switzerland 2016
K.L. Eckstrand, J.M. Ehrenfeld (eds.), *Lesbian, Gay, Bisexual, and Transgender Healthcare*,
DOI 10.1007/978-3-319-19752-4_20

## Controversies Surrounding Surgery

In 1953, media coverage of Christine Jorgensen's "sex-change surgery" captured the public's attention. While a few surgeons in Mexico, Casablanca, and South America were willing to perform reassignment surgery, most hospitals prohibited the procedure. Opposition to sex reassignment surgery arose rapidly, in tandem with Ms. Jorgenson's fame. The "Christine operation" generated legal controversies, religious opposition, and moral outrage. But it was the psychiatric community that was most vociferous in challenging the viability of surgery as a legitimate treatment [4].

## Ethical Objections to Surgery

Even as newly-formed gender clinics opened their doors to transsexual patients (in this chapter, the term transsexual applies to patients with gender dysphoria seeking gender-affirming surgeries), little was known about the condition they purported to treat. Many early opponents viewed sex reassignment surgery as "psychosurgery." Prominent psychiatrists claimed that the desire for surgery was a delusion, or a symptom of severe psychopathology. Some conceptualized it as a psychosis: "The transsexual is unconsciously motivated to discard bad and aggressive features and create in the fabric of the body a new idealized perfection" [5].

The inflammatory rhetoric of the debate escalated, and transsexualism was often conflated with homosexuality and transvestism. Sadly, many people with severe gender dysphoria requesting help were committed to mental institutions, where electroshock and aversion therapies were too often the default treatments [6].

Those surgeons who championed the therapeutic value of surgery were accused of removing healthy organs on the demand of a delusional patient, and threatened with legal consequences. The same year that Johns Hopkins opened its pioneer treatment program, 1966, saw an Argentinean surgeon convicted of assault for performing a "sex-change" operation [7]. One might presume that informed consent would constitute a better legal defense than that of therapeutic benefit. However, most courts held that informed consent was invalid if a patient was mentally incompetent. As the majority of professionals of that era believed that transsexual patients were suffering from psychopathology, the patient was viewed as incompetent in the eyes of the law. In 1978, a New York court deemed the operation "an experimental form of psychotherapy by which mutilating surgery is conducted on a person with the intent of setting his mind at ease" [7].

It was not only the medical and legal community that spoke out against surgical treatment for gender dysphoria. Negative public perception intensified as prominent individuals and religious spokespersons vigorously protested sex reassignment. Indeed, opposition arose from many sources. Janice Raymond, a cultural feminist, attacked the treatment on the grounds that it reinforced stereotypic gender roles and should be "morally mandated out of existence" [8]. Representatives of the Catholic Church insisted that chromosomes alone determine gender, and chromosomal composition remained unchanged after surgery.

By the late 1970s, many of the early gender clinics closed their doors, ceding to the myriad challenges and potential liability [4]. While it is standard surgical practice to remove diseased tissue and/or organs, or to alter structures to improve a patient's appearance, sex reassignment did not fit neatly into either category. Surgeons performing sex reassignment surgery were removing healthy tissue and altering normal structures. In some US states that constituted "mayhem"—a felony whereby one intentionally maims a person, rendering a body part useless [7].

## Financial Issues

With the advent of an evidence-based approach to medical treatment, a burgeoning body of research, and well-established standards of care, the scientific community advanced to endorse sex reassignment surgery as the appropriate and medically necessary treatment for intractable, severe gender dysphoria. But the question as to whether these surgeries are aesthetic or reconstructive is often still raised by third party payers.

Most cosmetic surgeries are not deemed medically necessary, and thus, are paid for by the patient. Reconstructive procedures, on the other hand, are considered medically necessary, and therefore paid, in part or full, by national health systems or insurance providers.

Genital surgery for affirmation purposes is reconstructive surgery. It is an intervention that relieves a medical condition, through removal of hormone-producing target organs. Nevertheless, there are still many insurers who regard these surgeries as "cosmetic" or "elective" and deny coverage.

The issue is more indeterminate in the case of non-genital gender-confirming surgeries. For instance, is surgical reduction of a prominent Adam's apple (chondrolaryngoplasty) in a male-to-female transperson a cosmetic procedure? If the cartilaginous structure is a telltale stigmata of masculinity, isn't surgical modification necessary to insure an authentic female presentation? The same rationale holds true for breast augmentation. Breast development—a visible secondary sex characteristic—confers a female-specific body profile that can be an essential component of gender transition. Most of these costly procedures however, are wholly dependent on the ability of the patient to finance them. The prohibitive expense of face and body surgery has led many desperate individuals to turn to high-risk alternatives, such as the injection of silicone and the engagement of disreputable providers.

## Gender-affirming Surgeries

Male-to-female (MTF) surgical procedures can include:

- Facial feminization surgeries, liposuction, lipofilling, voice surgery (thyroplasty), thyroid cartilage reduction (chrondrolaryngoplasty),

gluteal implants, and possibly other procedures (see also Chap. 21).
- Breast surgery: augmentation mammoplasty.
- Genital surgery: penectomy, orchiectomy, vaginoplasty, and clitoroplasty with reconstruction of the labia majora and minora [2].

Female-to-male (FTM) surgical procedures can include:

- Liposuction, lipofilling, pectoral implants, and possible other cosmetic procedures.
- Breast surgery: subcutaneous mastectomy
- Genital surgery: hysterectomy/oophorectomy, reconstruction of the urethra (sometimes performed with metaidoplasty or phalloplasty), vaginectomy, scrotoplasty, and implantation of testicular prosthesis and/or erectile prosthesis [9].

## Criteria for Providing Surgical Interventions

Medical governing bodies throughout the world, such as the World Health Organization, publish guidelines to protect consumers from undergoing operations that are experimental, useless, or generate unacceptably high rates of complications.

Three overarching conditions apply: First, and foremost, a surgical procedure must demonstrate a *therapeutic* effect [10]. Gender affirming surgeries meet this criterion. More than three decades of research confirms that gender affirming surgery is therapeutic, and an effective treatment for severe gender dysphoria. Indeed, while some transgender patients may not desire gender affirming surgery, surgery is the *only* effective treatment for others.

The therapeutic benefits of genital reconstruction are twofold: First, removal of the testicles eliminates the major source of testosterone in the body. Second, the patient attains body congruence resulting from normal appearing and functioning female genital and urinary structure.

In a 1998 meta-analysis, Pfafflin and Junge reviewed data from 80 studies, spanning 30 years, from 12 countries. They concluded that "reassignment procedures were effective in relieving gender dysphoria" [11]. Numerous subsequent studies confirm this conclusion. In 2007, Gijs and Brewayes analyzed 18 studies published between 1990 and 2007, encompassing 807 patients. The researchers concluded: "Summarizing the results from the 18 outcome studies of the last two decades, the conclusion that sex reassignment surgery is the most appropriate treatment to alleviate the suffering of extremely gender dysphoric individuals still stands: Ninety-six percent of the persons who underwent surgery were satisfied and regret was rare" [12].

Patient satisfaction is an important measure of effective treatment. Studies have shown that by relieving the suffering caused by severe gender dysphoria, virtually every aspect of a patient's life improves. This includes enhanced interpersonal relationships and improved social functioning [13–17], improvement in self-image and body-image [17, 18], better integration into the family [19], and improvement in initiating and sustaining intimate relationships [13, 17, 19–25].

A second criterion mandates that a surgical procedure must not be experimental or investigational. Surgery for gender dysphoria is not experimental. Such surgeries have been performed for decades, and are endorsed by the American Medical Association, the Endocrine Society, the American Psychological Association and other professional bodies. Resolution 122 (A-08) of the American Medical Association states that experts have "rejected the myth that these treatments are 'cosmetic' or 'experimental' and have recognized that these treatments provide safe and effective treatment for a serious health condition" [26].

Finally, a surgical procedure must be safe. Although there is an element of risk in any procedure, the benefit must outweigh the risk. Complications that arise from surgery must be relatively few and easily managed.

Gender affirming surgery satisfies this condition. The rate of complications occurring during and after genital surgery is relatively low, and most complications are minor [27, 28]. Lawrence investigated complications in 232 MTF patients who underwent affirmation surgery, and concluded that significant complications were "uncommon" [21]. A study comparing results during the period 1965–1995, revealed superior outcomes in those patients undergoing surgery after 1985 [29]. Clearly, improvements in surgical techniques advanced considerably thereafter, resulting in shortened hospital stays and improved post-operative care.

The literature regarding regret after surgery has remained remarkably consistent over time. Few people regret undergoing affirmation surgery. Among those who report remorse, poor surgical outcomes are a major factor in their dissatisfaction. In fact, quality of surgical results appears to be one of the best predictors of overall satisfaction with affirmation surgery and post-operative adjustment [30].

## WPATH Standards of Care

The first Standards of Care (SOC) for the treatment of gender dysphoria were published in 1979. At that time, the few professionals who offered care to the transgender population formed the Harry Benjamin International Gender Dysphoria Association, named for the endocrinologist who identified the condition. Concerned for the safety of patients compelled to pursue illicit or unsafe treatments, members drafted the first Standards of Care. Revised in 1980, 1981, 1990, 1998, 2001, and 2011, the frequent iterations reflected the rapid acceleration of scientific knowledge, the refinement of medical protocols, and the evolution in techno-cultural environments. Even the name of the organization was changed to World Professional Association for Transgender Health (WPATH), to acknowledge the diversity of gender identities and to reject a pathologizing ethos.

The WPATH Standards of Care are explicit in promulgating the necessary and sufficient criteria that must be met for surgical interventions:

## Criteria for Surgeries

### Criteria for Breast/Chest Surgery (One Referral Required)

### Criteria for Mastectomy and Creation of a Male Chest in FTM Patients

- Persistent, well-documented gender dysphoria;
- Capacity to make a fully informed decision and to consent for treatment;
- Age of majority in a given country (if younger, follow the SOC for children and adolescents);
- If significant medical or mental health concerns are present, they must be reasonably well controlled.

Hormone therapy is not a prerequisite.

### Criteria for Breast Augmentation (Implants/Lipofilling in MTF Patients)

- Persistent, well-documented gender dysphoria;
- Capacity to make a fully informed decision and to consent to treatment;
- Age of majority in a given country (if younger, follow the SOC for children and adoclescents);
- If significant medical or mental health concerns are present, they must be reasonably well controlled.

Although not an explicit criterion, it is recommended that MTF patients undergo feminizing hormone therapy (minimum 12 months) prior to breast augmentation surgery. The purpose is to maximize breast growth in order to obtain better surgical (aesthetic) results.

### Criteria for Genital Surgery (Two Referrals)

The criteria for genital surgery are specific to the type of surgery being requested.

### Criteria for Hysterectomy and Salpingo-Oophorectomy in FTM Patients and for Orchiectomy in MTF Patients

- Persistent, well-documented gender dysphoria;
- Capacity to make a fully informed decision and to consent to treatment;

- Age of majority in a given country;
- If significant medical or mental health concerns are present, they must be reasonably well controlled.
- 12 continuous months of hormone therapy as appropriate to the patient's gender goals (unless hormones are not clinically indicated for the individual).

The aim of hormone therapy prior to gonadectomy is primarily to introduce a period of reversible estrogen or testosterone suppression, before the patient undergoes irreversible surgical intervention.

These criteria do not apply to patients who are having these procedures for medical indications other than gender dysphoria.

### Criteria for Metoidoplasty or Phalloplasty in FTM Patients and Vaginoplasty in MTF Patients

- Persistent, well-documented gender dysphoria;
- Capacity to make a fully informed decision and to consent to treatment;
- Age of majority in a given country;
- If significant medical or mental health concerns are present, they must be reasonably well controlled.
- 12 continuous months of hormone therapy as appropriate to the patient's gender goals (unless hormones are not clinically indicated for the individual).
- 12 continuous months of living in a gender role that is congruent with their gender identity.

Although not an explicit criterion, it is recommended that these patients also have regular visits with a mental health or other medical professional [31].

**Helpful Hint**

Facial feminizing procedures and liposuction do not require letters from providers

# Surgery for the Male-to-Female Patient

## A History of MTF Genital Surgery

In the 1950s, surgeries for congenital aplasia and other genital anomalies were successfully executed, and reported in the literature. Such surgeries provided a template for the first attempts to create a vagina in MTF patients. The few surgeons who attempted the procedure did so in two stages. First, the male organs were removed. After a lengthy convalescence, the second stage was performed, where skin from the buttocks or thighs was harvested and grafted to construct a neovagina [2].

The publicity storm created by the Jorgensen case caused thousands of individuals to request these surgeries. Ms. Jorgensen received an avalanche of letters from individuals pleading for help and information. Having undergone surgery in Denmark, European doctors were besieged with requests for the procedure [4]. The thorny legal issues, and uncertainty regarding diagnostic criteria, caused surgeons to eschew the procedure. The deluge of mail became onerous, and created a problem for the Danish government:

> The doctors who converted the sex of ex-GI George Jorgensen to Christine Jorgensen have done four more such operations, the last within the year. Two men were in their forties. One was married. All were Danish. The Danish government will no longer permit surgery of foreigners. The wide-spread publicity given the Christine case is responsible for the decision. Since the Christine operation, the doctors have received about 2,000 letters from all over the world. About twenty-five per cent have come from the U.S. from individuals with assorted sex problems [32].

As a recourse, people in need of surgery flocked to Casablanca to enlist the services of Dr. Georges Burou, a French gynecologist. Borou became renowned for operating on several famous Parisian female impersonators. In 1973, after having performed 3000 reassignment surgeries, he presented his novel technique to an audience at Stanford University Medical School. Borou is credited with inventing the anteriorly pedicled penile skin flap inversion technique: With proper dissection of the penile skin, a sustainable graft is constructed to line the neovagina.

Variations of Borou's inversion technique are still in use today [2].

Due to the influence of Harry Benjamin, and his seminal work *The Transsexual Phenomenon*, and despite intense pressure, Johns Hopkins Clinic began to perform reassignment surgery, soon to be followed by Stanford and Chicago County Hospitals [4]. The Hopkins surgeons initially used partial skin grafts to line the neovaginal cavity, but later utilized penile skin, applied as a full thickness graft. Ultimately, they employed a variation of Borou's method, whereby the *posteriorly* pedicled penile skin was used to form the lining. The Chicago group utilized the *anteriorly* pedicled flap to line the neovagina [2].

While the techniques varied in these early surgeries, the goal of surgery did not. The aim was, and is, to create a perineum and genitalia that are normal in appearance and function. The surgeon must modify the urethra so that the urinary stream is appropriately directed, create a neovagina of sufficient depth to allow for sexual intercourse, and preserve sensation.

## Modern Surgical Techniques

### Vaginoplasty

Creation of the neovagina ideally involves producing a lining that is moist, hairless and flexible. There are five different techniques used to attain this result:

- *Non-genital skin grafts:* Skin is harvested from the abdomen and used as a full-thickness skin graft. This allows for ample depth and width and does not introduce the problem of hair within the neovagina. The scarring at the donor site however, is a drawback to this technique, as is the absence of lubrication and diminished sensation.
- *Penile skin graft:* This technique has several advantages. The skin is hairless, and there is no obvious scarring at the donor site. There is less shrinkage of the skin, when compared to non-genital grafts. However, grafts have a greater tendency to shrink than flaps, and this necessitates persistent dilation post-operatively to keep the neovagina patent.

- *Penile-scrotal skin flaps:* Currently, variations of this technique are employed routinely by most surgeons, and considered to be the "gold standard." There are distinct advantages to using penile skin flaps. They tend to contract less than grafts—although dilation is still necessary—and they are hairless. Additionally, sensation is maintained through innervation. The disadvantage is that there may be an inadequate amount of penile skin available. Therefore, scrotal skin flaps or grafts are also used which requires hair removal prior to surgery.
- *Non-genital skin flaps:* Use of skin from the thigh has been reported in the literature, but only in cases of revision surgery due to a previous unsatisfactory vaginoplasty. While there is less risk of skin contraction and a reduced necessity of dilation, there are many drawbacks to this approach. The procedure is technically complex, and there is scarring at the donor site. The new skin obtained is bulky in comparison to genital skin flaps.
- *Pedicled intestinal transplant:* The use of cecum and sigmoid (colocolpopoiesis) transplanted to line the neovagina was first reported in 1974. Laub employed this method routinely, and cited several advantages. For one, the length of the rectosigmoid provides ample depth and the texture of the tissue is similar to that of a natural vagina. This technique is the only one that allows for natural lubrication. There are drawbacks to the technique, however, which result from the invasion of another system—the intestinal system—which include bowel and colon complications as well as the potential for damage to the fragile colonic mucosa that forms the lining of the neovagina. Most surgeons concur that this technique is best utilized as a revision procedure when repairing a failed vaginoplasty [2] (see Fig. 20.1a–c).

---

**Helpful Hint**

The penile-scrotal skin flap technique is most frequently employed. In the case of a failed vaginoplasty, the rectosigmoid procedure is used to repair the vagina.

---

## Vulvoplasty

In the early era of affirmation surgery, the primary focus was on construction of a neovagina. As surgical acumen advanced, patients and surgeons sought refinements in the aesthetics of the labia complex and clitoris. When the common inversion technique is employed, labia majora are formed from the resected scrotal skin. Oftentimes, surgeons perform a "Zplasty" procedure after the vaginoplasty—a simple procedure that excises tissue and creates the anterior commissure covering the neoclitoris. Some surgeons feel that this procedure is best performed after the swelling and edema in the perineal complex have resolved.

Creation of a neoclitoris proved challenging to surgeons, and high rates of clitoral necrosis—33 %—occurred when tissue of the glans of the penis was utilized. Various grafts were tried in the search for an alternative functional neoclitoris. Presently, most surgeons use the dorsal portion of the glans penis and the dorsal neurovascular pedicle, but clitoroplasty and construction of labia minora remain difficult structures to construct surgically [2] (see Fig. 20.2).

## Post-surgical Considerations

Patients are typically discharged 5–7 days after surgery, and instructed on dilation schedules and care of the neovagina. Complications following surgery can include infection or poor healing with unresolved swelling and/or bleeding. A potential complication of vaginoplasty is a recto-vaginal fistula, as the wall of the rectum is thin and easily perforated during surgery. If this occurs, it requires surgical closure, and usually heals well.

### Breast Augmentation

Many patients request breast augmentation when feminizing hormones fail to produce sufficient or desired development. Anatomical differences in the natal male and natal female breast tissue and chest wall necessitates a somewhat different approach in MTF patients than that used in natal females seeking augmentation.

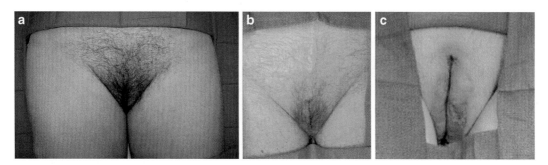

**Fig. 20.1** (**a–c**) Patients after undergoing vaginoplasty. Photographs by Loren S. Schechter, MD, FACS. Used with permission

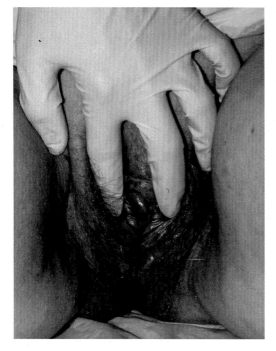

**Fig. 20.2** Patient after undergoing vaginoplasty, demonstrating clitoris. Photographs by Loren S. Schechter, MD, FACS. Used with permission

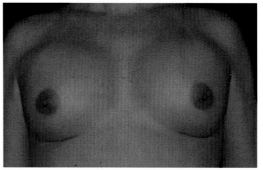

**Fig. 20.3** MTF patient after breast augmentation surgery. Photographs by Loren S. Schechter, MD, FACS. Used with permission

cage. This allows the prosthesis to be covered with more tissue and reduces the risk of capsular contraction [2].

Complications from this surgery are the same as for any surgical procedure: infection, poor wound healing, and/or bleeding. The augmentation mammoplasty is frequently performed at the same time as genital surgery (see Fig. 20.3).

## Other Feminizing Surgeries

### Facial Surgery

Gender presentation is non-verbally communicated largely via visual cues. The face and body habitus convey information that is intuitively and unconsciously processed. In the absence of cognitively conflicting evidence, a decision regarding a stranger's gender binary designation—male or female—is reached instantaneously.

Typically, natal males have a stronger pectoral facia and pectoralis muscle, and a smaller nipple and areola. Therefore, a periareolar incision is not the best choice, due to the smaller size of the areola. A pocket for the prosthesis is usually created behind the glandular tissue or behind the pectoralis muscle. Surgeons can choose between saline and silicone gel prostheses. Many surgeons implant the prosthesis in a retropectoral position, after detaching the muscle from the thoracic

Facial features and proportions are intimately connected with identity. For gender dysphoric individuals nothing is more important than looking in the mirror and seeing a congruent reflection.

One patient with severe gender dysphoria felt that a transition was impossible because her nose was "so big and manly." No feminizing process—not genital surgery or hormones—eliminated the dysphoria she experienced. In this case, rhinoplasty was the most important and the most therapeutic procedure performed.

Although there are quantitative analyses of the differences in measurements between natal male and natal female faces and skulls—such as facial height—there is no agreement regarding these indices, and ethnic variations make generalizations meaningless. Nevertheless, certain aspects of the face are reliably perceived as being either "male" or "female," and this consensual validation guides surgeons performing facial feminizing procedures. For more details, see Chap. 21: Otolaryngology for the Transgender Population.

## Forehead

The forehead is a feature that tends to differ in several aspects between natal male and natal female. Natal males have brow bossing, a prominent forehead with an arch, while natal females tend to have skulls that are convex, in all planes. Surgical alterations to the forehead can include bone contouring, complex alterations of the frontal sinus, forehead lift to position the brows higher, and/or scalp advancement to reduce the distance from the brows to the hairline. When the forehead is surgically altered it can produce a dramatic feminizing effect [2].

## Cheeks

Cheeks, in and of themselves, do not differ significantly in shape or prominence between natal male and natal female. However, prominent cheeks are universally viewed as attractive, and can impart a feminine dimension to the face. Surgeons often use implants or other fillers to provide volume in this area. In some cases, bone repositioning is performed.

## Nose

There is tremendous variation in nose shape and size amongst individuals. However, natal females tend to have less nasal prominence. Rhinoplasty can reduce the size and improve the contour of the nose. There are, of course, limitations as to the amount of reduction that is surgically possible, but an alteration of contour alone can result in a feminizing effect.

## Chin

The chin is a feature that does differ between natal male and natal female. Natal female chins tend to be pointier, narrower and shorter (vertically) than those in natal males. Modifications to the chin can truly feminize the lower face and can range from the relatively simple insertion of an implant to more complex bone cutting and repositioning [2].

## Jaw

The natal male jaw is typically more angular than that of a natal female. This is due to a larger and thicker masseter muscle. The masseter muscle can be reduced through the mouth, eliminating external excisions. The bone can also be reduced, which softens the angle of the mandible [2].

## Hair Transplantation

Natal male pattern scalp recession or balding vanquishes an attempt to appear natal female. Scalp advancement or hair transplantation can be successful in achieving a natal female hair pattern. Plugs and micrografts have been used to fill in areas, and in some cases scalp reductions have been useful. Totally or extensively bald individuals usually rely on a hairpiece.

## Adam's Apple Reduction and Voice Surgery

Several surgical techniques have been reported that raise vocal pitch. In general, these procedures shorten the vocal cords and increase vocal cord tension. While few patients undergo these procedures, in some cases natal male voice quality can cause psychological distress and dismantle an otherwise successful gender transition as in the following example:

Anita was a transwoman who, after several years of hormonal therapy, underwent surgical reassignment. Although she was attractive and pleased with her appearance, she was disturbed by her deep, "obviously male" voice, which she felt "outed" her. Ultimately, Anita stopped speaking when she was in public. If she were in a store, for example, she would get panicky, fearing that a clerk might ask her a question. She avoided her neighbors, not wanting to greet them verbally. She stated that the sound of her voice made her "feel sick."

In cases such as this, patients may be very pleased with the results of voice surgery, particularly if they have already tried speech therapy [33].

The reduction of the prominent thyroid cartilage is a relatively simple surgical procedure: The cartilage is exposed and resected. This can yield a great benefit as it eliminates the need to "hide" this feature with clothing that covers the neck. In patients who do undergo surgical vocal procedures, a chrondrolarygnoplasty can be performed at the same time [2].

## Surgery for the Female-to-Male Patient

### History of FTM Genital Surgery

Creating tissue and structures is much harder than removing them, which is the case with phalloplasty. This also explains why there are no documented surgeries to reduce gender dysphoria in FTM patients prior to the twentieth century. In 1957, Gillies reported the first use of a penile reconstructive technique in a transsexual patient [34].

### Modern Surgical Techniques

#### Phalloplasty

The surgeon who performs phalloplasty for the FTM patient aims to reconstruct an authentic-appearing and sensate neophallus. The patient must be able to urinate in a standing position and to have sexual intercourse. The scrotum should be reconstructed, and the procedure should be performed with minimal scarring or destruction at the donor site.

This is a tall order for the surgeon and it explains why so many variations of phalloplasty have been attempted throughout the last 30 years. In 1936, Bogoras performed the first penile reconstruction using a tubed abdominal flap. Subsequent attempts involved complex, multistage surgeries. As surgical techniques improved, particularly reconstructive and plastic surgery techniques, many refinements evolved, including the use of microsurgery. Such improvements allowed for the use of distant flaps and the joining of nerves from the donor site to nerves in the perineum. While many different flaps have been attempted and described in the literature, the radial forearm flap is most frequently employed [9].

### Radial Forearm Flap in Phalloplasty

In this technique, the patient has previously undergone hysterectomy and bilateral salpino-oophrectomy. After a minimum of 6 months, the genital reconstruction can be performed. Most often two surgical teams operate simultaneously. A urologist performs the vaginectomy and lengthening of the urethra. After removal of the mucosal lining of the vaginal cavity, the pelvic floor is reconstructed to prevent rectocele—herniation of the rectum into the vagina. The labia majora are then reconstructed into scrotum [9].

The plastic surgeon is simultaneously creating a flap from vascularized forearm tissue. The flap is tubed, thus creating a phallus, and a small skin flap and graft are used to create a corona and glans of the neophallus. The hollow tubular flap is transferred to the groin area for the coalescence of blood vessels, and a vein graft is used to connect arteries [9].

As one can imagine, the forearm is severely disfigured and must be repaired, usually with grafts harvested from the inner thigh. Postoperatively, patients remain in bed for 1 week, after which a catheter is removed. The average hospital stay for phalloplasty is usually two and a half weeks. Tattooing, insertion of testicular prostheses, and penile erection prosthesis require an additional surgery. This can only be performed after the top of the penis regains sensation, which usually requires at least 1 year [9].

Other techniques for penile creation have been reported, e.g. a thigh flap, and none are perfect. There are several advantages of the forearm technique, however: For one, the skin is pliable and allows for a tube within a tube to be constructed (the urethra within the penis). Additionally, the skin on the innermost aspect is hairless and can be used to line the urethra, and finally, the flap is well-vascularized, which aids in tactile sensation. Monstrey et al reports that all patients undergoing phalloplasty with a radial forearm flap are able—ultimately—to urinate standing. This has not been the case when other techniques have been used. A disadvantage of the radial forearm flap is that the flap can shrink over time [9].

## Complications

Fistulas and strictures and not uncommon complications in the genito-urinary tract after phalloplasty, and may require surgical repair. In addition to the usual complications that occur with any surgery, such as infection, vaginectomy is a difficult procedure with a high risk of excessive bleeding. Other potential complications occur as a result of vascular compromise of the flap and can cause arterial and/or venous thrombosis. Occasionally, there is a loss of skin or partial necrosis of the flap [9]. As smoking increases this risk, most surgeons will not perform phalloplasty on patients who do not quit smoking a year prior to genital surgery.

## Metoidoplasty

Phalloplasty is a complex, lengthy and costly surgery, and complications occur fairly often. Therefore, many patients opt for an alternative genital surgery that is less extensive and less expensive. As a result of testosterone, the clitoris enlarges allowing this structure to be reconstructed into a phallus. In metoidoplasty, the clitoral hood is lifted and the clitoris is detached from the pubic bone, causing the clitoris to extend. The urethra is extended, and scrotum are reconstructed from a flap of the labia majora. Some surgeons perform vaginectomy during metoidoplasty.

This procedure will usually allow an individual to void while standing, but sexual intercourse will not be possible. There is the advantage that there is no visible scarring on other areas of the body, and it is possible to perform phalloplasty at a late time if the patient so desires. Complications from metoidoplasty most commonly involve the urethra, and can include fistula or urethral obstruction [9].

## The Future of FTM Genital Surgery

The transfer of tissue from one body area to another, and the problems inherent in such transfer, is the major surgical obstacle in reconstructing an aesthetic and functional male urogenital complex. Improvements in phalloplasty will likely come from innovations in tissue transfer from adjacent and distant donor areas to the groin. The use of perforator flaps promises to be an important advancement [9].

Perforator flaps, so named because they are based on vessels that perforate or traverse a muscle, allow for a longer vascular pedicle for dissection. Perforators are composed of skin, fatty tissue, and tiny blood vessels. Unlike the flaps typically used in reconstructive surgery, they preserve the underlying musculature [35].

Use of a perforator flap in phalloplasty would diminish the scarring, possible disfigurement and morbidity at the donor site—typically the radial forearm—and has the potential to dramatically reduce recovery time and complications. The most promising perforator would be the anterolateral thigh. The thickness of this flap, however, makes it unsuitable for creating the tube within a tube—the urethra. If a solution to the problem of vascularizing the urethra can be found, the perforator flap would likely become the method of choice for phalloplasty [9, 35].

## Subcutaneous Mastectomy

For transmen, genital surgery is typically not the first, or even the most important gender-confirming surgical procedure they undergo. Subcutaneous mastectomy is the surgical intervention that allows one to live safely and comfortably as a male, without the telltale breasts that are anathema.

In the FTM patient, removal of the breasts is desired, but so is the creation of a male-contoured

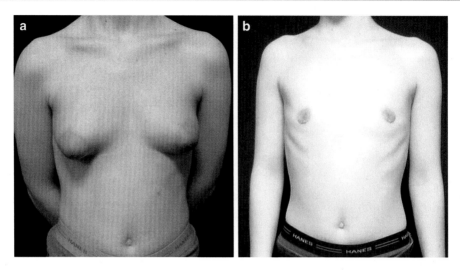

**Fig. 20.4** (**a**) FTM patient before chest surgery. (**b**) FTM patient after chest surgery. Photographs by Loren S. Schechter, MD, FACS. Used with permission

chest. Therefore, the surgical procedure employed differs from mastectomy in the case of disease. The goal of this surgery in reassignment is to remove breast tissue and excess skin, reduce the size of the nipple, ensure proper placement of the aerola, release the inframammary fold, and accomplish all with a minimum of scarring [9].

Various techniques are used to perform subcutaneous mastectomy, and there is no consensus on which technique produces the best outcome. Four factors are considered relevant in determining the most appropriate surgical technique. These are: breast volume, degree of excess skin, size and position of the nipple-areola complex, and skin elasticity. Some cases may require a free nipple graft, where the breasts are removed and the nipple-areola complex is grafted onto the chest wall [9].

Complications that can occur with subcutaneous mastectomy include the formation of abscesses and necrosis of the nipple. Some patients require a second surgery to improve the aesthetic outcome. Skin elasticity may be the most important factor in attaining a good outcome and is often sub-optimal due to prolonged breast binding [9]. The importance of a good aesthetic outcome is vital to an individual's body

image and therefore the surgeon's experience in performing this complex surgery cannot be minimized (see Fig. 20.4a, b).

## Collaborative Care

Long-term follow-up is essential for patients who undergo gender affirming surgeries. For patients who undergo phalloplasty, a urologist will figure largely in the ongoing care plan. The complexity of creating a urethra in the bladder of these patients demands vigilance over time, as urination through this tube can lead to future complications [9].

The surgeon is a vital member of the multidisciplinary team that provides care to the transgender population and brings essential technical expertise to the treatment. Hopefully, the surgeon also brings an abiding respect and deep understanding of the condition of gender dysphoria. The emotional status of the patient, before, during, and after surgery is an important determinant of the ultimate outcome. For this reason, it may be as important to consult and collaborate with the mental health professional as it is to work with the urologist, gynecologist and other surgical specialists.

# References

1. Edgerton M. The role of surgery in the treatment of transsexualism. Ann Plast Surg. 1984;13:473–81.
2. Monstrey S, Selvaggi G, Ceulemans P. Surgery: male-to-female patient. In: Ettner R, Monstrey S, Eyler AE, editors. Principles of transgender medicine and surgery. New York: Routledge; 2007.
3. Sadies S, editor. The new Grove dictionary of music and musicians. London: Macmillan; 1980.
4. Ettner R. Gender loving care. New York: WW Norton; 1999.
5. Lothstein LM. Psychological testing with transsexuals: a 30-year review. J Pers Assess. 1984;48(5):500–7.
6. Burke P. Gender shock. New York: Doubleday; 1996.
7. Belli M. Transsexual surgery: a new tort? JAMA. 1978;239(20):2143–8.
8. Raymond J. The transsexual empire: the making of the she-male. Boston: Beacon; 1979.
9. Monstrey S, Ceulemans P, Hoebeke P. Surgery: female-to-male patient. In: Ettner R, Monstrey S, Eyler AE, editors. Principles of transgender medicine and surgery. New York: Routledge; 2007.
10. Monstrey S, De Cuypere G, Ettner R. Surgery: general principles. In: Ettner R, Monstrey S, Eyler AE, editors. Principles of transgender medicine and surgery. New York: Routledge; 2007.
11. Pfafflin F, Junge A. Sex reassignment: thirty years of international follow-up studies after sex reassignment surgery, a comprehensive review. Stuttgart: Shattauer; 1992.
12. Gijs L, Brewaeys A. Surgical treatment of gender dysphoria in adults and adolescents: recent developments, effectiveness, and challenges. Annu Rev Sex Res. 2007;18:178–224.
13. Rehman J, Lazar S, Benet A, Schaefer L, Melman A. The reported sex and surgery satisfaction of 20 postoperative male-to-female transsexual patients. Arch Sex Behav. 1999;28(1):71–89.
14. Johansson A, Sundbom E, Hodjerback T, Bodlund O. A five-year follow-up of Swedish adults with gender identity disorder. Arch Sex Behav. 2010;39(6):1429–37.
15. Hepp U, Klaghofer R, Burkhard-Kubler R, Buddeberg C. Treatment follow-up of transsexual patients. A catamnestic study. Nervenarzt. 2002;73(3):283–8.
16. Ainsworth T, Spiegel H. Quality of life of individuals with and without facial feminization surgery or gender reassignment surgery. Qual Life Res. 2010;19:1019–24.
17. Smith Y, van Goozen S, Kuiper A, Cohen-Kettenis P. Sex reassignment: outcomes and predictors of treatment for adolescents and adult transsexuals. Psychol Med. 2005;35:89–99.
18. Lawrence A. Factors associated with satisfaction or regret following male-to-female sex reassignment surgery. Arch Sex Behav. 2003;32:299–315.
19. Lobato M, Koff W, Manenti C, Seger D, Salvador J, Fortes M, Henriques A. Follow-up of sex reassignment surgery in transsexuals: a Brazilian cohort. Arch Sex Behav. 2006;35(6):711–5.
20. Lawrence A. Sexuality before and after male-to-female sex reassignment surgery. Arch Sex Behav. 2005;34:147–66.
21. Lawrence A. Patient-reported complications and functional outcomes of male-to-female sex reassignment surgery. Arch Sex Behav. 2006;35:147–66.
22. Imbimbo C, Verze P, Palmieri A, Longo N, Fusco F, Arcaniolo D, Mirone V. A report from a single institute's 14-year experience in treatment of male-to-female transsexuals. J Sex Med. 2009;6(10): 2736–45.
23. Klein C, Gorzalka B. Sexual function in transsexuals following hormone therapy and genital surgery: a review. J Sex Med. 2009;6(11):2922–39.
24. Jarolim L, Sedy J, Schmidt M, Ondrej N, Foltan R, Kawaciuk I. Gender reassignment surgery in male-to-female transsexualism: a retrospective 3-month follow-up with anatomical remarks. J Sex Med. 2009;6:1635–44.
25. DeCuypere G, T'Sjoen G, Beerten R, Selvaggi G, De Sutter P, Hoebeke P, Rubens R. Sexual and physical health after sex reassignment surgery. Arch Sex Behav. 2005;34(6):679–90.
26. American Medical Association. Resolution 122 (A-08): Removing financial barriers to care for transgender patients; 2008.
27. Spehr C. Male to female sex reassignment surgery in transsexuals. Int J Transgend. 2007;10(1):25–37.
28. Amend B, Seibold J, Toomey P, Stenzl A, Sievert K. Surgical reconstruction for male-to-female sex reassignment. Eur Urol. 2012;64(1):141–9.
29. Eldh J, Berg A, Gustafsson M. Long term follow up after sex reassignment surgery. Scand J Plast Reconstr Surg Hand Surg. 1997;31:39–45.
30. Lawrence A. Sex reassignment surgery without a one-year real life experience: still no regrets. 2001. Paper presented at the XVII Harry Benjamin international symposium on gender dysphoria. Galveston, Texas.
31. Coleman E, Bockting W, Botzer M, Cohen-Kettenis P, DeCupere G, Feldman J. et al. Standards of care for the health of transsexual transgender and gender-non-conforming people. 7th version. World Professional Association for Transgender Health; 2012.
32. Science Digest. New York; Hearst Magazines; 1959.
33. Adler R, Hirsch S, Mordaunt M, editors. Voice and communication therapy for the transgender/transsexual client: a comprehensive guide. 2nd ed. San Diego: Plural Publishing; 2012.
34. Gillies H, Millard Jr DR. The principles and art of plastic surgery, vol. 2. London: Butterworth; 1957. p. 368–84.
35. Morris S. Perforator flaps: a microsurgical innovation. Medscape J Med. 2008;10(11):266.

Scott R. Chaiet

## Learning Objectives

- Understand the range of surgical procedures available for facial feminization surgery *(PC3)*
- Describe facial analysis and key differences between the biologic male and female facial structure *(PC3)*
- Review the best practices in surgical techniques for facial feminization surgery *(PC3)*

## Introduction

### Facial Feminization Surgery

Facial plastic and reconstructive surgical procedures performed on the male to female transgender patient have been grouped together in a relatively new field called facial feminization surgery. Popularized by anthropologic descriptions of Douglas Ousterhout in the 1980s and his more recent patient book, *Facial Feminization Surgery: A Guide for the Transgendered Woman*, many of these procedures are familiar to the facial plastic surgeon. Most are commonly performed throughout the United States on cisgender patients. Other procedures to manipulate the shape of thyroid cartilage, a tracheal shave procedure, may require specialized experience. This chapter will present a wide variety of procedures performed today in facial feminization surgery, outline an approach to facial analysis of a biologic male patient seeking surgical consultation for feminization, and describe technical pearls of wisdom found in the literature.

Before embarking on surgical alteration of the face, many transgender patients have initiated hormone therapy. The effects of hormonal supplementation with estrogen complement the surgical process of feminization by reducing facial hair, altering fat distribution, and changing skin appearance and texture [1] Estrogen also suppresses testosterone, reducing the rate of growth of male-pattern hair [2]. As stated elsewhere in this book, any surgical therapy on the male to female transgender patient should be performed in conjunction with a team of treatment professionals for mental and medical health.

Facial feminization surgery is an important step for many in the transgender community, and research demonstrates the significant quality of life impact. Patients score statistically higher on physical, mental, and social functioning outcome scales following facial feminization surgery compared to those without surgery, a finding also applicable to genital reassignment surgery [3]. Surgical care can

S.R. Chaiet, M.D., M.B.A. (✉)
Division of Otolaryngology – Head and Neck
Surgery, Department of Surgery, University of
Wisconsin School of Medicine and Public Health,
600 Highland Avenue, Madison,
WI 53792-7375, USA
e-mail: scottchaiet@yahoo.com

© Springer International Publishing Switzerland 2016
K.L. Eckstrand, J.M. Ehrenfeld (eds.), *Lesbian, Gay, Bisexual, and Transgender Healthcare*,
DOI 10.1007/978-3-319-19752-4_21

significantly aid in the transition from male to female and may be complemented with non-surgical interventions. For example, speech therapy alters voicing style where surgery raises the fundamental pitch. Data presented later in this chapter shows the importance of these auditory alterations congruent with feminine recognition.

Like other facial plastic surgery, proper preoperative patient counseling is imperative for successful outcomes including the management of expectations. Informed consent includes a discussion of risks, benefits, and alternates to the procedure and also reasonable expectations of outcomes. The transgender patient, however, may present with specific goals and photographs of a desired result, travel long distances for expert care, post photographs of the operative process in public forums such as the internet, and share the experience with others in the transgender community [4]. While these challenges should not deter a facial plastic surgeon from providing this care, careful thought and a mutual understand of expectations throughout the surgical process will result in a more meaningful experience.

> **Key Points**
> - Hormone therapy and mental health care complement surgical therapy of the male to female transgender patient. Patients who undergo facial feminization surgery score statistically higher on physical, mental, and social functioning outcome scales following surgery compared to those without surgery.
> - Proper pre-operative patient counseling and management of expectations are imperative for successful outcomes for all facial plastic procedures including facial feminization surgery.

## Recognition of Femininity

It may be overwhelming for the patient, surgeon, or both to embark on facial feminization surgery of the entire face. Where should the surgical process begin for a male to female transgender patient to create the most female appearance? Of course

patient preference is the first priority, but research by Jeffrey Spiegel, MD, FACS provides further information. To determine which aspects of the face are most associated with femininity, he feminized frontal and lateral photographs of biologic men in either the forehead, midface (nasal and lip modifications), or the jaw, digitally stimulating procedures discussed in this chapter. 100 adult research participants viewed 30 sets of three frontal photographs and 30 sets of three lateral photographs and ranked which alteration made to three photographs—forehead, midface, or jaw—resulted in the most feminine result. In both views, forehead modification was selected in all sets for the most stereotypically feminine appearance.

Spiegel also showed research participants horizontal thirds of the face of real photographs of biologic male patients, biologic female patients, and post-operative transgender facial feminization patients. Transgender patients who underwent surgery were identified as women in 82 %, 87 %, and 85 % of upper, mid, and lower facial photographs. Spiegel's landmark research showed that facial feminization procedures can result in recognition as a women 6 out of 7 times, and demonstrated the upper third of the face as a major determinant of femininity [5]. By no accident, this chapter discusses the face in a "top down" manner beginning with the upper face, proceeding to the midface and then the lower face and neck.

Although each facial subunit will be discussed in isolation, any procedure should maintain aesthetic facial proportions to other areas of the face. As a patient and physician embark on facial feminization procedures over few or many operations, maintaining facial proportions should guide the sequence of events [6].

> **Key Points**
> - Research by Jeffrey Spiegel, MD, FACS showed forehead modification results in the highest recognition of a stereotypically feminine appearance, more than changes to the middle or lower one thirds of the face.
> - Spiegel also demonstrated facial feminization surgical procedures result in feminine recognition.

## Facial Analysis

## Overview

Facial analysis of the male to female transgender patient interested in facial feminization surgery can be challenging, but the initial consultation is not dissimilar to other facial plastic surgery evaluations. Some patients will present with specific goals in mind for a segment or for the entire face, where others may express a general disliking of facial traits. After the initial history taking and discussion of goals, the next step in a thorough facial plastic surgery consultation is facial analysis, complemented by high quality imaging. Photographs should include the frontal view, right and left lateral views with the head in the Frankfort horizontal plane (a line drawn from the upper border of tragus to the infraorbital rim is parallel to the ground), right and left three quarter views, and the base view.

The literature contains many "normal" values of facial angles, proportions, widths and heights for each gender. The origin of many are from work by Powell and Humphreys in 1984 [7]. The authors provide an overview of the differences between a biologic male and female face:

> The male's bone structure is sterner, bolder and more prominent. The dominance of the forehead, nose, and chin is more striking than the females. The zygoma and mandible produce much stronger contours in the male as opposed to the female face.

Although there may be conflicting "normal" values since ethnic and racial variations are not represented, Powell and Humphreys provide a foundation for objective facial analysis [7]. It should be noted that this chapter will describe facial characteristics typical for each "gender" with reference to biologic sex.

> **Key Points**
> - Facial analysis of the male to female transgender patient is similar to other facial plastic surgery evaluations and includes high quality photography.
> - Many normal values of measurements of the biologic male and female face are based off work by Powell and Humphreys in the 1980s.

## Overview of Facial Analysis

The face is traditionally divided into five equal vertical segments and three equal horizontal segments, the "vertical fifths" and "horizontal thirds" (Fig. 21.1). The vertical segments are aligned with the medal and lateral canthi (corners of the eyelid opening) and the outer helical rims so that each fifth is equal to the width

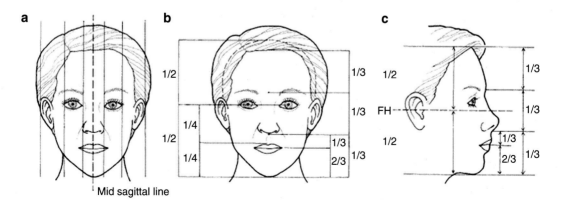

**Fig. 21.1** Facial analysis with "vertical fifths" (**a**); "horizontal thirds" and further division of the lower face showing upper and lower lip relationship (**b**); lateral view of horizontal thirds in Frankfort horizontal (FH) plane with line marked through the upper border of the tragus and infraorbital rim (**c**). With kind permission from Springer Science + Business Media: Morgan and Haug [8]

of one eye. Practically, the vertical fifths analysis is used as a starting point to measure the width of the base of the nose, identify asymmetry or variations within a face, and less for facial feminization surgery.

Landmarks for the horizontal thirds are the trichion (hairline), glabella (forehead prominence between the brows), subnasale, and menton (chin) [8]. Immediately, the relationship of the hairline to facial aesthetic balance is evident, particularly in the male to female transgender patient. The biologic male hairline is commonly higher [8]; there may also be male pattern baldness or a receding hairline, creating an elongated upper third of the face. Analysis of the upper face may also generate discussion of a prominent glabella and prominent supraorbital ridges, often called frontal bossing, seen on the biologic male forehead. The eyebrow position should be carefully examined by palpation, as the biologic male eyebrow rests below the bony supraorbital rim where the biologic female brow should lay at or above it. Hairline and brow position are intimately related in facial appearance and surgery can address both simultaneously.

The lower horizontal third can be further divided into horizontal segments to analyze the ratio of the upper lip to lower lip and chin, ideally one third to two thirds. An long vertical chin height is common in the biologic male jaw, often accompanied by upper lip deflation and elongation seen with aging.

A second method for lower facial analysis measures lips and chin projection and their harmony with the face. Although many chin measurements are reported in the literature, the Gonzalez-Ulloa method is often cited where a tangential line extends downward in the lateral view from the nasion (soft tissue depression above nose) perpendicular to the Frankfort horizontal plane. This line should transect the anterior soft tissue prominence of chin (pogonion) and may indicate over- or under-projection of the chin [9]. Alternately a line can be extended downward through the red-white vermillion lip borders of the upper and lower lips; anterior chin projection should rest behind this line in a biologic female chin where the biologic male chin may be at the line, or farther anterior.

**Key Points**
- Facial analysis using the "vertical fifths" and "horizontal thirds" provide a starting point to identify symmetry and facial proportions.
- The upper third of the face contains many key landmarks in facial feminization surgery such as hairline location, eyebrow position, and forehead projection.
- Multiple methods exist for lower facial analysis to describe the relationship of the upper and lower lips with the chin, but anterior chin projection should be less in the female chin.

## Facial Units

Moving to the central face, nasal analysis is particularly important when considering differences between biologic males and females. The nasolabial angle on lateral view is formed between lines along the nasal columella and the upper lip. The angle defines nasal tip rotation and has been reported as 90°–95° in biologic men and slightly more obtuse, 95°–110°, in biologic females [10]. In other words, the stereotypical feminine nasal tip looks turned slightly upwards. The width of the lower nose, the alar base, should align with the vertical fifths, although may be wider in a non-Caucasian nose.

Regarding the upper half of the nose, the male appearing nasal dorsum is stereotypically straight where the female dorsum has a slight concavity when viewed from the side. The biologic female nasofrontal angle measured between the nasal dorsum and forehead is also more obtuse [11, 12]. Cisgender female patients seek facial plastic surgery to reduce a dorsal convexity, a hump, to achieve a feminine nasal appearance. Hump reduction is often performed in conjunction with nasal tip surgery to create an asthetically balanced nose, called reductive rhinoplasty. Other nasal angles are defined in facial plastic surgery textbooks, but discussion of the tip and nasal dorsum will provide a foundation for nasal analysis and rhinoplasty surgery for the male to female transgender patient.

Finally, lower facial and neck analysis is made in a similar fashion to the "aging face" consultation, with careful attention to jowls, tissue laxity, neck fullness and neck skin redundancy. One aspect of the lower face unique to facial feminization surgery is the underlying bone structure of the jaw, particularly the prominence of the mandibular angles as well as anterior chin shape. Anthropologic studies show the chin is more pointed in a biologic female [12].

Although there are no standard bone measurements, the angles of the mandible (posterior inferior corners of the jawbone) are wider and lower creating a square shape in biologic males. Like jaw width, mid-face width is not a defined variable but important for facial feminization analysis. The biologic male zygomatic (cheek) bones have more bulk, but lack the prominence and height of the biologic female face [1]. Frontal photography aids in the evaluation of facial width. Drawing in the lines of vertical fifths may help visualize the bone structure as it relates to the face, and can aid in analysis of chin shape, jaw width, cheek width and contour of the mandible.

Finally, upper and lower lip projection can be measured, provided that chin projection is in harmony with the face. Lip fullness is measured as the distance from each lip to a line from subnasale (soft tissue depression under nose) to the anterior chin prominence (Fig. 21.2).

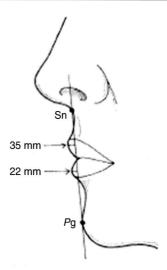

**Fig. 21.2** Ideal lip projection from a vertical line between the upper lip junction with the nose and anterior chin. With kind permission from Springer Science + Business Media: Morgan and Haug [8]

## Facial Feminization Surgery

### Surgery of the Upper Face and Hairline

Although the upper face may seem to have less interesting anatomy, it contains many key determinants for recognition of a stereotypically feminine face [5]. The landmarks include hairline position, eyebrow location relative to the underlying bony supraorbital rims, forehead height between the hairline and brows, and prominence seen best from the lateral view.

Browlifts are commonly performed in the United States, with the American Society for Aesthetic Plastic Surgery reporting nearly 30,000 operations in 2013 [14]. The procedure can be performed without addressing the hairline via an upper eyelid blepharoplasty incision, minimally invasive incisions hidden in the hairline, a long coronal incision across the head 2–3 cm behind the hairline, or less commonly in deep furrows of the forehead. None of these approaches address the distance between the hairline and brows, and may actually cause an unwanted elevation of the hairline.

**Key Points**
- The stereotypical female nose has an slightly upturned tip, concave nasal dorsum, and may have a slightly smaller shape.
- Lower facial and neck analysis looks at jowls, tissue laxity, neck fullness and neck skin redundancy in a similar fashion to the "aging face" consultation.
- The biologic male mandible is wider with a square shape, where the zygomatic (cheek) bones lack the prominence and height of the biologic female face.

Scalp advancement, or hairline lowering, can be combined with a browlift by placing a trichophytic incision along the hairline to approach both procedures. Once the brow has been elevated to a more feminized location, just above the bony supraorbital rims, excess non-hair bearing forehead skin and soft tissue may be excised, with or without relaxing incisions in the galea underneath the hair-bearing scalp for hairline advancement. Careful attention to surgical technique such as beveling the incision will improve post-operative outcome; also, limited hair transplanting can camouflage the incision and improve the aesthetic result along a new hairline [15, 16].

The male to female transgender patient with significant receding hairline may forego scalp advancement all together. Depending on hair quality and abundance, hair transplantation can create a new hairline. Hormone therapy with spironolactone may complement surgical procedures to diminish the male-pattern hair growth [2]. However a hairpiece may be more practical and economical if limited donor hair exists.

The biologic female eyebrow shows a higher peaked shape than the biologic male brow. The position of the peak was historically described above the lateral limbus (lateral border of the iris), but modern studies have shown the ideal peak is positioned above the lateral canthus [17]. During a browlift, aesthetic contouring of the eyebrow can be made by differential brow elevation medially and laterally to further feminize the upper face.

Forehead cranioplasty surgery can reduce supraorbital ridges and a prominent glabella, referred to as frontal bossing. Results provide excellent aesthetic change in facial feminization surgery. The trichophytic incision and coronal incisions both give surgical access for forehead reshaping (Fig. 21.3).

Because of the close relationship of the frontal sinuses under the frontal bone, multiple surgical approaches have been described to reduce complications. A forehead with a small prominence and thick anterior table (frontal bone anterior to the frontal sinus) can be addressed with burs to sculpt the forehead and orbital rims. Alternately, a traditional osteoplastic flap can be performed to remove the anterior table with an oscillating saw, re-shape the bone with burs and saws, and secured it back in place with miniplates to newly contoured supraorbital rims [18]. With either approach, care must be taken to avoid injury to the supratrochleal sensory nerves (Fig. 21.4).

Spiegel reported a third method, also common in Thailand, where the anterior table of the frontal sinus is thinned with burrs and set back as "islands" without mini-plating while preserving the underlying sinus mucosa. Due to complications of non-union and mobility of these fragments, this method was abandoned. The other approaches to forehead cranioplasty resulted in no other complications in his series of 168 forehead reductions [5].

**Fig. 21.3** A prominent supraorbital ridge amenable to reduction for upper facial feminization (**a**); a wide orbital rim can also be sculpted (**b**). With kind permission from Springer Science + Business Media: Habal [13]

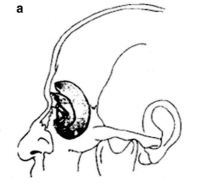
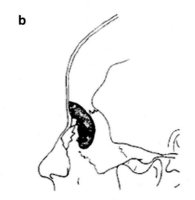

**Fig. 21.4** View from top of head of an osteoplastic flap of the frontal bone secured to newly contoured supraorbital rims with mini-plates after removal and shaping. With kind permission from Springer Science + Business Media: Cho and Jin [18]

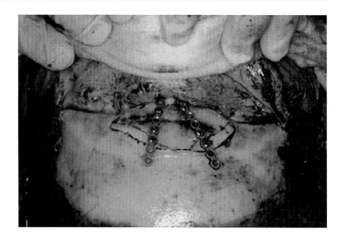

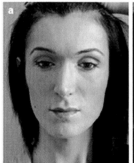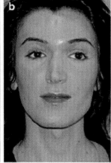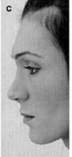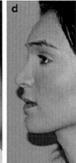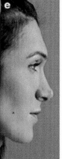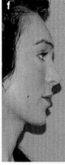

**Fig. 21.5** Pre-operative photographs of a male to female transgender patient with a prominent glabella (**a**, **c**, **e**); 15 month post-operative result after facial feminization surgery including forehead cranioplasty and hydroxyapatite cement placement (**d**, **e**, **f**). With kind permission from Springer Science + Business Media: Hoenig [19]

As an adjunct to any of the three methods, Ousterhout described contouring the forehead by filling in the concavity above the recontoured supraorbital rims with the bone filler methyl methacrylate [12]; today this has been largely replaced by hydroxyapatite cement due to rare infections with the former material [19].

As noted throughout this chapter, surgical alteration of the forehead such as brow elevation, eyebrow shape change, forehead cranioplasty, and scalp advancement can produce a dramatic feminizing effect (Fig. 21.5).

**Key Points**
- Scalp advancement can be added to a browlift procedure using a trichophytic incision along the hairline to reduce the height of the forehead.
- Forehead cranioplasty surgery can reduce a prominent glabella and prominent supra-orbital ridges but must be performed with care due to the underlying frontal sinuses and nearby sensory nerve branches.

## Nasal Surgery

Rhinoplasty surgery can result in a dramatic change to facial appearance for the male to female transgender patient. A full discussion of rhinoplasty surgery is beyond the scope of this chapter, however there are three items notable for facial feminization surgery. The stereotypically female nasal dorsum displays a slight concavity compared to the straight male dorsum and contains a supratip break. The nasofrontal angle is also wider at the junction of the nose and forehead. Secondly, the nasal tip is slightly upturned corresponding to a more obtuse nasolabial angle. After facial feminization rhinoplasty, a recent study showed an increased in the nasofrontal angle from 141.6° to 150.5°; the nasolabial angle increased from 107.4° to 115.2°; surgery also created a supratip break [11].

Lastly, nasal size should be congruent to the face. If a patient undergoes forehead reduction and mandibular angle contouring, reductive rhinoplasty techniques to the nasal dorsum and tip may be considered to maintain an aesthetic balance and create a more petite nose. Surgical considerations include nasal bone osteotomies, tip bulk reduction with suture techniques and cephalic trim of the lower lateral cartilages, and alar base reduction.

Patients considering nasal changes in conjunction with facial feminization surgery should seek consultation with a facial plastic surgeon experienced in rhinoplasty to create a nose in harmony with the feminized face and simultaneously preserve nasal breathing function.

> **Key Points**
> - Although a full discussion of rhinoplasty surgery is beyond the scope of this chapter, facial feminization surgery should address the tip, dorsum, and nasal size.
> - The nasolabial and nasofrontal angles are more obtuse on the stereotypically female nose.
> - A reductive rhinoplasty yields a smaller nose in proportion to the feminized face.

## Surgery of the Midface

Although the zygomas (cheekbones) have more bulk in the biologic male face, they lack the prominence to create the stereotypical feminine appearance of "high cheekbones". To contour the midface, alloplastic malar implants may be placed through oral incisions above the upper teeth, through which the implant can be secured to the underlying bone. Osteotomies and fixation of the bone, or bone grafts were historically performed to relocate the zygomas into more lateral positions but are less commonly performed today [1]. Changes to the underlying facial structure with bone or alloplastic implants will alter the topography of the overlying skin and soft tissue. When lifting the soft tissue of the midface does not provide enough contrast between the cheekbones and the contour beneath, excision of buccal fat has been described to provide a sub-malar concavity [16].

Alternately, non-surgical therapy such as autologous fat or injectable fillers can help achieve a similar feminizing change to the midface, providing volume to the cheeks and lifting the malar soft tissue. Non-surgical procedures have seen large increases in popularity across the world in recent years due to the limited down time and healing. Whether by surgical or non-surgical means, prominent cheeks and a slight hallowing of the sub-malar area under the cheekbones will result in the ideal feminine "heart-shaped" face [16, 20]. Chin shape alterations can complete the heart shape, and these will be discussed in the next section.

> **Key Points**
> - Cheek augmentation with implants, autologous fat or injectable fillers help to create feminine high cheekbones.
> - The ideal female face is "heart-shaped" with prominent, wide cheekbones and contrasting sub-malar concavities.

## Surgery of the Lower Face and Mandible

Depending on the age of the transgender patient, lower face and neck surgery can be quite similar to aging face procedures for cisgender patients. Although rhytidectomy (facelift) is a common procedure in the United States, the American Society for Aesthetic Plastic Surgery reported in 2013 that only 10 % are performed on biologic males [14]. Surgical considerations specific to the biologic male rhytidectomy are incision placement with regard to any remaining facial hair and with regards to post-operative hematoma, thought to be higher due to increased skin vascularity [21].

A unique aspect of lower facial surgery in facial feminization is the underlying shape of the mandible, particularly the prominence of the mandibular angles and the shape of the chin. As noted earlier, there are no specific defined measurements jaw width but the biologic male lower face is wider. Volume of the masseter muscles overlying the bone can further contribute to the width.

Bone reduction softens the prominence of both wide and square shaped mandibular angles. An oral incision lateral and posterior to the dentition provides access to the angles of the mandible. Once generous sub-periosteal dissection is made to retract and protect the soft tissue, bone can be removed using high speed burrs or by osteotomies using saws and a curved osteotomes [16] (Fig. 21.6).

Masseter muscle reduction, common also in Asian biologic female patients, can lessen the wide appearance of the jaw. In addition to direct surgical excision, botulinum toxin (Botox) injected into the masseter muscles results in muscle inactivity for 3–4 months and can reduce muscle bulk over time with repeated injections. Care is taken to inject posteriorly and inferiorly to prevent diffusion into muscles of facial expression such as the zygomatic smiling muscles [22].

The chin's distinct box shape can be modified in the male to female transgender patient to achieve a pointier shape, to complete the ideal feminine "heart-shaped" face. Genioplasty surgery can reposition bone pieces to create anterior projection and simultaneously reduce vertical height; chin shape alterations may also be accomplished with an alloplastic implant. For both procedures, care must be taken to avoid injury to the mental sensory nerves exiting the mandible and to fixate the implant/bone securely in place. If the pre-operative teeth alignment shows overbite or underbite, referral to an oral surgeon is recommended before surgery.

Lastly, alteration to lip volume may complement other facial feminization surgical procedures. Usually hyaluronic acid, the filler provides volume to the lips and is easily performed in the office setting with local anesthetic. Alternately, dermal or fat grafts can add volume the lips. The height of the upper red lip can be surgically lifted with a cheiloplasty (lip lift) which simultaneously

**Fig. 21.6** Reduction of a wide prominent mandible angle (**a**); and resultant decrease in mandibular vertical height (**b**). With kind permission from Springer Science + Business Media: Habal [13]

**a**   **b**

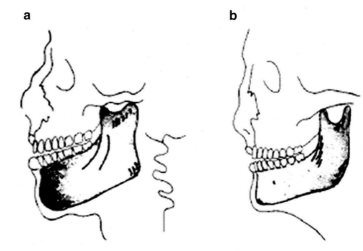

**Key Points**
- Reducing the width and square shape of the mandible will result in a more stereotypical female appearance.
- Masseter muscle hypertrophy contributes to lower facial width and can be reduced with Botox.
- Occlusion of the teeth should be carefully examined when considering genioplasty surgery to alter the appearance of the chin.

shortens a long upper white lip, but this is generally performed with additional anesthetic.

## Other Procedures

### Thyroid Cartilage (Adam's Apple) Alteration

The male to female transgender patient may desire laryngchondroplasty or a "tracheal shave" to reduce a prominent thyroid cartilage (Adam's apple). The vocal folds are attached to the midpoint of the underside of the thyroid cartilage. Those familiar with the complex anatomy of the larynx can safely remove a prominent thyroid notch by avoiding violation of the middle and lower thirds of the thyroid cartilage through a small horizantal incision in the anterior neck, commonly used for other laryngeal procedures (Fig. 21.7).

Conrad suggests an additional precaution of placement of a Keith needle through the thyroid cartilage into the laryngeal lumen, above the attachment of the vocal folds. Laryngoscopy confirms its placement at 2 or 3 mm above the anterior commissure. Cartilage superior to the needle is safely removed and contoured with a scalpel or even saw, depending on the degree of cartilage ossification. The endoscopic verification with the laryngoscope resulted in preservation of vocal function and maximal cartilage excision [23].

**Key Points**
- Laryngchondroplasty or "tracheal shave" can reduce a prominent Adam's apple.
- Placing a needle through the thyroid cartilage into the laryngeal lumen and verifying its position above the vocal fold attachment guides the surgeon to cartilage that can be safely reshaped.

**Fig. 21.7** Prominent thyroid cartilage (**a**); and flattened, more feminine appearance after anterior tracheal shave (**b**). With kind permission from Springer Science + Business Media: Habal [13]

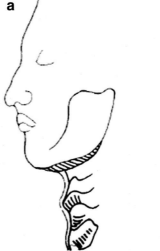
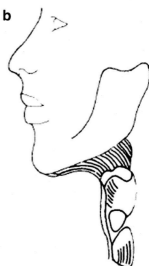

## Phonosurgery and Speech Therapy

Male to female transgender patients may also seek surgery to change their voice, as biologic females phonate in a higher fundamental frequency. Auditory perception of a lower biologic male fundamental frequency has been shown to negatively effect perception. Auditory recognition is so important, that observers rated "femaleness" the lowest when presented with an auditory only presentation of male to female trangender patients, compared to a visual presentation or when observers saw combined presentations [24].

To combat the dichotomy between a feminized visual appearance and male phonation, numerous phonosurgical procedures on the larynx have been reported to try and increase the pitch of phonation above 155 Hz. Higher fundamental frequencies are produced by increasing tension or decreasing mass of the vocal folds through procedures such as cricothyroid approximation to lengthen the vocal folds, scarring to increase stiffness, and vocal fold tissue reduction. A recent summary of phonosurgical procedures to raise pitch noted significant risks and disappointing outcomes [25]. Of note vocal fold elongation is a Type IV Thyroplasty with Isshiki's commonly used classification scheme; in contrast, the Type III Thyroplasty reduces the length of the vocal folds and decreases pitch for the female to male transgender patient [26].

Where surgical procedures to alter the voice have not shown impressive results, speech therapy is an important adjuvant to facial feminization surgery to change the voicing style. Non-surgical therapy alone may be superior to phonosurgical procedure given disappointing outcomes that are seen throughout the literature to raise the fundamental pitch. The transgender patient should consult with a qualified team of laryngologists and speech therapists for recommendations of voice alteration.

**Key Points**
- Vocal procedures or therapy can aid the male to female transgender patient with recognition of "femaleness".
- Phonosurgery alters the tension or mass of the vocal folds with the goal of raise the pitch of voicing to above 155 Hz.
- Speech therapy helps change the voicing style and consultation is should be considered before any procedures to the vocal folds.

## Conclusion

Facial feminization surgery is an important part of treatment for male to female transgender patients. Alterations of the face help transgender patients achieve recognition as a woman, and can result in better physical, mental, and social functioning outcomes following facial feminization surgery compared to those without surgery.

As in all facial plastic surgery, proper preoperative counseling and a mutual understand of expectations will result in a more meaningful experience.

Patients and physicians interested in further reading on facial feminization surgery are encouraged to read the excellent patient centered book by Douglas Ousterhout, *Facial Feminization Surgery: A Guide for the Transgendered Woman*, and also review the peer reviewed literature cited in this chapter.

**Conflicts of Interest and Sources of Funding** None.

## References

1. Becking AG, Tuinzing DB, Hage JJ, Gooren LJG. Transgender feminization of the facial skeleton. Clin Plast Surg. 2007;34(3):557–64.
2. Spack NP. Management of transgenderism. JAMA. 2013;309(5):478–84.

3. Ainsworth T, Spiegel JH. Quality of life of individuals with and without facial feminization surgery or gender reassignment surgery. Qual Life Res. 2010;19(7):1019–24.

4. Spiegel JH. Challenges in care of the transgender patient seeking facial feminization surgery. Facial Plast Surg Clin North Am. 2008;16(2):233–8.

5. Spiegel JH. Facial determinants of female gender and feminizing forehead cranioplasty. Laryngoscope. 2011;121(2):250–61.

6. Ousterhout DK. Facial feminization surgery: a guide for the transgendered woman. Omaha, Nebraska: Addicus Books; 2009.

7. Powell N, Humphreys B. Proportions of the aesthetic face. New York, NY: Thieme Medical Publishers; 1984.

8. Morgan JPI, Haug RH. Evaluation of the craniomaxillofacial deformity patient. In: Greenberg AM, Prein J, editors. Craniomaxillofacial reconstructive and corrective bone surgery. New York: Springer; 2002. p. 5–21.

9. Gonzalex-Ulloa M. Quantitative principles in cosmetic surgery of the face (profileplasty). Plast Reconstr Surg Transplant Bull. 1962;29:186–98.

10. Zimbler MS. Aesthetic facial analysis. In: Flint PW, Haughey BH, Lund VJ, Niparko JK, Richardson MA, Robbins KT, et al., editors. Cummings otolaryngology – head and neck surgery: head and neck surgery. 5th ed. Philadelphia, PA: Mosby Elsevier; 2010. p. 272–3.

11. Noureai SAR, Randhawa P, Andrews PJ, Saleh HA. The role of nasal feminization rhinoplasty in male-to-female gender reassignment. Arch Facial Plast Surg. 2007;9(5):318–20.

12. Ousterhout DK. Feminization of the forehead: contour changing to improve female aesthetics. Plast Reconstr Surg. 1987;79(5):701–13.

13. Habal MB. Aesthetics of feminizing the male face by craniofacial contouring of the facial bones. Aesthetic Plast Surg. 1990;14(2):143–50.

14. The American Society for Aesthetic Plastic Surgery. Cosmetic Surgery National Data Bank [Internet]. 2013. Available from: http://www.surgery.org/media/statistics

15. Ramirez AL, Ende KH, Kabaker SS. Correction of the high female hairline. Arch Facial Plast Surg. 2011;11(2):84–90.

16. Altman K. Facial feminization surgery: current state of the art. Int J Oral Maxillofac Surg. 2012;41(8): 885–94.

17. Roth JM, Metzinger SE. Quantifying the arch position of the female eyebrow. Arch Facial Plast Surg. 2003;5(3):235–9.

18. Cho S-W, Jin HR. Feminization of the forehead in a transgender: frontal sinus reshaping combined with brow lift and hairline lowering. Aesthetic Plast Surg. 2012;36(5):1207–10.

19. Hoenig JF. Frontal bone remodeling for gender reassignment of the male forehead: a gender-reassignment surgery. Aesthetic Plast Surg. 2011;35(6):1043–9.

20. Glasgold MJ, Glasgold RA, Lam SM. Volume restoration and facial aesthetics. Facial Plast Surg Clin North Am. 2008;16(4):435–42.

21. Downs BW, Wang TD. Midcheek and lower face/neck rejuvenation in the male patient. Facial Plast Surg Clin North Am. 2008;16(3):317–27.

22. Bentsianov B, Francis A, Blitzer A. Botulinum toxin treatment of temporomandibular disorders, masseteric hypertrophy, and cosmetic masseter reduction. Oper Tech Otolaryngol Neck Surg. 2004;15(2):110–3.

23. Conrad K, Yoskovitch A. Endoscopically facilitated reduction laryngochondroplasty. Arch Facial Plast Surg. 2003;5(4):345–8.

24. Van Borsel J, De Cuypere G, Van den Berghe H. Physical appearance and voice in male-to-female transsexuals. J Voice. 2001;15(4):570–5.

25. Spiegel JH. Phonosurgery for pitch alteration: feminization and masculinization of the voice. Otolaryngol Clin North Am. 2006;39(1):77–86.

26. Fakhry C, Flint PW, Cummings CW. Medialization thyroplasty. In: Flint PW, Haughey BH, Lund VJ, Niparko JK, Richardson MA, Robbins KT, Thomas JR, editors. Cummings otolaryngology – head and neck surgery: head and neck surgery. 5th ed. Philadelphia, PA: Mosby Elsevier; 2010. p. 904.

# Immigrant and International LGBT Health

# 22

Samantha J. Gridley and Vishesh Kothary

## Purpose

The purpose of this chapter is (1) to provide an overview of the unique healthcare needs of LGBT immigrants in the United States; (2) to highlight the political, legal, and social realities this population faces; and (3) to contextualize medical needs as they relate to patients' diverse backgrounds and countries of origin.

## Learning Objectives

- Discuss differences in terminology for sexual orientation and gender identity between Western and other cultures, and the benefit of adopting patients' preferred vocabulary during a medical encounter *(KP1, ICS1)*
- Describe how mental, physical, and interpersonal health concerns of LGBT patients may differ based on immigrant or asylum status *(PC5)*
- Describe the complex interactions between immigration, law enforcement, and healthcare systems that marginalize LGBT immigrants *(KP4, SBP1)*

S.J. Gridley, A.B. • V. Kothary, B.S. (✉)
Vanderbilt University School of Medicine,
Box 230, 215 Light Hall, Nashville, TN 37212, USA
e-mail: samantha.j.gridley@vanderbilt.edu; Vishesh.
kothary@vanderbilt.edu

## The Changing Demographics of U.S. Healthcare

As we progress into the twenty-first century, the population of the United States is changing in ways that will dramatically transform the delivery and management of healthcare systems. One major demographic trend is notable as part of this change: the increasing racial and ethnic diversification of the U.S. population driven by immigration and the higher number of children born to immigrants.

The Pew Research Center estimates that, if current trends continue, the U.S. population will increase from 324 million in 2015 to 441 million by 2065, and 88 % of this increase is attributed to new immigrants (both documented and undocumented) and their U.S.-born descendants. The country's foreign-born population is projected to rise from 45 million in 2015 to 78 million by 2065. The Hispanic community is currently the nation's largest immigrant group, expected to constitute 24 % of the population in 2065 compared to 18 % in 2015. The Asian population in the United States is expected to grow even more rapidly, and is projected to constitute 14 % of the population in 2065 compared to 6 % in 2015 [1]. These patterns of demographic change will impact healthcare delivery systems in myriad ways, from increased demand for multilingual and culturally competent healthcare providers to meeting the challenge of extending healthcare

© Springer International Publishing Switzerland 2016
K.L. Eckstrand, J.M. Ehrenfeld (eds.), *Lesbian, Gay, Bisexual, and Transgender Healthcare*,
DOI 10.1007/978-3-319-19752-4_22

coverage to new immigrants and their U.S.-born families. Undocumented immigrants, estimated to number 11.3 million in 2014, face numerous additional challenges in accessing healthcare services in a timely and affordable manner [2].

Comprehensive studies show that immigrants fare better than the U.S.-born on several health parameters such as better comprehensive health outcomes, lower disability and mortality rates, and higher life expectancy, with significant variation across immigrant racial/ethnic groups. However, immigrants fare substantially worse than the U.S.-born in health insurance coverage and access to preventive health services [3]. Within this complex and multifaceted picture of immigrant health, LGBT-identified immigrants provide an added layer of complexity that healthcare providers must effectively navigate in order to provide the highest standard of compassionate and culturally competent healthcare.

**Helpful Hint**
Immigrants fall under one of three legal categories: documented (lawfully present in the U.S. with proper legal authorization), undocumented (unlawfully present in the U.S. without government authorization or with expired authorization), and refugees/asylum seekers. The category under which a person falls has an enormous impact on that person's opportunities for employment, housing, freedom of movement, and access to healthcare and government services.

## What Percentage of U.S. Immigrants Identify as LGBT?

Confidently estimating the number of documented and undocumented LGBT immigrants in the U.S. is a formidable challenge. An excellent analysis of available data is presented in a report by the UCLA Law School's Williams Institute,

which compiles data gathered by The Pew Research Hispanic Center, Gallup Daily Tracking Survey and the U.S. Census Bureau's 2011 American Community Survey [4]. Key findings from the report include:

- There are 637,000 documented adult LGBT immigrants (2.4 % of documented adult immigrants), of whom 30 % are Hispanic, and 35 % are Asian or Pacific Islander.
- There are 267,000 undocumented adult LGBT immigrants (2.7 % of undocumented adult immigrants), of whom 71 % are Hispanic, and 15 % are Asian or Pacific Islander.
- Compared to foreign-born individuals in opposite-sex couples, foreign-born individuals in same-sex couples are more likely to be male, and have lower incomes despite attaining higher educational levels.

While it is even more challenging to accurately estimate the number of transgender immigrants, a report by the National Center for Transgender Equality estimates that of the approximately 267,000 undocumented LGBT immigrants present in the U.S., between 15,000 and 50,000 are transgender [5]. This number is most likely an underestimate due to the reluctance of many transgender individuals to identify as such before authorities. This unwillingness to publicly identify as transgender may be attributed to past instances of discrimination and prejudice in their homelands, and/or due to mistrust and continued fear of U.S. authorities. No data on the number of documented transgender immigrants is currently available.

An important sub-population, one that is perhaps the most vulnerable and most likely to encounter the healthcare system under adverse circumstances, is that of LGBT refugees and asylum seekers. Due to various factors discussed further in this chapter, LGBT individuals face a high risk of physical, mental, and sexual violence; political and legal persecution; and socio-cultural isolation and ostracization in many parts of the world. Since the mid-1990s asylum claims based on persecution due to sexual orientation and gender identity/expression have become increasingly commonplace, and U.S. Courts have consistently upheld the validity of these claims. There is no official data maintained either by the United Nations Human Rights Commission (UNHCR) or the United States Citizenship and Immigration Services (USCIS) on the numbers of LGBT asylum seekers and those granted asylum on this basis in the U.S. A report from the Heartland Alliance Rainbow Welcome Initiative [6] estimates that about 3,500 LGBT refugees arrive in the U.S. each year, and about 1,250 LGBT individuals are granted asylee status each year (based on data from 2010). It is important to keep in mind that many LGBT refugees will not disclose their identity, and others may not seek assistance from asylum agencies.

Another important subpopulation to consider is LGBT immigrants who are HIV positive and hence must routinely interact with the U.S. healthcare system. While there are no official statistics on this subpopulation, it is a well-established fact that gay men and transgender individuals—in the U.S. and globally—are at high risk of HIV/AIDS and carry a disproportionate burden of the epidemic [7]. Given the history of prejudice and discrimination against HIV positive people—a prejudice that is often legally enshrined—LGBT immigrants who are HIV positive are likely to face triple marginalization due to their status as immigrants (documented or undocumented), LGBT identification, and HIV seropositivity.

## Back Home: Anti-LGBT Laws and Attitudes Abroad

In order to provide sensitive and culturally competent care for LGBT immigrants here in the United States, it is important to have a basic understanding of the environment from which many of these patients come. While LGBT rights and safety vary significantly across the globe, a number of countries that will be discussed below have particularly harsh laws against LGBT persons. The criminalization of these citizens' actions and identities translates into fear of being exposed, aversion to health providers, and poorer

health outcomes. Even when immigrants from these countries are no longer bound by their laws, the anxiety and fear that these laws inculcated in them may carry over into their interactions with healthcare providers here in the U.S.

Of note, unprecedented progress has been made over the past decade domestically as well as globally in advancing the cause of LGBT equality, and many people have come to consider the LGBT rights struggle as the Civil Rights movement of our time. In many parts of the world that have been historically hostile to LGBT people, grassroots organizations as well as national campaigns have emerged to advocate for LGBT equality. While many legal, political, and social changes have been made all over the world, in some areas the increased visibility of the LGBT population has unfortunately led to a backlash against them.

A United Nations report from 2011 documents 76 countries in which consensual same-sex relationships are a crime, demonstrating just how pervasive anti-LGBT laws still are across the globe. In six of these countries—Mauritania, Sudan, Saudi Arabia, Yemen, Iran, and Shariah-governed northern Nigeria—same-sex sexual acts are punishable by death. Those in power often justify laws that criminalize same-sex acts and gender nonconforming behavior as a "necessary public health measure." (This stance was unsuccessfully argued in defense of a law criminalizing same-sex consensual conduct among men in the case of Toonen v. Australia in 1992 [8].) In reality, such laws infringe on the health rights of LGBT people because these laws engender fear of revealing unlawful conduct, which in turn discourages LGBT persons from seeking health care services. As a result, the available healthcare providers and services are ill-equipped to cater to this population's specific needs. Moreover, such laws make it difficult for organizations to promote LGBT health. For example, authorities in some countries have confiscated safer sex literature, thereby impairing HIV prevention efforts.

Even in countries where no formal anti-LGBT laws exist, pervasive homophobic attitudes, especially when espoused by healthcare providers, negatively impact the health of LGBT people.

Fear of being judged, chastised, or exposed through a breach of confidentiality may deter LGBT persons from seeking healthcare in these countries.

The 2011 UN report also draws attention to particular health issues that transgender persons across the globe face. Gender-affirming surgery and cross-gender hormone therapy are not available in many countries, and when they are, astronomical costs and lack of insurance coverage (or insurance policy exclusions) prohibit many patients from receiving the care they need. Other pervasive problems include lack of professional training on transgender health issues and insensitivity to the needs of transgender patients [9].

With these ripple effects of anti-LGBT laws and attitudes in mind, we provide you with a short summary of the politico-legal climates that foster oppression of LGBT persons in different regions of the world.

> **Helpful Hint**
> An understanding of anti-LGBT laws and attitudes abroad can help you understand and address the unique reservations your patient may have toward discussing their LGBT identity with healthcare professionals.

## Africa

Same-sex sexual acts are criminalized in 34 African countries. In many places, recent laws have been stricter and more oppressive than the laws that preceded them. The new, harsher laws are often precipitated by tacit encouragement from anti-LGBT American organizations. Here is a sampling of countries in Africa with such laws:

### Cameroon

In Cameroon, homosexual conduct is punishable with a fine and up to 5 years in jail. This law is vigorously enforced; Cameroon has arrested more homosexual persons (or persons perceived as such) than any other African country [10]. Unfortunately,

legislation condemning same-sex sexual acts is only the tip of the iceberg of LGBT antipathy in the country. A more demonstrative example of the palpable hostility toward LGBT Cameroonians is the torture and murder of Eric Ohena Lembembe, the most vocal and well-known LGBT rights activist in Cameroon, in 2013 [11].

### Uganda

Penalties for homosexuality in Uganda range from 14 years in jail to life imprisonment. The Anti-Homosexuality Bill proposed in 2009 sought to include the death penalty as punishment for same-sex sexual acts in particular circumstances [12]. The bill also endorsed imprisonment of anyone who becomes aware that a person is gay and fails to report that person within 24 h. The bill was temporarily tabled due to international pressure, but it was resurrected quickly with a few revisions. This revised version dropped the death penalty for persons who engage in same-sex sexual acts and replaced it with life in prison—a punishment that Uganda's Minister of Ethics and Integrity James Nsaba Buturo claimed would be more "helpful" than the death penalty because it "gives room for offenders to be rehabilitated" [13]. The bill intensified the criminalization of same-sex sexual acts both on Ugandan soil and for Ugandans who engage in same-sex sexual acts abroad. According to the bill, offenders in the latter category may be extradited for punishment back to Uganda. Penalties apply not only to individuals but also to groups who know and do not report gay people or who generally support gay rights. Ugandan President Yoweri Museveni signed the bill into an act on February 24, 2014 [14], but on August 1, 2014 the act was overturned by Uganda's constitutional court. Even with this judicial ruling, rampant violence has continued against LGBT people in Uganda.

### Democratic Republic of the Congo

In 2014, the Democratic Republic of the Congo (DRC) had a bill sponsored in Parliament that sought to criminalize same-sex sexual acts as "acts against nature" [10]. National Assembly Member Steve Mbikayi promoted the bill as a means to avoid "moral depravity" and to "preserve African values," which, he insisted, "have never tolerated romantic relationships between persons of the same sex" [10].

## Nigeria

In January 2014, Nigeria's president, Goodluck Jonathan, signed the Same Sex Marriage Prohibition Act, which punishes persons who attempt to enter into same-sex marriages with up to 14 years imprisonment. The law also prescribes up to a decade in prison for those who "directly or indirectly" make a "public show" of same-sex relationships [15]. In addition, the law incriminates LGBT rights advocacy groups and people witnessing or aiding same-sex relationships. The cultish drive to "morally sanitize" the country extends beyond jargon-filled laws—it permeates the mindset of countless citizens who say they "are ready to take the law into their own hands to combat homosexuality" [15]. Even in prison, gay inmates are kept isolated from other prisoners so that they do not "indoctrinate the other inmates" [15].

## Zimbabwe

In 2013, under the presidency of Robert Mugabe—who in one speech called for the beheading of homosexuals [16]—the "sexual deviancy law" passed, which extended crimes of same-sex behavior to include holding hands, hugging, or kissing.

## Middle East

### Iran

In Iran, the legal code is based on Islamic law. Death is a potential punishment for same-sex sexual acts, and kissing a person of the same sex may result in 60 lashes. In March 2013, the secretary general of Iran's high council for human rights described homosexuality as "an illness and malady"; in May 2013, homosexual identity, beyond specific acts, was criminalized and deemed punishable by lashes as well [17]. Given this politically sanctioned description of gay persons as intrinsically diseased at the core of their being, one can extrapolate that LGB Iranians face numerous hostilities when accessing healthcare

services. Interestingly, the political, religious, and medical authorities in Iran recognize "Gender Identity Disorder" as a valid medical diagnosis and the government even provides financial support for cross-gender hormone therapy and sex reassignment surgery. However, since homosexuality is criminalized, the government often forces LGB individuals who are not transgender to undergo sex reassignment therapies against their will or risk being penalized for having a same-sex relationship [29].

### Qatar

The law in Qatar categorizes same-sex sexual acts as an offense that is punishable by up to 7 years in jail [18]. Curiously, only homosexual acts between males are deemed criminal acts by the law, whereas same-sex sexual acts between adult females are not illegal in Qatar.

### Yemen

Same-sex sexual acts are punishable by death in Yemen, and the official position held by the government is that "there are no gays in Yemen" [18]. LGBT websites are censored, and there are no public spaces in which LGBT people can congregate. The invisibility of LGBT culture and persons in Yemen renders LGBT-specific health care nonexistent.

## Asia

### Russia

During the 2014 Winter Olympics, Russia fell under international scrutiny for its anti-LGBT legislation. In June 2013, a new law was passed banning the "propaganda of non-traditional sexual relationships" to minors, and subjecting distributors of these materials to lofty fines [19]. Foreigners breaking this law are subject to even heavier penalties: they are fined more severely and may be subject to 15 days in prison and deportation from Russia. This law serves as an amendment to the previously existing federal law mandating that children be protected from "information that can bring harm to their health and wellbeing" [20].

## Kyrgyzstan

In March 2014, a draft bill that criminalizes spreading information about LGBT issues was published by Kyrgyzstan's national parliament. In June 2015, the bill passed a second reading in parliament, with 90 members voting in favor and only 2 members voting against it. If the bill passes a third reading and is signed by the president, it will become a law. The bill has been criticized internationally as homophobic and blatantly discriminatory against LGBT people [21].

## The Americas

Despite a recent trend toward LGBT-protective laws being passed in the Americas, some countries still maintain their anti-LGBT laws.

## Belize

The Belize Criminal Code criminalizes "carnal intercourse against the law of nature," describing any sexual act carried out without the intent to procreate [22]. A case arguing for removal of this law, citing its unconstitutionality, was heard in the Supreme Court in 2013. As of 2015, a decision is still pending.

## Caribbean

Same-sex sexual acts can be penalized with imprisonment in Antigua and Barbuda, Barbados, Dominica, Grenada, Jamaica, Saint Kitts and Nevis, Saint Lucia, Saint Vincent and the Grenadines, and Trinidad and Tobago. Jamaica was labeled "the most homophobic place on earth" in a 2006 TIME magazine article [23].

## New Home: Recent Victories in LGBT Immigrant Rights in the U.S.

While the United States has not always been at the forefront of advancing LGBT equality, the past two decades have seen unprecedented progress in this area, both in terms of politico-legal changes as well as socio-cultural shifts in public opinion regarding LGBT people. Some important highlights that have dramatically expanded the rights of LGBT immigrants and their access to healthcare services include [5]:

- In 2009, the Obama administration ended a 22-year-old policy banning HIV positive individuals from traveling to or immigrating to the United States. Enacted in 1987 amidst a climate of fear and ignorance regarding HIV, the policy lacked any scientific or medical basis and prevented international AIDS conferences from coming to the U.S. It had a detrimental effect on gay men and transgender individuals (who continue to carry a disproportionate burden of the AIDS epidemic) engaged in binational relationships or seeking to come to the U.S. for medical treatment.
- In 2011, the Department of Homeland Security issued prosecutorial discretion guidelines to halt deportations of individuals with significant family relationships in the United States, including those with "long-term same-sex partners".
- In 2011, United States Citizenship and Immigration Services (USCIS) issued guidance to all refugee and asylum officers on adjudicating LGBT refugee and asylum claims; in the past, these officers lacked formal guidance and training in working with LGBT populations.
- In March 2012, the DHS released new detention standards titled "Performance-Based National Detention Standards" that seek to improve the treatment of LGBT detainees. Among other provisions, the standards mandate that strip searches of transgender detainees be conducted in private and allow transgender immigrants to continue to receive medically necessary hormone therapy if they received it prior to being detained. Immigration officials may also not determine a transgender detainee's housing based solely on their physical anatomy but instead must house detainees in accordance with their gender identity. The new detention standards also require that "all FDA-approved medications necessary for the treatment of HIV/

AIDS" are accessible to HIV-positive detainees [24].

- In April 2012, USCIS adopted new policy guidelines to clarify the eligibility of transgender people and their partners for family-based immigration benefits, including changing one's gender on immigration documents.
- In December 2012, the Department of Homeland Security (DHS) proposed regulations to implement the Prison Rape Elimination Act of 2003 in immigration detention. The rules propose standards for officials to be trained by to prevent, detect, and respond to sexual abuse and assault in detention facilities. This training includes teaching officials "how to communicate effectively and professionally with detainees, including gay, bisexual, transgender, intersex, or gender nonconforming detainees". These rules were finalized in February 2014 [24].
- In 2013, the U.S. Supreme Court struck down a major provision of the Federal Defense of Marriage Act (D.O.M.A.). The Federal government now recognizes same-sex marriages performed in states and foreign countries where such unions are legal. Over 1100 legal protections of marriage that were denied to same-sex couples formerly have now been extended to all married couples including immigration benefits such as the ability to sponsor a foreign same-sex spouse for legal U.S. residency, access to a same-sex spouse's health insurance coverage, and numerous other benefits. These legal changes will go a long way in ensuring unity of binational LGBT families and improving access to healthcare services for LGBT immigrants.
- In 2015, the United States Supreme Court in Obergefell v. Hodges legalized same-sex marriage in all states of the U.S [28]. This landmark decision will allow LGBT immigrants to lawfully marry their partners and gain greater access to health insurance as well as the ability to establish lawful permanent residence ("green card") in the U.S.

## Addressing the Double-Marginalization of LGBT Immigrants and Refugees

Heartland Alliance, a leading anti-poverty and human rights organization, has produced a comprehensive guide to resettling LGBT refugees titled *Rainbow Response*. This guide identifies LGBT immigrants and refugees as a vulnerable patient population that merits extra care from health care providers. While non-LGBT refugees are usually fleeing oppressive governments, LGBT refugees are often seeking asylum from both discriminatory laws *and* violence committed by their own families, friends, and neighbors [6]. Not only is this population new to the U.S., but they may also face the same isolation within their ethnic community here that they dealt with in their home country. For this reason, Heartland Alliance deems LGBT refugees "doubly marginalized". Health care providers are called upon to make these patients feel respected and welcome at a time when they feel like outsiders on all fronts.

## Looking Through a Non-Western Lens

It is critically important that a physician caring for LGBT immigrant/refugee patients be aware that Western conceptions of sexuality and gender identity may not align with their patient's terminology for describing non-heteronormative behaviors or identities. The culturally competent physician will resist imposing Western labels onto these patients. Instead, you should ask nonjudgmental and open-ended questions about the patient's health behaviors; then use the patient's chosen terminology to shape the discussion. Be sure to document in the medical record what the preferred term means to the patient. Remember, every patient has the right to identify as they choose. Working within the patient's lexicon will help you present your medical advice in a way that best gets through to the patient. Doing so will also minimize the risk of alienating the patient with labels that carry stigmatizing connotations in their mind.

**Helpful Hint**
Different cultures ascribe different labels to non-heteronormative actions. Work within your patient's preferred terminology to help them feel comfortable and respected.

*Rainbow Response* captures one reason why patients from different countries may dissociate same-gender sexual activity from LGBT identity: "Not everyone who has same-sex sexual partners identifies as gay, lesbian, or bisexual; there are often other cultural and societal implications for identifying as a member of the LGBT community. Consequences may include endangering oneself, bringing shame or dishonor to one's family, and experiencing difficulty in securing employment" [6]. As we noted earlier in "Back Home: Anti-LGBT Laws and Attitudes Abroad", many patients carry with them the stigma and fear of non-heteronormative labels even after they have left the country that ingrained these associations in their mind. For this reason, physicians should adopt vocabulary that the patient prefers and allow these terms to evolve only when the patient feels comfortable utilizing different labels.

Because terms used to describe different sexual behaviors vary across cultures, the culturally competent healthcare provider will not make assumptions about sexual behavior based on a patient's relationship status or how a person self-identifies. For example, in Iraq, identifying as LGBT is "taboo, in part because it poses an immediate threat to the family unit... the foundation on which many communities are built" [6]. In Latin American countries, power dynamics within same-sex sexual acts color the terminology describing those involved: "Men who penetrate other men are not considered to be gay; only their male partners who are penetrated are... Active partners are perceived as masculine and often have wives. Receptive partners are [perceived as] more feminine and typically do not partner with women" [6].

One study examining the context and dynamics of same-sex sexual experiences among rural youth in India found that disparities existed between reported sexual activities and self-identified sexuality. About one fifth of the sexually active young men in the study reported same-sex sexual experiences, but a substantial subgroup of these same young men did not self-identify as homosexual or bisexual. It was found that the group reporting same-sex sexual experiences "begin their sexual careers early, engage with a higher number of sexual partners, both male and female; and are more likely to report inconsistent condom use, as compared to their heterosexually active peers" [25]. Each of these factors contributes to a higher risk for acquiring STIs, including HIV. Given the disconnect between same-sex sexual acts and identities in this population, in order to adequately address associated risk factors the provider should ask these patients about specific sexual acts. Within their cultural context, one cannot accurately deduce sexual behaviors from self-identified sexuality alone.

Another point to consider when asking patients about their sexual practices is that the terms homosexual, heterosexual, bisexual, or transgender may not translate into the patient's native language. However, the absence of labels that correspond to Western vocabulary does not imply that varying sexual behaviors do not exist in other parts of the world; there is no culture in which a spectrum of gender and sexual identities does not exist [6]. Avoid miscommunication by asking whether the patient has sex with men, women, or both, in addition to asking how they self-identify.

**Helpful Hint**
Be specific! In addition to asking how the patient self-identifies, be sure to ask whether they have sex with men, women, or both. Do not assume that the way a patient labels their sexuality encompasses all you need to know about their sexual behavior.

## Let's Get Comfortable

One of the biggest ways in which you as a medical provider can cultivate a trusting relationship with your LGBT immigrant/refugee patients is to confront any discomfort you may have with LGBT identity before a patient walks in the door. These patients may come from areas where LGBT status is so stigmatized that they have had to hide or suppress their identity out of fear for their safety or the safety of their loved ones. With such vulnerable patients, it is important to refrain from expressing discomfort with LGBT identity lest we deter them from continuing to seek healthcare in the future.

At the start of the first clinic visit with an LGBT immigrant/refugee patient, it is a good idea to reiterate that the conversations you have with them are strictly confidential. Stress that your goal is to provide them with the best medical care possible, and explain that answering questions about their background and lifestyle helps you to tailor your care to their individual needs. Confidentiality is not something that all LGBT immigrants and refugees will automatically assume exists when they seek healthcare. *Rainbow Response* highlights the fact that distrust is a natural consequence of many LGBT refugee/asylees' past experiences: "The fear of their sexual orientation or gender identity/expression being discovered is very real; many have experienced breaches of trust and confidentiality in the past, which often led to arrest, abuse, and torture. While repercussions such as these are not likely to occur in the United States, providers must honor their feelings and appreciate the sensitive nature of these issues" [6].

These patients' fear of breached confidentiality in a healthcare setting is not limited to providers' role as confidants—interpreters represent another group that may be seen as potentially untrustworthy to an LGBT immigrant patient. If you are using an interpreter during a clinical encounter, reassure the patient that the interpreter is obligated to protect confidentiality in the same way that you are.

If your facility has the benefit of professional interpreters, always utilize a professional rather than a friend or relative of the patient as an interpreter. Employing the services of someone who does not know the patient ensures anonymity and encourages honesty from the patient. In the presence of a family member, the patient might

omit potentially embarrassing or stigmatizing components of their history, and such omissions work to the detriment of their healthcare. Use of an interpreter both improves patient understanding and affords the patient the freedom to speak about confidential issues without fear of loved ones listening.

An additional benefit of professional interpreters is that they are trained to minimize their presence during the clinical encounter and to repeat everything that is said. This interpretation technique allows the conversation to flow naturally between provider and patient. Ideally, the interpreter will create a situation in which you and the patient feel as though you are speaking to each other *through* the interpreter rather than talking *at* the interpreter. Patients' family members who interpret will likely be less competent in facilitating an interaction like this during the visit.

## LGBT Immigrant/Refugee Patients and Intimate Partner Violence

All providers should be on the lookout for signs of intimate partner violence (IPV) in a patient's history or physical exam. IPV comes in many forms: physical, emotional, psychological, verbal, and sexual violence are a few examples (see Chap. 5 for details).

LGBT survivors of abuse face "compound discrimination—prejudice against their same-sex relationship and shame associated with domestic violence" [6]. Some LGBT individuals affected by abuse may not seek help because they fear doing so will show a lack of solidarity within the LGBT community [26]. They may also be afraid that if they report domestic violence, society will assume that LGBT relationships are inherently dysfunctional or abusive [26]. Individuals with this fear may remain silent in an attempt to protect the public image of the broader LGBT community.

Adding immigrant or refugee status into the picture makes reporting domestic violence an even more complex decision for LGBT individuals affected by abuse. *Rainbow Response* offers two additional reasons why this population may abstain from reporting: (1) concern that their immigration status will be affected, and (2) threats by the abuser "to 'out' her/his partner if s/he were to report" [6]. Fear of being "outed"—either as LGBT, undocumented, or both—is often exploited by abusive partners as a power play.

> **Helpful Hint**
> Detailing ways in which your clinic or hospital works to protect individuals affected by abuse from retaliation by their abuser can help patients feel safe enough to report abuse they may have suffered.

## Addressing Barriers to Successful Care

LGBT patients, regardless of immigration status, have unique health concerns that differ from those of the general population, as highlighted in Chap. 2. Limited knowledge about the U.S. healthcare system further compounds the health risks that LGBT immigrant/refugee patients face [6]. They may also not feel comfortable advocating for themselves when they do have medical appointments, or they may be ashamed to reveal that they do not fully understand what their provider has told them [6]. They may come from cultures in which talking about sexual practices is not appropriate, even in the context of medicine [6]. In such cultures it is likely that comprehensive sex education is lacking, in which case the patient may have limited knowledge about safe sex practices and risks of STIs. Below is a list of strategies to overcome these challenges that arise in serving LGBT immigrant/refugee patients.

- *Referrals:* You must carefully consider the providers to whom you refer your LGBT immigrant/refugee patients for specialty care. Fortunately, *Health Professionals Advancing LGBT Equality* provides a free directory of LGBT-friendly healthcare providers across the country at www.glma.org. If you would like to be included in this directory, you can sign up for free at the same website.

- *Patient understanding:* Remind your patient that they are free to ask questions and that you *want* them to ask for clarification when they do not understand something. Some patients may come from cultures in which it would be rude or disrespectful to ask questions to their doctor, or they may be embarrassed about not understanding something. Encourage them to speak up! In addition, remember that interpreters are crucial to facilitating patient understanding if the patient is not fluent in English.

- *Accommodations:* Explain that the patient has a right to request accommodations (within reason) to make them feel comfortable during their appointment. *Rainbow Response* offers the example that LGBT refugees/asylees may wish to request care from a provider of the same or opposite sex [6]. Keep in mind that medical care delves into intimate areas of people's lives and bodies, and it is important to respect cultural norms as much as possible.

- *Privacy:* Reiterate to your patient that they have a right to see their provider alone (without family members present) if they want. They can also request that their family members remain in the room if they prefer.

- *Past trauma and physical exams: Rainbow Response* calls upon providers to take special care to explain each step of the physical exam for LGBT immigrants and to be prepared to address triggers of past trauma: "LGBT refugees and asylees are far more likely to be survivors of torture and/or to have suffered from other forms of life-threatening violence. They may feel uncomfortable during physical examinations; breast exams, gynecological exams, pap smears, and colorectal exams are particularly sensitive procedures that could trigger past traumatic events. Medical staff should know that to make LGBT patients more comfortable, they should move through each procedure slowly, explaining the purpose of each step" [6].

- *Infectious disease concerns:* LGBT refugee/immigrant patients may not have had prior access to STI education or testing. Consider offering STI screening if your patient is at risk. To demonstrate the lack of adequate sexual healthcare in some regions of the world, consider these findings in a study evaluating STI treatment services available to transgender patients in Pakistan: "Fewer than 45 % of private and public sector general practitioners [in Pakistan] had been trained in STI treatment after the completion of their medical curriculum, and none of the traditional healers had received any formal training or information on STIs" [27]. Moreover, the study found that WHO guidelines for STI management were being followed by only 29 % of public and private sector doctors and a mere 5 % of traditional healers. Cost of STI drugs, diagnostic fees, and consultations fees were found to be further barriers to treatment. These findings exemplify one country in which healthcare for patients with or at risk for STIs is sub-par, but many other regions also have healthcare systems that are poorly equipped to care for at-risk patients, especially those within the LGBT population.

- In addition, keep in mind that refugee patients who are HIV positive are more likely to have been exposed to TB and other latent infectious diseases before coming to the U.S. [6]. Be sure to screen for such infections if your LGBT immigrant/refugee patient is HIV positive.
- *Non-allopathic Medicine:* Be sure to ask about prior medical practices, treatments, and medications that your patient may have utilized in their home country. This includes home remedies and supplements.

and sexual abuse; and often violent persecution in many parts of the world. Many such individuals enter the United States scarred by a traumatic past, habituated to suppressing their LGBT identity, and deeply mistrustful of government agencies and other institutions. It is imperative that as a healthcare provider you are aware of the unique challenges faced by such patients and are well-equipped to treat them with the empathy, understanding, and compassion that they deserve. For many of these patients, revealing their LGBT identity or HIV seropositivity could have had fatal consequences in their home countries, and it is understandably not easy for them to readily confide in their healthcare providers in the U.S. given the unequal power differential inherent in the provider-patient relationship.

> **Helpful Hint**
> Transgender immigrants, LGBT refugees/asylum seekers, and HIV positive immigrants (many of whom also identify as LGBT) are especially marginalized, and many have suffered from physical, emotional, and sexual violence in their home countries as well as in the U.S. immigration detention system. Acquaint yourself with the unique issues faced by these groups so you can better empathize with these patients and provide culturally competent care to them.

## Mental Health and LGBT Immigrants

Psychological and emotional well-being, and coping with past trauma/abuse are important issues to consider when interacting with immigrant patients, especially with vulnerable groups such as transgender immigrants, LGBT refugees/asylum seekers, and HIV positive immigrants. Individuals belonging to these groups routinely face discrimination; prejudice; physical, emotional,

## LGBT Refugees/Asylum Seekers

As discussed earlier in the chapter, many countries around the world have laws that foster institutionalized oppression of LGBT people. When LGBT identity and/or same-sex sexual acts are criminalized, it opens the doors to persecution of LGBT people by police, military, and government officials; judiciary, public, and private agencies; and even one's own family, community, and religious institutions. An environment that engenders discrimination and prejudice against LGBT individuals can be detrimental to physical and mental health. Such traumatic experiences can leave a lasting impact on one's psyche and increase the risk for post-traumatic stress disorder (PTSD), substance abuse disorders, generalized and social anxiety, and other psychological illnesses. Often, clinicians in the U.S. who work with refugee populations are the first to identify these problems, and thus it is imperative that you have the requisite background knowledge and training to work with at-risk LGBT immigrant populations.

## Transgender Immigrants

Transgender immigrants, especially those who are undocumented, have lower rates of health insurance coverage than the general population [5]. Even those who are insured may lack coverage for trans-related health issues such as cross-gender hormone therapy and gender-affirming surgery. These barriers to quality health insurance coverage and affordable healthcare contribute to significant disparities in physical and mental health for transgender immigrants. The National Transgender Discrimination Survey found that undocumented transgender immigrants reported twice the rate of physical assault in a medical setting compared to the overall sample of transgender adults (4 % vs. 2 %). The report also found a higher HIV prevalence rate among transgender immigrants compared to the overall U.S. transgender population (6.96 % of undocumented transgender immigrants and 7.84 % of documented transgender immigrants compared to 2.64 % for the overall sample). Moreover, undocumented transgender immigrants were half as likely to know their HIV status compared to the overall sample [5]. Healthcare providers working with transgender immigrant patients should be mindful of these socio-economic difficulties and systemic barriers to optimum health faced by their patients.

In conclusion, LGBT immigrants routinely face the challenges of double marginalization and encounter numerous difficulties while navigating the complexities of the U.S. immigration, law enforcement, and healthcare systems in order to receive access to quality healthcare. All healthcare providers should familiarize themselves with the diverse backgrounds, politico-legal challenges, and unique health needs of LGBT immigrants in order to provide compassionate, quality, and culturally competent healthcare to this population.

## Resources

- Immigration Equality is a major national non-profit organization that works in policy development and advocacy for LGBT immigrants. Their website is an excellent resource for more information, and patients who need legal assistance related to immigration can also be referred to them.
- http://immigrationequality.org/
- Heartland Alliance Rainbow Welcome Initiative "supports the resettlement of Lesbian, Gay, Bisexual, and Transgender (LGBT) refugees and asylees by offering technical assistance to service providers and disseminating critical resources relevant to both resettlement staff and refugees and asylees. The Rainbow Welcome Initiative is committed to ensuring the successful integration of LGBT refugees and asylees as they establish new lives in this country and pursue new possibilities."
- http://rainbowwelcome.org/– Gay Men's Health Crisis Inc. Immigration projecthttp://www.immigrationadvocates.org/nonprofit/legaldirectory/organization.393220-Gay_Mens_Health_Crisis_Inc_Immigration_Project

## References

1. Pew Research Center, 2015. "Modern Immigration Wave Brings 59 Million to U.S., Driving Population Growth and Change Through 2065: Views of Immigration's Impact on U.S. Society Mixed." Washington, D.C.: September.
2. Passel, Jeffrey S., and D'Vera Cohn. "Unauthorized Immigrant Population Stable for Half a Decade." Pew Research Center. 22 July 2015.
3. Singh GK, Rodriguez-Lainz A, Kogan MD. Immigrant health inequalities in the United States: use of eight

major national data systems. Scientific World Journal. 2013:512313.

4. Gates G. LGBT adult immigrants in the United States. Los Angeles, CA: The Williams Institute at UCLA Law School; 2013.

5. Jeanty J, Tobin HJ. Our moment for reform: immigration and transgender people. Washington, DC: National Center for Transgender Equality; 2013.

6. Heartland Alliance for Human Needs and Human Rights. Rainbow response: a practical guide to resettling LGBT refugees; 2014. Retrieved from: http://www.rainbowwelcome.org/uploads/pdfs/Rainbow%20Response_Heartland%20Alliance%20Field%20Manual.pdf

7. Lambda Legal. When health care isn't caring: Lambda Legal's survey of discrimination against LGBT people and people with HIV. New York; 2010. Retrieved from: www.lambdalegal.org/health-care-report

8. United Nations Human Right Committee, Toonen v. Australia, U.N. Doc. CCPR/C/50/D/488/1992 (2014, Jun 7), at http://www.globalhealthrights.org/health-topics/health-care-and-health-services/toonen-v-australia/

9. United Nations High Commissioner for Human Rights (2011, Nov 17). Discriminatory laws and practices and acts of violence against individuals based on their sexual orientation and gender identity. United Nations General Assembly Human Rights Council. Retrieved from: http://www2.ohchr.org/english/bodies/hrcouncil/docs/19session/A.HRC.19.41_English.pdf

10. Nzioka D (2014, Feb 26). Africa: a look at Africa's anti-gay laws. All Africa. Retrieved from: http://allafrica.com/stories/201402281416.html

11. Kordunsky A (2013, Aug 14). Russia not only country with anti-gay laws. National Geographic. Retrieved from: http://news.nationalgeographic.com/news/2013/08/130814-russia-anti-gay-propaganda--law-world-olympics-africa-gay-rights/

12. The Anti Homosexuality Bill, Uganda; 2009. Retrieved from: http://nationalpress.typepad.com/files/bill-no-18-anti-homosexuality-bill-2009.pdf

13. Biryabarema E (2009, Dec 23). Uganda government softens proposed anti-gay law. Thomson Reuters. Retrieved from: http://af.reuters.com/article/topNews/idAFJOE5BM0EQ20091223

14. The Anti-Homosexuality Act, Uganda; 2014. Retrieved from: http://wp.patheos.com.s3.amazonaws.com/blogs/warrenthrockmorton/files/2014/02/Anti-Homosexuality-Act-2014.pdf

15. Nossiter A (2014, Feb 8). Nigeria tries to 'sanitize' itself of gays. The New York Times. Retrieved from: http://www.nytimes.com/2014/02/09/world/africa/nigeria-uses-law-and-whip-to-sanitize-gays.html?_r=0

16. Littauer D (2013, Jul 26). Zimbabwe president calls for the beheading of gays. Coalition for Advancement of Lesbian Business in Africa. Retrieved from: http://www.calbia-foundation.org/zimbabwe-president-calls-for-the-beheading-of-gays/

17. Dehghan SK (2013, Mar 14). Iranian human rights official describes homosexuality as an illness. Guardian News and Media. Retrieved from: http://www.theguardian.com/world/iran-blog/2013/mar/14/iran-official-homosexuality-illness

18. Marriage Equality USA (2013, Aug 25). Marriage equality in the Middle East. Retrieved from: http://www.marriageequality.org/middle-east

19. The Council for Global Equality. The facts on LGBT rights in Russia; 2013. Retrieved from: http://www.globalequality.org/newsroom/latest-news/1-in-the-news/186-the-facts-on-lgbtrights-in-russia

20. Russian LGBT Network. The state Duma passed the bill on "non-traditional sexual relations"; 2013. Retrieved from: http://www.lgbtnet.ru/en/content/state-duma-passed-bill-non-traditional-sexual-relations

21. Human Rights Watch (2014, Mar 27). Kyrgyzstan: withdraw draconian homophobic bill. Retrieved from: https://www.hrw.org/news/2014/03/27/kyrgyzstan-withdraw-draconian-homophobic-bill

22. Glickhouse R, Keller M (2013, May 16). Explainer: LGBT rights in Latin America and the Caribbean. Americas Society/Council of the Americas. Retrieved from: http://www.as-coa.org/articles/explainer-lgbt-rights-latin-america-and-caribbean#Without_Protections

23. Padgett T (2006, Apr 12). The most homophobic place on earth? TIME Magazine. Retrieved from: http://content.time.com/time/world/article/0,8599,1182991,00.html

24. Burns C, Garcia A, Wolgin P. Living in shadows: LGBT undocumented immigrants. Washington, DC: Center for American Progress; 2013.

25. Singh AK, Mahendra VS, Verma R. Exploring context and dynamics of homosexual experiences among rural youth in India. J LGBT Health Res. 2008; 4(2–3):89–101.

26. Center for American Progress (2011 Jun 14). LGBT domestic violence fact sheet. Retrieved from: http://www.americanprogress.org/wp-content/uploads/2012/12/domestic_violence.pdf

27. Rahimtoola M, Hussain H, Khowaja SN, Khan AJ. Sexually transmitted infections treatment and care available to high risk populations in Pakistan. J LGBT Health Res. 2008; 4(2–3):103–10.

28. "Obergefell v. Hodges". Encyclopædia Britannica. Encyclopædia Britannica Online.Encyclopædia Britannica Inc., 2015. Web. 24 Oct. 2015 <http://www.britannica.com/event/Obergefell-v-Hodges>.

29. Terman, Rochelle. "Trans[ition] in Iran." World Policy Journal, 2014. Web. 27 Oct. 2015. <http://www.worldpolicy.org/transition-iran>.

# Differences of Sex Development/Intersex Populations

# 23

Matthew A. Malouf and Amy B. Wisniewski

## Learning Objectives

- Define culturally competent language for discussing differences of sex development (DSD) and intersexuality with practitioners and affected individuals and families *(KP1)*
- Describe the unique etiologies resulting in differences of sex development including underlying genetics and endocrine function *(KP2)*
- Discuss the context and challenges, both individual/family and systemic/cultural, in which DSD are diagnosed and treated *(KP4, PBLI1, ICS1, SBP5, IPC1)*
- Describe the medical and surgical treatments for DSD, and models in which these treatments are provided *(PC3, PC6, KP5, SBP6)*
- Describe the medical, surgical and psychological outcomes for individuals affected by DSD and appreciate the intersections of these outcomes *(PC6)*
- Identify at least three strategies that providers can assist and advocate for those affected by a DSD *(SPB5, PBLI1, PBLI2, Pr2)*

M.A. Malouf, Ph.D. (✉)
Connecticut Children's Medical Center, Hartford
Hospital, University of Connecticut Health,
Hartford/Farmington, CT, USA
e-mail: mmaloufphd@gmail.com

A.B. Wisniewski, Ph.D.
University of Oklahoma Health Sciences Center,
Oklahoma City, OK, USA
e-mail: amy-wisniewski@ouhsc.edu

## Why Learn About DSD?

Congenital conditions in which chromosomal, gonadal, hormonal and/or anatomical sex is discordant within a person or vary from binary definitions of sex are collectively known as disorders or differences of sex development [1]. Historically, people affected by DSD were not told about their condition or associated medical and surgical treatments. This paternalistic approach is no longer acceptable, and as a result, more and more people affected by DSD know about their conditions and are seeking answers from physicians about their health and treatment options. Additionally, some types of DSD that are life-threatening now have effective therapies so that affected individuals are surviving into adulthood. The net result of both of these changes is that physicians of all kinds are increasingly likely to have patients affected by some type of DSD under their care.

Contrary to experiences of some transgender people who have historically been denied medical and surgical therapies, some people with DSD report harm from undesired medical and surgical treatments they received during childhood. Starting in the 1950s, physicians who treated people affected by DSD followed the "optimal gender policy" that supported gender assignment within the context of optimizing reproductive and sexual function, as well as supporting stable gender development [2]. Unfortunately, many

© Springer International Publishing Switzerland 2016
K.L. Eckstrand, J.M. Ehrenfeld (eds.), *Lesbian, Gay, Bisexual, and Transgender Healthcare*,
DOI 10.1007/978-3-319-19752-4_23

people who were patients under this era were not informed of their DSD status nor of the accompanying medical and surgical treatments employed to stabilize gender development. Thus, as unwanted side effects of such treatments revealed themselves over time, many patients learned of their medical histories as adolescents or adults without the benefit education or counseling. The result has been dissatisfaction with care, distrust of the medical community, and a call for change in the medical approach to DSD [3].

## An Introduction for the Busy Practitioner

What is DSD? The term DSD resulted from the 2006 Chicago Consensus meeting and replaced outdated terminology such as "intersex" and "hermaphrodite." For the most part, "DSD" has been adopted by physicians and scientists; however, this new terminology has not been universally accepted by affected people [4]. Thus, when working with affected individuals and their families it is important to determine how they themselves wish to describe their unique experience with sex differentiation and development.

To understand DSD, it is necessary to appreciate how sex development and differentiation typically proceeds, where multiple aspects of sex consistently follow a male or female pathway (see Table 23.1). During fetal development, bipotential gonads are established early. If a fetus possesses the SRY gene encoded on the Y chromosome, then the bipotential gonads differentiate into testes. This explains why most fetuses with a 46,XY chromosomal complement develop testes. Fetal testes are physiologically active dur-

ing gestation and also for the first few months of postnatal life and produce 2 signals—the peptide hormone Müllerian Inhibiting Substance (MIS) and the steroid hormone testosterone. These hormones then drive the remainder of male differentiation including development of internal male reproductive structures, penis and scrotum. In contrast, when a fetus does not possess the SRY gene as a result of having a 46,XX chromosomal complement, the bipotential gonads differentiate into ovaries that are physiologically quiescent during gestation and postnatal life. Thus, in the absence of MIS and testosterone production, female fetuses develop internal female reproductive structures, a clitoris, labia and outer portion of the vagina [5]. For most people, genetic sex (XY), gonadal sex (testes), hormonal sex (MIS and testosterone) and anatomical sex (internal male reproductive structures, penis and scrotum) are concordant.

A person affected by DSD experiences a different path in their sex development and differentiation resulting in discordance between their genetic sex, gonadal sex, hormonal sex and/or anatomic sex. For example, a person may possess a 46,XY chromosome complement and testes, but due to atypical or incomplete development of their testes they are unable to produce the hormones MIS and testosterone. This person would then experience development of their internal reproductive structures and external genitalia that is not male-typical. As a result of this discordance, this person has a DSD. Because sex differentiation is a complex process, atypical development can occur due to multiple causes and result in variable presentations at the genetic, gonadal, hormonal and anatomic levels. With this heterogeneity of DSD in mind, it is not surprising

**Table 23.1** Multiple levels of sex associated with typical male and female differentiation

|  | Chromosomal sex | Gonadal sex | Hormonal sex | Internal anatomical sex | External anatomical sex |
|---|---|---|---|---|---|
| Male | XY | Testes | MIS, testosterone | Prostate, epididymides, vas deferens | Penis, scrotum |
| Female | XX | Ovaries | None | Uterus, fallopian tubes, cervix, upper vagina | Clitoris, labia, outer vagina |

that a single nomenclature to describe how people perceive DSD remains elusive.

Along with the new terminology of DSD to describe differences in sex development and differentiation is also a new nomenclature to categorize DSD conditions according to sex chromosome complement and gonadal differentiation [1]. For example, "46,XY DSD" refers to situations where a person possesses a 46,XY chromosome complement but does not experience full masculinization of their internal reproductive structures and/or external genitalia as a result of (1) an inability to produce MIS and/or testosterone, (2) an inability of target tissues to respond to the hormones due to nonfunctioning hormone receptors, or (3) atypical timing of testicular differentiation or hormone production (i.e., a timing defect). Other classifications of DSD are 46,XX DSD and sex chromosome DSD.

While the prevalence of every etiology underlying DSD is not well established, in general, the prevalence of DSD including atypical genital development at birth is reported to be 1 in 4500 [1]. For people with a type of DSD that does not include genital ambiguity, presentation of their condition may occur around the time that puberty is expected to occur. Adolescents who present to clinic with DSD typically do so in 1 of 3 ways; (1) girls with primary amenorrhea, (2) girls who virilize at puberty and (3) boys with delayed puberty [6]. The education and mental health approach to such adolescents and their families will differ from that of parents of newborns with genital ambiguity.

The understanding of sex in general, and treatment for DSD specifically, has evolved over the decades. The "true sex" conceptualization of two sexes—male and female—determined solely by biology was replaced by the "optimal-gender policy" of John Money in the mid-twentieth century. This newer theory posited that behavioral sex could be influenced by learning, independent of biological sex. Early genital surgery to remove anatomical ambiguity of affected children was part of the management plan under which the optimal-gender policy was employed for DSD treatment [7]. More recently, the "full-consent" treatment plan for DSD has been suggested

whereby no elective genital surgeries should be performed on any persons with DSD until such individuals are old enough to provide informed consent for such procedures [8]. Finally, providing mental health support to parents who make medical decisions for their child with DSD [9] as well as integrating patient- and family-centered care for DSD within the larger context of congenital, chronic medical conditions [3] and service systems [10] are also recent suggestions for improving DSD care as our appreciation of sex and gender development expands.

## Linguistic and Cultural Competency around DSD

Over the last decade, cultural and linguistic competency (CLC) has emerged as a growing force in the promotion of health equity [11]. In relation to LGBT health, CLC may be defined as the capacity to address the healthcare needs of individuals who identify as LGBT and their families (adapted from [12]. Tools for conducting organizational assessments [13] and measuring individual competency [14] for providing services to LGBT populations have been developed. Intersex-identified individuals and/or those diagnosed with a DSD and their families stand to benefit from these tools and increasing emphasis on provider competence. Since DSD are somewhat rare and often poorly understood both by health professionals and consumers, a competency-based model allows providers who may not have had previous focused training on DSD to still provide quality care to individuals. Additionally, CLC promotes social justice aims by challenging individual biases and assumptions and emphasizing language and communication around sex and gender. A competent provider can also effectively model skills for families and individuals who engage in a similar process as they learn to manage societal biases and linguistic barriers when communicating about DSD to others in their lives.

A key component of competency is an appreciation for both the communicator and the audience's values and attitudes. Thus, it is essential to ask families about their background and to attend to intersecting aspects of culture. Families' decision-making around DSD will be shaped by their expectations, experiences and understanding of sex and gender within the religious and cultural context of their social networks [15].

As noted in the introduction, while "DSD" has been adopted by physicians and scientists [4], there are a variety of terms used in conjunction with this population so it is important to allow individuals and families to self-label and to be mindful of several nuances. For example, it is important to differentiate between language used to describe a physical phenomenon, an observed behavior or an identity. "Disorder or difference of sex development" should be used to describe medical conditions only. Additionally, person-first language is recommended and it is preferable to use the specific DSD diagnosis if it is known (e.g. a child with congenital adrenal hyperplasia). In terms of behavior, "gender non-conforming (GNC)" or "gender variant" generally refers to behaviors or statements which do not clearly match or follow societal gender roles. Not all individuals with a DSD will exhibit GNC behaviors or identify as such, though, in some cases, individuals may describe themselves using similar language (e.g. as a gender non-conforming teenager). "Intersex" is used by some individuals to self-label and can be used to describe their diagnosis, their gender, their identity or any other aspect of themselves. It serves as an alternative to and challenges the socially-constructed sex binary.

When barriers to using preferred language exist (e.g. medical billing), it is recommended that these be openly discussed with patients so they understand the intent of any communication that uses non-preferred language. Be mindful that communication between providers may unintentionally be shared with consumers. For new diagnoses, it is the job of the provider to help educate families and individuals about DSD. It is important to realize that an individual's understanding of biological sex may be very different than a medical definition and time may need to be spent

explaining these varying aspects of language in lay terms.

> **Helpful Hint**
> Transgender is an identity label that refers to the experience of one's internal gender identity not matching one's sex of rearing. Some individuals with DSD may identify as transgender. DSM-5 criteria for Gender Dysphoria (GD) in Children (302.6) and in Adolescents and Adults (302.85) have been revised. DSD is no longer an exclusion criteria for GD and is instead coded as a specifier.

## Etiologies of DSD (Fig. 23.1)

1. The category 46,XX DSD encompasses many congenital conditions in which ovarian development is atypical, genitalia are masculinized due to excess androgen exposure in utero, and/or female reproductive structures develop differently than expected for unknown reasons [1]. In terms of number of cases, congenital adrenal hyperplasia (CAH) due to 21-hydroxylase (21-OH) deficiency is the most common presentation of 46,XX DSD.

2. The category 46,XY DSD also encompasses many congenital conditions in which testicular development is atypical, genitalia are demasculinized due to insufficient androgen exposure in utero, and/or male reproductive structures develop differently than expected for unknown reasons [1]. Unlike 46,XX DSD no single etiology of 46,XY DSD constitutes the majority of presentations. Additionally, the etiology underlying 46,XY DSD remains undetermined in approximately half of all cases of 46,XY DSD including ambiguous external genitalia [16].

3. Sex Chromosome DSD is a category that encompasses any condition in which the sex

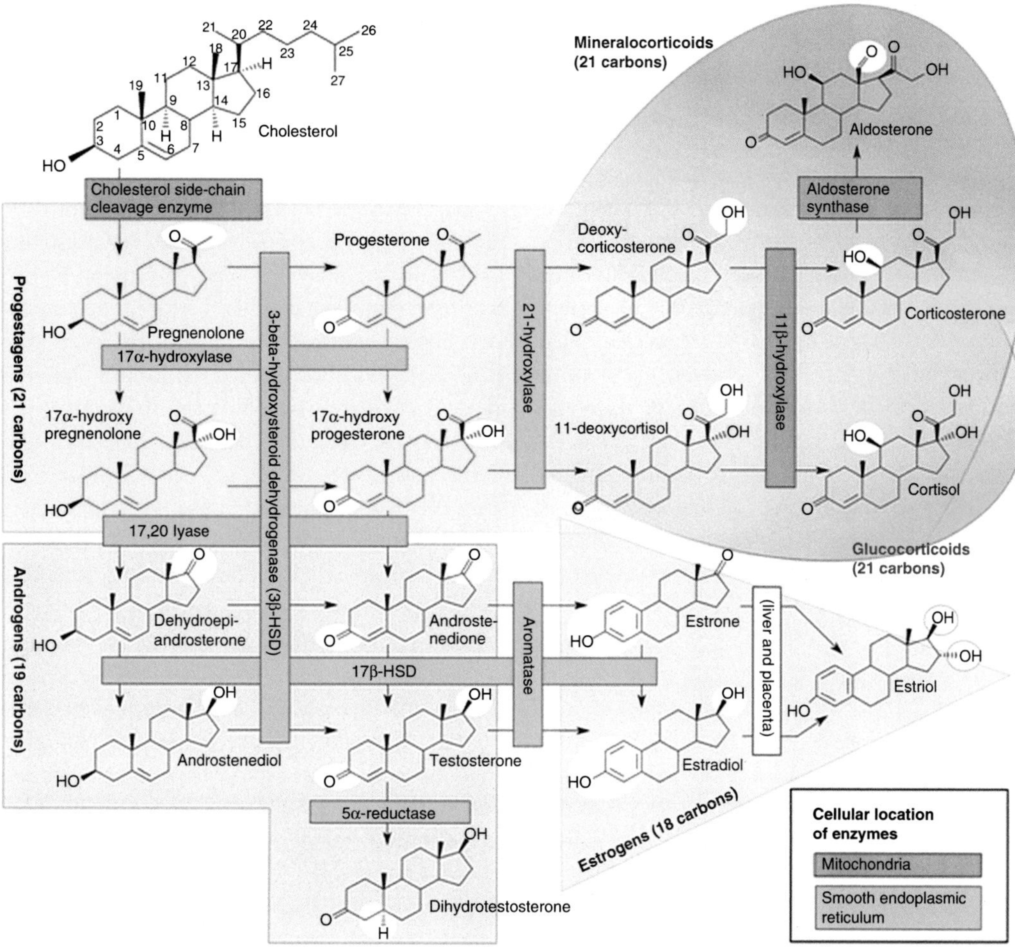

**Fig. 23.1** Enzymes, substrates and products in human steroidogenesis ["Steroidogenesis" by David Richfield (User:Slashme) and Mikael Häggström. Derived from previous version by Hoffmeier and Settersr. In external use, this diagram may be cited as: Häggström M, Richfield D (2014). "Diagram of the pathways of human steroidogenesis". Wikiversity Journal of Medicine 1(1). DOI:10.15347/wjm/2014.005. ISSN 20018762.—Self-made using bkchem and inkscape. Licensed under Creative Commons Attribution-Share Alike 3.0 via Wikimedia Commons—http://commons.wikimedia.org/wiki/File:Steroidogenesis.svg#mediaviewer/File:Steroidogenesis.svg]

chromosome complement is neither 46,XX nor 46,XY. For example, a person with a 45,X/46,XY complement would be categorized as having a Sex Chromosome DSD [1]. The most common presentations in this category are Turner Syndrome (45,X) and Klinefelter Syndrome (47,XXY).

**Helpful Hint**
Although the nomenclature for DSD is based largely upon sex chromosomal complement, genetic sex is thought to exert a small impact, if any impact at all, on gender development.

## Practice Guidelines

Recommendations for the treatment of people affected by DSD are inherently multi-disciplinary in nature and reflective of the range of outcomes of concern, e.g. medical, surgical, quality of life, mental health and psychosocial. All processes surrounding treatment of DSD, from evaluation and diagnosis to surgical decision-making must involve parents and, to an age-appropriate extent, the patient. In all cases of DSD, general clinical goals include anticipating likely medical problems and determining timing of any necessary interventions, understanding the underlying etiology and educating the family and the affected individuals [6, 17, 18]. In the majority of cases where a DSD is diagnosed at birth or in infancy, initial clinical goals also include deciding on a sex of rearing.

As DSD represents a large group of heterogenous conditions with different causes and natural histories, we will touch only on generalities of medical management here. Hughes et al. offer detailed information on medical evaluation specific to particular types of DSD [19]. Worth noting, is that there has been a shift toward rearing more infants with 46,XY DSD as male [20]. In terms of timing, the 2006 Consensus states that gender assignment should only occur after medical evaluation for newborns, and for older children gender should not be reassigned unless the child requests it [1]. Delaying assignment past birth may represent a shift in thinking for both families and medical staff but is an important one that can help set a paced tone for further evaluation and treatment. Medical evaluation should occur with an experienced multidisciplinary team that will likely include genetics, pediatric endocrinology, pediatric urology, pediatric surgery, adolescent gynecology and mental health professionals. The 2006 Consensus states that, once the evaluation has occurred, all patients should receive a gender assignment if they have not already received one. Some, but not all, children will require sex hormone replacement to induce puberty and maintain secondary sex characteristics in adolescence and adulthood. Depending on the type of DSD, some children will require other

types of hormone replacement such as cortisol and growth hormone. Finally, transitioning medical treatment for people with DSD from pediatrics to adult-oriented care remains as a challenge but is increasingly being recognized for optimizing health outcomes [21, 22].

Surgery as part of DSD treatment is controversial, and some people have called for a moratorium of these procedures [23]. At present, parents can represent their child by proxy in the surgical decision-making process, particularly when there is no clear evidence that the outcomes of surgical interventions are worse than not doing surgery at all, and also when the interest of the present-day child and future adult are not identical [8]. However, claims that modern surgical techniques for DSD procedures result in better cosmetic and functional outcomes have not been substantiated with peer-reviewed data [20]. A description of unsatisfactory cosmetic and functional outcomes of surgical procedures for DSD employed in the past is provided later in this chapter. If surgeries are part of an affected individuals treatment plan, then a thorough anatomical assessment is necessary to guide surgical management [24] The most common types of surgery for DSD are removal of gonadal tissue that has an elevated risk for developing cancer, genitoplasty to create male or female external genitalia that appear more typical, and vaginoplasty to allow for vaginal intercourse and/or menstruation.

At the heart of DSD care is the interface between multidisciplinary teams and families. Guidelines for developing and implementing DSD teams exist, including a sample operational pathway, proposed goals for multidisciplinary team meetings, and a proposed timeline of multidisciplinary care visits [25–28]. Further recommendations include auditing clinical activity, conducting clinical research, and building collaborative working partnerships with other DSD teams to optimize team performance [6]. Additional guidelines for teams and individual providers are provided in Table 23.2.

Throughout medical management, family members must take part in the decision-making, including gender assignment [1]. As noted above, raising a child with a DSD may represent

**Table 23.2** Guidelines and resources on management of DSD

| Target audience | Organization | Guideline/Resource |
|---|---|---|
| All providers, Endocrinology | Society for Endocrinology | UK guidance on the initial evaluation of an infant or an adolescent with a suspected disorder of sex development. |
| All providers | ISNA/ACCORD Alliance | Clinical Guidelines for the Management of Disorders of Sex Development |
| All providers | Pediatric Endocrine Society and the European Society for Paediatric Endocrinology | Hughes et al. [1] statement on management of intersex disorders |
| Urology | European Association of Urology; European Society for Paediatric Urology | Disorders of sex development. In: Guidelines on paediatric urology (2009) |
| Counseling (MA-level) | American Counseling Association | ALGBTIC Competencies for Counseling LGBQQIA Individuals |
| Psychology | American Psychological Association | Answers to Your Questions About Individuals With Intersex Conditions (2006) |
| All providers | World Professional Association for Transgender Health | Standards of Care for the Health of Transsexual, Transgender, and Gender-Nonconforming People, Version 7 |
| All providers, medical ethics | German Network of Disorders of Sex Development (DSD)/Intersexuality | Ethical principles and recommendations for the medical management of differences of sex development (DSD)/intersex in children and adolescents (2010) |
| VA providers | Department of Veterans Affairs | VHA Directive 2013-003: Providing Healthcare for Transgender and Intersex Veterans |
| Policy makers, Justice/Corrections | U.S. Department of Justice: National Institute of Corrections | Policy Review and Development Guide Lesbian, Gay, Bisexual, Transgender, and Intersex Persons In Custodial Settings (2013) |

a shift in families' understanding of sex and gender. Prior to learning of their child's diagnosis, many parents will never have heard of DSD [29] and, as a result, face a steep learning curve requiring support through decision making. Informed consent models of decision making, which often rely on single-episode consent and emphasize individual autonomy, are problematic, especially for families of children with DSD since DSD are complex and have the potential to impact many family members [30]. The latter is an important consideration since parents often struggle with their own reactions to their child's illness. They may view surgical decisions as a sole solution, or alternatively, surgical decisions made by parents may, in-turn, impact their own mental health [31–34]. To better support families through this process, a model of shared decision making has been proposed for surgical decisions but may also be valuable at all stages of DSD treatment [35]. An alternative to informed consent, it places emphasis on collaboration between families and multidisciplinary teams and takes into account the emotions that families experience as well as each individual's value- and belief-system. Similarly, as more and more young people are educated about their DSD, it is essential to include them in the decision-making process and acknowledge their own values and beliefs [36].

An important assumption of shared decision making is that, with support, families are able to manage their own reactions in order to make decisions focused on long-term, child-centered outcomes. Therefore, providing families with psychosocial support and assessing their understanding of such outcomes is essential and must be the responsibility of the entire team [37]. Beyond medical decision making, psychosocial support can also assist families as they raise a child with a DSD and help them navigate disclosing medical history and treatment to their child [10]. While outside therapists and support groups may play a valuable role in this process, there may be additional stigma associated with getting such support. Specific guidance on finding a support group or connecting with a mental health clinician are provided later in this chapter. Furthermore, the multidisciplinary team is ultimately responsible for following the child across the life-span and can best assess family functioning at any given point. Best practices recommend the inclusion of a mental health representative and, where possible, an affected individual or parent, on the team from the start to reduce associated stigma and provide families with an initial psychosocial support contact [6, 10, 17].

## Medical Outcomes

Fertility potential varies with type of DSD. If a person with 46,XX DSD, 46,XY DSD or Sex Chromosome DSD possesses normally functioning gonads, then their fertility potential can be high. For instance, women with 46,XX DSD due to 21-OH deficiency who receive appropriate medical management are capable of maintaining pregnancies and delivering healthy babies [38]. Men with 46,XY DSD due to 5α-reductase deficiency have fathered children [39] and men with Sex Chromosome DSD as a result of Klinefelter Syndrome are able to father children with assisted reproductive technology [40].

In general, people with 46,XX DSD due to 21-OH deficiency have the same life expectancy as unaffected individuals, provided they receive appropriate cortisol replacement and maintain a healthy lifestyle. People with some types of 46,XY DSD that include maldeveloped organs such as the kidneys can have a decreased life expectancy despite healthy habits; however, most people with 46,XY DSD are expected to have a typical life expectancy. Individuals with Sex Chromosome DSD do experience early mortality, usually due to cardiovascular problems associated with Turner Syndrome and Klinefelter Syndrome. Women with Turner Syndrome also have a higher than average chance of developing hypothyroidism and celiac disease than unaffected women. Finally, people with any type of DSD who are unable to produce sex steroids at puberty are at risk for developing osteopenia and osteoporosis if left untreated [5].

Surgeries for DSD include removal of gonadal tissue that is at risk for developing gonadoblastomas, clitoroplasty, vaginoplasty, hypospadias repair and scrotoplasty. Reduced genital sensitivity in women with CAH who received clitoroplasty [41] and dissatisfaction with cosmetic outcomes for men and women with ambiguous genitalia who received genitoplasty as young children [42] are typical of reports in the literature. Men with DSD report greater satisfaction with genital function following genitoplasty than women. Thus, just as the etiologies and natural histories of DSD are varied, so too are patients' perceptions of genitoplasty. Despite these poor outcomes, some people with DSD report that infancy or childhood is the best time to receive surgery for DSD [43]. More studies are required to understand such disparate perceptions of genitoplasty among people with DSD. Additionally, information about how children with ambiguous genitalia who do not receive genitoplasty develop is needed to assess the costs and benefits of these irreversible procedures.

## Psychological and Emotional Outcomes

Differences of sex development have the potential to impact aspects of psychological and emotional functioning, particularly mental health and self-concept. The rarity of these conditions as well as the variation between and within specific DSD, make it hard to generalize across groups. As a result, outcomes vary from study to study and between DSD sub-groups. Additionally, cohort effects due to treatment models and changing societal beliefs related to secrecy around sex/gender non-conformity could influence individual experiences and outcomes. The studies referenced in the following sections have primarily examined adult samples with mean ages ranging from early twenties to early thirties and include participants as young as 18 years of age and up to their early 50s. While contemporary advances in treatment and changes to treatment models may have occurred prior to the birth of or during the lifetime of many of these participants, their data may not be reflective of the latest treatment guidelines [17]. Furthermore, research has not examined whether current guidelines have been widely adopted and implemented, so individuals in younger cohorts may still receive care typical of past treatment models. Therefore, providers are encouraged to assess both families and patients within the context of their illness, their unique treatment history, cultural influences and family dynamics, and other psychosocial or environmental stressors.

## Mental Health

Approximately 40 % of children affected by a DSD in one study met diagnostic criteria for a psychiatric illness and an additional 20 % reported mild but non-clinical psychological concerns [44]. However, adolescents affected by DSD did not differ from controls on a measure of psychological functioning [45] and girls diagnosed with CAH did not differ from controls on a measure of psychological functioning [46].

Data on adult outcomes are similarly inconclusive. More than half of the participants in a sample of individuals affected by DSD met clinical cutoffs for psychological distress, with a particularly high incidence of mental health concerns (80 %) in the CAIS subsample [47]. Studies on women with CAH have also documented broad concerns related to mental health [48] and, specifically, increased anxiety compared to controls [49]. Other samples of individuals with DSD have not differed from controls on broad measures of mental health, PTSD and depression [50] including those with CAIS [51] and CAH [46, 52]. One study on 58 women with MRKH noted higher levels of anxiety but no differences in depression compared to a standardized sample [53]. Despite the heterogeneity of findings, it is recommended that providers be mindful of the potential for poor psychological outcomes in these populations and work to prevent and/or ameliorate their impact through appropriate psychological and psychosocial support.

Findings surrounding suicide and self-injury also warrant concern due to both the prevalence of lethality in DSD populations and the relative constancy of these findings within the literature. Rates of suicidal ideation in one DSD sample were comparable to control trauma groups groups who had experienced either sexual or physical trauma or both, with self-harm behaviors most prevalent in 46,XY individuals, male- or female-identifying [47]. Women with CAH and 46,XX- and 46,XY-virilized females have also reported increased suicidal ideation and mental health service use compared to controls [49]. Additionally, over one third of participants in a study of 46,XX women with CAH reported a history of a suicide attempt [48]. It is recommended that all providers screen their patients for lethality concerns, even in the absence of other stated or documented mental health history.

## Self-Concept

In addition to the impact of DSD on mental health, these conditions have the potential to profoundly influence self-concept including: gender, sexuality and dating, and self-esteem and body image. Though the majority of individuals affected by a DSD do not experience gender dysphoria (GD), rates of GD are somewhat higher than in general population and certain conditions (e.g. PAIS, 5-$\alpha$ reductase, 17 $\beta$ hydroxysteroid dehydrogenase) have higher rates of GD than other types of DSD (e.g. CAH, CAIS; see

Sandberg et al. [54] for review). Some data also suggest that girls with and women with CAH have more typically-masculine personality traits than unaffected peers [46, 55, 56] but gender variance is distinct from gender dysphoria [57] and conformity to gender stereotypes is not a viable treatment outcome. Instead, families and individuals should be supported in understanding that variation in interests and personality is normal and that societal expectations for behavior (i.e. gender role) evolve over time and vary across cultures. Similarly, parents may be concerned about their child's future sexual orientation, and there is some data to support greater variation of sexual orientation within some DSD populations [58, 59]. Akin to gender conformity, a non-heterosexual orientation is not pathological and is not a treatment goal. This is consistent with policy statements from multiple professional organizations including the American Academy of Pediatrics, the American Psychiatric Association and the American Psychological Association warning that interventions to change non-heterosexual sexual orientation are contraindicated in practice [60]. Instead, parents should realize that non-heterosexuals can have equally fulfilling lives as heterosexuals and that parent support is a critical factor in outcomes for lesbian, gay and bisexual youth [61].

However, individuals affected by a DSD may have other concerns related to sexual and/or gender identity. Some women with AIS have described feeling like their womanhood has been comprised and fear devaluation by others [62]. Women with CAH have also expressed concerns related to fears of romantic rejection and have poor body image and lower self-esteem [50, 63]. Women and girls with DSD are also less likely to have been in romantic relationships [45, 49, 64], and while this is not inherently pathological, it may be reflective of concerns surrounding self-worth.

Though much of the research has focused on women affected by a DSD, research including boys affected by a DSD found that they had more negative body image than controls [45]. Surprisingly, the girls in the study affected by a DSD did not differ from unaffected peers. This finding was most pronounced in individuals who do not spontaneously enter puberty. Research on

timing of puberty in non-DSD-affected populations has suggested that precocious puberty is associated, in varying patterns, with poor psychosocial outcomes for both boys and girls [65, 66] while delayed puberty generally has more negative impact for boys than girls [67, 68]. It is possible that sex differences related to poor body image in DSD populations [45] are moderated by delays in puberty.

Finally having a DSD can feel isolating [48, 69]. This isolation may reinforce feelings of abnormality or inadequacy and make it hard for individuals to have realistic appraisals of themselves in comparison to other individuals, both affected and unaffected. Providers should be mindful of the language they use around sex and gender and work to help families and individuals normalize their experiences and construct their own definitions of femininity and masculinity.

## Exercise: Boy or Girl?!

Now that you understand key language, the underlying biology, and potential treatments and outcomes for DSD, let's try to apply this understanding.

Imagine you are a healthcare provider seeing a 3-month old who has a 46,XY DSD owing to a partial unresponsiveness to androgenic hormones resulting in a moderate degree of genital ambiguity (AKA partial androgen insensitivity syndrome). This is your fourth follow-up and, medically, the patient is doing well. The parents are still in the process of making surgical decisions and there is some disagreement between them about sex of rearing. Just as you are about to conclude your visit, mom asks you for help. She has been invited to a holiday celebration at her cousin's house and she knows she will see a lot of extended family who she has purposely been avoiding since the baby was born. She is hesitant to go since she is afraid of how people will react to her child's diagnosis and she doesn't know how to explain it. This is atypical for her since she and her spouse are both recent immigrants and their extended family has been a strong support system for them previously.

They have decided to go but to leave the baby with another relative.

What would you council mom to do if a family member asks her about the sex of the baby?

Choose the best answer, given what you know about this family:

1. She should explain that sex is not binary but is a spectrum comprised of many characteristics and that their baby has some differences that are not all that uncommon but is otherwise healthy and well cared for.
2. She should say things are too complicated to explain and asks them to read a book on DSD and then talk later.
3. She should avoid answering the question by taking out a picture and gushing over how cute the new baby is.
4. She should pretend to take a phone call and then join a different conversation.
5. They should just decide to skip the party but keep the baby-sitter and go out to a nice dinner, just the two of them.

**Correct Answer** All of the above could be correct depending upon the parent's comfort with the individual they are speaking to and their confidence in their ability to manage the disclosure. It is important to remind parents and individuals that having boundaries is healthy but that boundaries can also be flexible. It will take practice to adapt them to new settings and situations. It is important for the family to find ways to engage their natural supports to reduce isolation and to practice disclosing to others. It is also valuable to link them with additional supports, including other families who are dealing with similar diagnoses. The following section describes strategies to help individuals disclose their condition in safe, affirming and empowering ways and in a range of contexts.

## Advocating for Competent Care

It is essential that families and affected individuals be able to advocate for competent and ethical care and support in a variety of settings. In order to effectively do so, individuals and families must become comfortable with and skilled at disclosing their/their child's condition. This is challenging for many people, especially when they are still coming to terms with a DSD diagnosis [29, 69] so it is recommended that they proceed slowly and with support and modeling from their health providers. Individuals may benefit from choosing to first disclose to someone they believe will be understanding and supportive. This could include extended family members or close friends, or, in cases where these are not safe people, a support group, a therapist, a religious leader, or another individual affected by a DSD or parents of an affected child.

Deciding what to disclose ahead of time can also make this task easier and allow individuals to enforce healthy boundaries. For example, for school-age children, parents may need to share certain aspects of their child's medical history with the school, especially if a school nurse needs to provide medication (e.g. stress dosing for CAH). Any information provided to the school should be tailored to the needs of the child. In this example, the school nurse does not need to know any surgical history and questions about genitalia are a violation of the student's privacy. If the child is old enough to understand, the parent should also let them know what information has been disclosed and to who. Many health providers are happy to write a letter which families can share with the school system to assist in disclosing this information. Similarly, providers can help write letters for adults to employers, colleges, etc. as warranted.

## Medical Care

Families and individuals should be encouraged to seek out specialized, multidisciplinary care consistent with current best practices [1, 6, 70] when possible. These are often located in major medical centers that have the necessary clinical and research support. Therefore, not all individuals will have convenient access to these teams or access may change following relocation for work, school, etc. In cases where DSD specialists are not available, medical providers should be directed to both general DSD and specialty-specific resources as described in the prior section on practice guidelines. Families can facilitate care by keeping copies of medical records and signing consents to allow providers to share information with one another. Similarly, for adolescents and adults, it is important that they be able to communicate any medical needs or complications they have due to their condition with providers they may be seeing for other reasons. Support groups can also be helpful in guiding families and individuals to competent providers and many groups keep provider listings on their website or provide them via listservs.

---

**Helpful Hint**

Physicians can be patient advocates too! To ensure that family and patient voices are at the center of care, help coordinate meetings between patients and all providers (including primary care and specialties). This can occur even outside of formal DSD teams. These meetings should be distinct from medical visits and focus on making sure families and patients understand their options and that providers understand decisions that are made by families and patients. These can also be used to identify gaps in knowledge or support for both patients and providers and to develop a plan to address them.

---

## Support Groups

When looking for a support group, it is important to remember that each group varies depending upon several factors: emphasis, audience, leadership and format. Some groups emphasize disease specific issues (e.g. CARES) while others include individuals with diverse diagnoses (e.g. AIS-DSD). Some groups primarily target parents while others have an adult-focus. In terms of leadership and structure, it is important that consumers be intentional. If they

are seeking medical advice, it may be most prudent to contact a group that has a medical advisory board associated with it and regularly updates the information they share to reflect current findings. For other individuals who are primarily seeking peer-support, joining a group that is organized by affected individuals can be affirming and empowering. Finally, groups communicate through varying ways; some groups meet regularly in person while others function primarily via online message boards. Both have benefits and drawbacks. In either case it is important to realize that each member of any group has had a different experience and personality and to couch their communications in that context. The same holds true for other online resources (e.g. personal websites, blogs, youtube videos) which are often valuable resources but must be considered within their context.

## Therapists, Psychologists and Psychiatrists

Finding a mental health clinician who is trained to work with issues related to sex development may seem challenging at first. However, many therapists are trained to work around broader issues of sex, gender and sexual orientation and/or around health conditions, and could be competent and comfortable working with individuals affected by DSD even if this is not their specialty. When asked about the kind of therapist they would find most helpful, women with CAH prioritized basic therapeutic skills (listening, empathy, and acceptance) over CAH-specific knowledge [10]. It is therefore possible to find a therapist who may be effective even without expertise on DSD. However, it is important to note that if the individual or family finds that time spent educating their therapist on DSD detracts from their sessions or serves only to satisfy the therapist's curiosity, it is appropriate to let the therapist know this and suggest the therapist consult with colleagues or gain education on DSD from an expert or professional organization. The focus of therapy should be on the individual's and/or the family's presenting issues.

Therapeutic interventions for DSD vary across the lifespan. At time of diagnosis, therapists should work to help the family and/or individual process their emotions, use positive coping strategies, understand medical information, participate in decision-making, manage disclosure as needed, and engage DSD-specific psychosocial support. The next critical tasks when working with families are to help them disclose age-appropriate information to their child about diagnosis and treatment and to help the family maintain social connections with other parents of DSD children. This is critical as affected individuals enter puberty and begin to learn more about their body, about sex and increasingly compare themselves to peers. In adolescence, therapists can help the individual make meaning of their diagnosis and integrate it into their identity through exploration, education and engagement in social support groups with peers and mentors. Finally, for adults with DSD, therapists can help them further understand their diagnosis and treatment history, navigate interpersonal relationships and issues of disclosure and, if present, validate and treat any depression, anxiety, negative self-worth, shame or other mental health concerns associated with their diagnosis or treatment history.

> **Helpful Hint**
> Remember that individuals and families might want to talk to a therapist about topics that are unrelated to DSD but are equally important to treat, especially since premorbid psychological issues may present a risk for poor DSD-related outcomes.

## Schools, Social Services, Insurance and Legal Issues

In some cases, families and individuals may need support around other institutional issues like insurance coverage, adoption, custody and child welfare, school, or other social services. Medical providers can be strong advocates for their patients/clients but, in more complex cases, it is helpful to involve social workers or legal aid on the team [1, 6]. When possible, it is recommended that providers have face-to-face multidisciplinary team meetings which include representatives from involved agencies. Do not assume that agencies will document these meetings. Ideally, the team should have met in advance so that they can clearly and uniformly articulate any recommendations or requests and provide a sound rationale for them. Always, gain consent from families and individuals and review limits of confidentiality and protections of privacy prior to disclosing information to outside parties. Additionally, at least one organization specializes in providing legal counsel and advocacy on issues related to DSD (e.g. aiclegal.org), however, other organizations that deal with broader sex, sexuality and gender advocacy (e.g. www.lambdalegal.org, www.aclu.org) may also be valuable resources.

## Conclusion

As readers have likely gathered from this chapter's discussion of the etiologies, treatments and outcomes for DSD, these conditions are not homogenous and require multidisciplinary treatment tailored to the individual. Current models of care emphasize the importance of supporting families through decision-making and helping them develop a plan that addresses their child's medical and psychosocial needs across the lifespan. Cultural values and beliefs about sex and gender must be discussed as part of routine care. The language providers use when discussing these conditions plays an essential role, not only in helping families' understand various conditions and treatment options, but also for affected individuals to understand their treatment history, to integrate their condition into their identity in a way that has meaning to them, and to believe in their potential to grow into healthy, happy adults.

# References

1. Hughes IA, Houk C, Ahmed SF, Lee PA. Consensus statement on management of intersex. Arch Dis Child. 2006;91(7):554–63.
2. Meyer-Bahlburg HFL. Gender assignment in intersexuality. J Psychol Hum Sex. 1998;10:1–21.
3. Sandberg D, Mazur T. A noncategorical approach to the psychosocial care of persons with DSD and their families. In: Kreukels BPC et al., editors. Gender dysphoria and disorders of sex development: progress in care and knowledge, focus on sexuality research. New York City, NY: Springer Science + Business Media; 2014. p. 93–114.
4. Davis G. The power in a name: diagnostic terminology and diverse experiences. Psychol Sex. 2013;5(1):15–27.
5. Wisniewski AB, Chernausek SD, Kropp BP. Disorders of sex development: a practical guide for parents and physicians. Baltimore, MD: The Johns Hopkins University Press; 2012.
6. Ahmed SF, Acherman JC, Arlt W, Balen AH, Conway G, Edwards ZL, et al. UK guidance on the initial evaluation of an infant or an adolescent with a suspected disorder of sex development. Clin Endocrinol. 2011;75:12–26.
7. Meyer-Bahlburg HFL. Sex steroids and variants of gender identity. Endocrinol Metab Clin N Am. 2013;42:435–52.
8. Wiesemann C, Ude-Koeller S, Sinnecker GHG, Thyen U. Ethical principles and recommendations for the medical management of differences of sex development (DSD)/intersex in children and adolescents. Eur J Pediatr. 2010;169:671–9.
9. Tamar-Mattis A, Baratz A, Baratz Dalke K, Karkazis K. Emotionally and cognitively informed consent for clinical care for differences of sex development. Psychol Sex. 2013;5(1):44–55.
10. Malouf MA, Baratz A. Youth and families affected by disorders of sex development. In: Fisher SK, Poirier JM, Blau GM, editors. Addressing the needs of youth who are lGBT and their families: a system of care approach. Baltimore, MD: Brookes Publishing; 2012. p. 67–86.
11. Goode TD, Dunne MC, Bronheim S, Commonwealth Fund. The evidence base for cultural and linguistic competency in health care. New York, NY: Commonwealth Fund; 2006.
12. Poirier JM, Martinez KJ, Francis KB, Denney T, Roepke SL, Caycee-Gibson NA. Providing culturally and linguistically competent services and supports to address the needs of LGBT youth and their families. In: Fisher SK, Poirier JM, Blau GM, editors. Addressing the needs of youth who are LGBT and their families: a system of care approach. Baltimore, MD: Brookes Publishing; 2012. p. 9–24.
13. Goode TD, Fisher SK. Self-assessment checklist for personnel providing services and supports to lgbtq youth and their families. In: Fisher SK, Poirier JM, Blau GM, editors. Improving emotional and behavioral outcomes for LGBT youth: a guide for professionals. Baltimore, MD: Brookes Publishing; 2012. p. 25–32.
14. Bidell MP. The Sexual Orientation Counselor Competency Scale: assessing attitudes, skills, and knowledge of counselors working with lesbian, gay, and bisexual clients. Couns Educ Superv. 2005;44(4):267–79.
15. Warne G, Raza J. Disorders of sex development (DSDs), their presentation and management in different cultures. Rev Endocr Metab Disord. 2008;9(3):227–36.
16. Ahmed SF, Bashamboo A, Lucas-Herald A, McElreavey K. Understanding the genetic aetiology in patients with XY DSD. Br Med Bull. 2013;106:67–89.
17. Lee PA, Houk CP, Ahmed SF, Hughes IA, International Consensus Conference on Intersex organized by the Lawson Wilkins Pediatric Endocrine Society and the European Society for Paediatric Endocrinology. Consensus statement on management of intersex disorders. International Consensus Conference on Intersex. Pediatrics. 2006;118(2):488–500.
18. Schweizer K, Brunner F, Handford C, Richter-Appelt H. Gender experience and satisfaction with gender allocation in adults with diverse intersex conditions (divergences of sex development, DSD). Psychol Sex. 2013;5(1):56–82.
19. Hughes IA, Morel Y, McElreavey K, Rogol A. Biological assessment of abnormal genitalia. J Pediatr Urol. 2012;8:592–6.
20. Lee PA, Houk CP. Key discussions from the Working Party on Disorders of Sex Development (DSD) evaluation, Foundation Merieux, Annecy, France, March 14-17, 2012. Int J Pediatr Endocrinol. 2013;2013:12.
21. Liao LM, Tacconelli E, Wood D, Conway G, Creighton SM. Adolescent girls with disorders of sex development: a needs analysis of transitional care. J Pediatr Urol. 2010;6:609–13.
22. Hullmann SE, Chalmers LJ, Wisniewski AB. Transition from pediatric to adult care for adolescents and young adults with a disorder of sex development. J Pediatr Adolesc Gynecol. 2012;25(2):155–7.
23. Creighton SM, Michala L, Mushtaq I, Yaron M. Childhood surgery for ambiguous genitalia: glimpses of practice changes or more of the same? Psychol Sex. 2013;5(1):34–43.
24. Malone PS, Hall-Craggs MA, Mouriquand PDE, Caldamone AA. The anatomical assessment of disorders of sex development (DSD). J Pediatr Urol. 2012;8:585–91.
25. Brain CE, Creighton SM, Mushtaq I, Carmichael PA, Barnicoat A, Honour JW, Larcher V, Achermann MB. Holistic management of DSD. Best Pract Res Clin Endocrinol Metab. 2010;24(2):335–54.
26. Moran ME, Karkazis K. Developing a multidisciplinary team for disorders of sex development: planning, implementation, and operation tools for care providers. Adv Urol. Vol. 2012:12 pages.

27. Palmer BW, Wisniewski AB, Schaeffer TL, Mallappa A, Tryggestad JB, Krishnan S, Chalmers LJ, et al. A model of delivering multi-disciplinary care to people with 46 XY DSD. J Pediatr Urol. 2012;8(1):7–16.

28. Schaeffer TL, Tryggestad JB, Mallappa A, Hanna AE, Krishnan S, Chernausek SD, Chalmers LJ, et al. An evidence-based model of multidisciplinary care for patients and families affected by classical congenital adrenal hyperplasia due to 21-hydroxylase deficiency. Hindawi Publishing Corporation; 2010, 13 pages.

29. Crissman HP, Warner L, Gardner M, Carr M, Schast A, Quittner AL, Kogan B, et al. Children with disorders of sex development: a qualitative study of early parental experience. Int J Pediatr Endocrinol. 2011;1:10–2.

30. Kegley JA. Challenges to informed consent. EMBO Rep. 2004;5(9):832–6.

31. Hullmann SE, Fedele DA, Wolfe-Christensen C, Mullins LL, Wisniewski AB. Differences in adjustment by child developmental stage among caregivers of children with disorders of sex development. Int J Pediatr Endocrinol. 2011;2011(1):16.

32. Sanders C, Carter B, Goodacre L. Parents' narratives about their experiences of their child's reconstructive genital surgeries for ambiguous genitalia. J Clin Nurs. 2008;17(23):3187–95.

33. Sanders C, Carter B, Goodacre L. Searching for harmony: parents' narratives about their child's genital ambiguity and reconstructive genital surgeries in childhood. J Adv Nurs. 2011;67(10):2220–30.

34. Sanders C, Carter B, Goodacre L. Parents need to protect: influences, risks and tensions for parents of prepubertal children born with ambiguous genitalia. J Clin Nurs. 2012;21:3315–23.

35. Karkazis K, Tamar-Mattis A, Kon AA. Genital surgery for disorders of sex development: implementing a shared decision-making approach. J Pediatr Endocrinol Metab. 2010;23(8):789–805.

36. Liao L-M, Green H, Creighton SM, Crouch NS, Conway GS. Service users' experiences of obtaining and giving information about disorders of sex development. BJOG. 2010;117(2):193–9.

37. Magritte E. Working together in placing the long term interests of the child at the heart of the DSD evaluation. J Pediatr Urol. 2012;8(6):571–5.

38. Reichman DE, White PC, New MI, Rosenwaks Z. Fertility in patients with congenital adrenal hyperplasia. Fertil Steril. 2014;101:301–9.

39. Cai LQ, Fratianni CM, Gautier T, Imperato-McGinley J. Dihydrotestosterone regulation of semen in male pseudohermaphrodites with 5 alpha-reductase-2 deficiency. J Clin Endocrinol Metab. 1994;79:409–14.

40. Aksglaede L, Juul A. Testicular function and fertility in men with Klinefelter syndrome: a review. Eur J Endocrinol. 2013;168:R67–76.

41. Crouch NS, Liao LM, Woodhouse CRJ, Conway GS, Creighton SM. Sexual function and genital sensitivity following feminizing genitoplasty for congenital adrenal hyperplasia. J Urol. 2008;179:634–8.

42. Köhler B, Kleinemeier E, Lux A, Hiort O, Grüters A, Thyen U, The DSD Network Working Group. Satisfaction with genital surgery and sexual life of adults with XY Disorders of Sex Development: results from the German Clinical Evaluation Study. Endo Res. 2012;97:577–88.

43. Meyer-Bahlburg HF, Migeon CJ, Berkovitz GD, Gearhart JP, Dolezal C, Wisniewski AB. Attitudes of adult 46, XY intersex persons to clinical management. J Urol. 2004;171:1615–9.

44. Slijper F, Drop SLS, Molenaar J, Keizer-Schrama SMP. Long-term psychological evaluation of intersex children. Arch Sex Behav. 1998;27(2):125–44.

45. Kleinemeier E, Jürgensen M, Lux A, Widenka PM, Thyen U, Disorders of Sex Development Network Working Group. Psychological adjustment and sexual development of adolescents with disorders of sex development. J Adolesc Health. 2010;47(5):463–71.

46. Berenbaum SA, Korman BK, Duck SC, Resnick SM. Psychological adjustment in children and adults with congenital adrenal hyperplasia. J Pediatr. 2004;144(6):741–6.

47. Schützmann K, Brinkmann L, Schacht M, Richter-Appelt H. Psychological distress, self-harming behavior, and suicidal tendencies in adults with disorders of sex development. Arch Sex Behav. 2009;38(1):16–33.

48. Malouf MA, Inman AG, Carr AG, Franco J, Brooks LM. Health-related quality of life, mental health and psychotherapeutic considerations for women diagnosed with a disorder of sexual development: congenital adrenal hyperplasia. Int J Pediatr Endocrinol. 2010;2010;11 pages.

49. Johannsen TH, Ripa CP, Mortensen EL, Main KM. Quality of life in 70 women with disorders of sex development. Eur J Endocrinol. 2006;155(6):877–85.

50. Warne G, Grover S, Hutson J, Sinclair A, Metcalfe S, Northam E, Freeman J, … others in the Murdoch Childrens Research Institute Sex Study Group. A Long-term outcome study of intersex conditions. J Pediatr Endocrinol Metab. 2005;18(6):555–68.

51. Hines M, Ahmed SF, Hughes IA. Psychological outcomes and gender-related development in complete androgen insensitivity syndrome. Arch Sex Behav. 2003;32(2):93–101.

52. Morgan JF, Murphy H, Lacey JH, Conway G. Long term psychological outcome for women with congenital adrenal hyperplasia: cross sectional survey. Br Med J. 2005;7487:340.

53. Liao LM, Conway GS, Ismail-Pratt I, Bikoo M, Creighton SM. Emotional and sexual wellness and quality of life in women with Rokitansky syndrome. Am J Obstet Gynecol. 2011;205(2):117.e1–6.

54. Sandberg DE, Gardner M, Cohen-Kettenis PT. Psychological aspects of the treatment of patients with disorders of sex development. Semin Reprod Med. 2012;30(5):443–52.

55. Mathews GA, Fane BA, Conway GS, Brook CGD, Hines M. Personality and congenital adrenal hyperplasia:

possible effects of prenatal androgen exposure. Horm Behav. 2009;55(2):285–91.

56. Pasterski V, Hindmarsh P, Geffner M, Brook C, Brain C, Hines M. Increased aggression and activity Level in 3- to 11-year-old girls with Congenital Adrenal Hyperplasia (CAH). Horm Behav. 2007;52(3):368–74.

57. American Psychiatric Association. Diagnostic and statistical manual of mental disorders: DSM-5. Washington, DC: American Psychiatric Association; 2013.

58. Malouf MA, Wisniewski AB, Migeon CJ. Gender and reproduction in women with congenital adrenal hyperplasia. Pediatr Res. 2003;53:828.

59. Migeon CJ, et al. Ambiguous genitalia with perineo-scrotal hypospadias in 46, XY individuals: long-term medical, surgical, and psychosexual outcome. Pediatrics. 2002;110(3):e31.

60. Just the Facts Coalition. Just the facts about sexual orientation and youth: A primer for principals, educators, and school personnel. Washington, DC: American Psychological Association; 2008. Retrieved from www.apa.org/pi/lgbc/publications/justthefacts.html.

61. Ryan C, Russell ST, Huebner D, Diaz R, Sanchez J. Family acceptance in adolescence and the health of lgbt young adults. J Child Adolesc Psychiatr Nurs. 2010;23(4):205–13.

62. Alderson J, Madill A, Balen A. Fear of devaluation: understanding the experience of intersexed women with androgen insensitivity syndrome. Br J Health Psychol. 2004;9:81–100.

63. Cull ML. Commentary: a support group's perspective. Br Med J. 2005;330(7487):341.

64. Kuhnle U, Bullinger M. Outcome of congenital adrenal hyperplasia. Pediatr Surg Int. 1997;12(7):511–5.

65. Mensah FK, Bayer JK, Wake M, Carlin JB, Allen NB, Patton GC. Early puberty and childhood social and behavioral adjustment. J Adolesc Health. 2013;53(1):118–24.

66. Mendle J, Turkheimer E, Emery RE. Detrimental psychological outcomes associated with early pubertal timing in adolescent girls. Dev Rev. 2007;27(2):151–71.

67. Lindfors K, Elovainio M, Wickman S, Vuorinen R, Sinkkonen J, Dunkel L, Raappana A. Brief report: the role of ego development in psychosocial adjustment among boys with delayed puberty. J Res Adolesc. 2007;17(4):601–12.

68. Schwab J, Kulin HE, Susman EJ, Finkelstein JW, Chinchilli VM, Kunselman SJ, Liben LS, et al. The role of sex hormone replacement therapy on self-perceived competence in adolescents with delayed puberty. Child Dev. 2001;72(5):1439–50.

69. MacKenzie D, Huntington A, Gilmour JA. The experiences of people with an intersex condition: a journey from silence to voice. J Clin Nurs. 2009;18(12):1775–83.

70. Moshiri M, Chapman T, Fechner PY, Dubinsky TJ, Shnorhavorian M, Osman S, Bhargava P, et al. Evaluation and management of disorders of sex development: multidisciplinary approach to a complex diagnosis. Radiographics. 2012;32(6):1599–618.

## Ignatius Bau and Kellan Baker

## Purpose

The purpose of this chapter is to provide an overview of how federal and state legislation, regulations, and other public policies affect LGBTI health.

## Learning Objectives

- List trends in policy related to LGBT health on the governmental (federal and state) and nongovernmental levels. *(KP4, SBP1)*
- Describe how specific policy issues, including standards for medical education and data collection, affect LGBT people and families. *(KP4, SBP1, ICS3)*
- Identify at least 2 ways in which the Affordable Care Act impacts LGBT communities. *(KP4, SBP1)*
- Identify at least 3 ways in which LGBT civil rights priorities such as nondiscrimination and marriage equality relate to LGBT health and wellbeing. *(KP4, SBP1)*

I. Bau (✉)
Independent Consultant, San Francisco, CA, USA
e-mail: ignatius.bau@gmail.com

K. Baker
Senior Fellow, LGBT Research and Communications Project, Center for American Progress, Washington, DC, USA
e-mail: kbaker@americanprogress.org

## Discrimination in Health Care against LGBTI Patients and Their Families

When considering legal and policy issues related to lesbian, gay, bisexual, transgender, and intersex (LGBTI) patients and their families, it is important to remember that LGBTI individuals across the United States continue to face discrimination on the basis of their sex, sexual orientation, and gender identity in many areas of their lives, including from health care providers and in health care delivery settings. In many situations, no law prohibits such discrimination, and the individuals harmed have few legal remedies. Numerous surveys, studies, and reports have documented both the widespread extent of the discrimination experienced by LGBTI patients and their families in health care settings and the effect that discrimination has on the health and wellbeing of LGBTI individuals.

### Discrimination and Gay, Lesbian, and Bisexual Health

In a 2009 national survey conducted by Lambda Legal with nearly 5000 respondents, 29 % of lesbian, gay, and bisexual (LGB) respondents reported that they believe health care providers will treat them differently because of their sexual

© Springer International Publishing Switzerland 2016

421

K.L. Eckstrand, J.M. Ehrenfeld (eds.), *Lesbian, Gay, Bisexual, and Transgender Healthcare*,
DOI 10.1007/978-3-319-19752-4_24

orientation, and 9 % believed providers will refuse them treatment because of their LGB status [1]. These fears are well-founded: Overall, nearly one in ten LGB respondents reported actually being refused needed medical care because of their sexual orientation; 11 % reported that health care providers had used harsh or abusive language with them, and 4 % reported that providers had been physically rough or abusive.

Even professional medical associations have formally participated in sexual orientation discrimination. In the mid-2000s, for instance, the California Medical Association (CMA) filed a legal brief defending the right of a California physician to deny fertility services to a lesbian because the physician disapproved of her sexual orientation. Fortunately, the CMA ultimately reversed its position and filed a new brief supporting the patient's right to equal access to health care services, regardless of her sexual orientation [2]. The California Supreme Court eventually ruled in favor of the patient and established a statewide legal precedent prohibiting discrimination by health care providers based on sexual orientation [3]. Despite the positive outcome of this case, however, concerns remain in jurisdictions across the country that providers may be able to invoke so-called "conscience clauses" to evade legal bans on discrimination on the basis of sexual orientation or gender identity.

---

**Selected Court Decisions Relevant to LGBT Health**

Discrimination by health care providers based on sexual orientation prohibited:

*North Coast Women's Care Medical Group v. San Diego County Superior Court*, 44 Cal. 4th 1145 (2008)

Federal constitutional right to marriage equality for same-sex couples

*United States v. Windsor*, 570 U.S. ___, 133 S. Ct. 2675 (2013)

*Obergefell v. Hodges*, 576 U.S. ___, 135 S. Ct. 2071 (2015)

---

In another well-publicized case in 2007, Florida's Jackson Memorial Hospital rejected legal documents authorizing visitation and powers of attorney for health care decisions between a lesbian couple [4]. When Lisa Pond collapsed with a brain aneurysm during a family vacation in Florida, hospital staff denied her partner Janice Langbehn and their children access to Lisa's bedside, telling Janice that they were in an "anti-gay state." The ensuing years of controversy and publicity over this case eventually prompted President Barack Obama to issue a presidential memorandum in 2010 directing the Centers for Medicare and Medicaid Services (CMS) to use its regulatory authority to require all hospitals receiving federal funding to recognize same-sex couples and other patient-designated support persons as family members for purposes of visitation and health care decision-making [5]. Since almost all hospitals receive some federal funding through programs such as Medicare and Medicaid, this regulation should be implemented by most hospitals in the United States [6]. Nonetheless, this policy development highlights the importance of efforts to educate LGBTI individuals about having advance legal directives for health care decision-making, including powers of attorney for health care decisions, advance directives, and physician orders for life-sustaining treatment.

The CMS regulations notwithstanding, it remains a challenge to ensure that all health care facility employees, including providers and other staff, recognize and respect the rights of same-sex couples and LGBTI patients in general. Every year, the Human Rights Campaign Foundation compiles the Healthcare Equality Index (HEI), which documents voluntary responses by health care organizations to a survey about their LGBT-inclusive policies and practices [7]. The HEI documents whether participating facilities have implemented LGBT-inclusive nondiscrimination policies, including visitation policies that recognize LGBT families, as well as training for employees on LGBT health issues. In 2014 more than 1500 health care organizations from every state and the District of Columbia participated, including hospitals, community health centers, and Veterans Administration medical centers.

The HEI is a useful tool to monitor the implementation of inclusive visitation policies.

Concerns about health care discrimination and health disparities on the basis of sexual orientation are not confined to gay and lesbian individuals. A 2011 report from the San Francisco Human Rights Commission thoroughly documented the health disparities experienced by bisexual women and men and the barriers they face in accessing appropriate health care services [8]. In comparison to heterosexuals, lesbian women, and gay men, bisexual people are more likely to suffer from depression and other mood or anxiety disorders and to report higher rates of hypertension, poor or fair physical health, smoking, and substance use. Bisexual women in particular also experience higher rates of domestic violence compared to other women, and they are significantly less likely to have health insurance coverage and more likely to experience financial barriers to appropriate health care services. A 2014 report from Centers for Disease Control and Prevention (CDC) using data from the 2013 National Health Interview Survey also revealed significant health disparities among bisexual women in comparison to both heterosexual women and gay and lesbian women [9].

## Discrimination and Transgender Health

Lambda Legal's 2009 survey also found endemic discrimination against transgender and gender-nonconforming people in health care settings. Three-quarters (73 %) of transgender respondents reported fears that health care providers would treat them differently because of their gender identity, and half (52 %) believed providers would refuse them treatment because they are transgender or gender-nonconforming [1]. More than 25 % of transgender respondents—substantially higher even than the 8 % incidence of discrimination on the basis of sexual orientation highlighted by the same survey—reported being refused needed medical care because of their gender identity. Worse, 21 % of transgender respondents reported that health care providers had used harsh or abusive language with them, and 8 % reported physically rough or abusive treatment.

A 2011 national survey conducted by the National Center for Transgender Equality and National Gay and Lesbian Task Force similarly uncovered catastrophic rates of health-related discrimination against transgender and gender-nonconforming people: Roughly one-quarter of the more than 6400 respondents reported being denied needed treatment, being harassed in health care settings, or postponing medical care because of discrimination from providers [10]. These encounters with discrimination are correlated with significant health disparities in the transgender population, including a lifetime risk of suicide attempts up to 26 times higher than the general population and an HIV prevalence among transgender women of color that is among the world's highest [11].

This survey also highlighted the pervasive problem of health insurance discrimination against transgender individuals. As discussed in more detail in the section "State Policy Related to LGBTI Health", private and public health insurance plans, including most plans offered by health insurance marketplaces, most employer-sponsored health insurance plans, and many state Medicaid programs, routinely use exclusions to deny coverage to transgender insureds for medically necessary health care services that are covered for other enrollees on the same plan [12]. Such rampant insurance discrimination has helped perpetuate the estrangement of many transgender people from the health care system and exacerbates the already severe health disparities that the transgender population experiences.

## Discrimination and Intersex Health

A 2005 report from the San Francisco Human Rights Commission documents a pervasive lack of awareness and understanding about intersex conditions [13], also known as differences of sex development (DSD) [14]. Overall, intersex conditions are much more common than typically expected: Estimates of the frequency of intersex conditions range from one in 2000 up to one in 150 births and, according to the University of

California at San Francisco, 40 genital surgeries are performed annually in the city of San Francisco alone to assign a binary male or female sex to an infant born with "ambiguous" or "abnormal" sexual anatomy.

The Commission report found no evidence that intersex children benefit from "normalizing" interventions, and other data suggest that the long-term consequences of "normalizing" genital surgeries are quite negative. Many intersex adults report that the endocrine treatments and/or surgeries they were subjected to as infants, children, or adolescents—in most cases, without their informed consent—cause scarring, pain, diminished or absent sexual function, and other physical harm, as well as psychological problems such as post-traumatic stress disorder, depression and anxiety, poor body image, and suicidal ideation. Thus, a major policy principle for adult intersex individuals and advocates is that, barring true medical emergencies, a child's anatomy and identity should not be determined in infancy by health care providers or parents. Rather, individuals with intersex conditions should be able to exercise autonomy over their own bodies and identities and should be free to make their own decisions about gender, sexuality, and major medical interventions such as irreversible surgeries.

## LGBTI Inclusion in Health Care Education, Training, and Practice

A major barrier to more consistent integration of LGBTI issues in health care settings is a lack of provider and other staff training on LGBTI health issues [15, 16]. Studies have documented that LGBTI health issues are rarely included in medical school curricula and, when they are, that the majority of the 5 average hours of study time spent on LGBTI health are devoted almost exclusively to HIV/AIDS [17, 18]. Further, according to the 2014 HEI, 14 % of surveyed facilities still did not provide even a minimum of employee training on LGBTI health issues. The training requirements of the HEI are not especially onerous, suggesting that an easy way for these facili-

ties to take steps toward meeting them is to explore the use of standard Continuing Medical Education (CME) sessions and other professional training modules that are becoming increasingly widely available about LGBTI health issues. Recognizing the importance of CME in incentivizing learning and training, California has expanded state-mandated CME cultural competency requirements to include "understanding and applying cultural and ethnic data to the process of clinical care, including, as appropriate, information pertinent to the appropriate treatment of, and provision of care to, the lesbian, gay, bisexual, transgender, and intersex communities[1].

**Selected LGBTI Cultural Competency Resources**
American Association of Medical Colleges—*Implementing Curricular and Institutional Climate Changes to Improve Health Care for Individuals Who Are LGBT, Gender Nonconforming, or Born with DSD: A Resource for Medical Educators* (2014): www.aamc.org/lgbtdsd.

U.S. Office of Minority Health—*Culturally and Linguistically Appropriate Services (CLAS) Standards* and *Implementation Blueprint* (2013): www.thinkculturalhealth.hhs.gov/Content/clas.asp and www.thinkculturalhealth.hhs.gov/pdfs/EnhancedCLASStandardsBlueprint.pdf.

Centers for Medicare & Medicaid Services—*Special Populations Help (LGBT)*: https://marketplace.cms.gov/technical-assistance-resources/special-populations-help.html

Agency for Healthcare Research and Quality—*Innovations Exchange* https://innovations.ahrq.gov/search/node/LGBT

Health Resources and Services Administration—*LGBT Cultural*

---

[1] http://leginfo.legislature.ca.gov/faces/billNavClient.xhtml?bill_id=201320140AB496

*Competency Resources*: http://www.hrsa.gov/lgbt

Substance Abuse and Mental Health Services Administration—*LGBT Cultural Competency Resources*: http://samhsa.gov/lgbt/curricula.aspx

The Fenway Institute and Center for American Progress—*Do Ask, Do Tell: A Toolkit for Collecting Data on Sexual Orientation and Gender Identity in Clinical Settings*: www.doaskdotell.org.

GLMA: Health Professionals Advancing LGBT Equality—*Cultural Competency Webinar Series* (2013): http://www.glma.org/index.cfm?fuseaction=Page.viewPage&pageId=1025&grandparentID=534&parentID=940&nodeID=1

GLMA: Health Professionals Advancing LGBT Equality—*Recommendations for Enhancing the Climate for LGBT Students and Employees in Health Professional Schools* (2013): http://healthcareguild.com/Recommendations%20for%20Enhancing%20LGBT%20Climate%20in%20Health%20Professional%20Schools.pdf

Fenway Institute—*Affirmative Care for Transgender and Gender Non-Conforming People: Best Practices for Front-line Health Care Staff* (2013): www.lgbthealtheducation.org/wp-content/uploads/13-017_TransBestPracticesforFrontlineStaff_v6_02-19-13_FINAL.pdf

The Joint Commission—*Advancing Effective Communication, Cultural Competence, and Patient- and Family-Centered Care for the Lesbian, Gay, Bisexual, and Transgender (LGBT) Community: A Field Guide* (2011): www.jointcommission.org/assets/1/18/LGBTFieldGuide.pdf

Further, institutional climates around LGBTI issues at both health professional schools and health care facilities are strongly affected by the degree to which LGBTI-identified staff themselves are comfortable and visible in leadership positions. While the number continues to grow, as of 2014 there were few "out" LGBT medical school faculty at schools across the United States [19] and only a handful of LGBT student organizations at any health profession school in the country [20].

Fortunately, there are promising developments in changing the institutional climate in medical and other health professional education institutions to be more supportive of LGBTI health. For example, prompted by the Group on Student Affairs and the Organization of Student Representatives [21], the leadership of the Association of American Medical Colleges (AAMC) has publicly endorsed support for LGBTI students and faculty [22] and published a comprehensive curriculum guide for medical schools on addressing LGBTI health issues[2]. The AAMC also established the LGBT & DSD-Affected Patient Care Advisory Committee in 2012 and is actively collecting curricular tools for teaching about LGBTI health issues in MedEdPORTAL [23]. In recent years, LGBTI health-focused programs have been established at several medical schools and other health professions schools [24–27].

## State Policy Related to LGBTI Health

Under the U.S. system of government, the states are an important source of health-related law and regulation. Particularly in states where progressive social attitudes around LGBTI issues have historically been dominant, substantive legislation has been enacted to prohibit discrimination based on sexual orientation and/or gender identity in the delivery of health care and health-related services, in line with prohibitions against discrimination in other state-governed or state-funded programs and services. California, for example, enacted legislation in 2006 prohibiting discrimination based on sexual orientation and gender identity in all state programs and services, including health care [28], and in 2008 the state required training on LGBT health issues in all

---

[2] www.aamc.org/lgbtdsd

nursing homes and senior care facilities [29]. In 2012, California became the first state to prohibit mental health providers from engaging in so-called reparative therapy to attempt to change a patient's sexual orientation, [30] and as of 2015, three other states and the District of Columbia have enacted similar bans [31].

After several unsuccessful attempts, California enacted legislation in 2015 requiring its Departments of Health Care Services, Public Health, Social Services, and Aging to collect data about sexual orientation and general identity [32]. Efforts to expand health-related data collection about sexual orientation and gender identity—whether at the level of population health surveys, administrative forms for health programs, or medical records—continue to be a priority in other states and at the federal level. New York, for example, moved administratively in 2014 to launch a statewide initiative coordinating new LGBT data collection efforts across a range of state agencies, including the Departments of Health, Corrections and Community Supervision, Mental Health, and Children and Family Services, among others [33]. While most legislative activity in the states to date has involved sexual orientation and gender identity rather than intersex status, there may be future opportunities in states such as California to advance public policies that support the autonomy of individuals with DSD [34].

## Marriage Equality and LGBT Health

Though states such as California and New York have more progressive histories on LGBTI issues than many other U.S. states, these examples will likely be instructive for similar efforts in other states as momentum in support of LGBT rights, led largely by public acceptance of marriage equality for same-sex couples, gains strength across the country. In 2013, the U.S. Supreme Court struck down the provision of the so-called Defense of Marriage Act (DOMA) that prohibited the federal government from recognizing marriages between people of the same sex [35], and in 2015, the Court affirmed a federal constitutional right to marriage equality, striking down all the remaining state prohibitions on same-sex marriage and establishing marriage equality throughout the United States [34].

Marriage equality is good news for health. In the early 2000s, Dr. Ilan Meyer used the term "minority stress" to describe the mechanism whereby the stressors of social stigma and prejudice become embodied as poorer health outcomes for members of a targeted group such as LGBT individuals [36]. And indeed, studies have shown that anti-gay legislation, such as state laws denying the benefits and protections of marriage to same-sex couples, provoke increased incidence of mental and behavioral health disorders such as depression, anxiety, and substance abuse among lesbian, gay, and bisexual populations [37]. A lack of marriage equality has also historically contributed to elevated rates of uninsurance among same-sex couples. Legalizing marriage for same-sex couples, on the other hand, not only improves health and access to health coverage and care for these couples but also helps mitigate minority stress by contributing to a more affirming and healthier social environment for LGBT people generally [38–40].

## Insurance Coverage for Transgender Health Needs

California was also the first state to specifically prohibit insurance discrimination against transgender people. In 2012 and 2013, the California Department of Insurance [41] and Department of Managed Health Care [42] (which has regulatory authority over managed care health plans doing business in California) issued regulations and legal guidance implementing a 2005 insurance nondiscrimination law that includes gender identity [43] and clarifying that insurers may not use exclusions that specifically deny transgender people coverage for care that is covered for non-transgender people [44]. Most, if not all, of the treatments that transgender people may need to medically transition are covered for non-transgender people for a variety of conditions, including endocrine disorders, cancer prevention or treatment, and reconstructive surgeries following an injury [45]. Under transgender-specific insurance exclusions, however, transgender individuals have frequently faced denials of coverage not only for care that related to gender transition, such as hormone therapy and gender-confirming surgeries, but also for "gendered" preventive screenings such as Pap tests and mammograms, and sometimes for any care at all [46].

Expert medical bodies such as the American Medical Association (AMA), American Psychiatric Association, American Psychological Association, American Academy of Family Physicians, American Congress of Obstetricians and Gynecologists, and Endocrine Society have all affirmed the medical necessity of health care services related to gender transition or Gender Dysphoria, which is the diagnostic term sometimes used to describe a transgender identity. (The diagnosis of Gender Dysphoria replaced the older diagnosis of Gender Identity Disorder in the DSM-5, which was published in 2013.) The AMA in particular has specifically taken the policy position that health care services related to gender transition should be covered by health insurance plans [47], and a 2012 assessment from the California Department of Insurance showed that access to transition-related care significantly improves the health of transgender individuals on indicators such as mental health and HIV treatment adherence [48].

In addition to California, insurance commissioners in nine other states plus the District of Columbia issued bulletins between 2012 and 2015 prohibiting transgender exclusions in insurance [49–56]. In 2015, the Office for Civil Rights at the U.S. Department of Health and Human Services followed suit by clarifying that Section 1557 of the Affordable Care Act, the health reform law's primary civil rights provision, prohibits insurance plan exclusions that categorically deny transgender individuals access to health care services related to gender transition. In implementing these requirements that plans remove transgender exclusions, future challenges at the state and federal levels will include ensuring that health plans actually cover all of the health care services that are medically necessary for their transgender enrollees and that there are enough providers nationwide who provide primary and specialty care related to gender transition.

## Health Care in Detention Settings

A particular challenge in the provision of health care services for transgender people, as well as for the LGBTI population generally, is detention facilities such as jails, prisons, and immigration detention [57, 58]. Numerous reports have documented the barriers transgender people in detention settings experience in trying to access transition-related health care, even when they have a diagnosis of Gender Dysphoria or are already being prescribed hormone therapy when they enter detention [59, 60]. Similarly, people living with HIV report difficulties in accessing anti-retroviral medications in detention settings, and most of these facilities do not permit the distribution of prevention and harm reduction aids such as condoms or clean needles [61]. Finally, in addition to the mental health consequences of detention, LGBTI people in these facilities are at substantial risk of sexual assault, particularly transgender women, who are frequently and inappropriately housed with the male inmate population [62].

## Federal Policy Related to LGBTI Health

In addition to the states, all three branches of the federal government—the executive, legislative, and judicial—play an important role in making and interpreting policy that affects the health of LGBTI populations. In the realm of the courts, for instance, the U.S. Supreme Court's 2013 *Windsor* decision on DOMA prompted the Internal Revenue Service (IRS), the U.S. Office of Personnel Management (OPM), and the U.S. Department of Health and Human Services (HHS) to issue a raft of new guidance relating to the recognition of same-sex marriages for purposes such as federal income taxes [63], qualified retirement plans [64], and programs such as the Federal Employees Health Benefits Program [65], Medicare [66], Medicare Advantage [67], and Medicaid [68]. Similar guidance will follow the 2015 *Obergefell* decision that extended marriage equality nationwide.

## LGBTI Health at the U.S. Department of Health and Human Services

Among the Executive Branch agencies, HHS in particular has emerged as a leader on LGBTI issues and a key player in LGBTI health policy. During Bill Clinton's presidency, there were unprecedented initiatives at HHS such as the release of an Institute of Medicine report on lesbian health [69], the beginning of efforts to initiate a more effective federal response to HIV and AIDS among gay and bisexual men and other men who have sex with men (MSM), the convening of the first-ever agency-wide steering committee on health disparities related to sexual orientation (expanded in practice to include gender identity), and the inclusion of sexual orientation (though not gender identity) as a disparity factor of concern in *Healthy People 2010*, the federal government's blueprint for a healthier nation between 2000 and 2010.

This momentum continued for the first few months of 2001, when the National Institutes of Health (NIH) released the first program announcement offering funding for research on "lesbian, gay, bisexual, transgendered [sic], and related populations" [70], and HHS supported the publication of the *Companion Document for Lesbian, Gay, Bisexual, and Transgender Health* as part of *Healthy People 2010* [71]. Throughout the remainder of the George W. Bush Administration, however, LGBTI health was sidelined at HHS. Some programs, such as support for LGBTI-related research at NIH, even attracted politically motivated attacks that had a chilling effect on the development of the field [72].

Not until the start of the Obama Administration did HHS again began to undertake policymaking related to LGBTI health. Two substantive overviews of LGBT health issues serve as cornerstones of this work: In 2010, HHS released *Healthy People 2020* with a new LGBT Health topic area that discussed a range of LGBT health disparities in the context of discrimination and minority stress [73]. And in 2011, the Institute of Medicine released a comprehensive, NIH-commissioned report on LGBT health, *The Health of Lesbian, Gay, Bisexual, and Transgender People: Building a Foundation for*

*Better Understanding* [74]. In response, NIH took steps such as compiling its own report and portfolio analysis [75], reissuing its funding opportunity announcement on LGBTI health research [76], and convening several listening sessions between NIH senior leadership and LGBTI health stakeholders to inform the development of an NIH-wide strategic plan on advancing LGBTI health research [77].

> **Recommendations from the 2011 Institute of Medicine Report on LGBT Health**
>
> 1. NIH should implement a research agenda designed to advance knowledge and understanding of LGBT health.
> 2. Data on sexual orientation and gender identity should be collected in federally funded surveys administered by HHS and in other relevant federally funded surveys.
> 3. Data on sexual orientation and gender identity should be collected in electronic health records.
> 4. NIH should support the development and standardization of sexual orientation and gender identity measures.
> 5. NIH should support methodological research that relates to LGBT health.
> 6. A comprehensive research training approach should be created to strengthen LGBT health research at NIH.
> 7. NIH should encourage grant applicants to address explicitly the inclusion or exclusion of sexual and gender minorities [LGBT] in their samples.

Also in 2010, shortly after CMS released the hospital visitation regulations described in the section "Discrimination in Health Care Against LGBTI Patients and Their Families" [5], Secretary of Health and Human Services Kathleen Sebelius convened an HHS LGBT Coordinating Committee co-chaired by senior HHS officials. Throughout Secretary Sebelius's tenure, the HHS LGBT Coordinating Committee and other internal and external stakeholders collaborated on a range of LGBTI health initiatives, and in 2011 the committee began to release annual reports outlining the previous year's activities and laying out objectives for the next year [78]. Among others, these activities included:

- Collaborating with the White House on an LGBT health summit [79].
- Establishing the National Resource Center on LGBT Aging [80].
- Incorporating sexual orientation and gender identity into the Office of Minority Health's revised Culturally and Linguistically Appropriate Services (CLAS) Standards, which serve as the federal government's de facto definition of cultural competency [81].
- Funding the National LGBT Health Education Center through the Health Resources and Services Administration (HRSA) to help community health centers serve LGBT patients [82].
- Updating the Substance Abuse and Mental Health Services Administration's (SAMHSA) 2001 guide to substance abuse treatment for LGBT individuals [83].
- Establishing a joint HRSA/SAMHSA committee to identify and promote effective LGBT cultural training modules (see [84, 85]).
- Publishing a new resource toolkit on LGBT health issues [86].
- Addressing disparities related to sexual orientation and gender identity in high-profile annual reports such as the *National Healthcare Disparities Report* [87, 88], *Women's Health USA* [89], and the CDC's *Health Disparities and Inequalities Report* [90, 91].
- Including sexual orientation and gender identity in federal strategies around issues such as multiple chronic conditions [92], HIV/AIDS [93], and racial and ethnic disparities [94].
- Partnering with the Out2Enroll initiative [95] to ensure that the benefits of the Affordable Care Act reach LGBT communities.
- Publishing a report documenting the scientific evidence against so-called conversion therapy [96].

In another key advance, in 2014 an independent Departmental Appeals Board at HHS lifted the exclusion in Medicare that had barred the program from covering "transsexual surgery" for more than 30 years [97].

## Congressional Actions on LGBT Health

The Congressional record on LGBT health is significantly thinner than the portfolio of agency activities. The first substantive legislative effort on LGBT health did not come until 2009, when then-Representative Tammy Baldwin (D-WI) introduced the Ending LGBT Health Disparities Act (ELHDA) [98]. This omnibus bill sought to advance LGBT health priorities such as promoting LGBT-inclusive research and data collection; encouraging the routine incorporation of LGBT cultural competency in programs across HHS; establishing LGBT-inclusive nondiscrimination policies in federal health programs such as Medicaid, Medicare, the Federal Employees Health Benefits Program, and health services provided by the Veterans Administration; and creating an Office of LGBT Health within the HHS Office of Minority Health.

Though ELHDA was never passed, it represents a pivotal moment in Congressional attention to LGBT health. Prior to this bill, no federal legislation had proposed to specifically address LGBT health disparities. In 2007, for instance, then-Representative Hilda Solis (D-CA) introduced the Health Equity and Accountability Act (HEAA) [99] to guide and improve federal efforts in areas such as data collection, culturally and linguistically appropriate health care, health workforce diversity, high-impact minority diseases, nondiscrimination, and the social determinants of health and health disparities. This groundbreaking legislation on racial and ethnic minority health disparities did not include, however, any reference to sexual orientation or gender identity.

But following the introduction of ELHDA in 2009, each biennial iteration of the HEAA has reflected a deeper understanding of intersectional health disparities and recognized that racial, ethnic, and other disparities cannot be fully addressed in isolation from the disparities associated with stigmatized sexual orientation and gender identity [100]. The HEAA is an essential statement of the importance of addressing health disparities, and it is a key source of health equity provisions that can be incorporated into other legislation or enacted administratively.

## The Affordable Care Act and LGBTI Populations

A major piece of enacted legislation that has significant relevance for LGBT health is the Patient Protection and Affordable Care Act of 2010, commonly known as the Affordable Care Act (ACA) [101]. Though the term "sexual orientation" appears only once in the law, in a section about cultural competency training for mental health care providers [102], and the term "gender identity" does not appear at all, the law provides numerous opportunities for advocates to advance LGBT health priorities with the states and with HHS, the lead federal agency charged with implementing the law [103]. According to Secretary Sebelius, "the Affordable Care Act may represent the strongest foundation we have ever created to begin closing LGBT health disparities" [104, 105].

**Resources on the ACA and LGBTI Populations**
Out2Enroll [95] is a nationwide campaign launched in 2013 to provide information for LGBT people about their insurance options under the Affordable Care Act and train health insurance enrollment assistance personnel to work effectively with LGBT individuals and families.

Center for American Progress—*Moving the Needle: The Impact of the Affordable Care Act on LGBT Communities* (2014): https://www.americanprogress.org/issues/lgbt/report/2014/11/17/101575/moving-the-needle.

Out2Enroll—*Key Lessons for LGBT Outreach and Enrollment under the*

*Affordable Care Act* (2014): http://out2enroll.org/out2enroll/wp-content/uploads/2014/07/O2E_KeyLessons_FINAL.pdf.

Kaiser Family Foundation—*Health and Access to Care and Coverage for Lesbian, Gay, Bisexual, and Transgender Individuals in the U.S.* (2014, updated 2015): http://kff.org/disparities-policy/issue-brief/health-and-access-to-care-and-coverage-for-lesbian-gay-bisexual-and-transgender-individuals-in-the-u-s/.

Center for American Progress and National Coalition for LGBT Health—*Changing the Game: What Health Care Reform Means for Lesbian, Gay, Bisexual, and Transgender Americans* (2011): http://cdn.americanprogress.org/wp-content/uploads/issues/2011/03/pdf/aca_lgbt.pdf

### Closing the Coverage Gap

A central premise of the ACA is expanding the availability and quality of health insurance coverage. Before the ACA's coverage reforms took full effect, almost 50 million Americans were uninsured [106], including more than 24 % of LGBT people [107]. In particular, one in three (34 %) of LGBT people with incomes under $45,000 per year were uninsured [108]. Almost half of LGBT people in this income range had put off going to a doctor for medical care they needed in the last year because they could not afford it, and 31 % had unpaid medical debt, rising to 43 % for parents [109–113].

The ACA has significantly expanded access to insurance coverage across the United States. As of November 2015, 17.6 million people have gained coverage under the ACA, reducing the uninsurance rate to 9 %—the lowest rate of uninsurance in U.S. history and a drop of 45 % since 2010 [149]. Uninsurance among low- and middle-income LGBT adults declined by a quarter between 2013 and 2014 (from 34 % uninsured in 2013 to 26 % uninsured in 2014) [150], and the ACA cut unisurance almost in half among LGB adults—from 21.7 % to 11.1 %—in all income ranges between 2013 and 2015 [151].

The ACA facilitates access to affordable health insurance coverage in two main ways: It requires the states to open Medicaid eligibility to everyone making up to 138 % of the Federal Poverty Level (FPL), and it establishes new health insurance marketplaces in every state to offer financial assistance in the form of sliding-scale tax credits [114].

Because of the Supreme Court decision on the ACA in June 2012, the states do not have to expand their Medicaid programs as the law originally required [115]. As of November 2015, 30 states and the District of Columbia had expanded their Medicaid programs [116], making it possible for LGBT people who previously would not have met traditional Medicaid's stringent eligibility criteria to gain coverage. Expansion Medicaid also eliminates the problem that individuals with HIV would not get Medicaid coverage for HIV treatment until their health had deteriorated to the point where they became disabled by AIDS [117]. In states that do not expand Medicaid, however, the health reform law no longer offers new options to help people with incomes under the poverty line access insurance coverage [118].

There is no deadline for states to decide to move forward with the expansion, though states that delay lose substantial amounts of federal funding: The federal government pays 100 % of the costs of expansion between 2014 and 2016, and this percentage drops slightly before settling at 90 % in 2020 and beyond. Overall, this financing arrangement means that the states pay only approximately 7 % of the cost of closing the coverage gap through Medicaid expansion [119].

The other major coverage initiative under the Affordable Care Act is the system of health insurance marketplaces in every state. The marketplaces are intended to foster competition in insurance markets by allowing people to shop for private health insurance plans through a single streamlined interface that allows for easy comparisons between different products [120]. The ACA's marketplaces provide income-based financial assistance in the form of tax credits that people can use to offset the cost of their monthly premiums.

The intent of the ACA was that the states would operate their own marketplaces, but the political environment around the reform effort led a majority of states to leave marketplace governance to HHS. This has led to a system in which the federal government runs the majority of the marketplaces through HealthCare.gov, while a handful of states such as California and New York run their own marketplaces [121].

## Nondiscrimination Under the ACA

The Affordable Care Act extends the nondiscrimination protections of existing federal civil rights laws to any entity established under Title I of the ACA, administered by a federal executive agency, or receiving federal funds—including providers and facilities participating in Medicare or Medicaid. The protected classes enumerated in ACA Section 1557 include HIV status through the Rehabilitation Act and sex through Title IX, and HHS clarified in regulations that the sex protections of Section 1557 include gender identity and sex stereotypes, such as expectations that women or men must dress or behave a certain way or that an individual can only be in a marriage or other relationship with a person of a different sex [122]. These regulations also prohibit categorical insurance exclusions targeting transgender individuals; require facilities such as hospitals to treat transgender people according to their gender identity in policies such as room assignments; and require insurance carriers and health care providers to make medically necessary health care services equally available to transgender and cisgender (that is, non-transgender) individuals, including preventive health care screenings that are typically associated with only one sex.

Further, the ACA prohibits marketplaces, their employees, the plans sold through them (known as "qualified health plans," or QHPs), and individuals and organizations providing consumer assistance with enrollment from discriminating on bases that include sexual orientation, gender identity, and health status. QHPs and other plans subject to the ACA's requirements must also meet a variety of other new standards. These standards prohibit practices such as medical underwriting, gender rating, pre-existing condition exclusions, annual and lifetime limits on coverage, and arbitrary withdrawal of insurance coverage [123]; they also require plans to treat same- and different-sex married couples equally in access to family and spousal coverage, allow young people to stay on their parents' insurance plans until age 26, and require most plans to cover the "essential health benefits" (EHBs) [124, 125]. The EHBs are services and procedures across 10 broad categories of care:

1. Ambulatory patient services
2. Emergency services
3. Hospitalization
4. Maternity and newborn care
5. Mental health and substance use disorder services, including behavioral health treatment
6. Prescription drugs
7. Rehabilitative and habilitative services and devices
8. Laboratory services
9. Preventive and wellness services and chronic disease management
10. Pediatric Services, including oral and vision care

With regard to coverage for people living with HIV, insurance plans in several states have engaged in questionable practices such as placing HIV medications in restrictive tiering arrangements that require patients to pay high out-of-pocket costs and refusing to accept Ryan White Comprehensive AIDS Resources Emergency (CARE) Act dollars to pay premiums for plans purchased through the marketplaces. These and other concerns about the continuing potential for discriminatory practices in insurance make federal and state enforcement of the ACA's nondiscrimination protections an ongoing policy priority [126].

## Federal and State Data Collection

Section 4302 of the ACA calls on all HHS-funded surveys and programs to collect data on several disparity factors, such as race and eth-

nicity [127]. Importantly, it also grants HHS authority to collect "any other demographic data as deemed appropriate by the Secretary regarding health disparities" [128]. In 2011, Secretary Sebelius released the "LGBT Data Progression Plan" through the HHS Office of Minority Health to guide the agency in adding sexual orientation and gender identity to its data collection efforts [129].

In 2013, HHS added a new sexual orientation question to its flagship health and demographics instrument, the National Health Interview Survey [9, 130]. Later that year the CDC approved a sexual orientation and gender identity question module that 19 states plus Guam began using on their Behavioral Risk Factor Surveillance System (BRFSS) questionnaires in 2014. In many states the youth corollary of the BRFSS, the Youth Risk Behavioral Survey, has also asked questions related to sexual orientation, sexual behavior, and transgender status, and CDC used these data to publish a report on health disparities among sexual minority youth in 2011 [131]. In 2015, HHS proposed new objectives for Healthy People 2020 that would measure progress on these and other state activities to collect data about sexual orientation and gender identity [132].

## From Coverage to Care

The ACA contains numerous provisions aimed at bridging the gap between coverage and care, particularly preventive services. In addition to including prevention and wellness services as one of the 10 essential health benefits most insurance plans must cover, the law requires insurance carriers to cover a range of preventive services, including depression screening and HIV testing, without cost, and provides free annual checkups. Insurance carriers must also provide appropriate preventive screenings for transgender individuals, such as mammograms and prostate exams for transgender women and cervical Pap tests for transgender men, regardless of the individual's sex assigned at birth, gender identity, or the gender marker on their insurance card.

Under the ACA, the Surgeon General chairs a National Prevention Council that brings together representatives from 17 Cabinet agencies to assess opportunities for government initiatives in fields such as criminal justice, transportation, and housing to partner in helping prevent illness and injury and promote health and wellbeing. The Council compiles an annual report that recognizes sexual orientation and gender identity as factors that contribute to disparities and that require particular attention in prevention and wellness initiatives. The law also established a $15-billion-dollar Prevention and Public Health Fund that supports initiatives such as the Racial and Ethnic Approaches to Community Health (REACH) grants program and the Community Transformation Grants program, which contributed more than $370 million between 2011 and 2013 to nutrition, exercise, and anti-smoking programs serving 130 million people [133, 134].

With regard to the provision of health care services, the ACA tripled the size of the National Health Service Corps, which places newly qualified physicians in medically underserved areas; established an $11-billion fund to support the maintenance and expansion of community health centers; and allocated millions of dollars to health centers to assist in outreach, education, and enrollment related to the new insurance coverage options available through Medicaid and the health insurance marketplaces [135]. The ACA also established a "negotiated rulemaking committee" to make recommendations to the Secretary of Health and Human Services regarding an update to the "medically underserved population" designation used to define Health Professional Shortage Areas and determine whether health centers are eligible for funding through the Federally Qualified Health Center program. The committee's 2011 report recommended that the unmet health care needs of LGBT people should qualify the LGBT population as a medically underserved population [136, 137].

On the other hand, while the law significantly increased funding for community health centers, it also relied on projections of expanded insurance coverage to cut funding for safety net public hospitals that predominantly serve the uninsured, including undocumented immigrants and other populations that include low-income LGBTI individuals [138]. The law may also have unintended negative consequences for LGBTI people as a result of the uncertainty it introduces around the future of condition- and population-specific funding such as the Ryan White CARE Act for HIV care [139] and the Title X Family Planning Program for family planning and reproductive health services [140]. Finally, despite significant decreases in uninsurance for LGB adults, research indicates that problems with access and affordability remained higher for LGB adults than for non-LGB adults in winter 2014–15 [141], and many concerns remain regarding access to appropriate health care services for transgender individuals.

## National Quality Improvement Standards and Policies

As attention shifts from the expansion of health insurance coverage through the ACA to longer-term reform of the U.S. health care delivery system, there are numerous opportunities to integrate the improvement of LGBTI health into national quality improvement standards, policies, and practices. Common frameworks for national quality improvement include the six aims of safety, timeliness, effectiveness, efficiency, patient-centeredness, and equity set forth by the Institute of Medicine [142], and the "triple aim" of improved patient experiences of care, improved population health outcomes, and reduced costs developed by the Institute for Healthcare Improvement [143, 144].

Under the IOM framework, the aims of patient-centeredness and equity provide numerous opportunities to integrate LGBTI health improvement into overall quality improvement. For example, two leading national organizations supporting quality improvement, The Joint Commission and the Patient-Centered Outcomes Research Institute (PCORI), have both recognized the connection between patient-centeredness and LGBTI health. The Joint Commission published a field guide in 2011 on improving effective communication, cultural competence, and patient-

and family-centered care for LGBT patients and families [145], and in 2013 PCORI made its first award investigating improvement of patient-centered outcomes for LGBTI patients through data collection in a clinical setting [146]. The aim of equity further provides the opportunity to highlight and address LGBTI health disparities as part of efforts to address the needs of diverse patient populations [147–149].

LGBTI health can be advanced within the triple aim framework by not only by addressing LGBTI disparities as part of broad efforts to improve population health outcomes but also by initiatives that focus on improving LGBTI people's experiences of care [150]. Given the context of continuing discrimination LGBTI individuals encounter in health care settings, for instance, initiatives combining LGBTI nondiscrimination policies and more inclusive institutional practices such as those recommended by The Joint Commission's LGBT field guide with enhanced provider LGBTI cultural competency can be important drivers for improved experiences of care among the LGBTI population.

The National Committee on Quality Assurance also released new standards in 2014 for patient-centered medical homes (PCMH). Echoing the updated Office of Minority Health's CLAS Standards [151], these standards direct practices to evaluate the diversity of their patient populations as part of a comprehensive health assessment, defining "diversity" as "a meaningful characteristic of comparison … that accurately identifies individuals within a non-dominant social system who are underserved. These characteristics of a group may include, but are not limited to, race, ethnicity, gender identity, sexual orientation, and disability" [152].

Collecting data on sexual orientation and gender identity is an important first step in designing effective interventions for improving quality of care and health care outcomes for LGBTI populations [153–156]. A key area for advancing LGBTI data collection in clinical settings is electronic health records (EHRs). On the national policy level, electronic data collection in clinical settings is the focus of a major multi-stage initiative, the Incentive Program for the Meaningful Use of Electronic Health Records (known as "Meaningful Use"). This program was launched under the Health Information Technology for Economic and Clinical Health (HITECH) Act in 2009 and is being overseen by HHS through CMS and the Office of the National Coordinator for Health Information Technology (ONC). In October 2015, ONC and CMS issued regulations requiring all EHR systems certified under Stage 3 of Meaningful Use to have the capacity to collect sexual orientation and gender identity data [157]. Importantly, this does not require providers to collect SO/GI information. Rather, the requirement applies to vendors who are building certified EHR systems and health institutions and practices that are using these systems as part of their participation in the Meaningful Use program.

Large health care organizations, such as Vanderbilt, the University of California at Davis, the Veterans Administration, and Kaiser Permanente are using their EHR systems to collect demographic data that include sexual orientation and gender identity. Many community health centers, such as New York City's Callen-Lorde and Boston's Fenway Health, already collect sexual orientation and gender identity information, and some are starting to mine their EHRs as part of research projects looking at LGBT health disparities, quality of care, and patient outcomes. The Center for American Progress and the Fenway Institute developed a toolkit, "Do Ask, Do Tell: A Toolkit for Collecting Data on Sexual Orientation and Gender Identity in Clinical Settings," that collects best practices and provides resources for health care organizations that want to integrate sexual orientation and gender identity data collection into their record systems.

In addition to sexual orientation and gender identity data collection and the use of patient data to help identify and reduce health disparities, there are a variety of strategies and interventions for integrating LGBTI health improvement into quality improvement and disparities reduction frameworks. For example, patient-centered medical homes could be tailored to address the prevention and care needs of LGBTI individuals and their families, particularly transgender and intersex people and people living with HIV. In addition, value-based purchasing models that achieve the triple aim of improving population health outcomes, improving patient experiences of care, and reducing health care costs can be used to develop health care delivery systems that address the needs of LGBTI populations. Applying principles of continuous and iterative quality improvement to test, spread, and evaluate the effectiveness of interventions to reduce LGBTI health disparities and improve quality outcomes for LGBTI patients, families, and communities will require ongoing commitment and institutional resources.

## References

1. Lambda Legal. When health care isn't caring; 2010, accessed at: http://www.lambdalegal.org/publications/when-health-care-isnt-caring
2. Storrow RF. Medical conscience and the policing of parenthood. William and Mary J Women and Law. 2010;16(2):369–393.
3. North Coast Women's Care Medical Group v. San Diego County Superior Court, 44 Cal. 4th 1145; 2008, accessed at: http://www.lambdalegal.org/sites/default/files/legal-docs/downloads/benitez_ca_20080818_decision-ca-supreme-court.pdf
4. Parker-Pope T. Kept from a dying partner's bedside. New York Times (May 18, 2009), accessed at: http://www.nytimes.com/2009/05/19/health/19well.html?_r=0
5. Centers for Medicare and Medicaid Services. Changes to the hospital and critical access hospital conditions of participation to ensure visitation rights for all patients, 75 Fed. Reg. 70831 (November 19, 2010), accessed at: http://www.gpo.gov/fdsys/pkg/FR-2010-11-19/pdf/2010-29194.pdf
6. The Joint Commission, the leading accreditation organization for hospitals, also has included the requirement of equal visitation rights in its accreditation standards. New and revised hospital EPs to improve patient-provider communication. Joint Commission Perspectives. 2010; 30(1):5–6..
7. Human Rights Campaign Foundation. Healthcare equality index; 2014, accessed at: http://www.hrc.org/hei
8. San Francisco Human Rights Commission. Bisexual invisibility: impacts and recommendations; 2011, accessed at: http://www.sf-hrc.org/modules/showdocument.aspx?documentid=989
9. Ward BW, Dahlhamer JM, Galinsky AM, Joestl SS. Sexual orientation and health among U.S. adults: National Health Interview Survey, 2013. Natl Health Stat Rep. 2014;(77), accessed at: http://www.cdc.gov/nchs/data/nhsr/nhsr077.pdf
10. National Gay and Lesbian Task Force and National Center for Transgender Equality. Injustice at every turn: a report of the national transgender discrimination survey; 2011, accessed at: http://www.thetaskforce.org/reports_and_research/ntds
11. Baral SD, Poteat T, Stromdahl S, Wirtz AL, Guadamuz TE. Worldwide burden of HIV in transgender women: a systematic review and meta-analysis. Lancet. 2013;13(3):214–22.
12. Cray A, Baker KE. Health insurance needs for transgender Americans. Center for American Progress; 2012, accessed at: http://www.americanprogress.org/wp-content/uploads/2012/10/TransgenderHealth.pdf
13. San Francisco Human Rights Commission. A human rights investigation into the "normalization" of intersex people; 2005, accessed at: http://www.sf-hrc.org/modules/showdocument.aspx?documentid=1798
14. Accord Alliance. Clinical guidance for the management of disorders of sex development in childhood; 2008, accessed at: http://www.accordalliance.org/dsdguidelines/clinical.pdf
15. Dorsen C. An integrative review of nurse attitudes towards lesbian, gay, bisexual, and transgender patients. Can J Nurs Res. 2012;44(3):18–43.
16. Eliason MJ, Dibble SL, Robertson PA. Lesbian, gay, and transgender (LGBT) physicians' experiences in the workplace. J Homosex. 2011;58(10):1355–71.
17. Obedin-Maliver J, Goldsmith ES, Stewart L, White W, Tran E, Brenman S, Wells M, Fetterman DM, Garcia G, Lunn MR. Lesbian, gay, bisexual, and transgender-related content in undergraduate medical education. JAMA. 2011;306(9):971–7.
18. Snowdon S. The medical school curriculum and LGBT health concerns. AMA J Ethics. 2010;12(8):638–43.
19. University of California San Francisco Out List, accessed at: http://lgbt.ucsf.edu/out_outlist.html
20. Snowdon S. Recommendations for enhancing the climate for LBGT students and employees at health professional schools, GLMA: health professionals advancing LGBT equality; 2013, accessed at: http://www.glma.org/_data/n_0001/resources/live/Recommendations%20for%20Enhancing%20LGBT%20Climate%20in%20Health%20Professional%20Schools.pdf
21. Association of American Medical Colleges Group on Student Affairs and Organization of Student Representatives. Institutional programs and educational activities to address the needs of lesbian, gay, bisexual and transgender students and patients; 2007, accessed at: https://www.aamc.org/download/157460/data/institutional_programs_and_educational_activities_to_address_th.pdf
22. AAMC's Marc Nivet on Developing LGBTI Competencies, Josiah Macy Foundation News and Commentary; 2012, accessed at: http://macyfoundation.org/news/entry/aamcs-marc-nivet-on-developing-lgbti-competencies-in-medical-school-curricu

23. Association of American Medical Colleges. Lesbian, gay, bisexual, transgender and/or disorders of sex development-affected patient care project, accessed at: https://www.aamc.org/initiatives/diversity/porfolios/330894/lgbt-patientcare-project.html; see also https://www.mededportal.org/icollaborative/about/initiatives/lgbt

24. Vanderbilt University School of Medicine Program for LGBT Health, accessed at: https://medschool.vanderbilt.edu/lgbti/about-us

25. George Washington University LGBT Health Graduate Certificate, accessed at: http://programs.columbian.gwu.edu/lgbt/

26. Drexel University School of Public Health, Program for Lesbian, Gay, Bisexual & Transgender Health, accessed at: http://publichealth.drexel.edu/lgbthealth/

27. University of California San Francisco LGBT Resource Center, accessed at: http://lgbt.ucsf.edu

28. California Senate Bill 1441; 2006, accessed at: http://www.leginfo.ca.gov/pub/05-06/bill/sen/sb_1401-1450/sb_1441_bill_20060828_chaptered.pdf

29. California Senate Bill 1729; 2008, accessed at: http://www.leginfo.ca.gov/pub/07-08/bill/sen/sb_1701-1750/sb_1729_bill_20080928_chaptered.pdf

30. California Senate Bill 1172; 2012, accessed at https://leginfo.legislature.ca.gov/faces/billNavClient.xhtml?bill_id=201120120SB1172

31. National Center for Lesbian Rights, http://www.nclrights.org/cases-and-policy/cases-and-advocacy/anti-lgbt-conversion-therapy

32. California Assembly Bill 959; 2015, accessed at: http://www.leginfo.ca.gov/pub/15-16/bill/asm/ab_0951-1000/ab_959_bill_20151007_chaptered.pdf

33. Tamar-Mattis A. Sterilization and Minors with Intersex Conditions in California. The Circuit, Paper 40 (2012). Available from http://scholarship.law.berkeley.edu/clrcircuit/40

34. California Senate Bill 416; 2011, accessed at: http://www.leginfo.ca.gov/pub/11-12/bill/sen/sb_0401-0450/sb_416_bill_20110913_enrolled.pdf

35. United States v. Windsor, 570 U.S. ___, 133 S. Ct. 2675 (2013) and Obergefell v. Hodges, 576 U.S. ___, 135 S. Ct. 2071 (2015)

36. Mayer I. Prejudice, social stress, and mental health in lesbian, gay, and bisexual populations: conceptual issues and research evidence. Psychol Bull. 2003; 129(5):674–97.

37. Hatzenbuehler ML, O'Cleirigh C, Grasso C, Mayer K, Safren S, Bradford J. Effect of same-sex marriage laws on health care use and expenditures in sexual minority men: a quasi-natural experiment. Am J Public Health. 2012;102(2):285–91.

38. Gay and Lesbian Medical Association. Same-sex marriage and health; 2008, accessed at: http://www.lgbthealthinitiative.com/pdf/Same-Sex_Marriage_and_Health.GLMA.08%5B1%5D.pdf

39. Gonzales G. Same-sex marriage: a prescription for better health. N Engl J Med. 2014;370(15):1373–6.

40. Stephenson R. Could same-sex marriage improve the nation's health? The Health Care Blog (November 11, 2012), accessed at: http://thehealthcareblog.com/blog/2012/11/11/could-same-sex-marriage-improve-the-nation's%C2%A0heal/

41. California Department of Insurance, California Code of Regulations, Title 10, Chapter 5, Subchapter 3, Section 15.1. Gender nondiscrimination in health insurance, accessed at: http://www20.insurance.ca.gov/epubacc/REG/167830.htm

42. California Department of Managed Health Care. Gender nondiscrimination requirements; 2013, accessed at: http://transgenderlawcenter.org/wp-content/uploads/2013/04/DMHC-Director-Letter-re-Gender-NonDiscrimination-Requirements.pdf

43. California Assembly Bill 1586; 2005, accessed at: http://www.leginfo.ca.gov/pub/05-06/bill/asm/ab_1551-1600/ab_1586_bill_20050929_chaptered.pdf

44. Baker KE, Minter SP, Wertz K, Wood M. A new approach to health care equality for transgender people: California's insurance gender non-discrimination act. LGBTQ Policy J. 2012;2.

45. Baker KE, Cray A. Why gender identity nondiscrimination in insurance makes sense. Center for American Progress; 2013, accessed at http://cdn.americanprogress.org/wp-content/uploads/2013/05/BakerNondiscriminationInsurance-6.pdf

46. Hong KE. Categorical exclusions: exploring legal responses to health care discrimination against transsexuals. Columbia J Gend Law. 2002;11:88–126.

47. American Medical Association House of Delegates. Removing financial barriers to care for transgender patients; 2008, accessed at http://www.tgender.net/taw/ama_resolutions.pdf

48. California Department of Insurance. Economic impact assessment: gender nondiscrimination in health insurance; 2012, accessed at: http://transgenderlawcenter.org/wp-content/uploads/2013/04/Economic-Impact-Assessment-Gender-Nondiscrimination-In-Health-Insurance.pdf

49. Oregon Department of Consumer and Business Services. Insurance Division Bulletin INS 2012-1 (2012), accessed at: http://www.cbs.state.or.us/external/ins/bulletins/bulletin2012-01.pdf

50. Colorado Department of Regulatory Agencies. Division of Insurance Bulletin No. B-4.49; 2013, accessed at: http://www.one-colorado.org/wp-content/uploads/2013/03/B-4.49.pdf

51. Vermont Department of Financial Regulation. Division of Insurance Bulletin No. 174; 2013, accessed at: http://www.dfr.vermont.gov/sites/default/files/Bulletin_174.pdf

52. District of Columbia Department of Insurance. Securities and Banking, Bulletin 13-IB-01-30/15 Revised; 2014, accessed at: http://disb.dc.gov/sites/default/files/dc/sites/disb/publication/attachments/Bulletin-ProhibitionDiscriminationBasedonGenderIdentityorExpressionv022714.pdf

53. Connecticut Insurance Department. Bulletin IC-34 (2013), accessed at: http://www.ct.gov/cid/lib/cid/Bulletin_IC-37_Gender_Identity_Nondiscrimination_Requirements.pdf

54. Massachusetts Office of Consumer Affairs and Business Regulation. Division of Insurance Bulletin 2014-03; 2014, accessed at: http://www.mass.gov/ocabr/docs/doi/legal-hearings/bulletin-201403.pdf

55. Washington Office of Insurance Commissioner. Letter to Health Insurance Carriers in Washington State; 2014, accessed at: http://www.insurance.wa.gov/about-oic/news-media/news-releases/2014/documents/gender-identity-discrimination-letter.pdf

56. Illinois Department of Insurance. Company Bulletin 2014-10, accessed at: http://insurance.illinois.gov/cb/2014/CB2014-10.pdf

57. Mogul JL, Ritchie AJ, Whitlock K, editors. Queer (In)Justice: the criminalization of LGBT people in the United States. Boston: Beacon; 2011.

58. Gruberg S. Dignity Denied: LGBT immigrants in U.S. immigration detention. Center for American Progress; 2013, accessed at: http://cdn.americanprogress.org/wp-content/uploads/2013/11/ImmigrationEnforcement.pdf

59. Brown GR, McDuffie E. Health care policies addressing transgender inmates in prison systems in the United States. J Correct Health Care. 2009;15(4):280–91.

60. Lambda Legal. Transgender prisoners in crisis (n.d.), accessed at: http://www.lambdalegal.org/sites/default/files/publications/downloads/transgender_prisoners_in_crisis.pdf

61. Human Rights Watch. Ensure access to condoms in U.S. prisons and jails; 2007, accessed at: http://www.hrw.org/sites/default/files/reports/condoms0307web.pdf

62. National Center for Transgender Equality. LGBT People and the Prison Rape Elimination Act; 2012, accessed at: http://www.prearesourcecenter.org/sites/default/files/library/preajuly2012.pdf

63. Internal Revenue Service. Revenue Ruling 2013-17, accessed at: http://www.irs.gov/pub/irs-drop/rr-13-17.pdf

64. Internal Revenue Service. Notice 2014-19, accessed at: http://www.irs.gov/pub/irs-drop/n-14-19.pdf

65. Office of Personnel Management. Benefits Administration Letter Number 13-203; 2013, accessed at: https://www.opm.gov/retirement-services/publications-forms/benefits-administration-letters/2013/13-203.pdf

66. Centers for Medicare and Medicaid Services. Important information for individuals in same-sex marriages, accessed at: http://medicare.gov/sign-up-change-plans/same-sex-marriage.html

67. Centers for Medicare and Medicaid Services. Letter to Medicare Advantage Organizations, (August 29, 2013), accessed at: http://www.cms.gov/Medicare/Health-Plans/HealthPlansGenInfo/Downloads/HPMS_Memo_US_vs_Windsor_Aug13.pdf

68. Centers for Medicare and Medicaid Services. State Health Officer and State Medicaid Director Letter, SHO#13-006 (September 27, 2013), accessed at: http://medicaid.gov/Federal-Policy-Guidance/Downloads/SHO-13-006.pdf

69. Institute of Medicine. Lesbian health: current assessment and directions for the future; 1999, accessed at: http://www.ncbi.nlm.nih.gov/books/NBK45100/

70. National Institutes of Health. Program announcement for behavioral, social, mental health, and substance abuse research with diverse populations; 2001, accessed at: https://grants.nih.gov/grants/guide/pa-files/PA-01-096.html

71. Healthy people 2010 companion document for lesbian, gay, bisexual, and transgender health; 2001, accessed at: http://www.glma.org/_data/n_0001/resources/live/HealthyCompanionDoc3.pdf

72. Scout. How far has LBGT health research progressed since Bush-era 'Big Chill'? (December 19, 2013), accessed at: http://www.huffingtonpost.com/scout-phd/how-far-have-we-come-in-l_b_4468902.html

73. U.S. Department of Health and Human Services. Healthy people 2020 LGBT health topic area; 2010, accessed at: http://healthypeople.gov/2020/topicsobjectives2020/overview.aspx?topicid=25

74. Institute of Medicine. The health of lesbian, gay, bisexual, and transgender people: building a foundation for better understanding; 2011, accessed at: http://www.iom.edu/Reports/2011/The-Health-of-Lesbian-Gay-Bisexual-and-Transgender-People.aspx

75. National Institutes of Health LGBT Research Coordinating Committee. Consideration of the institute of medicine report on the health of lesbian, gay, bisexual and transgender individuals; 2013, accessed at: http://report.nih.gov/UploadDocs/LGBT%20Health%20Report_FINAL_2013-01-03-508%20compliant.pdf

76. National Institutes of Health. Funding opportunity announcement PA-12-111: research on the health of LGBTI populations [RO1] (2012-2015), accessed at: http://grants.nih.gov/grants/guide/pa-files/PA-12-111.html

77. McManus R. NIH holds 'listening session' for LGBTI health issues, NIH record (July 19, 2013), accessed at: http://nihrecord.nih.gov/newsletters/2013/07_19_2013/story1.htm

78. The reports can be found at http://www.hhs.gov/lgbt/index.html

79. White House Conference on LGBT Health; 2012, accessed at: http://jdc.jefferson.edu/lgbt_white_house_summit/2012/ and http://www.hhs.gov/secretary/about/speeches/sp20120216.html

80. Services and Advocacy for GLBT Elders (SAGE) National Resource Center on LGBT Aging, accessed at: http://www.sageusa.org/programs/nrc.cfm

81. U.S. Office of Minority Health. Enhanced national standards for culturally and linguistically appropriate services; 2013, accessed at: https://www.thinkculturalhealth.hhs.gov/Content/clas.asp. The CLAS Standards themselves do not reference any specific population groups, but the accompanying implementation document describes how LGBT populations fit into the CLAS framework: https://www.thinkculturalhealth.hhs.gov/pdfs/EnhancedCLASStandardsBlueprint.pdf

82. Fenway Institute National LGBT Health Education Center, accessed at: http://www.lgbthealtheducation.org

83. Substance Abuse and Mental Health Services Administration. A provider's guide to substance abuse treatment for lesbian, gay, bisexual, and transgender individuals; 2011, accessed at: http://store.samhsa.gov/shin/content//SMA12-4104/SMA12-4104.pdf

84. http://samhsa.gov/lgbt/curricula.aspx

85. http://www.hrsa.gov/lgbt

86. Substance Abuse and Mental Health Services Administration. Top health issues for LGBT populations information & resource kit; 2012, accessed at: http://store.samhsa.gov/shin/content/SMA12-4684/SMA12-4684.pdf

87. Agency for Healthcare Research and Quality. National healthcare disparities report, chapter 10 priority populations; 2013, accessed at: http://www.ahrq.gov/research/findings/nhqrdr/nhdr11/chap10a.html#lgbt

88. Agency for Healthcare Research and Quality. National healthcare disparities report, chapter 11 priority populations; 2014, accessed at: http://www.ahrq.gov/research/findings/nhqrdr/nhdr13/2013nhdr.pdf

89. Health Resources and Services Administration. Women's health USA, 2011, accessed at: http://mchb.hrsa.gov/whusa11/hstat/hssp/pages/234lbw.html

90. Centers for Disease Control and Prevention. Health Disparities and Inequalities Report, Morb Mortal Wkly Rep, vol. 60 (Supplement), January 14, 2011, accessed at: http://www.cdc.gov/mmwr/pdf/other/su6001.pdf

91. Centers for Disease Control and Prevention. Health Disparities and Inequalities Report, Morb Mortal Wkly Rep, vol. 62 (Supplement), November 22, 2013, accessed http://www.cdc.gov/mmwr/pdf/other/su6203.pdf

92. U.S. Department of Health and Human Services. Multiple chronic conditions: a strategic framework; 2010, accessed at: http://www.hhs.gov/ash/initiatives/mcc/mcc_framework.pdf

93. National HIV/AIDS Strategy for the United States (2010), accessed at: http://www.whitehouse.gov/sites/default/files/uploads/NHAS.pdf

94. U.S. Department of Health and Human Services. Action plan to reduce racial and ethnic health disparities; 2011, accessed at: http://minorityhealth.hhs.gov/npa/files/Plans/HHS/HHS_Plan_complete.pdf

95. www.out2enroll.org

96. http://www.samhsa.gov/newsroom/pressannouncements/201510150630

97. http://www.hhs.gov/dab/decisions/dabdecisions/dab2576.pdf

98. https://www.govtrack.us/congress/bills/111/hr3001

99. https://www.govtrack.us/congress/bills/110/hr3014

100. https://www.govtrack.us/congress/bills/113/hr5294/text

101. Pub. L. No.111-148; 2010, codified at 124 Stat. 119-1025

102. Patient Protection and Affordable Care Act Section 5306

103. Baker KE. Where do we go from here? Incorporating LGBT-inclusive health policies in affordable care act implementation. LGBTQ Policy J. 2012;2:61.

104. The Honorable Kathleen Sebelius. Speech to the national coalition for LGBT health (October 17, 2011), accessed at: http://www.hhs.gov/secretary/about/speeches/2011/sp20111017.html

105. U.S. Department of Health and Human Services. The Affordable Care Act and LGBT Americans, accessed at: http://www.healthcare.gov/news/factsheets/2011/01/new-options-for-lgbt-americans.html

106. http://kff.org/uninsured/fact-sheet/key-facts-about-the-uninsured-population/

107. Gates GJ. In U.S., LGBT more likely to be uninsured than non-LGBT, Gallup Well-Being (August 26, 2014), accessed at: http://www.gallup.com/poll/175445/lgbt-likely-non-lgbt-uninsured.aspx

108. Baker KE, Durso LE, Cray A. Moving the Needle: The Impact of the Affordable Care Act on LGBT Communities. Center for American Progress (2014), accessed at: https://www.americanprogress.org/issues/lgbt/report/2014/11/17/101575/moving-the-needle

109. Durso LE, Baker K, Cray A. LGBT communities and the Affordable Care Act: findings from a national survey, Center for American Progress; 2013, accessed at: http://www.americanprogress.org/wp-content/uploads/2013/10/LGBT-ACAsurveybrief1.pdf

110. http://aspe.hhs.gov/basic-report/health-insurance-coverage-and-affordable-care-act-september-2015

111. http://www.cdc.gov/nchs/data/nhis/earlyrelease/insur201511.pdf

112. https://www.americanprogress.org/issues/lgbt/report/2014/11/17/101575/movingthe-needle/

113. http://hrms.urban.org/quicktakes/Uninsurance-Rate-Nearly-Halved-for-Lesbian-Gay-and-Bisexual-Adults-since-Mid-2013.html

114. Baker KE, Cray A, Gates GJ. Infographic: how new coverage options affect LGBT communities (September 12, 2103), accessed at: http://www.americanprogress.org/issues/lgbt/news/2013/09/12/74029/infographic-how-new-coverage-options-affect-lgbt-communities/

115. National Federation of Independent Business v. Sebelius, 567 U.S. ___, Slip Opinion No. 11-393 (June 28, 2012).

116. Kaiser Family Foundation. Status of state medicaid expansion decisions (2014), accessed at: http://kff.org/health-reform/slide/current-status-of-the-medicaid-expansion-decision/

117. Kates J, Garfield R, Young K, Quinn K, Frazier E, Skarbinski J. Assessing the impact of the affordable care act on health insurance coverage of people with HIV. Kaiser Family Foundation (2014), accessed at:

http://kaiserfamilyfoundation.files.wordpress.com/2013/12/8535-assessing-the-impact-of-the-affordable-care-act-on-health-insurance-coverage.pdf

118. White House Council of Economic Advisors. Missed opportunities: the consequences of state decisions not to expand Medicaid (July 2014), accessed at: http://www.whitehouse.gov/sites/default/files/docs/missed_opportunities_medicaid.pdf

119. Holahan J, Buettgens M, Carroll C, Dorn S. The cost and coverage implications of the ACA Medicaid expansion: national and state-by-state analysis. Kaiser Family Foundation (2012), accessed at: http://kaiserfamilyfoundation.files.wordpress.com/2013/01/8384.pdf

120. Butler SM. Assuring affordable health care for all Americans. Washington, DC: The Heritage Foundation; 1989.

121. Kaiser Family Foundation. State Marketplace Decisions; 2014, accessed at: http://kff.org/health-reform/slide/state-decisions-for-creating-health-insurance-exchanges/

122. Letter from U.S. Department of Health and Human Services Office of Civil Rights to National Center for Lesbian Rights (July 12, 2012), accessed at: http://transgenderlawcenter.org/archives/1433

123. Centers for Medicare and Medicaid Services. Center for consumer information and insurance oversight, frequently asked question on coverage of same-sex spouses (March 14, 2014), accessed at: https://www.cms.gov/CCIIO/Resources/Regulations-and-Guidance/Downloads/frequently-askedquestions-on-coverage-of-same-sex-spouses.pdf

124. Centers for Medicare and Medicaid Services. Center for consumer information and insurance oversight, health insurance market reforms; 2014, accessed at: http://www.cms.gov/CCIIO/Programs-and-Initiatives/Health-Insurance-Market-Reforms/

125. Centers for Medicare and Medicaid Services. Center for consumer information and insurance oversight, essential health benefits standards: ensuring quality, affordable health coverage; 2013, accessed at: http://www.cms.gov/CCIIO/Resources/Fact-Sheets-and-FAQs/ehb-2-20-2013.html

126. Keith K, Lucia KW, Monahan CH. Nondiscrimination Under the Affordable Care Act, Georgetown University Health Policy Institute (July 1, 2013), accessed at: http://ssrn.com/abstract=2362942

127. Patient Protection and Affordable Care Act Section 4302 adds "Title XXXI—Data Collection, Analysis, and Quality" to the Public Health Service Act (42 U.S.C. 201 et seq.), accessed at: http://www.gpo.gov/fdsys/pkg/CREC-2009-11-19/pdf/CREC-2009-11-19-pt1-PgS11607-3.pdf#page=127

128. Public Health Service Act Section 3101(a)(1)(D)

129. U.S. Office of Minority Health. Plan for health data collection on lesbian, gay, bisexual and transgender populations; 2011, accessed at: http://minority-health.hhs.gov/templates/browse.aspx?lvl=2&lvlID=209

130. National Center for Health Statistics. Development of sexual identity question for national health interview survey, accessed at: http://wwwn.cdc.gov/qbank/report/Miller_NCHS_2011_NHIS%20Sexual%20Identity.pdf

131. Kann L, Olsen EO, McManus T, Kinchen S, Chyen D, Harris WA, Wechsler H. Sexual identity, sex of sexual contacts, and health-risk behaviors among students in grades 9-12: Youth Risk Behavior Surveillance, Selected Sites, United States, 2001-2009. MMWR. 2011;60(SS07):1–133, accessed at: http://www.cdc.gov/mmwr/preview/mmwrhtml/ss6007a1.htm

132. http://www.healthypeople.gov/2020/proposed-objective-landing-page/lesbian-gay-bisexual-and-transgender-health

133. U.S. Department of Health and Human Services. Prevention and public health fund; 2014, accessed at: http://www.hhs.gov/open/recordsandreports/prevention/

134. Centers for Disease Control and Prevention. Community transformation grants; 2014, accessed at: http://www.cdc.gov/nccdphp/dch/programs/communitytransformation/

135. Patient Protection and Affordable Care Act Sections 5601 and 10503, as amended by Health Care and Education Affordability Reconciliation Act Section 2303.

136. The Fenway Institute, Center for American Progress, Human Rights Campaign, and GLMA: Health Professionals Advancing LGBT Equality. The case for designating LGBT people as a medically underserved population and health professional shortage area population group; 2014, accessed at: http://thefenwayinstitute.org/wp-content/uploads/MUP_HPSA-Brief_v11-FINAL-081914.pdf

137. Negotiated Rulemaking Committee on the Designation of Medically Underserved Populations and Health Professions Shortage. Final report to the secretary (2011), accessed at: http://www.hrsa.gov/advisorycommittees/shortage/nrmcfinalreport.pdf

138. Patient Protection and Affordable Care Act Section 3133.

139. Pub. L. 101-381, codified at 104 Stat. 576; see Kates J, Garfield R, Young K, Quinn K, Frazier E, Skarbinski J. Assessing the impact of the affordable care act on health insurance coverage of people with HIV. Kaiser Family Foundation; 2014, accessed at: http://kaiserfamilyfoundation.files.wordpress.com/2013/12/8535-assessing-the-impact-of-the-affordable-care-act-on-health-insurance-coverage.pdf

140. 42 U.S.C. Sections 300-300a-6.

141. http://content.healthaffairs.org/content/34/10/1769.full.html

142. Institute of Medicine. Crossing the quality chasm; 2001, accessed at: http://www.iom.edu/Reports/2001/Crossing-the-Quality-Chasm-A-New-Health-System-for-the-21st-Century.aspx

143. Berwick DM, Nolan TW, Whittington J. The triple aim: care, health and cost. Health Aff. 2008;27(3): 759–69.
144. The triple aim framework is used in the U.S. Department of Health and Human Services *National Strategy for Quality Improvement in Health Care*; 2011, accessed at: http://www.ahrq.gov/workingforquality/nqs/nqs2011annlrpt.htm
145. The Joint Commission. Advancing effective communication, cultural competence, patient- and family-centered care for the lesbian, gay, bisexual, and transgender community: a field guide; 2011, accessed at: http://www.jointcommission.org/lgbt/
146. Patient-Centered Outcome Research Institute. Patient-centered approaches to collect sexual orientation/gender identity information in the emergency department; 2013, accessed at: http://pfaawards.pcori.org/node/20/datavizwiz/detail/3980
147. Wilson-Stronks A. A call to action for healthcare professionals to advance health equity for the lesbian, gay, bisexual and transgender community. Human Rights Campaign Foundation; 2011, accessed at: http://www.hrc.org/files/assets/resources/health_calltoaction_HealthcareEqualityIndex_2011.pdf
148. Krehely J. How to close the LGBT health disparities gap. Center for American Progress; 2009, accessed at: http://www.americanprogress.org/wp-content/uploads/issues/2009/12/pdf/lgbt_health_disparities.pdf
149. Krehely J. How to close the LGBT health disparities gap: disparities by race and ethnicity. Center for American Progress; 2009, accessed at: http://www.americanprogress.org/wp-content/uploads/issues/2009/12/pdf/lgbt_health_disparities_race.pdf
150. Ard KL, Makadon HJ. Improving the health care of lesbian, gay, bisexual, and transgender people: understanding and eliminating health disparities. The Fenway Institute; 2012, accessed at: http://www.lgbthealtheducation.org/wp-content/uploads/12-054_LGBTHealtharticle_v3_07-09-12.pdf
151. https://www.thinkculturalhealth.hhs.gov/pdfs/EnhancedCLASSStandardsBlueprint.pdf
152. 2014 PCMH Standard 2: Team-Based Care, Element C: Culturally and Linguistically Appropriate Services, Factor 1 (diversity); 2014 PCMH Standard 3: Population Health Management, Element C: Comprehensive Health Assessment, Factor 2 (family/social/cultural characteristics). Available from www.ncqa.org
153. Cahill S, Makadon H. Sexual orientation and gender identity data collection in clinical settings and in electronic health records: a key to ending LGBT health disparities. LGBT Health. 2013;1(1):1–8.
154. Institute of Medicine. Collecting sexual orientation and gender identity data in electronic health records; 2012, accessed at: http://www.iom.edu/Reports/2012/Collecting-Sexual-Orientation-and-Gender-Identity-Data-in-Electronic-Health-Records.aspx
155. Office of National Coordinator for Health Information Technology, 2015 Edition Health IT Certification Criteria, 80 Fed. Reg. 62602-62759 (October 16, 2015)
156. Cahill S, Singal R, Grasso C, King D, Mayer K, Baker KE, Makadon H. Asking patients questions about sexual orientation and gender identity in clinical settings. Center for American Progress and The Fenway Institute; 2013, accessed at: http://www.lgbthealtheducation.org/wp-content/uploads/COM228_SOGI_CHARN_WhitePaper.pdf
157. http://doaskdotell.org/ehr/toolkit/policyissues

# Common LGBT Sexual Health Questions

25

Keith Loukes

## Purpose

This chapter will assist providers in discussing the problematic area of sexual behaviours with their patients by outlining contextual considerations and by providing examples of commonly asked questions along with possible responses.

**Helpful Hint**
- Patient anatomy and behaviors should guide your discussions, not labels or the various ways patients self-identify.
- Have educational material easily accessible in the clinical space and waiting rooms. A pre-printed list of relevant websites may also be a useful tool.
- When discussing sensitive issues like sexual activity, think about timing, setting, and the language you use.

## Learning Objectives

- Identify at least 5 ways in which the environment, language and appropriate questioning can influence sensitive interactions about sexuality with patients *(KP1, ICS1, ICS2)*
- Define common terms (slang) which patients may use *(KP1)*
- Discuss common questions LGBT patients may ask their healthcare providers and their answers *(PC4, PC6, ICS1, ICS2)*

## Preamble

This chapter is not about best evidence-based practice, nor is it a detailed review of specific subject matter. Quite simply, this chapter is about talking to patients, particularly LGBT patients, and providing a script of answers to questions they may commonly present to you about sex.

I do have a few take-home points, which are essential from my own personal experience:

### Use the Right Language

The language in this question-and-answer format is kept as basic as possible. As physicians, it is easy to forget that the person sitting before you

K. Loukes, M.D., M.H.Sc., F.C.F.P. (✉)
Department of Family Medicine, University of Toronto, Toronto, ON, Canada
e-mail: keith_loukes@yahoo.com

© Springer International Publishing Switzerland 2016
K.L. Eckstrand, J.M. Ehrenfeld (eds.), *Lesbian, Gay, Bisexual, and Transgender Healthcare*,
DOI 10.1007/978-3-319-19752-4_25

likely did not go to medical school. (Perhaps never had any formal education.) Or even just learned English. So unless the person receiving your conversation has the same background as you, never presume it is acceptable to use medical words without explanation—it can be intimidating and seen as a way of dominating the conversation. Finding common-denominator language is essential to build rapport and trust. (A quick list of common slang is included as an appendix to the chapter.)

Slang is a challenging area for providers because it can be seen as unprofessional. If you can become comfortable with using slang, it can be a useful tool to connect with patients. Through small talk you can usually gauge what kind of language people prefer and may even ask what words patients are comfortable in using during your discussion. For example, some people are put off by the word "penis" and "vagina" and that can immediately yield resistance and unease. Substituting words like "dick" and "pussy" might be a better fit for patients and yield a more relaxed and connected interaction. Another example would be when talking about ano-receptive sex in MSM contact: "bottoming" is much more understandable for most gay men.

For example, I usually start off with the following sentence from my personal toolbox:

> I have to ask some personal questions and apologize if that makes you uncomfortable, but it is important for me to know everything I can in order to help. I just want to touch base with what words you feel more comfortable with—we use the words vagina/penis between doctors/nurses, but which words are you more comfortable with?

Notice I start with a sentence about impending personal questions to break the ice… I find that personally very effective. In MSM sexual situations you can then follow up with:

> When having sex with men, do you bottom, top or both?

This will have much more impact than using clinical words which may require further explanation.

## Choose the Right Environment

Where you initiate conversation and gather history is key. Although having patients draped and gowned (or positioned in stirrups) ready for clinicians may be an efficient time-saver, it is the worst place to have a conversation and get a proper medical history from. The more relaxed you can make apprehensive patients, the better the outcome will be. Wearing their own clothes and sitting in a comfortable chair under non-institutional lighting and casual artwork or posters on the wall are good tools to promote honest and effective communication. However, some providers may have no control over the physical features of the space they are in. Hospital examination rooms and Emergency Department stretchers can be a particular challenge. It is helpful to identify in advance areas that may be more appropriate for delicate history taking. Try and take advantage of rooms set aside for counseling or quiet rooms for families before moving the patient to a clinical room for appropriate physical examination.

## Ask the Right Questions

Talking to patients about sex is akin to the childhood game "ten questions"—you usually only have so many chances to ask about personal details before the person shuts off and becomes unreceptive. Therefore asking the right questions is important. Focus your questions about activity, not about preferences. What behaviors people do with their anatomy is much more important than what they would prefer to be doing. Avoid assumptions—just because someone identifies as gay or lesbian does not mean they are having physical contact only with the same sex, or even having sex at all. I always ask questions like:

> Do you have intimate contact with men, women, or both?
> Do you have any sexual partners at the present or had any in the last 3 months?

Remember that "sex" means different things to different people and is a word that should be avoided. "Do you have sex" could mean anything from coitus to physical contact.

## Male Questions

## General Questions

### Penis Size

#### What Is the Average Penis Size? What Can I Do to Make My Penis Bigger?

There is a social demand for bigger male genitalia—in gay culture, some men put high value in finding a partner who has a larger than average penis. A study of over 1400 American men self-reported an average of 14.15 cm (5.6 inches) while erect. Media including pornography probably skews our expectation of what "average" should be, and drives some men to desire greater size.

If you have a partner unhappy with your size, you may want to find another partner. Many other men and prospective partners do not care about size and probably will help your low self-image. Being with someone who is critical of your physical attributes can contribute to unhealthy  body image issues. But should you wish to pursue options for bigger apenis:

*Pumps* rely on suction and can cause temporary enlargement by engorgement of the penile tissues—by drawing more blood into the penis causing it to swell larger than number. The effect disappears shortly thereafter as the blood returns to the body. Caution should be used as blood vessels may break and cause bruising or discomfort.

*Pills and creams.* There is no pill to date that causes penis growth. Or cream. Despite large promises and larger price tags, there is no evidence these are effective.

*Surgery.* The only generally acceptable surgery is where they release the ligament inside the body, which provides a modest (even minimal) increase in length. Most urologists will only recommend this procedure in extreme cases.

## Prostate Enlargement

### What Is an Enlarged Prostate?"

The prostate is a gland in the male urinary tract that lies between the bladder and the urethra, the passage where urine exits through penis and is responsible for producing a significant portion of the fluid contained in ejaculate. Because it sits in front of the bladder and surrounds part of the urethra, if it swells or gets larger, the prostate can slow or stop the flow of urination, the most common complaint due to this condition.

The main cause of an enlarged prostate is simple aging. As we get older, our prostate gradually swells, a medical condition called "hypertrophy". We call this Benign Prostatic Hypertrophy (BPH for short) because it is a natural process not due to serious illness and therefore 'benign'. With BPH, some men can experience difficulty peeing. Less frequently, the prostate can eventually block the bladder completely, requiring emergency intervention. Most men, however, have few or no symptoms, and their BPH is of no consequence.

A urinary tract infection can also cause enlargement of the prostate. Such cases often happen quickly, are very painful, and can be treated with antibiotics. A third and less frequent cause of a larger prostate is prostate cancer, which can grow inside the gland causing its size to increase. Consult your doctor for recommendations when you should start routine screening for this.

## Erectile Dysfunction

### What Can I Do If I Am Having Difficulty with My Erections? What Can I Do to Get Better Erections?

Unfortunately, this is not an uncommon complaint and can interfere significantly in people's sex lives. There are many causes of ED, including normal aging. It can also be seen with conditions like depression/anxiety, diabetes, and neurological diseases like multiple sclerosis. Other frequent culprits of sexual dysfunction are things we put into our bodies like alcohol, recreational drugs, and prescription medications (blood pressure medicines, anti-depressants, anti-anxiety pills to name a few). In younger persons, stress and drugs/alcohol are more likely culprits.

A doctor needs to do a careful history and a physical that includes a neurological and genital exam, along with some blood tests to assess if have other diseases which need to be dealt with first. If everything to that point looks ok, erectile dysfunction drugs can be tried to try and ease "performance anxiety"—a condition where you worry so much about being able to achieve an erection, you are unable to get an erection.

Erectile dysfunction drugs can be costly and should never be used when using amyl nitrate (poppers). Always check with your doctor before taking to help you choose which one is right for you.

# STI

## Warts

### What Are Anal/Genital Warts? How Do I Know If I Have Them and How Are They Treated?

Anal and genital warts are caused by a virus called the Human Papilloma Virus (HPV), a virus which has many different strains which can have different effects on different individuals—skin changes, lesions and sometimes no effect at all.

Although they are generally harmless they can cause lesions which could progress to cancer if left untreated. These changes or lesions are the main reason why women undergo pap smears to detect problems which could lead to cancer of the cervix. Similar changes can also occur in the anus of men who have sex with men leading to increased risk of anal cancer, particularly those HIV+, thus an "anal pap smear" has been developed.

Besides increased cancer risk, the lesions are a nuisance—and contagious. They can be treated by burning or freezing them off, or by applying medications (or both) until the lesions are gone.

## Oral Sex

### What Infections Can I Get from Oral Sex?

Gonorrhea, chlamydia, HPV and even syphilis can infect your mouth and throat—and therefore passed on to a partner if you perform oral sex on them. Condoms may reduce the risk but are rarely used for oral sex.

Always make sure you get your mouth and throat checked (and swabbed) when you get your STI screening done.

## Barebacking

### What Is Barebacking?

Barebacking is the common term used to describe anal sex without condoms.

Decreasing condom use has been the focus of many AIDS service organizations and this rising trend is a huge area of debate in itself. Some say that the community doesn't fear contracting HIV disease like they used to, as they perceive HIV infection to be benign with all of the treatments we have available. Others hypothesize that the abundance of public education out there has encouraged thrill-seekers to "live on the edge."

### What is PrEP?

Pre-exposure prophylaxis or PrEP is a recent development in sexual medicine which reduces the transmission of the HIV virus. It consists of HIV medication taken on a regular basis by a *non-infected person* to reduce their chances of contracting the virus. Although it seems to be quite effective, in can be costly and may cause adverse side effects, and therefore is not for everyone. We also recommend the continued usage of condoms to prevent the transmission of other STIs like syphillis, gonorrhea or chlamydia.

### Is Barebacking Riskier for the Bottom or the Top?

Barebacking is likely to carry higher risk to the person receiving (bottom) since the skin in the anus and rectum is more fragile than the skin on the penis. However, the risk to the top is still significant, because it only takes one small nick or scratch on the top's genitals for the HIV virus to be transmitted if you the person you are with is HIV positive.

## What Infections Can I Get from Sex Without Condoms?

Preventing infection is the main reason why condoms are recommended for use. Some of these infections like gonorrhea, chlamydia and ordinary urinary tract infections can be cured with antibiotics but if left undetected can cause serious illness or damage. Other infections like hepatitis, HIV, and herpes are chronic infections and cannot be cured—despite having treatments to control these infections, the best treatment is still prevention.

## Why Should I Get Hepatitis Vaccines?

Viral hepatitis is a group of viruses that cause inflammation of the liver. They are transmitted through your digestive tract or through your blood. Some cause acutely to become quite sick and then you recover while others can cause ongoing (chronic) infections which can have serious health consequences and put you at risk for cancer. Two forms of viral hepatitis, A and B, have vaccines which can prevent you from catching it if exposed. Hepatitis C, a chronic virus, currently has no vaccine.

## Sexual Activity

## Anal Sex

## How Should I Prepare for Anal Sex So the Mess Is Minimal?

Firstly, mess is normal. It usually cannot be avoided. So have a towel handy. That being said, if you want to minimize the mess go to the toilet before sex then gently clean the anus and rectum with soap and water. Prepackaged moist wipes work better but are costly. Additionally, some men choose to anal douche (clean stool out of the rectum) using either a shower attachment or a

small bulb-syringe (which can be purchased in most large drug stores). Finally, lay a towel down to protect your sheets and to wipe your hands.

## What Is Anal Douching? Is It Risky?

Anal douching is a common practice for bottom (anoreceptive) partners, usually coming from the wish to be "clean" and prevent any "mess" that may result from anal penetration. Douching is certainly not necessary before or after anal sex, and many couples don't bother. Those who choose to douche can use female douching products or enema kits (insertion of water into the colon by tubing). The easiest to transport and use are probably the bulb syringes, soft plastic ball-shaped devices with a hard plastic tip designed to rinse the rectum with water. Lubricate the tip well and insert into the rectum, rinsing several times before sex. The small amount of water used is less irritating and less likely to cause long-term problems.

Frequent douching in theory can lead to constipation. It should be warned that douching may cause minor irritation or even trauma (cuts or scratches) that facilitate HIV or hepatitis transmission.

The prepared female douches should be avoided since they often contain scents and other chemicals designed to make a woman feel more "fresh." (In fact, many gynecologists will recommend that women avoid them as well.)

## Why Does It Hurt When I (Receive) Anal Sex?

Pain during anal sex is something to pay attention to as it can sometimes be a warning sign that something "down there" isn't right. Or sometimes the anus may just be too tight to allow penetration by your partner.

If tightness is the issue, the key is to relax and become comfortable—take your time. Squeezing or bearing-down with your sphincter (for as long as you can hold it) just prior to insertion may fatigue the muscle and allow easier entry. Some guys will use muscle relaxants they buy from pharmacies. The benefit from this is minimal and has drowsiness as a major side effect. Some people use alcohol to relax before sex which may help, however you don't want your sex life to depend on alcohol. In addition, should you drink too much, while intoxicated you may cause injury that you are not aware during sex. Remember that excessive alcohol use can also impair your judgement around safe sex practices and other safety issues.

Physical examination by a medical provider will rule out anything that might be causing pain in your rectum. Then start anal activities with your partner, using *plenty* of lubrication, inserting small things like fingers to begin with. Build up gradually to larger items, using discomfort as your guide: if it hurts, stop and try something smaller again. Eventually you will train your body to be able to take larger items, including your partner's penis.

### What Is a Butt Plug?

The word "plug" is not a plug to hold things in, like one in a sink. A butt plug is a sex toy similar to a dildo; it is often bulb-shaped, tapered into a smaller tip. It can be used for anal stimulation or to gently stretch the rectum in preparation for penetration and/or intercourse. It is important to only use one shaped in such a way that it can't be lost inside the rectum (like having a wide, flat base). Should you experience pain or bleeding, you should immediately stop and follow up with a doctor if the pain or bleeding persists.

### Fisting

#### What Is Fisting? Is It Dangerous?

Fisting is a sexual activity where a partner inserts their fist into the other person's rectum. While this seems dangerous, the lining of the rectum is actually quite resistant and tough; it has to be as its primary function is for storage and passage of stool. Your rectum and lower bowel is basically a hose-shaped layer of special membrane that absorbs water from what you have eaten. This membrane or *mucosa* is surrounded by layers of muscle and tissue that propel the waste through. This makes for a relatively tough, resistant structure.

Of course injury is still possible should too much force occur leading to injury, resulting in tearing and bleeding. Always make sure that before taking anything into your rectum, it is big enough to stretch around that object, otherwise serious injury may occur. The ability to fist safely actually takes months to years of gentle stretching to be able to accommodate something as wide in diameter as a fist.

### Oral Sex

#### What Can I Do to Avoid Gagging During Oral Sex?

A common problem is the gag reflex (medically known as the pharyngeal reflex) and a frequent complaint by partners trying to perform oral sex on their partners. Some people have very brisk reflexes while others have none. You gag when the sides and back of your throat are touched by something other than the swallowing of food. (This is why some people stick their fingers in their throats when they want to vomit.) This is to protect you from choking on food or other objects which are not supposed to be in your mouth.

So avoiding contact with these areas in your throat is key so try repositioning first. The important thing is to keep the penis centered in your mouth to avoid touching the gag areas. One largely successful strategy is to lie on your back with the head hanging over the edge of the bed, so that the neck and head are tilted backwards. (This is a position similar to that used by sword swallowers!). Other positions may work too so experiment to find which ones are best.

Throat sprays and lozenges with topical anesthetic in them, marketed to treat sore throats, can also be useful. These work by numbing your throat, and therefore decrease activation of the gag reflex. The down side is that you can't feel or taste anything, two potential motivators for performing oral sex in the first place. You may also inadvertently numb your partner's penis.

Lastly, concentrating on the part of the penis you can get into your mouth without gagging. This is the most sensitive part of the penis anyway, especially the head (glans). Use of the hands can compliment oral stimulation and feel nice for the receiving without having to swallow his whole erection.

## Cock-Rings

### What Are Cock Rings? Are they Dangerous and Could Cause Damage?

"Cock rings" are ring-shaped objects designed to encircle the penile base and scrotum, retaining blood in the penis and therefore maximizing erections (by keeping the blood inside the expandable tissues causing the penis to stay engorged and stiff). They also stimulate these sensitive areas and enhance pleasure for many men.

Like anything, cock rings can be dangerous if not used properly. Since they act by strangulating the penis, it also restricts new blood from entering and prolonged use of cock rings can cause damage to the nerves and blood vessels. (Imagine wrapping a tight elastic band around your hand.) They should therefore be used carefully, ensuring they are not too tight, and only for short periods at a time.

## Poppers

### What Are Poppers? Do They Really Help with Anal Sex? And Are They Safe?

"Poppers" is the layman's term for amyl nitrate, a chemical that is sold as a liquid and inhaled as vapor. To avoid attention, it is often sold as room deodorizers or leather cleaner. (Amyl nitrate is actually good for neither.) Like many nitrogen-based chemicals or drugs, it causes smooth muscle in the body to relax—including the muscles which surround your anus and rectum (sphincter muscles). This can help bottoming.

Most common side effects include dizziness, headache and erectile dysfunction. It can burn if spilled on the skin. It some rare cases it can cause serious eye damage or heart problems. It should never be combined with erectile dysfunction drugs like Viagra and Cialis as this can cause serious drops in blood pressure.

## Female Questions

## General Health

### Vaginal Cleaning

### What Are the Facts About Vaginal Douching? Is It Bad for Me?

Douching is the practice of cleansing out the vaginal area with liquid for the purpose of cleaning or removal of odor. Products can be purchased in the pharmacy or some women will make their own (using things like vinegar, baking soda, soaps and fragrances). The practice seems to have a bit of a controversial and stormy past, especially due to links to pelvic inflammatory disease, ectopic pregnancy and other possible problems including the increased risk of getting an STI. It has also been linked to Bacterial Vaginosis, a common and treatable vaginal infection in women.

In woman who have sex with women (WSW) there is much less known. In general, most gynecologists recommend against the practice because of the above reasons. If you want to clean your vagina, the best practice is gentle application with warm water. If soap must be used, a small amount of a simple, unscented soap is best.

## Breast Cancer

### Why Should I Be Concerned About Breast Cancer? What Should I Be Doing?

Studies have shown that WSW (women who have sex with women) have higher rates of breast cancer, likely because of lowered screening rates and the presence of risk factors. It has been shown that lesbians are less likely to see their doctor out of fear of discrimination, money/insurance issues or previous bad experiences with health care providers (HCP). WSW also tend to cluster some known or suspected risk factors for the cancer like overweight/obesity, non-use of oral contraceptive pills, alcohol, and later-in-age pregnancies. Some woman are also higher risk due to genetic traits or family histories.

Know your breasts and report any changes immediately to your HCP. Average risk women between the age of 50 and 74 should be receiving mammograms (a special x-ray of the breast) every two years. Ultrasound screening may also be requested by your HCP if there are specific concerns.

## STI

### STIs and WSW

#### What Sexually Transmitted Infections Are WSW at Risk for?

WSW sexual activity is generally considered low risk and infections are seen at much lower rates than other women. Any STI is still possible, particularly if there is a history of sex with men— such as HIV, herpes, warts, gonorrhea, syphilis, trichomoniasis, chlamydia, hepatitis. Periodic screening should be based on past history with men, other specific risk factors like IV drug use or developing any suspicious symptoms.

### HIV

#### What Is the HIV Risk for Women (Who Have Sex with Women)?

Women who have sex with women (WSW) are at less risk for HIV contraction through sexual activity. There are no well-documented cases to date of HIV transmission from woman to woman through sex. HIV infection generally occurs in the WSW community through needle-sharing and sex with infected men. And there may be some hypothetical risk with sharing of toys.

HIV virus is also present in menstrual blood so this may increase your risk of infection if exposed, particularly if you have open sores or cuts. Protect yourself and minimize your risk: avoid menstrual blood, do not share needles, use condoms when sleeping with men, and always properly clean toys before using or sharing.

### Bacterial Vaginosis

#### What Is Bacterial Vaginosis? How Do You Get It?

Bacterial Vaginosis, or BV, is a common vaginal infection where the wrong bacteria overpowers healthy background bacteria causing symptoms like discharge, odor, itching and/or burning. It is

easily treated and cured with antibiotics. Exactly how or why some women get this infection is unclear but according to the CDC website some activities like douching, frequent vaginal sex or multiple partners may increase your risk.

BV is mostly risky because it may increase your risk of catching STIs—particularly HSV, HIV, gonorrhea, and chlamydia. Or can cause problems if occurs during a pregnancy.

### Trichomoniasis

#### What Is Trichomoniasis?

Trichomoniasis, commonly called "trich", is caused by an organism called *trichomonas vaginalis*, a parasite that usually lives in the vagina, urethra or on the vulva. In men, it can inhabit the inside of the penis of urethra. Vaginal sex with male partners are the main source of infection, although some experts believe that it can be spread vagina to vagina.

Most people with infection do not have symptoms and know they have it. It can elevate your risk for HIV and other STIs and should therefore be treated if discovered.

### Oral Sex

#### What Infections Can I Get from Receiving Oral Sex?

It is unclear exactly how risky this activity is, although it is considered to be much less than sexual activity with men. Any infections present on your partner's face or inside her mouth and throat may be transmitted to your genitals and cause infection. Herpes (cold sores) of the face are a particular concern, although in theory gonorrhea and chlamydia can be spread as well.

### Sexual Activity

#### Female Ejaculation

#### Why Do Some Women Produce a Lot of Liquid When They Orgasm?

Female ejaculation is a subject of debate in the medical community—both gynecologists and urologists cannot seem to agree. Men have glands like the prostate gland that produce most of their fluid on ejaculation, but women lack these or anything similar. Because of this, some experts will argue that a large female ejaculation has to be the involuntary release of urine. There is conflicting evidence around this (minimal research exists at all, actually).

Why some women do and others do not is part of the mystery. But it's important to remember that while people have similar blueprints, we all function a bit differently. Like men, when women orgasm the difference in the amount of fluid produced can vary greatly, from none at all to volumous amounts—all of which is normal.

## Vaginal Dryness

### Why Do I Have a Problem with Vaginal Dryness and What Can I Do?

Vaginal lubrication varies between women but also decreases as women age, especially during and after menopause. This is caused by decreased hormone levels in the body. A doctor should do a regular check-up including a quick exam to ensure there are no vaginal problems and your overall health is good.

Hormone Replacement Therapy (HRT) can be helpful for vaginal dryness by replacing these hormones, but at the current time it is not as popular since it might be more harmful for women than once thought (linked to increases in heart disease, stroke and breast cancer). Local hormone creams might be a safer option, but good old-fashioned lubrication should be tried first. Some lubrication can be irritating, so avoid those containing nonoxyl and glycerine (glycerol). Both chemical compounds have frequently caused problems for women.

## Trans/Other Gender

### General Health

### Am I Transgender?

Yes, if your gender identity does not match your assigned sex. Gender identity is how you identify based on how you feel inside and how you

express that, while your "sex" is what is assigned to you based on what you were born with.

Most people have gender identities and sexes that match—someone who identifies as female and was born with a female body for example. However, if you feel like your "insides" do not match your "outsides"—then you fit the "transgender" label, whether or not you choose to express it.

## STI

### Can Transgender Persons Get Infections from Sex?

Infections do not discriminate. You can get any STI like anyone else—depending on who your partners are, what you are doing with them, and what your current anatomy is.

## Genderless Questions

### Relationship

### What Is an Open Relationship?

Open relationships are agreements between two partners where other sexual partners are permitted. Many couples have these understandings but develop certain rules around when it can occur (i.e. only when traveling, no barebacking, one-time only, etc.). A 2010 study reported 45 % of San Francisco couples were in agreed monogamous relationships.

## STIs

### Herpes

### Can I Get Genital Herpes from Someone's Lips?

Yes. Oral herpes or "cold sores" is caused by a variant of the virus that causes genital herpes and is called "herpes simplex virus" or HSV for short. HSV 1 is found mostly on the face and/or mouth, while HSV 2 is a virus typically seen on the genitals or anus. But both viruses have the same ability to penetrate sensitive tissues, so both can affect either place.

While generally not harmful, the worst part about herpes is that there is no cure. Most of the time it is not visible and hides in your nervous system, periodically reappearing as blister-like lesions in the affected area. Caution should be used if you're having an outbreak, or if you feel the presence of one coming on, since most people complain of tingling or discomfort in the area prior to it's appearance. Barriers such as condoms or dental dams and abstinence during break-outs are the best ways of minimizing the transmission of herpes.

If you or your partners have herpes, know that there are medications available that you can take to treat outbreaks (decrease the duration of your "flare") or even prevent them happening (suppression). This may help reduce infecting others as well.

## Glossary: Common Slang

**Ass/Asshole** anus

**Bag** scrotum

**Barebacking** having anal sex without condoms

**Blowing/Blow job** performing oral sex on the penis

**Boner** erection

**Bottom/Bottoming** the sexual partner who receives penetration, usually referring to males

**Box** vagina

**Clap** gonorrhea

**Cock** penis

**Cock-Ring** Ring or band wrapped around the base of the penis and scrotum

**Crabs** pubic lice

**Cunt** vagina (usually considered to be offensive)

**Cum/Cumming** ejaculation

**Dick** penis

**Dry-humping** rubbing against your partner with your clothes on

**Fingering** stimulating and/or inserting a digit into the anus or vagina

**Fisting** inserting a fist into the rectum or vagina during sexual play

**Fuck/Fucking** penetrative sex

**Getting off** reaching orgasm

**Head** oral sex, usually on the penis

**Hand Job** physical manipulation of the penis

**Jack off/Jerking off** physical manipulation of the penis

**Jism (sometimes spelled Gism)** ejaculate

**Lube** lubrication used for sexual penetration

**Nuts** testicles

**PNP or Party and Play** refers to having sex under the influence of drugs, usually methamphetamine

**Poppers** amyl nitrate or similar chemical, inhaled to relax the anal sphincter muscles or induce pleasure

**Pussy** vulva/vagina

**Rimming** anal cunilingus or licking the anus

**Sack/Nut-Sack** scrotum

**Seeding** ejaculating inside the receptive partner

**Sucking off** performing oral sex on the penis

**Taint** perineum

**Tits** breasts

**Top/Topping** the sexual partner who penetrates, usually referring to males

**Toys** sexual aids usually used for stimulation, like dildos, nipple clamps, etc.

**Twat** vagina/vulva

# Appendix A: Chapter Learning Objectives in Competency-Based Medical Education

## Kristen L. Eckstrand

Competency-based medical education (CBME) as an educational framework utilizing teaching curricula and assessments supporting the acquisition of health practitioner's competence in clinical practice. General physician competencies are already described [1], and have been adapted by the Association of American Medical Colleges (AAMC) Advisory Committee on Sexual Orientation, Gender Identity, and Sex Development to describe the key features of competence in caring for individuals who are lesbian, gay, bisexual, and transgender (LGBT), gender nonconforming, and/or born with a difference of sex development (DSD) [2].

The learning objectives in this book are mapped to the *Professional Competencies to Improve Health Care for People Who Are or May Be LGBT, Gender Nonconforming, and/or Born with DSD*. This is denoted in each chapter next to each learning objective using the following abbreviations for the competency domains:

- KP = Knowledge for Practice
- PC = Patient Care
- PBLI = Practice-Based Learning and Improvement
- ICS = Interpersonal and Communication Skills
- Pr = Professionalism
- SBP = Systems-Based Practice
- IPC = Interprofessional Collaboration
- PPD = Personal and Professional Development

1. Englander R, Cameron T, Ballard AJ, Dodge J, Bull J, Aschenbrener CA. Toward a common taxonomy of competency domains for the health professions and competencies for physicians. Acad Med. 2013;88(8):1088–94.
2. Eckstrand KL, Leibowitz SL, Potter J, Dreger AD. Professional competencies to improve health care for people who are or may be LGBT, gender nonconforming, and/or born with DSD. In: Hollenbach A, Eckstrand KL, Dreger AD, editors. Implementing curricular and institutional climate changes to improve health care for individuals who are LGBT, gender nonconforming, or born with DSD: a resource for medical educators. Washington, DC: Association of American Medical Colleges; 2014.

## Professional Competencies to Improve Health Care for People Who Are or May Be LGBT, Gender Nonconforming, and/or Born With DSD

### AAMC Advisory Committee on Sexual Orientation, Gender Identity, and Sex Development

### Competency Domain: Patient Care

*Gather essential and accurate information about patients and their conditions through history taking, physical examination, and the use of laboratory data, imaging, and other tests by:*

1. Sensitively and effectively eliciting relevant information about sex anatomy, sex development, sexual behavior, sexual history, sexual orientation,

© Springer International Publishing Switzerland 2016
K.L. Eckstrand, J.M. Ehrenfeld (eds.), *Lesbian, Gay, Bisexual, and Transgender Healthcare*,
DOI 10.1007/978-3-319-19752-4

sexual identity, and gender identity from all patients in a developmentally appropriate manner.

2. Performing a complete and accurate physical exam with sensitivity to issues specific to the individuals described above at stages across the lifespan. This includes knowing when particulars of the exam are essential and when they may be unnecessarily traumatizing (as may be the case, for example, with repeated genital exams by multiple providers).

*Make informed decisions about diagnostic and therapeutic interventions based on patient information and preferences, up-to-date scientific evidence, and clinical judgment by:*

3. Describing the special health care needs and available options for quality care for transgender patients and for patients born with DSD (e.g., specialist counseling, pubertal suppression, elective and nonelective hormone therapies, elective and nonelective surgeries, etc.)

*Counsel and educate patients and their families to empower them to participate in their care and enable shared decision-making by:*

4. Assessing unique needs and tailoring the physical exam and counseling and treatment recommendations to any of the individuals described above, taking into account any special needs, impairments, or disabilities.
5. Recognizing the unique health risks and challenges often encountered by the individuals described above, as well as their resources, and tailoring health messages and counseling efforts to boost resilience and reduce high-risk behaviors.

*Provide health care services to patients, families, and communities aimed at preventing health problems or maintaining health by:*

6. Providing effective primary care and anticipatory guidance by utilizing screening tests, preventive interventions, and health care maintenance for the

populations described above (e.g., screening all individuals for inter-partner violence and abuse; assessing suicide risk in all youth who are gender nonconforming and/or identify as gay, lesbian, bisexual and/or transgender; and conducting screenings for transgender patients as appropriate to each patient's anatomical, physiological, and behavioral histories).

## Competency Domain: Knowledge for Practice

*Apply established and emerging biophysical scientific principles fundamental to health care for patients and populations by:*

1. Defining and describing the differences among: sex and gender; gender expression and gender identity; gender discordance, gender nonconformity, and gender dysphoria; and sexual orientation, sexual identity, and sexual behavior.
2. Understanding typical (male and female) sex development and knowing the main etiologies of atypical sex development.
3. Understanding and explaining how stages of physical and identity development across the lifespan affect the above-described populations and how health care needs and clinical practice are affected by these processes.

*Apply principles of social–behavioral sciences to the provision of patient care, including assessment of the impact of psychosocial and cultural influences on health, disease, care seeking, care compliance, and barriers to and attitudes toward care by:*

4. Understanding and describing historical, political, institutional, and sociocultural factors that may underlie health care disparities experienced by the populations described above.

*Demonstrate an investigatory and analytic approach to clinical situations by:*

5. Recognizing the gaps in scientific knowledge (e.g., efficacy of various interventions for DSD in childhood; efficacy of various inter-

ventions for gender dysphoria in childhood) and identifying various harmful practices (e.g., historical practice of using "reparative" therapy to attempt to change sexual orientation; withholding hormone therapy from transgender individuals) that perpetuate the health disparities for patients in the populations described above.

## Competency Domain: Practice-Based Learning and Improvement

*Identify strengths, deficiencies, and limits in one's knowledge and expertise by:*

1. Critically recognizing, assessing, and developing strategies to mitigate the inherent power imbalance between physician and patient or between physician and parent/guardian, and recognizing how this imbalance may negatively affect the clinical encounter and health care outcomes for the individuals described above.
2. Demonstrating the ability to elicit feedback from the individuals described above about their experience in health care systems and with practitioners, and identifying opportunities to incorporate this feedback as a means to improve care (e.g., modification of intake forms, providing access to single-stall, gender-neutral bathrooms, etc.).

*Locate, appraise, and assimilate evidence from scientific studies related to patients' health problems by:*

3. Identifying important clinical questions as they emerge in the context of caring for the individuals described above, and using technology to find evidence from scientific studies in the literature and/or existing clinical guidelines to inform clinical decision making and improve health outcomes.

## Competency Domain: Interpersonal and Communication Skills

*Communicate effectively with patients, families, and the public, as appropriate, across a broad range of socioeconomic and cultural backgrounds by:*

1. Developing rapport with all individuals (patient, families, and/or members of the health care team) regardless of others' gender identities, gender expressions, body types, sexual identities, or sexual orientations, to promote respectful and affirming interpersonal exchanges, including by staying current with evolving terminology.
2. Recognizing and respecting the sensitivity of certain clinical information pertaining to the care of the patient populations described above, and involving the patient (or the guardian of a pediatric patient) in the decision of when and how to communicate such information to others.

*Demonstrate insight and understanding about emotions and human responses to emotions that allow one to develop and manage interpersonal interactions by:*

3. Understanding that implicit (i.e., automatic or unconscious) bias and assumptions about sexuality, gender, and sex anatomy may adversely affect verbal, nonverbal, and/or written communication strategies involved in patient care, and engaging in effective corrective self reflection processes to mitigate those effects.
4. Identifying communication patterns in the health care setting that may adversely affect care of the described populations, and learning to effectively address those situations in order to protect patients from the harmful effects of implicit bias or acts of discrimination.

## Competency Domain: Professionalism

*Demonstrate sensitivity and responsiveness to a diverse patient population, including but not limited to diversity in gender, age, culture, race, religion, disabilities, and sexual orientation by:*

1. Recognizing and sensitively addressing all patients' and families' healing traditions and beliefs, including health-related beliefs, and understanding how these might shape reac-

tions to diverse forms of sexuality, sexual behavior, sexual orientation, gender identity, gender expression, and sex development.

*Demonstrate respect for patient privacy and autonomy by:*

2. Recognizing the unique aspects of confidentiality regarding gender, sex, and sexuality issues, especially for the patients described above, across the developmental spectrum, and by employing appropriate consent and assent practices.

*Demonstrate accountability to patients, society, and the profession by:*

3. Accepting shared responsibility for eliminating disparities, overt bias (e.g., discrimination), and developing policies and procedures that respect all patients' rights to self-determination.
4. Understanding and addressing the special challenges faced by health professionals who identify with one or more of the populations described above in order to advance a health care environment that promotes the use of policies that eliminate disparities (e.g., employee nondiscrimination policies, comprehensive domestic partner benefits, etc.).

## Competency Domain: Systems-Based Practice

*Advocate for quality patient care and optimal patient care systems by:*

1. Explaining and demonstrating how to navigate the special legal and policy issues (e.g., insurance limitations, lack of partner benefits, visitation and nondiscrimination policies, discrimination against children of same-sex parents, school bullying policies) encountered by the populations described above.

*Coordinate patient care within the health care system relevant to one's clinical specialty by:*

2. Identifying and appropriately using special resources available to support the health of

the individuals described above (e.g., targeted smoking cessation programs, substance abuse treatment, and psychological support).
3. Identifying and partnering with community resources that provide support to the individuals described above (e.g., treatment centers, care providers, community activists, support groups, legal advocates) to help eliminate bias from health care and address community needs.

*Participate in identifying system errors and implementing potential systems solutions by:*

4. Explaining how homophobia, transphobia, heterosexism, and sexism affect health care inequalities, costs, and outcomes.
5. Describing strategies that can be used to enact reform within existing health care institutions to improve care to the populations described above, such as forming an LGBT support network, revising outdated nondiscrimination and employee benefits policies, developing dedicated care teams to work with patients who were born with DSD, etc.

*Incorporate considerations of cost awareness and risk-benefit analysis in patient and/or population-based care by:*

6. Demonstrating the ability to perform an appropriate risk/benefit analysis for interventions where evidence-based practice is lacking, such as when assisting families with children born with some forms of DSD, families with prepubertal gender nonconforming children, or families with pubertal gender nonconforming adolescents.

## Competency Domain: Interprofessional Collaboration

*Work with other health professionals to establish and maintain a climate of mutual respect, dignity, diversity, ethical integrity, and trust by:*

1. Valuing the importance of interprofessional communication and collaboration in providing culturally competent, patient-centered care to the individuals described above and

participating effectively as a member of an interdisciplinary health care team.

## Competency Domain: Personal and Professional Development

*Practice flexibility and maturity in adjusting to change with the capacity to alter one's behavior by:*

1. Critically recognizing, assessing, and developing strategies to mitigate one's own implicit (i.e., automatic or unconscious) biases in providing care to the individuals described above and recognizing the contribution of bias to increased iatrogenic risk and health disparities.

# Appendix B: Glossary of Terms

## Carolina Ornelas and Laura Potter

| Term | Definition[a] |
|---|---|
| Androgyne | Someone whose gender identity is both male and female, or neither male nor female. A person might present as androgynous, and/or as sometimes male and sometimes female, and might choose to use an androgynous name. Pronoun preference typically varies, including alternately using male or female pronouns, using the pronoun that matches the gender presentation at that time, or using newly developed gender-neutral pronouns (e.g., hir, zie). |
| Autogynephilic | Being sexually aroused by the thought or image of oneself as a woman. |
| Behaviorally bisexual women | Women who have sex with both men and women. |
| Beyond binary | See "Gender bender". |
| Bi-gender | See "Gender bender". |
| Birth defect | Some people who suffer or have suffered with gender dysphoria may refer to their medical condition as a "birth defect" or a "variation from the norm". |
| Bisexual | One whose sexual or romantic attractions and behaviors are directed at members of both sexes to a significant degree. |
| Body mass index | A statistical measure of the weight of a person scaled according to height, used to estimate whether a person is underweight or overweight. BMI is weight in kilograms divided by the square of height in meters ($kg/m^2$). |
| Boi/tranny-boi | People assigned female sex at birth who feel that "female" is not an accurate or complete description of who they are. Other similar terms include "Butch", "Boychick", "Shapeshifter", and "Boss Grrl". |
| Bottom surgery | See "Surgery". |
| Cisgender, cissexual | People whose gender identity and gender expression align with their assigned sex at birth (i.e., the sex listed on their birth certificates). Cisgender is a newer term that some people prefer when writing and speaking about transgender and non-transgender people, with the non-transgender people being referred to as "cisgender". In this manner, a transgender person is not singled out as being different or not normal. A similar pair of words is "cissexual" and "transsexual". |
| Coming out | The process of accepting and disclosing one's theretofore hidden gender identity, gender affirmation, or sexual orientation. |
| Cross-dresser | People who wear clothing, jewelry, and/or make-up or adopt behaviors not traditionally or stereotypically associated with their anatomical sex, and who generally have no intention or desire to change their anatomical sex. Cross-dressing is more often engaged in on an occasional basis and is not necessarily reflective of sexual orientation or gender identity. Reasons for engaging in cross-dressing may include a need to express femininity/masculinity, artistic expression, performance (e.g., drag queen/king), or erotic enjoyment. Note: In the case of persons coming to terms with their gender dysphoria, they may start wearing clothing that matches their gender identity, which some people mistakenly say is the "cross-dressing phase" of their coming out process. These people are not cross-dressing and, therefore, should not be referred to as cross-dressers, because they are wearing the clothing that matches their gender identity. |

(continued)

© Springer International Publishing Switzerland 2016
K.L. Eckstrand, J.M. Ehrenfeld (eds.), *Lesbian, Gay, Bisexual, and Transgender Healthcare*,
DOI 10.1007/978-3-319-19752-4

(continued)

| Term | Definition[a] |
|---|---|
| Differences of sex development (DSD) | A spectrum of conditions involving anomalies of the sex chromosomes, gonads, reproductive ducts, and/or genitalia. The most traditional definition of intersex refers to individuals born with both male and female genitalia, genitalia that vary from typical male or female genitalia, or a chromosomal pattern that varies from XX (female) or XY (male). A person may have elements of both male and female anatomy, have different internal organs than external organs, or have anatomy that is inconsistent with chromosomal sex. This condition is sometimes not identified until puberty, when the person either fails to develop certain expected secondary sex characteristics, or develops characteristics that were not expected. According to the DSM-IV-TR, Gender Identity Disorder is not an appropriate diagnosis when a strong and persistent cross-gender identification is concurrent with a physical intersex condition. However, people born with certain intersex conditions may be more likely than the general population to feel their gender assignment at birth was incorrect. The term "disorders of sex development" (DSD) is currently recommended where the medical care of infants is considered. Sometimes written as "disorders of sexual development" or "disorders of sex differentiation". These terms are controversial and not widely accepted. Some people suggest that a better term is "variation in sex development" or "variability in sex development" (VSD), thus eliminating the negative connotation of the word "disorder". Some people suggest that gender-dysphoric people may be intersex or have a variation in sex development because their anatomical sex does not match their gender identity, perhaps as a result of cross brain feminization or masculinization. |
| Discrimination | Differential treatment of a person because of group membership, such as sexual- or gender-minority status. |
| Drag king | An anatomical female who cross-dresses as male primarily for performance or show. Drag kings generally identity as female and do not wish to change their anatomical sex. The term is sometimes used as an insult toward a transman. |
| Drag queen | An anatomical male who cross-dresses as a woman primarily for performance or show. Drag queens generally identity as male and do not wish to change their anatomical sex. The term is sometimes used as an insult toward a transwoman. |
| Facial feminization surgery (FFS) | See "Surgery". |
| Female to male (FTM) | See "Transman". |
| Gay | An attraction and/or behavior focused exclusively or mainly on members of the same sex or gender identity; a personal or social identity based on one's same-sex attractions and membership in a sexual-minority community. |
| Gender affirmation | Many people view their coming out as an affirmation of the gender identity they have always had, rather than a transition from one gender identity to another. They may prefer to call themselves "affirmed females" (or just "females") or "affirmed males" (or just "males") rather than "transgender" or "transsexuals" because the "trans" prefix suggests they have changed, rather than accepted, their true gender identity. This is consistent with the concept that people do not need to have any surgery in order to affirm their gender. Related terms are "process of gender affirmation"; "gender-affirmed female" (or just "affirmed female"); and "gender-affirmed male" (or just "affirmed male"). |
| Gender bender | Any gender variation other than the traditional, dichotomous view of male and female. People who self-refer with these terms may identify and present themselves as both or alternatively male and female, as no gender, or as a gender outside the male/female binary. Similar terms include "bi-gender", "beyond binary", "gender fluid", "gender outlaw", "pan gender", "polygender". |
| Gender confirmation surgery (GCS) | See "Surgery". |

(continued)

(continued)

| Term | Definition[a] |
|------|---------------|
| Gender dysphoria | Distress resulting from conflicting gender identity and sex of assignment. Some people prefer this term over "gender identity disorder" because it has a less stigmatizing impact. |
| Gender expression | The external manifestation of a person's gender identity, which may or may not conform to the socially- and culturally-defined behaviors and external characteristics that are commonly referred to as either masculine or feminine. These behaviors and characteristics are expressed through carriage (movement), dress, grooming, hairstyles, jewelry, mannerisms, physical characteristics, social interactions, and speech patterns (voice). |
| Gender fluid | See "Gender bender". |
| Gender identity | A person's innate, deeply-felt psychological identification as a man, woman, or something else, which may or may not correspond to the person's external body or assigned sex at birth (i.e., the sex listed on the birth certificate). "Sexual identity" should not be used as a synonym for, or as inclusive of, "gender identity". |
| Gender identity disorder (GID) | According to DSM-IV-TR, Gender Identity Disorder is the diagnosis used when a person has (1) a strong and persistent cross-gender identification and (2) persistent discomfort with his or her sex or sense of inappropriateness in the gender role of that sex, and the disturbance (2) is not concurrent with physical intersex condition and (4) causes clinically significant distress or impairment in social, occupational, or other important areas of functioning. According to DSM-IV-TR, gender identity disorder not otherwise specified can be used for persons who have a gender identity problem with a concurrent congenital intersex condition. Many people prefer the term "gender dysphoria", developed in an attempt to eliminate the negative connotation of the word "disorder"; however, some people find "dysphoria" to have a negative connotation as well. |
| Gender minority | A term to describe people whose gender expression and/or gender identity does not match traditional societal norms. "Sexual minority" should not be used as a synonym for, or as inclusive of, "gender minority". |
| Gender non-conforming | A term to describe people whose gender expression is (1) neither masculine nor feminine or (2) different from traditional or stereotypic expectations of how a man or woman should appear or behave. |
| Gender outlaw | See "Gender bender". |
| Gender reassignment surgery (GRS), gender realignment surgery (GRS) | See "Surgery". |
| Gender role conformity | The extent to which an individual's gender expression adheres to the cultural norms prescribed for people of his or her sex. |
| Gender role nonconformity | Nonconformity with prevailing norms of gender expression. |
| Gender/gender role | The traditional or stereotypical behavioral differences between men and women, as defined by the culture in which they live, in terms of, among other things, their gender expressions, the careers they pursue, and their duties within a family. |
| Genderqueer | An umbrella term that includes all people whose gender varies from the traditional norm, akin to the use of the word "queer" to refer to people whose sexual orientation is not heterosexual only; or a term to describe a subset or individuals who are born anatomically female or male, but feel their gender identity is neither female nor male. |
| Gender-variant children | Children who are gender role nonconforming. |

(continued)

(continued)

| Term | Definition[a] |
|------|---------------|
| Genital reassignment surgery (GRS), genital reconstruction surgery (GRS), genital surgery (GS) | See "Surgery". |
| Getting clocked/read/spooked | When people are not perceived as the gender they are presenting (e.g., based on their dress and mannerisms matching according to social norms). For example: an anatomical male dressed as a female who is perceived by others as male (e.g., a stranger says "that's a man in a dress"), or a transman who is perceived as a woman. |
| Hermaphrodite | Previously used to describe intersex; now considered pejorative and outdated. |
| Heterosexual | A term to describe individuals who identify as "straight" or whose sexual or romantic attractions and behaviors focus exclusively or mainly on members of the other sex or gender identity. |
| Homophobia | The various manifestations of sexual stigma, sexual prejudice, and self-stigma based on one's homosexual or bisexual orientation. |
| Homosexual | As an adjective, used to refer to same-sex attraction, sexual behavior, or sexual orientation identity; as a noun, used as an identity label by some persons whose sexual attractions and behaviors are exclusively or mainly directed to people of their same sex. |
| Intersectionality | A theory used to analyze how social and cultural categories intertwine. |
| Intersex | See "Differences of sex development" |
| Intimate partner violence | Physical, sexual, or psychological harm inflicted by a current or former partner or spouse. |
| Lesbian | As an adjective, used to refer to female same-sex attraction and sexual behavior; as a noun, used as a sexual orientation identity label by women whose sexual attractions and behaviors are exclusively or mainly directed to other women. |
| LGBT | Acronym for "lesbian, gay, bisexual, and transgender". |
| LGBTIQQAA | One of numerous variations of the basic LGBT acronym used by some people in order to be more inclusive, with "I" for intersex, "Q" for queer and/or questioning, and "A" for asexual and/or ally. |
| Lower surgery | See "Surgery". |
| Male to female (MTF) | See "Transwoman". |
| Neo-vagina | The technical term for when a vagina is surgically created. This term is suitable for use when having a discussion with another medical professional, but it is not a term that should be used with a client during routine office visits or routine gynecological examinations. A clinician need not remind a female client that she has a neo-vagina and may instead simply say "vagina". |
| Nulliparity | The condition of being nulliparous, or not bearing offspring. |
| Outing | The unauthorized disclosure by one person of another person's theretofore hidden gender identity, gender affirmation, or sexual orientation. |
| Pan gender | See "Gender bender". |
| Passing | When people are perceived as the gender they are presenting in (e.g., based on their dress and mannerisms matching according to social norms). For example: an anatomical male dressed as a female who is perceived by others as female, or a transman who is perceived as a man. |
| Polygender | See "Gender bender". |

(continued)

(continued)

| Term | Definition[a] |
|---|---|
| Queer | In contemporary usage, an inclusive, unifying sociopolitical, self-affirming umbrella term for people who are gay; lesbian; bisexual; pan-sexual; transgender; transsexual; intersexual; genderqueer; or of any other nonheterosexual sexuality, sexual anatomy, or gender identity. Historically, a term of derision for gay, lesbian, and bisexual people. |
| Real life experience (RLE), real life test (RLT) | Generally accepted guideline, from the Standards of Care for Gender Identity Disorders, that requires clients to live outwardly in the gender that matches their gender identity for a specified period of time (typically 1 year) prior to being eligible for genital surgery. Less often referred to as the "real life test" (RLT), which is considered a misleading and offensive term and, therefore, should be avoided. |
| Serostatus (HIV serostatus) | Blood test results indicating the presence or absence of antibodies the immune system creates to fight HIV. A seropositive status indicates that a person has antibodies to fight HIV and is HIV-positive. |
| Sex | (1) In a dichotomous scheme, the designation of a person as birth as either "male" or "female" based on their anatomy (genitalia and/or reproductive organs) and/or biology (chromosomes and/or hormones). Sometimes "sex" and "gender" are used interchangeably. For clarity, it is better to distinguish sex, gender identity, and gender expression from each other. Sex is typically assigned at birth based on the appearance of the external genitalia; only when this appearance is ambiguous are other indicators of sex assessed to determine the most appropriate sex assignment. (2) All phenomena associated with erotic arousal or sensual stimulation of the genitalia or other erogenous zones, usually (but not always) leading to orgasm. |
| Sex change, sex change operation, sex change surgery | These terms are considered by some to be pejorative and, therefore, should be avoided. See "Surgery". |
| Sex reassignment surgery (SRS), sex realignment surgery (SRS) | The term "sex reassignment surgery" and the lesser-used term "sex realignment surgery" are increasingly falling into disuse. See "Surgery". |
| Sexual minority | This term describes people whose sexual orientation is not heterosexual only. |
| Sexual orientation | A person's enduring physical, romantic, emotional, and/or spiritual attraction to another person. May be lesbian, gay, heterosexual, bisexual, pansexual, polysexual, or asexual. Sexual orientation encompasses attraction, desire, behavior, and personal and social identity but is distinct from sex, gender identity, and gender expression. Most researchers studying sexual orientation have defined it operationally in terms of one or more of its components. Defined in terms of behavior, sexual orientation refers to an enduring pattern of sexual or romantic activity with men, women, or both sexes. Defined in terms of attraction (or desire), it denotes an enduring pattern of experiencing sexual or romantic feelings for men, women, or both sexes. Identity encompasses both personal identity and social identity. Defined in terms of personal identity, sexual orientation refers to a conception of the self based on one's enduring pattern of sexual and romantic attractions and behaviors toward men, women, or both sexes. Defined in terms of social (or collective) identity, it refers to a sense of membership in a social group based on a shared sexual orientation and a linkage of one's self-esteem to that group. A person's sexual orientation should not be assumed based on the perceived sex of that person's partner(s). For example, a man who identifies himself as heterosexual may have sexual relationships with men and women. "Affectional orientation" is sometimes used as a more encompassing term. |
| Stealth | When a transgender person who has transitioned into a different sex or gender does not divulge the fact of transition. When a person has gone through gender affirmation and does not disclose that fact to others. The risk or fear of being "outed" may be very distressing to a person who is living stealth. Some people who considered themselves transgender prior to transition believe that after they transition that are no longer transgender and, therefore, no longer have anything to reveal. Many people believe the information about their medical treatments and surgeries is private and does not need to be divulged any more than anyone else divulges their medical histories to others. Clinicians need to treat such medical information with the same required degree of confidentiality as they would for all of their other clients. |

(continued)

(continued)

| Term | Definition[a] |
|------|---------------|
| Stigma | The inferior status, negative regard, and relative powerlessness that society collectively assigns to individuals and groups that are associated with various conditions, statuses, and attributes. |
| Surgery | Persons with gender dysphoria may or may not have surgery and, if they have surgery, they may have one or more types of surgery, depending upon their circumstances. Numerous terms are used to describe the genital surgeries that some people may undergo, including "gender affirmation surgery" (GAS), "gender reassignment surgery" (GRS), "genital reassignment surgery" (GRS), "genital reconstruction surgery" (GRS), "genital surgery" (GS), and "sex reassignment surgery" (SRS). The foregoing terms are purposely listed in alphabetical order in view of the strong feelings some people have with respect to what is the right or better term to use; clinicians should listen to their clients to see which terms they prefer. Sometimes, though very infrequently, "realignment" is used instead of "reassignment" or "reconstruction". "Sex reassignment surgery" is increasingly falling into disuse as many people find the term offensive. In discussion with clients, all a clinical really needs to say is "genital surgery". Some clients may prefer to use the term "bottom surgery". Others may call this "lower surgery", stating that they "did not have surgery on their bottoms". It is best to ask clients what terminology they prefer. Some people may have an orchiectomy. Some people may have a hysterectomy and a bilateral salpingo-oophorectomy. Some people may have breast augmentation. "Top surgery" is a term most often used by transmen to refer to the removal of breast tissue, relocation and resizing of nipple complexes, and chest reconstruction to a male chest structure. Some people may have "facial feminization surgery" (FFS). Some people may have a chondrolaryngoplasty ("trach shave" or Adam's apple reduction). Some people may have surgeries to alter the pitch of their voice. Surgery is not essential for some people to resolve their gender dysphoria. Moreover, for some people, surgery is a relatively minor aspect of their gender affirmations. Some people cannot have surgery because of, among other reasons, financial constraints and health reasons. In the United States, in most states and for federal government purposes, gender-affirmed people (transsexuals) cannot get the sex marker (i.e., "male" or "female") changed on their identity papers (e.g., birth certificates, drivers' licenses) without proof of some form or surgery. In many cases, the employees of government agencies may not be familiar with the other terms discussed in this Glossary and, therefore, clinicians may have no choice but to use the term "sex reassignment surgery" in any affidavits they sign for submission to the agencies. A few states, such as Massachusetts and New Jersey, will allow changes to drivers' licenses with medical documentation short of surgery. Clinicians may want to ask their clients for a copy of the governing legal regulations and/or forms their clients must submit to the government to confirm what terminology the government is currently requiring in order to minimize problems and embarrassment to their clients at the time they submit the forms. Many people consider "sex change", "sex change operation", "sex change surgery", "pre-op", and "post-op" as pejorative and, therefore, these terms should be avoided. |
| Top surgery | See "Surgery". |
| Tranny, trans | Short for a transgender person. Its use is similar to the use of the word "queer" by some LGBT people. Some people consider the terms tranny, trans, and/or queer derogatory, especially when used by someone who is not transgender or lesbian, gay, or bisexual. |
| Trans | See "Transgender". |
| Trans community | See "Gender minority". |
| Transgender | An umbrella term for people whose gender identity and/or gender expression differs from their assigned sex at birth (i.e., the sex listed on their birth certificates). Some groups define the term more broadly (e.g., by including intersex people) while other people define it more narrowly (e.g., by excluding "true transsexuals"). Transgender people may or may not choose to alter their bodies hormonally and/or surgically. While "transgender" is a popularly used word and generally seems to be a safe default term to use, some people may find the term offensive as a descriptor of themselves. It is best to ask clients which terms, if any, they use or prefer. Use "transgender", not "transgendered". |

(continued)

(continued)

| Term | Definition[a] |
|---|---|
| Transgenderist | An individual who lives full time in the cross-gender role and who may also take hormones, but does not desire sex reassignment surgery. |
| Transition | The process that people go through as they change their gender expression and/or physical appearance (e.g., through hormones and/or surgery) to align with their gender identity. A transition may occur over a period of time, and may involve coming out to family, friends, co-workers, and others; changing one's name and/or sex designation on legal documents (e.g., drivers' licenses, birth certificates); and/or medical intervention. Some people find the word "transition" offensive and prefer terms such as "gender affirmation" or "process of gender affirmation". |
| Transman | A term to describe a person who was identified female at birth but who identifies and portrays his gender as male. People will often use this term after taking some steps to express their gender as male, or after medically transitioning. Some, but not all, transmen male physical changes through hormones or surgery. Some people will refer to themselves as men of transgender experience. Some transmen do not use FTM (female-to-male) to describe themselves because they do not think of themselves as having transitioned from female to male. Some people prefer to be referred to as men rather than transmen or transgender men. Alternate terms: affirmed male, FTM, gender-affirmed male, man. |
| Transphobia | Dislike of, or discomfort with, people whose gender identity and/or gender expression do not conform to traditional or stereotypic gender roles. |
| Transsexual | People whose gender identity differs from their assigned sex at birth (i.e., the sex listed on their birth certificates). People who, often on a full-time basis, live their lives as a member of the sex opposite of their birth-designated sex. They may or may not (1) take hormones or have surgery or (2) be gender dysphoric. Use of the term "transsexual" remains strong in the medical community because of the DSM's prior use of the diagnosis "transsexualism" (changed to "gender identity disorder" in DSM-IV). Some people suggest that "transsexual" includes only those people who are in the process of changing, or who have changed, their anatomical sex to realign with their gender identity. In order writings, such people were referred to as "true transsexuals" when they had moderate to high intensity gender dysphoria. Some people use "primary transsexual" or "early transitioner" to refer to people who have not had a significant adult life in their birth gender because they started or completed their gender affirmations during their teen years (or earlier) or at the latest in young adulthood. These people also use "secondary transsexual" or "late transitioner" for those people who start their transitions after the age of 30. [These distinctions] have resulted in some very heated discussions and are considered offensive to many people. It is highly recommended that clinicians not use these terms unless their clients bring them up in discussions. The term "transsexual" is hotly debated, and it is not certain whether people will use or reject this term. For some, it is disliked in the same way "homosexual" has become disfavored. Many people find both transsexual and homosexual pejorative. "Transsexual" is considered by some to be a misnomer inasmuch as the underlying medical condition is related to gender identity and not sexuality. It is safer for clinicians not to use the term "transsexual" unless and until they are sure that it is a term their clients are comfortable with. When in doubt, clinicians should ask their clients which terms they would like the clinicians to use. |
| Transvestite (TV) | Previously used to describe a cross-dresser; now considered pejorative and outdated. See "Cross-dresser". |
| Transwoman | A term to describe a person who was identified male at birth but who identifies and portrays her gender as female. People will often use this term after taking some steps to express their gender as female, or after medically transitioning. Some, but not all, transwomen make physical changes through hormones or surgery. Some people will refer to themselves as women of transgender experience. Some transwomen do not use MTF (male-to-female) to describe themselves because they do not think of themselves as having transitioned from male to female. Some people prefer to be referred to as women rather than transwomen or transgender women. Alternate terms: affirmed female, gender-affirmed female, MTF, woman. |

(continued)

(continued)

| Term | Definition[a] |
|------|---------------|
| Two spirit, two-spirited | Adopted in 1990 at the third annual spiritual gathering of GLBT Natives, the term derives from the northern Algonquin word niizh manitoag, meaning "two spirits." and refers to people who display characteristics of both male and female genders. Sometimes referred to as a third gender or "the male-female gender," Two Spirit also means a mixture of masculine and feminine spirits living in the same body. This term also represents self-identity description used by many Native American gay men who do not identify as cross-gendered or transgender. |
| Vaginoplasty | A surgical procedure to construct a vagina. |

[a]All definitions were combined and paraphrased from the following two sources:

National Research Council. The health of lesbian, gay, bisexual, and transgender people: building a foundation for better understanding. Washington, DC: National Academies Press; 2011. http://blog.lib.umn.edu/sonweb/onrs/NIH-LGBT-Report_01.2013.pdf

Fenway Health. "Glossary of gender and transgender terms." January 2010 Revision. http://www.lgbthealtheducation.org/wp-content/uploads/Handout_7-C_Glossary_of_Gender_and_Transgender_Terms__fi.pdf

# Appendix C: Resource List and Position Statements

Laura Potter and Carolina Ornelas

© Springer International Publishing Switzerland 2016
K.L. Eckstrand, J.M. Ehrenfeld (eds.), *Lesbian, Gay, Bisexual, and Transgender Healthcare*,
DOI 10.1007/978-3-319-19752-4

| Medical society/organization | Title | Resource type | Target/subject population |
|---|---|---|---|
| Agency for Healthcare Research and Quality | Inclusive Policies, Communication Protocols and Ongoing Training Lead to Culturally Competent Care for Lesbian, Gay, Bisexual, and Transgender Patients | Provider resources | LGBT |
|  | Easily Accessible, Welcoming Center Enhances Access to Medical and Social Services for Lesbian, Gay, Bisexual, and Transgender Homeless Youth | Provider resources | LGBT |
|  | Culturally Tailored Cessation Program for Lesbian, Gay, Bisexual, and Transgender Smokers Enhances Access and Patient Satisfaction | Provider resources | LGBT |
|  | Centers for Disease Control and Prevention's Division of Adolescent and School Health: Sexual Risk Behavior Publications and Resources | Provider resources | LGBT |
|  | Heritage Month Toolkit | Provider resources | LGBT |
|  | LGBTQ Communities: Motivation to Quit Smoking Quitguide | Provider resources | LGBT |
|  | REALtalkDC | Provider resources | LGBT |
|  | The National Women's Health Information Center, womenshealth.gov | Provider resources | L |
|  | Hospital HIV Clinic Offers Convenient, Proactive Screening for Anal Cancer, Enabling Identification and Treatment of Precancerous Lesions | Provider resources | G |
|  | Multiagency Collaboration Improves Access to Culturally Sensitive Care and Support Services for Lesbian, Gay, Bisexual, and Transgender Seniors | Provider resources | LGBT |
|  | Community Health Centers Integrate Rapid HIV Screening Into Routine Primary Care, Leading to Significant Increases in Testing Rates | Provider resources | LGBT |
|  | Countywide Partnership Promotes Culturally Appropriate Outreach and Education, Leading to Increased Breast Cancer Screening and Earlier Detection in Underserved Minorities | Provider resources | L |
|  | Adapting Your Practice: Treatment and Recommendations for Homeless Patients with HIV/AIDS | Provider resources | LGBT |
| Accord Alliance | AccordAlliance.org | Provider resources, patient resources, national recommendations | I |

| Organization | Title | Resource type | 1. T / 2. LB / 3. G / 4. LGBT |
|---|---|---|---|
| American Academy of Family Physicians | Care of Special Populations—LGBT | Provider resources, national recommendations | 1. T<br>2. LB<br>3. G<br>4. LGBT |
| | Adolescent Health Care, Sexuality and Contraception | National recommendations | LGBT |
| | Reparative Therapy | National recommendations | LGBT |
| | Recommended Curriculum for Family Practice Residents—LGBT Health | Provider resources, national recommendations | LGBT |
| | Gay, Lesbian, Bisexual, and Transgender | Provider resources | LGBT |
| American Academy of Pediatrics | Sexual Orientation and Adolescents | National recommendations | LGBT |
| | Office based care for LGBT Youth | Provider resources | LGBT |
| | A Newborn Infant With a Disorder of Sexual Differentiation | Provider resources | I |
| | Coparent or Second-Parent Adoption by Same-Sex Parents | National recommendations | LGBT |
| | Reducing the Risk of HIV Infection Associated With Illicit Drug Use | Provider resources, recommendations | LGBT |
| American Academy of Child and Adolescent Psychiatry | Children, Adolescents, and HIV | Patient resources | LGBT |
| | Gay, Lesbian, and Bisexual Adolescents | Patient resources | LGB |
| American Psychiatric Association | Position Statement on Therapies Focused on Attempts to Change Sexual Orientation (Reparative or Conversion Therapies) | National recommendations | LGBT |
| | Position Statement on Discrimination Against Transgender and Gender Variant Individuals | National recommendations | T |
| | Position Statement on Access to Care for Transgender and Gender Variant Individuals | National recommendations | T |
| American Psychological Association | Appropriate Therapeutic Responses to Sexual Orientation | National recommendations | LGBT |
| | Transgender, Gender Identity, & Gender Expression Non-discrimination | National recommendations | T |
| American Congress of Obstetricians and Gynecologists | Transgender Health Resource Guide | Provider resources | T |
| | WEBTREATS: Transgender Health | Provider resources | T |
| | WEBTREATS: Lesbian & Bisexual Health | Provider resources | LB |
| | Lesbian Health Resources | Provider resources, patient resources | L |
| | Health Care for Lesbians and Bisexual Women | National recommendations | LB |
| | Health Care for Transgender Individuals | National recommendations | T |

(continued)

(continued)

| Medical society/organization | Title | Resource type | Target/subject population |
| --- | --- | --- | --- |
| American Society for Reproductive Medicine | Counseling Issues for Gay Men and Lesbians Seeking Assisted Reproductive Technologies | Patient resources | LG |
| | Access to fertility treatment by gays, lesbians, and unmarried persons: a committee opinion | Provider resources | LG |
| The American Academy of Otolaryngology—Head and Neck Surgery | Appendix of Resources for Clinicians and Patients | Provider resources, patient resources, national recommendations | LGBTI |
| American Society of Clinical Oncology | Awareness of HPV and its vaccine among lesbian, gay, bisexual, transgender, and queer (LGBTQ) populations | Provider resources | LGBT |
| American College of Nurses-Midwives | Transgender/Transsexual/Gender Variant Health Care | National recommendations | T |
| American Civil Liberties Union (ACLU) | Know Your Rights: A Guide for Trans and Gender Nonconforming Students | Patient resources | T |
| | Know Your Rights—Transgender People and the Law | Patient resources | T |
| | Non-Discrimination Laws: State by State Information—Map | Provider resources, patient resources | LGBT |
| American Academy of Physical Medicine & Rehabilitation | Impacts of the Affordable Care Act on LGBT Communities | Provider resources | LGBT |
| American College of Emergency Physicians | Sexual Assault ebook | Provider resources | LGBT |
| American Medical Association | GLBT Health Resources | Provider resources, national recommendations | LGBT |
| American Medical Directors Association | Gay Elders Face Uncomfortable Realities in LTC | Provider resources | G |
| Bisexual Resources Center | Books on Bisexuality | Patient resources | B |
| | How to Be an Ally to a Bisexual Person | Patient resources | B |
| Blue Cross Blue Shield of Minnesota | LGBT Quit Guide | Patient resources | LGBT |
| Centers for Disease Control and Prevention (CDC) | LGBT Health | Provider resources, patient resources | LGBT |
| COLAGE | Resources | Provider resources, patient resources | LGBT |
| Community Preventive Services Task Force | The Guide to Community Preventive Services | Provider resources | G |
| | The Guide to Community Preventive Services | Provider resources | LGBT |

| | | | |
|---|---|---|---|
| The Endocrine Society | Priorities for Care and Research in Disorders of Sex Development/Intersex Conditions | National recommendations | I |
| | Endocrine Treatment of Transsexual Persons: An Endocrine Society Clinical Practice Guideline | National recommendations | T |
| Fenway Health Center and Fenway Institute | Center for Population Research in LGBT Health | Provider resources | LGBT |
| | LGBT Aging Project | Provider resources, patient resources | LGBT |
| | National LGBT Health Education Center | Provider resources | LGBT |
| Gender Identity Research and Education Society | Information for medical professionals | Provider resources, patient resources, national recommendations | LGBTI |
| Gay and Lesbian Medical Association (GLMA) | Guidelines for care of LGBT patients | National recommendations | LGBT |
| | Transgender Health Resources | Provider resources, patient resources | T |
| | Cultural Competence Webinars | Provider resources | LGBT |
| | Top 10 Things to discuss with Healthcare Providers | Patient resources | LGBT |
| | Provider Directory | Patient resources | LGBT |
| Gender Spectrum | Resources for Mental Health Providers | National recommendations | T |
| | Resources for Medical Providers | National recommendations | T |
| | 10 Tips for Working with Transgender Individuals: A Guide for Health Care Providers from the Transgender Law Center | National recommendations | T |
| | Clinical management of gender identity disorder in adolescents: a protocol on psychological and paediatric endocrinology aspects | Provider resources | T |
| | Transgender Youth: Providing Medical Treatment for a Misunderstood Population | Provider resources | T |
| GLBT National Help Center | GLBT National Hotline & GLBT National Youth Talkline | Patient resources | LGBT |
| | The GLBT National Resource Database | Patient resources | LGBT |
| Gay, Lesbian & Straight Education Network (GLSEN) | GLSEN.org | Patient resources, national recommendations | |
| Human Rights Campaign (HRC) | Tips to Coming Out to Your Doctor | Patient resources | LGBT |

(continued)

(continued)

| Medical society/organization | Title | Resource type | Target/subject population |
|---|---|---|---|
| Infectious Diseases Society of America | Public Health Service Guideline for Reducing Transmission of Human Immunodeficiency Virus (HIV), Hepatitis B Virus (HBV) and Hepatitis C Virus (HCV) through Solid Organ Transplantation | Provider resources | LGBT |
|  | HIVMA Comments on LGBT Research Committee Report | National recommendations | LGBT |
| Institute of Medicine of the National Academies | The Health of Lesbian, Gay, Bisexual, and Transgender People: Building a Foundation for Better Understanding | Provider resources | LGBT |
| Intersex Society of North America | ISNA.org | Provider resources, patient resources | I |
| The Joint Commission | Advancing Effective Communication, Cultural Competence, and Patient- and Family-Centered Care for the Lesbian, Gay, Bisexual, and Transgender (LGBT) Community: A Field Guide | Provider resources, national recommendations | LGBT |
| Lambda Legal | Our Work | Patient resources, national recommendations | LGBT |
| Lesbian Health and Research Center (LHRC) | Resources & Research | Provider resources, patient resources, national recommendations | LBT |
| National AIDS Hotline | Hotline: (800) 342-AIDS Spanish: (800) 344-7432 TTY Service: (800) 243-7889 | Patient resources | General |
| National LGBT Cancer Network | Cultural Competence Training, Reexamining LGBT Healthcare | Provider resources | LGBT |
| National Center for Lesbian Rights (NCLR) | Navigating the System: A Know-Your-Rights Guide for Lesbian, Gay, Bisexual, and Transgender Elders in California | Patient resources | LGBT |
|  | Asserting Choice: Health Care, Housing, and Property—Planning for Lesbian, Gay, Bisexual, and Transgender Older Adults | National recommendations | LGBT |
| National Center for Transgender Equality (NCTE)), & National Gay and Lesbian Task Force | Injustice at Every Turn: A Report of the National Transgender Discrimination Survey | Provider resources | T |
| National Resource Center on LGBT Aging | Providing Quality Care to LGBT Clients with Dementia, How to Gather Data on Sexual Orientation and Gender Identity in Clinical Settings | Provider resources, patient resources, national recommendations | LGBTI |

| Organization | Resource | Resource type | Population |
|---|---|---|---|
| National Runaway Safeline | Safeline: (800) RUNAWAY, 1800 runaway.org | Patient resources | General |
| National Center for Transgender Equality (NCTE) | National Transgender Discrimination Survey Reports | Provider resources, patient resources | T |
| Out2Enroll | Out2Enroll Q&A Topics | Patient resources | LGBT |
| Our Family Coalition | Information and Resources | Patient resources | LGBT |
| Parents, Friends and Family of Lesbians and Gays (PFLAG) | More Resources for GLBT Persons | Patient resources | LGBT |
| | Coming out Help for Families, Friends, and Allies | Patient resources | LGBT |
| | Be Yourself | Patient resources | LGBT |
| | Our Daughters and Sons | Patient resources | LGBT |
| | Welcoming our Trans Family and Friends | Patient resources | T |
| Physicians for Reproductive Choice and Health, Adolescent Reproductive and Sexual Health Education Project (ARSHEP) | Module on Caring for Transgender Adolescents, Module on Gay, Lesbian, Bisexual, Transgender, and Questioning Youth | Provider resources | LGBT |
| Project TurnAround Foundation (PTF) | PTFGA.org, info@projectturnaroundga.org | Patient resources | LGBT |
| Services and Advocacy for GLBT Elders (SAGE) | Resources, Publications | Provider resources, patient resources, national recommendations | LGBTI |
| Strong Families | Where to Start, What to Ask: A Guide for LGBT People Choosing Health Care Plans | Patient resources | LGBT |
| | Resource List | Patient resources | LGBTI |
| | LGBT Kids/Youth | Patient resources | LGBT |
| | Transgender Healthcare | Patient resources | T |
| The Center for Substance Abuse Prevention (CSAP) of the Substance Abuse and Mental Health Services Administration (SAMHSA) | A Provider's Introduction to Substance Abuse Treatment for Lesbian, Gay, Bisexual, and Transgender Individuals | Provider resources, national recommendations | LGBT |
| Vancouver Coastal Health's Transgender Health Information Program | Transgender Health Information Program | Provider resources, patient resources | T |
| Tom Waddell Health Center | Protocols for Hormonal Reassignment of Gender | National recommendations | T |

(continued)

(continued)

| Medical society/organization | Title | Resource type | Target/subject population |
|---|---|---|---|
| Transgender Law Center (TLC) | Resources | Provider resources, national recommendations | T |
| US Department of Health and Human Services | U.S. Department of Health and Human Services Recommended Actions to Improve the Health and Well-Being of Lesbian, Gay, Bisexual, and Transgender Communities | National recommendations | LGBT |
| Center of Excellence for Transgender Health at UCSF | Primary Care Protocol for Transgender Patient Care | National recommendations | T |
| | Learning Center: Guidelines and Reports | Provider resources | T |
| | LGBT Resource Center | Provider resources, patient resources | LGBT |
| World Professional Association for Transgender Health (WPATH) | Standards of Care for the Health of Transsexual, Transgender, and Gender Nonconforming People | National recommendations | T |
| Trevor Project | Trevor Lifeline, TrevorChat, TrevorText, TrevorSpace, Ask Trevor | Patient resources | LGBT |
| | Resources | Provider resources, patient resources, national recommendations | LGBT |

# Index

© Springer International Publishing Switzerland 2016
K.L. Eckstrand, J.M. Ehrenfeld (eds.), *Lesbian, Gay, Bisexual, and Transgender Healthcare*,
DOI 10.1007/978-3-319-19752-4

Printed in the United States
By Bookmasters